Obstetrics
and
Gynecology

Obstetrics
and
Gynecology

J. Robert Willson, M.D.

Adjunct Professor
Department of Obstetrics and Gynecology
University of New Mexico School of Medicine
Albuquerque, New Mexico

Elsie Reid Carrington, M.D.

Adjunct Professor
Department of Obstetrics and Gynecology
University of New Mexico School of Medicine
Albuquerque, New Mexico

Associate Editors

Russell K. Laros, Jr., M.D.

Professor and Vice Chairman
Department of Obstetrics, Gynecology and Reproductive Sciences
University of California School of Medicine
San Francisco, California

William J. Ledger, M.D.

Given Foundation Professor of Obstetrics and Gynecology
Cornell University Medical College;
Obstetrician and Gynecologist in Chief
The New York Hospital
New York, New York

John H. Mattox, M.D.

Director
Obstetrics and Gynecology
Good Samaritan Regional Medical Center
Phoenix, Arizona;
Clinical Professor
Obstetrics and Gynecology
University of Arizona
Tucson, Arizona

9th Edition

with 385 *illustrations*

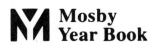

**Mosby
Year Book**

St. Louis   Baltimore   Boston   Chicago   London   Philadelphia   Sydney   Toronto

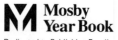

Mosby
Year Book
Dedicated to Publishing Excellence

RG
101
.W75
1991

Editor: Stephanie Manning
Assistant Editor: Anne Gunter
Project Supervisor: Lilliane Anstee
Book Design: Liz Fett

9th Edition

Mosby–Year Book, Inc.
11830 Westline Industrial Drive, St. Louis, Missouri 63146

Library of Congress Cataloging-in-Publication Data

Willson, J. Robert (James Robert), 1912-
    Obstetrics and gynecology / J. Robert Willson, Elsie Reid
Carrington. — 9th ed. / associate editors, Russell K. Laros, Jr.,
William J. Ledger, John H. Mattox.
        p.   cm.
    Includes bibliographical references.
    Includes index.
    ISBN 0-8016-5542-0
    1. Gynecology.   2. Obstetrics.   I. Carrington, Elsie Reid, 1912-
. II. Laros, Russell K., 1936-   .   III. Ledger, William J., 1932-
. IV. Mattox, John H.   V. Title.
    [DNLM: 1. Genital Diseases, Female.   2. Obstetrics.   WP 100
W742o]
RG101.W75   1991
618—dc20
DNLM/DLC
for Library of Congress   90-13589
                                                            CIP

CL/MY/MY   9   8   7   6   5   4   3   2   1

Contributors

Elsie Reid Carrington, M.D.
Adjunct Professor
Department of Obstetrics and Gynecology
University of New Mexico School of Medicine
Albuquerque, New Mexico

Lisa M. Fromm, Ph.D.
Assistant Professor of Obstetrics and Gynecology and
    Psychiatry
University of New Mexico School of Medicine
Albuquerque, New Mexico

Michael P. Hopkins, M.D.
Associate Professor
Department of Obstetrics and Gynecology
Northeastern Ohio University College of Medicine
Akron, Ohio

Russell K. Laros, Jr., M.D.
Professor and Vice Chairman
Department of Obstetrics, Gynecology and
    Reproductive Sciences
University of California School of Medicine
San Francisco, California

William J. Ledger, M.D.
Given Foundation Professor of Obstetrics and
    Gynecology
Cornell University Medical College;
Obstetrician and Gynecologist in Chief
The New York Hospital
New York, New York

John H. Mattox, M.D.
Director
Obstetrics and Gynecology
Good Samaritan Regional Medical Center
Phoenix, Arizona;
Clinical Professor
Obstetrics and Gynecology
University of Arizona
Tucson, Arizona

Teresita A. McCarty, M.D.
Assistant Professor of Psychiatry
University of New Mexico School of Medicine
Albuquerque, New Mexico

Kate Moffitt Musello, M.D.
Chief, Obstetrics and Gynecology
Santa Fe Indian Hospital
Santa Fe, New Mexico

Melissa Schiff, M.D.
Chief Resident
Department of Obstetrics and Gynecology
University of New Mexico School of Medicine
Albuquerque, New Mexico

J. Robert Willson, M.D.
Adjunct Professor
Department of Obstetrics and Gynecology
University of New Mexico School of Medicine
Albuquerque, New Mexico

Preface

To prepare a textbook in obstetrics-gynecology that provides basic information for medical students and that also serves as a reference for beginning residents and practicing physicians in several specialties is a challenging project. It is difficult to strike an appropriate medium between a brief outline of the material and a comprehensive, all-inclusive text which contains not only basic material, but that which is necessary for the practicing specialist. We have once more resisted the temptation to expand the book. In fact, we have reduced its size by eliminating repetitious material and those portions of the text that added little to the understanding of the conditions under discussion. We have, however, retained the concept of isolating material that is not essential for medical student education, but which may be helpful to those with more advanced knowledge and skills. Much of the material concerning treatment—particularly that which may be too advanced for medical students and junior residents—is in the latter category. As was true of previous editions the emphasis is on reproductive physiology and on the diagnosis and management of conditions that do not require the expertise of a specialist obstetrician-gynecologist.

Outdated illustrations and those that added little to understanding the text have been deleted. Others have been redrawn to make them more informative and many new ones have been added.

The references include comprehensive review articles, which contain extensive bibliographies for those who are interested in advanced study, as well as reports of recent research. A number of classical papers have been included in the references.

Each chapter has been extensively revised or completely rewritten by contributors with expertise in specific areas. Russell K. Laros, Jr., assumed responsibility for much of the material concerning pregnancy and its complications, John H. Mattox supervised the chapters on reproductive endocrinology and infertility, and Michael Hopkins oversaw those on oncology. Following the untimely death of Dr. M.J. Daly, Lisa M. Fromm, Teresita A. McCarty, and Melissa Schiff revised the chapters on the female life cycle and sexual physiology and dysfunction.

An addition that we hope will be helpful to medical students are objectives for each chapter. The objectives, which are modeled after the Instructional Objectives developed by the Educational Committee of the Association of Professors of Gynecology and Obstetrics, define the minimum information that seems appropriate for medical students. Those who wish to learn more can study the advanced material presented and the papers listed in the references.

Once more we hope that *Obstetrics and Gynecology* will continue to serve as a basic textbook for the undifferentiated medical student, for beginning residents in obstetrics-gynecology and those in other programs, and for practicing physicians who treat women patients.

J. Robert Willson
Elsie Reid Carrington

Contents

Obstetrics
and
Gynecology

1

J. Robert Willson

Introduction

Objectives

RATIONALE: Although there have been significant improvements in obstetric care, injuries to and deaths of many mothers, fetuses, and newborn infants are from preventable causes.

The student should be able to:

A. Define *birthrate* and describe changes that have occurred in the birthrate since 1930.

B. Define *maternal death, fetal death, neonatal death,* and *perinatal mortality,* and for each describe how the rate is calculated.

C. List three important causes of maternal, fetal, and neonatal deaths.

D. Describe the potential problems associated with births to unmarried women and to teenagers.

It might appear that physicians who confine their professional activities to the treatment of pregnant women (obstetrics) and patients with dysfunctioning genital organs (gynecology) are limiting their practice rather severely. On the contrary, obstetricians and gynecologists must be familiar with many fields of medicine because their patients vary in age from those newly born to senescent women. It is possible for women with medical conditions such as hypertension, tuberculosis, rheumatic heart disease, diabetes, multiple sclerosis, and a host of others to conceive; and all manner of acute medical and surgical conditions may develop during pregnancy.

Gynecologists must be pediatricians, internists, endocrinologists, and surgeons because they treat females of all ages and often are the first persons consulted because of symptoms that arise in structures other than the genital organs. They must also be familiar with the basic principles of psychiatry and be able to recognize the emotional problems that so frequently manifest themselves in sexual disorders.

Obstetrician-gynecologists often provide considerable amounts of general medical care for their own patients. A survey of Fellows of the American College of Obstetricians and Gynecologists indicated that 57% of those responding serve

1

as principal providers of medical care for at least half of their patients, and 36% serve as providers for more than half. This is not surprising, as an obstetrician-gynecologist often has provided care for an individual patient before her marriage, during pregnancies, and at regular periodic examinations after childbearing is completed.

Unfortunately, physicians cannot respond adequately to the steadily increasing demands for obstetric-gynecologic care. In fact, they cannot even cope with all serious problems. For example, in 1989 about 7000 women died with cancer of the cervix, a disease that can be diagnosed so early that it can be eradicated almost without exception. The deaths occurred because these women were not screened for early cellular changes. An additional 3000 died of other malignant uterine tumors; most of them might have been treated successfully had they consulted their doctors early. In the same year, 43,000 women died of breast cancer, another malignancy that can be diagnosed in its earliest stages by effective techniques that are not yet readily available to all women.

Unfortunately, lung cancer, a preventable disease, is increasing in women. In 1989 about 49,000 women died of this disease, an increase from about 36,000 in 1984. Lung cancer has surpassed breast cancer as a cause of death in women.

In 1987 there were 251 maternal deaths, most of them preventable; 24,627 neonatal deaths; and 29,349 fetal deaths, many of these also preventable. There are vast unmet needs in general nutrition and health care and in health education, notably in sex and family living.

Obstetric-gynecologic care can be improved and made more available and acceptable to women of any economic or social class through the development of *health care teams* composed of obstetrician-gynecologists, nurse-midwives, obstetric-gynecologic nurse practitioners, and specially trained aides. Each can be made responsible for the area of care that is appropriate on the basis of training and ability. For example, the nurse-midwife can provide much of the prenatal care

and education for *all* pregnant women and delivery and the care after delivery for those in whom normal deliveries are anticipated. Nurse-midwives or trained obstetric-gynecologic nurses can provide contraceptive counseling, perform periodic health examinations on well women, diagnose and treat minor gynecologic conditions such as vaginitis, and be responsible for a comprehensive health education program. With such capable associates, physicians could concentrate on women with high-risk pregnancies and with gynecologic problems that require their special skills; they would serve as immediately available consultants to associates working in their offices and be responsible for women who require special care during labor and delivery and for gynecologic operations.

Such teams can extend care into areas where there are no physicians, with nonphysician workers serving as screening and triage agents who refer women needing special care to an appropriate physician. It is essential that such a system be organized to deliver medical care to women of all socioeconomic classes. The model is not one that is appropriate only for poor women.

FACILITIES FOR OBSTETRIC CARE

Most births occur in hospitals, but more and more women are requesting out-of-hospital confinement. In 1940 1,043,631 births occurred outside hospitals. By 1980 this number was reduced to 35,888 and by 1987 to 35,288. More out-of-hospital births are now conducted by midwives and fewer by physicians than in years past. In 1980 11,093 of these births were conducted by midwives and 11,992 by physicians; for 12,776 the attendant was not stated. Comparable figures for 1987 were 15,465 by midwives, 8,132 by physicians, and 11,691 by "others."

HOSPITAL OBSTETRIC SERVICES

The remarkable decreases in maternal and perinatal mortality and morbidity were achieved not only by increasing the number of skilled obstetrician-gynecologists but also by simultaneously improving hospital obstetric services that in the past had been unorganized and in which obstetric practice was unregulated. Most hospital obstetric services are now organized; staff privileges are awarded on the basis of competence, and most hospitals make available essential services and equipment designed to make labor and delivery safe.

A national survey of maternity care by the American College of Obstetricians and Gynecologists pointed out several important inadequacies in hospitals in which infants are delivered. As a general rule the facilities provided by hospitals in which fewer than 2000 infants are delivered yearly are less adequate than those with larger services. Constant 24-hour coverage of the labor-delivery area was provided by registered nurses in almost all large services but in only 40% of hospitals with fewer than 250 deliveries each year. In 93% of hospitals with large services, emergency cesarean section could be performed in less than 40 minutes; this was possible in only 63% of hospitals with small services. In addition, intensive newborn care by experienced pediatricians was more readily available in larger hospitals.

In recent years perinatal centers, which have the facilities and personnel to manage the most complicated pregnancies, have been developed. More and more physicians, both family practitioners and obstetrician-gynecologists, are using such centers. They either perform deliveries in facilities in which consultation is readily available or transfer women with problems that cannot be managed safely in smaller hospitals. The end result is an improved outcome for both mothers and their infants.

An example of the change is indicated in a report of the outcome of obstetric care in Iowa hospitals of several levels of sophistication. Level Ia maternity units, in which fewer than 500 deliveries are conducted each year, are staffed by family physicians. Obstetricians and pediatricians staff level Ib institutions. All level I hospitals are designed to serve only low-risk obstetric patients and healthy newborn infants. Level II maternity units serve patients at moderate risk, and intensive obstetric and perinatal care is available in level III hospitals. Although 37% of deliveries are now conducted in level I units, the percentage of neonatal deaths in these hospitals has declined substantially. Neonatal mortality rates were 2.7/ 1000 live births in level Ia hospitals, 4.6 in level Ib hospitals, 5.5 in level II hospitals, and 17.6 in level III hospitals. More and more mothers with serious complications are being transferred to hospitals that are better equipped to manage the problems. Transfers can be made during pregnancy when a condition such as diabetes or hypertension is recognized or during labor when the need for a higher level of care becomes necessary.

ALTERNATIVE BIRTH CENTERS

The increasing use of technologic innovations during normal labor has led many women to seek less complicated alternative methods of obstetric care. They reason that a completely normal pregnancy and delivery can be managed successfully by a qualified nurse-midwife, without interference and without mechanical monitoring equipment, both of which are used frequently in scientifically oriented labor-delivery suites.

Alternative birth centers are specifically designed for women whose pregnancies have been uncomplicated and for whom normal labor and delivery is anticipated. The centers are alike in that the atmosphere is more like that of a home than a hospital. The patients labor and deliver in a comfortable bed where they remain with the newborn infant until they are discharged, usually within a few hours. Their families can be with them. The centers are staffed by personnel who are both well trained and experienced in providing care during labor and who support the concept of helping the perfectly normal pregnant woman have her baby as naturally as possible. The labor can be managed by nurse-midwives or physicians, and either can conduct the delivery.

Hospital-based centers are usually located near or within the regular labor-delivery area, which permits prompt consultation with a physician whenever it is necessary and immediate transfer when a complication arises. Freestanding centers have agreements with physicians and nearby hospitals that permit the immediate transfer of patients when a complication develops. They also are prepared to provide emergency care during transfer. Such precautions are essential because from 15% to 25% of carefully screened patients develop complications during labor or after delivery that require more sophisticated care than can be provided in an alternative birth center.

Many of the problems that arise during labor can be anticipated and prevented by careful patient selection. Only women in whom completely normal pregnancy, labor, and delivery are anticipated should be selected for care at a center. Some of them will be transferred during pregnancy, for example, when the membranes rupture prematurely, if an abnormal position is diagnosed, if hypertension is recognized, if bleeding occurs, or if labor begins prematurely. The most common reasons for transfer during labor are failure to progress, abnormal fetal position, and fetal distress.

The results of delivery in alternative birth centers in which patients are properly screened, in which meticulous care is provided during labor and delivery, and from which patients with complications are transferred to hospitals promptly are excellent. The overall intrapartum and neonatal mortality rate in 11,814 women who were admitted for labor and delivery in 84 birth centers was 1.3 per 1000 births. About 16% were transferred to a hospital because of intrapartum or early postpartum complications. The cesarean section rate was 4.4%. There were no maternal deaths.

Because the cost of obstetric care for women with normal pregnancies in birth centers is about half that for hospital delivery, it seems likely that more women will seek care in low-risk units.

HOME DELIVERY

Conversely, home delivery is far from safe. Neither the necessary safety support nor an adequate number of competent attendants is available, and transfer to a hospital when a complication arises is usually delayed. Few trained midwives or physicians will agree to perform deliveries in the home. This has led to the appearance of untrained birth attendants who are willing to do so. In many instances their only qualifications are that they have had children themselves or that they have assisted others in having babies. As might be anticipated, the results can be disastrous. In the states that maintain statistics concerning outcome of delivery, perinatal mortality is from two to five times higher in home than in hospital delivery.

BIRTHRATES

The *birthrate,* the number of live births per 1000 population, varies from year to year, depending on a multitude of factors. The rate fell progressively from 30 in 1910 to 18.4 in 1933. It is interesting that this low rate was attained before the present sophisticated contraceptive methods were available and undoubtedly represents a calculated mass decision to prevent pregnancy because of the severe financial depression.

Most couples were forced to delay starting their families because of World II, but the birthrate started upward in 1940 and rose steeply after 1945, reaching a peak of 26.6 in 1947. It was 25 with 4,254,784 births in 1957 and 23.3 with 4,268,326 births in 1961. The birthrate continued to fall, reaching 17.8 with 3,520,959 births in 1967.

An increase in the number of births was anticipated because of the large number of young people who were born during the "baby boom" years. The number of women between the ages of 15 and 45 years increased from 42,336,000 in 1970 to about 56,000,000 in 1985. However, the anticipated increase in births did not occur. By 1975 the birthrate had decreased to 14.8 with 3,144,198 births. In recent years total births have increased slightly, but the birthrate appears to have stabilized. In 1980 the birthrate was 15.9, and 3,612,258 live births were registered. Comparable figures for 1987 were 15.7 and 3,809,394.

There is no certain way of predicting the reproductive rates for the future, but some increase in the *number* of births is inevitable. Even though birthrates remain low, an increasing number of women will enter the childbearing years. In addition, the births may increase because women who have postponed pregnancy and are now in their late twenties and thirties will become pregnant and because a slight increase in family size may again become popular.

The *fertility rate,* the births per 1000 women between the ages of 15 and 45 years, is a better indication of reproductive patterns than the birthrate. It, too, is decreasing.

Even the fertility rate does not provide complete information concerning pregnancy because it does not include spontaneous and induced abortions.

BIRTHS TO UNMARRIED WOMEN

Both the number and ratio (number of births per 1000 unmarried women) of births to unmarried women are increasing. In 1950 there were 141,600 (ratio 39.8); in 1960, 224,300 (ratio 52.7); in 1970, 398,700 (ratio 106.9); and in 1977, 515,700 (ratio 155). The numbers continue to increase. In 1987 933,013 unmarried women bore children (ratio 244.9). Of these, 498,645 were white (ratio 166.6), and 399,144 were black (ratio 622.1).

The reported births represent only a small fraction of total out-of-wedlock conceptions. Estimates based on correlating the wedding date with the date the first child is born indicate that more than 50% of women of all ages are already pregnant at the time of their marriage. In addition, many births to unmarried women are not reported as such.

The availability of contraception and elective abortion has neither reduced the problem nor prevented recurrence. In 1987 474,631 unmarried women had their first child, 234,398 their second, 124,716 their third, 55,172 their fourth, and 39,851 their fifth or more.

TEENAGE PREGNANCY

Pregnancy in an unmarried woman is a problem at any age, but it may be disastrous to a teenager. Before legal abortion became available, the alternatives were to remain pregnant and either marry, give the baby up for adoption, or in some cases, keep the baby. None of these alternatives was a satisfactory solution in most instances. Teenage marriages, particularly those forced by pregnancies, are notoriously unsuccessful, and the alternative of remaining pregnant is often considered unacceptable or impossible by most young women. Whatever the choice, the result was disrupted education, which too often was not resumed; broken marriages; and often repeated pregnancies.

Fetal, neonatal, and postneonatal death rates are higher in teenage pregnancies than in those of mature married women. The highest mortalities occur in young women of the lowest socioeconomic groups, those who have had the least education, and those who have had more than one baby before they reach the age of 20 years.

The solution is far more complex than a simplistic approach of making contraceptives available to all girls entering their teens. Most young girls have little accurate and useful information concerning reproduction and, in many communities, no way of learning more. Parents are likely to avoid sexual discussions; and either there are no effective sex education courses in schools, or they do not include instruction in contraception. Some girls may be forced into premature sexual activity by the pressure of their peers; others are seeking love and attention, which they think they can get in no other way. Some have unprotected coitus because they know little about contraception and counseling is not available to them. Others fail to use contraceptives because of an unconscious wish to become pregnant to fill an emotional need. Pregnancy in more mature unmarried women often is a result of carelessness in the use of contraception.

The obvious solution, and it will not come soon, is basic and effective sex education at home and in schools, opportunities to discuss personal problems of sex and reproduction with understanding parents and counselors, and readily available contraception for those who are sexually active.

Counseling also is important for teenage girls who already have conceived. The initial decision is between abortion and remaining pregnant. Those who choose the latter must be permitted to continue their education. They, as well as those who select abortion, need continuing counseling and the best medical care.

An important objective in counseling is to provide the patient with an understanding of why she became pregnant and to help her develop the motivation to prevent a recurrence. Without such motivation, as many as 50% of teenagers will be pregnant within a year after delivery. Teenagers are more likely to conceive soon after a pregnancy than are more mature women.

MATERNAL MORTALITY

A *maternal death* is the death of any woman from any cause during pregnancy or within 42 days of the termination of pregnancy, irrespective of the duration of pregnancy or its site. A *direct obstetric death* is one resulting from a complication of pregnancy itself—from intervention, from omissions of or incorrect treatment, or from a chain of events resulting from any of the preceding. An example is a death from postpartum hemorrhage. An *indirect obstetric death* is one resulting from a disease that had existed previously or that developed during pregnancy, but the course of which was aggravated by the physiologic effects of pregnancy. An example is serious rheumatic heart disease with decompensation during the period of maximum cardiac stress. A *nonobstetric death* is one resulting from an incidental cause unrelated to pregnancy. Examples of

nonobstetric death are one resulting from injuries sustained in an automobile accident or death from a brain tumor.

The *maternal mortality* is the number of maternal deaths from direct causes per 100,000 live births as indicated in the following equation:

$$\frac{\text{Number of direct maternal deaths}}{\text{Total live births}} \times 100{,}000 = \text{Maternal mortality}$$

Maternal death rates vary considerably in different parts of the country and with different classes of patients. The mortality is higher in nonwhite patients than in either white nonprivate or white private patients. This undoubtedly occurs because the nonwhite patients include the most impoverished and least educated people in the United States. There is a higher incidence of medical complications such as essential hypertension, anemia, malnutrition, and preeclampsia-eclampsia among this group of patients, and these conditions often remain untreated. The patients frequently do not seek prenatal care and enter the hospital only after labor has begun; if they do register in clinics, they often appear late in pregnancy, attend irregularly, and cannot afford adequate diets and medications.

The death rate is highest in urban communities and in the southeastern states, where the concentration of nonwhite patients and those of low economic status is greatest. Maternal mortality is lowest in the Northwest, parts of New England, and the upper Midwest, where the population is more homogeneous with fewer blacks and less poverty and malnutrition. Reduction in maternal mortality therefore must be a concern of educators, sociologists, and economists, as well as physicians.

The maternal mortality in 1930 was more than 600/100,000 live births. The rate has fallen steadily to a level of 36.9 in 1961, 18.8 in 1971, 8.5 in 1981, and 7.2 in 1986. The causes of the 272 maternal deaths in 1987 are listed in Table 1-1.

Tabulations of causes of maternal mortality do

TABLE 1-1 Causes of maternal deaths (1987)

Cause	Total number
Puerperal complications	75
Toxemia	40
Ectopic pregnancy	36
Hemorrhage	27
Abortion	15
Other direct causes	59
Indirect causes	20

not reflect the overlap of all responsible contributing factors because they include only the primary cause listed on the death certificate. For example, most deaths listed as "abortion" are caused by infection; and many women who die of puerperal sepsis also had hemorrhage following delivery, which may represent a major factor in their deaths. In addition, indirect and nonobstetric deaths may be listed under specific causes such as heart disease and may not appear as deaths of pregnant or recently delivered women.

The reduced maternal death rate is a result of many factors, which include an increase in hospital deliveries, the development of perinatal centers, the availability of blood, and the ability to treat infection effectively. In addition, there are many more highly trained and skillful obstetricians in all parts of the United States with whom general practitioners can consult when a complication develops. Most hospital staffs are organized and have established rules by which obstetric practice in the institution is governed. Those without special training and experience are required to seek consultation for serious complications and for abnormalities of labor. This is in contrast to the previous situation, when any staff member, regardless of ability, was permitted to perform any type of operative procedure or manage any complication without seeking help.

An important factor in the reduction of maternal mortality was the development of state and local Maternal Mortality Review Committees in the early 1930s. The complete care of each pregnant woman who dies is reviewed by a committee of obstetrician-gynecologists who determine the cause and assign responsibility for the death to the primary physician, the consultant, the patient, the institution, or the community. The principal reason for these committees is physician education, and the result has been a dramatic reduction in maternal mortality. Maternal Mortality Review Committees represent the first organized peer review system to be developed in the United States.

Maternal mortality can be reduced even further. It should be possible at least to eliminate deaths from hemorrhage and infection, both of which can be prevented or treated if they occur. Deaths from abortion can be reduced to a minimum by making reliable contraceptive methods and legal abortion available to everyone who wants them. There may be an irreducible minimum of obstetric deaths, but it can only be reached if every physician concentrates on preventing or detecting and correcting potentially lethal abnormalities and if the facilities in which pregnant women are treated are optimal.

PERINATAL MORTALITY (Fig. 1-1)

A *fetal death* is the death before or during birth of a fetus weighing 500 g or more. No heartbeat, cord pulsation, respiratory activity, or movement of voluntary muscle can be detected after birth. If the weight is unknown, fetal death is diagnosed if the pregnancy duration is of 20 completed weeks or more as measured from the first day of the last normal menstrual period.

A *liveborn infant* is one in which signs of life, including breathing, cord pulsation, heartbeat, or voluntary muscle movement, can be detected after its complete expulsion from the vagina. A *neonatal death* is the death within the first 28 days of life of a liveborn infant weighing at least 500 g or after 20 completed weeks of pregnancy. A *hebdomadal death* is the death within the first 7 days of life of a liveborn infant weighing 500 g or more.

The term *perinatal death* is an inclusive one, indicating the death of a fetus weighing 500 g or more before or during labor and of a liveborn infant within the first 28 days of life.

The *fetal mortality* is the number of fetal deaths per 1000 births of liveborn *and* dead-born infants.

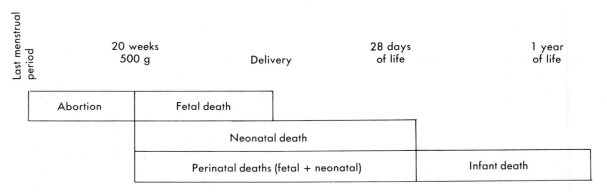

Fig. 1-1 Abortion, perinatal, and infant mortality.

The *neonatal mortality* is the number of deaths per 1000 births of *liveborn* infants. The *perinatal mortality* is the number of fetal plus the number of neonatal deaths per 1000 births of live and dead infants. *Infant mortality* includes deaths that occur between the twenty-eighth day and the end of the first year of life.

Most states require that the deaths of all infants born after 20 or more weeks of pregnancy be reported; in some states it is necessary to report deaths from pregnancies of less than 20 weeks' duration.

There are many reasons for perinatal deaths; some deaths, such as those associated with hypertension and other acute and chronic diseases in the mother, complications of labor, infections, and birth injuries, can often be prevented. Those caused by congenital malformation, cord entanglement, and certain disorders of placental function cannot yet be controlled. The latter, however, are in the minority.

Fetal deaths. The World Health Organization has recommended the term *fetal death* to replace the older terms, *stillbirth* and *abortion.* Fetal deaths are classified as follows:

Group I: Early fetal deaths—less than 20 completed weeks of pregnancy

Group II: Intermediate fetal deaths—20 to 27 completed weeks of pregnancy

Group III: Late fetal deaths—28 or more completed weeks of pregnancy

Group IV: Unclassified

In 1987 there were 29,349 fetal deaths of 20 weeks or more. The *fetal mortality ratio* was 7.7/1000 births.

The total number of fetal deaths cannot be determined accurately because most states do not require the reporting of deaths from pregnancies of less than 20 weeks' duration; 10% to 15% or more of all pregnancies terminate in spontaneous abortion.

The most common causes of fetal deaths are *anoxia* (many of these deaths are associated with abruptio placentae, placenta previa, hypertension, maternal diabetes, prolapsed cord, and abnormal labor), *congenital anomalies,* and *infection.* In one third to one half of fetal deaths no cause can be determined, even though an autopsy is performed.

Neonatal deaths. In 1987, 24,627 liveborn infants died during the first 28 days after birth. The *neonatal mortality rate* was 6.5.

The reduction in the number of neonatal deaths has been less spectacular than that of maternal deaths. The neonatal mortality fell from 39.7 between 1920 and 1924 to 28.8 in 1940, to 20 in 1951, and to 10.9 in 1976.

Because most perinatal deaths occur in low-birth-weight infants, there are two possible causes for the relatively rapid improvement in recent years: a lower incidence of prematurity and improved care for small infants. The latter is the more likely cause because there has been little decrease in the premature delivery rate.

Clearly, the principal reason for the improvement is that more women with pregnancy complications are now being treated in perinatal centers where specially trained teams provide intensive care both for mothers during pregnancy and labor and for their newborn infants.

Prevention of neonatal mortality. Approximately half of all neonatal deaths occur in premature infants who are unable to cope with the hazards of an independent existence. The most obvious way to reduce neonatal mortality therefore is to reduce the premature delivery rate. Although it is possible to accomplish this in certain patients, our understanding of many of the causes of premature labor is as yet incomplete, and we cannot always prevent it.

Most neonatal deaths occur with *high-risk pregnancies;* therefore it is essential that women with conditions associated with increased perinatal mortality be given special attention during pregnancy and labor. The principal problems of delivery are breech and other malpresentations, prolapsed cord, placenta previa, and abruptio placentae. *High-risk pregnancies are best managed in perinatal centers.*

Pregnancies in unmarried women and pregnancies at the extremes of the reproductive years are accompanied by increased prematurity and fetal and neonatal death rates. It is essential therefore that sexually active teenagers and women who want no more children be provided with reliable contraceptive methods.

Socioeconomic factors in perinatal mortality. Perinatal mortality from all causes is higher in poor women than in middle- and upper-class women. The general health of more affluent women is better, they are better nourished, they have relatively easy access to physicians, and they know how to use medical care facilities.

Poor women are likely to be congenitally malnourished and anemic, and they live in unfavorable environments. They are more likely to have more pregnancies at short intervals than are upper-class women. Medical care facilities available to poor women may be limited and inappropriate, and access to these facilities may be difficult. As a consequence, they use the facilities principally for serious acute illnesses rather than for health maintenance.

Adequate prenatal care alone, although obviously important in determining the outcome of high-risk pregnancies, is only a partial solution for the reproductive problems associated with poverty. Poor women must first be adequately fed and housed so they will no longer need to think only in terms of day-to-day existence. Physicians have little control over these aspects of the total problem, but they do have the responsibility of making certain that appropriate medical care facilities are made available and that acceptable educational programs, designed to help women learn to use these facilities, are instituted. Better general health alone will improve the outcome of pregnancy, but even this cannot be accomplished without concomitant social and economic advances.

NONLETHAL EFFECTS OF THE BIRTH PROCESS

Not all infants who are born alive are normal. Approximately 7% of all liveborn infants have structural or functional defects. Less than half of these defects are diagnosed during the early postnatal period; the rest appear weeks or even years later.

It is difficult to determine how many of these conditions could have been prevented by better obstetric care, because many are caused by unrecognized chromosomal conditions or teratogenic stimuli during pregnancy. Many individuals, however, might have been normal had they not been born prematurely, been injured during labor and delivery, or suffered hypoxia. Improvements in these figures must await more information concerning the prevention of premature labor, sensitive instruments that will detect early intrauterine hypoxia, precise methods for determining the need for delivery, and improvements in the treatment of respiratory distress following delivery.

SUGGESTED READING

Apgar V: Birth defects: their significance as a public health problem, JAMA 204:79, 1968.

Barton JJ, Rovner S, Puls K, and Read PA: Alternative birthing center: experience in a teaching obstetric service, Am J Obstet Gynecol 137:377, 1980.

Burnett CA III, Jones JA, Rooks J, Chen CH, Tyler CW Jr., and Miller CA: Home delivery and neonatal mortality in North Carolina, JAMA 244:2741, 1980.

Fox LP: A return to maternal mortality studies: a necessary effort, Am J Obstet Gynecol 152:379, 1985.

Fuchs VR: Expenditures for reproduction-related health care, JAMA 255:76, 1986.

Hein HA: The status and future of small maternity services in Iowa, JAMA 255:1899, 1986.

Kiely JL, Paneth N, and Susser M: Fetal death during labor: an epidemiologic indicator of level of obstetric care, Am J Obstet Gynecol 153:721, 1985.

Potter EL: Pathology of the fetus and newborn, Chicago, 1952, Year Book Medical Publishers, Inc.

Rooks JP, Weatherby NL, Ernst ERM, and others: Outcomes of care in birth centers: the National Birth Center Study, New Engl J Med 321:1804, 1989.

2

John H. Mattox

Diagnostic methods in obstetrics and gynecology

Objectives

RATIONALE: In addition to the knowledge of disease requisite to the practice of obstetrics and gynecology, it is critical to be able to conduct a patient-specific history and physical exam including the pelvic examination. Special laboratory tests and procedures may be required, being careful not to overutilize or underutilize these important tools in the assessment. Communication skills must be learned and developed to be an excellent practitioner.

The student should be able to:
A. Obtain an appropriate history of a woman in the reproductive age.
B. Enumerate the steps in the performance of pelvic examination.
C. Formulate a management plan utilizing the appropriate diagnostic studies.

The Oslerian admonition to listen to the patient is no less applicable today in spite of the advanced technology in medicine. An accurate medical history accompanied by a complete physical examination is as important for the obstetric or gynecologic patient as for patients with medical or surgical disorders. Although obstetrician-gynecologists function as specialists to patients with unique problems who are referred from physicians outside of their discipline, they also act as the primary care providers for the majority of women in their practice. Therefore, an evaluation may be *problem oriented,* focusing upon the history and physical exam required to address that problem, for example, infertility, in detail, or the patient assessment can be conducted in a broader sense, such as the periodic health screen or *annual examination.*

HISTORY

The patient should be encouraged to tell her story in her own words, even though this may be a prolonged process. Details can be filled in by questions that provide the additional information necessary to complete the recital. Questions should be phrased simply in words the patient can

TOPIC OUTLINE FOR HISTORY*

I. **Identifying information**
   A. Age
   B. Parity
   C. Marital status
   D. Current contraceptive
   E. Last menstrual period
   F. Last Pap smear
   G. Breast self-examination

II. **Chief complaint(s)**
   A. List in order
   B. Duration
   C. Characterization
      1. Location
      2. Self-administered remedies
      3. Prior episodes
      4. Prior testing
      5. Relation to menses

III. **Menstrual history**
   A. Pubertal sequence
   B. Menarche
   C. Periodicity
   D. Duration flow
   E. Pain
   F. Abnormal bleeding
   G. Perimenstrual symptoms

IV. **Obstetric data**
   A. Pregnancies
   B. Outcome
   C. Complications

V. **Gynecologic data**
   A. Contraceptives
   B. Surgery

   C. Sexual history (including potential for physical and verbal abuse)
   D. Prior lower/upper genital tract infections
   E. Pelvic pain
   F. Vaginal drainage

VI. **Significant past history**
   A. Serious medical illness and sequelae
   B. Surgical procedures
   C. Hospitalizations

VII. **Personal data**
   A. Occupation
   B. Weight change
   C. Medications
   D. Smoking
   E. Drug use
   F. Alcohol intake
   G. Allergies or drug sensitivities
   H. Exercise

VIII. **Family history**
   A. Health problems of first-degree relatives
   B. Problems with diabetes mellitus, heart attack at an earlier age, breast cancer
   C. Birth defects, mental retardation, pregnancy losses

IX. **Review of systems (special emphasis)**
   A. Genitourinary
   B. Gastrointestinal
   C. Musculoskeletal
   D. Bleeding disorders
   E. Psychiatric

*The information can be obtained in any sequence, and some of the headings may require in-depth questioning.

understand easily; too many patients answer "no" to questions they cannot understand rather than display what they presume to be ignorance. Although this chapter's purpose is not to discuss in detail each segment of a thorough history, a suggested outline can be seen in the box above. Physicians, attired appropriately, should always introduce themselves to the patient and avoid familiarity until they have the patient's permission to use her first name or until time and previous visits warrant closer rapport. In addition to obtaining historical medical information, physicians should make a conscious effort during the interview to evaluate the patient's dress and demeanor. The patient may wish to discuss other serious problems such as weight loss or gain or alcohol, substance, or sexual abuse. She needs to be made secure and may respond only with some sensitive probing, such as, "During the course of this visit I noticed that you seem worried. Is there anything else you wish to discuss?"

Present illness. A *chronologic account* is the most useful. Integrate information concerning any testing or therapy even though the patient may not remember all of the medical terms. Pertinent data from any of the categories in 2.1 should be incorporated into this section. *At the end of the interview, inquire if the patient wishes to include any additional information.*

Menstrual history. The menstrual history should include the age at which periods began and the type of flow at *onset* (regular, irregular, interval), preparation for menstruation and reaction to its onset, *frequency* and *duration* of periods and amount of bleeding (number of well-saturated or stained pads, clots, color), *pain* (type, when it began, how long it lasts, how much interference with activity, what medications required for relief), date of onset of the last *normal menstrual* period, and any *abnormal bleeding.*

Vaginal discharge. Information concerning vaginal discharge should include how long it has been present; its relation to menses, coitus, or other stimuli; bleeding; irritation; odor; and previous treatment.

Obstetric history. Each pregnancy should be listed chronologically with information concerning prenatal complications, duration of pregnancy, outcome, complications of labor, and puerperium; sex and weight of infants and their subsequent development; and patient's reactions to pregnancy and her evaluation of labors.

Sexual and marital history. This important topic is covered in greater detail in Chapter 5.

PHYSICAL EXAMINATION

A complete general physical examination should be performed on new patients with perhaps the exception of those referred from other physicians only for gynecologic evaluation. The *basic gynecologic examination* includes recording the weight and blood pressure, palpation of the breasts, and abdominal, vaginal, and rectal examinations.

Maintaining a comfortable milieu is highly de-

sirable for performing an adequate examination. When the ambient temperature is too cool or too warm, the patient is left alone in a dressing gown for a prolonged period of time, the physician is too harried during the conduct of the exam, or the examination room appears untidy or dreary, the impression is created that the physician is insensitive to patient needs.

Breast examination. This topic is discussed in detail in Chapter 12.

Abdominal examination. In most instances abdominal tenderness caused by painful lesions of the pelvic structures is located low in the abdomen. Tenderness in the upper abdomen, near the umbilicus, in the region of the cecum, and along the course of the descending colon is less characteristic of disease in the pelvic organs.

Pelvic examination. The pelvic examination is customarily performed with the patient in lithotomy position, suitably draped with a sheet, her feet in stirrups or using leg rests, and her buttocks hanging just over the lower end of the table. Unless the physician wishes to obtain a specimen of urine by catheter or to check for urinary control, the patient should void immediately before the examination.

Also, being told step by step what to anticipate during the examination helps the patient relax.

After the physician has gloved both hands, the patient's external genitals are inspected in a good light and then palpated. Note should be made of developmental anomalies, hair distribution, clitoral size, skin changes, discharge, irritation, new growths, and enlargements of Bartholin's glands.

A single digit placed inside the introitus and gentle pressure is applied to the posterior perineal muscles to provide the examiner some insight into the patient's comfort and the size of speculum to use (Fig. 2-1). Different specula should be used, depending upon the patient's age, parity, and size of the vaginal introitus.

A *warmed speculum* moistened with water is gently inserted into the vagina to expose the cervix. Lubricating jelly may interfere with accurate evaluation of vaginal and cervical secretions. The

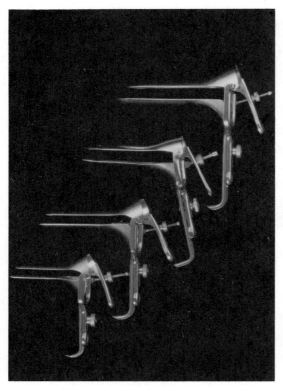

Fig. 2-1 Metal specula vary from the small size for young females to a larger one for obese, parous women.

labia minora and majora are separated with thumb and index finger to expose the introitus. As the tip of the speculum is inserted into the vaginal opening, downward pressure is exerted posteriorly to expand the size of the introitus enough to admit the speculum with a minimum of discomfort. The urethral meatus is the most sensitive structure in the area; hence every precaution must be made to protect it. Pain produced by the speculum may make the rest of the examination much more difficult. Material is collected from the cervix for cytologic examination, and, when indicated, a sample is obtained for culture.

Then the exposed cervix should be wiped clean with dry cotton; a note is made of its color, size, and configuration; any obvious lesions are described minutely. As the speculum is slowly withdrawn, the vaginal walls are inspected.

One or two fingers, usually of the examiner's left hand, are then inserted into the vagina to depress the posterior wall as the patient is requested to bear down. If the muscular supports of the bladder and rectum have been damaged, these structures will bulge through the open introitus, *cystocele,* or *rectocele* as intraabdominal pressure is increased. The uterus also may be forced downward if its supports have been weakened, *decensus.*

Although it is not possible to visualize the body of the uterus and the adnexal structures, their size, shape, position, mobility, and sensitivity can usually be determined by *bimanual examination* (Figs. 2-2 and 2-3), in which a well-lubricated index finger alone or the index and second fingers of one hand are inserted into the vagina while those of the other hand palpate through the abdominal wall. The accuracy with which bimanual examination can be performed is determined by the thickness of the abdominal wall, the patient's ability to relax her voluntary muscles, and whether a painful lesion is present. Nothing can be done about obesity, but it is possible to perform pelvic examinations on most women, even virgins, without causing undue pain. Two fingers can usually be inserted into the vagina of most multiparous women, but this is not often possible when the hymen is intact. If one learns to perform pelvic examination using only the index finger, one can examine almost anyone without causing pain.

The *consistency* of the cervix and the *direction in which it points* are determined, and the cervix and uterus are pushed upward and from side to side to determine whether it is mobile or fixed and to detect pain produced by motion. The body of the uterus is located; and *its size, shape, and consistency* are determined by palpating it between the finger in the vagina and the fingers pushing the abdominal wall structures inward.

The uterine corpus weighs about 60 to 100 g

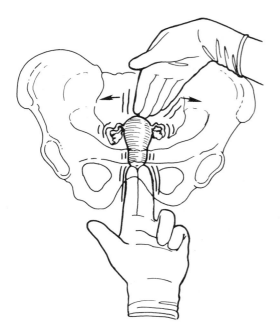

Fig. 2-2 Bimanual palpation of uterus. The hands are moved to the right or the left to palpate the adnexa.

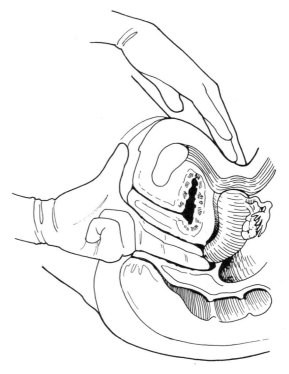

Fig. 2-3 Bimanual palpation of uterus.

and is usually palpable in one of three positions: anteflexed, in the vaginal axis, or retroflexed (Fig. 2-4).

An attempt is then made to feel the tube and ovary between the fingertips of the vaginal and abdominal hands. The right adnexum can be outlined most accurately with the fingers of the right hand in the vagina and those of the left hand palpating abdominally. The left adnexum can be felt best with the fingers of the left hand in the vagina. Normal tubes cannot be felt as distinct structures, and it may be difficult to feel normal ovaries unless the patient is very thin or the abdominal wall is relaxed; but she may experience momentary discomfort as the ovary is squeezed between the tips of palpating fingers. Adnexal masses can usually be felt if the patient can relax her abdominal muscles and if she is not too obese. For the woman with a rigid abdomen or obesity, *a pelvic ultrasound* may be considered as a means of assessing the pelvic structures.

The posterior surfaces of the uterus and broad ligaments, the uterosacral ligaments, the posterior cul-de-sac, and the structures on the lateral pelvic walls can be felt more accurately by rectal than by vaginal palpation. Rectocele and other lower bowel lesions such as polyps and carcinoma can also be felt. *A rectal or rectovaginal examination should be attempted as a part of every pelvic examination.*

Above the age of 35 the risks of polyps or malignancy increases; thus the rectal examination is critical. Stool obtained on the examining glove can be examined for *occult blood*. In a few young women a rectoabdominal exam produces so much discomfort as to negate its value. Additional lubricating jelly around the anus facilitates the patient's comfort.

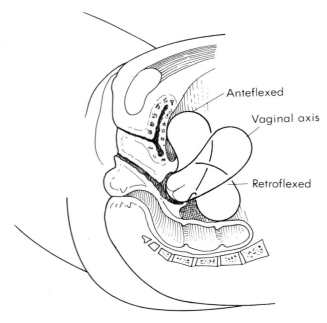

Anteflexed

Vaginal axis

Retroflexed

Fig. 2-4 A retroflexed corpus is found in about 15% to 20% of women. It is abnormal if it is tender or nonmobile.

After the exam is completed, the thoughtful examiner offers the patient some tissue to wipe away the lubricating jelly and allows her time to dress before the discussion of findings and any testing required.

DIAGNOSTIC TESTS

In many women the information obtained from the history and the physical examination is enough to indicate what treatment, if any, is required. In others, further study is necessary before a treatment plan can be developed. Most organic gynecologic disorders are caused by infection, endocrine dysfunction, tumor growth, and the late effects of childbirth injury; of these the last can usually be diagnosed without difficulty by physical examination alone, but it is necessary to perform certain laboratory studies to identify the type of tumor, the infecting organism, or the hor-

mone disorder. Many diagnostic tests are simple, can be performed in the physician's office, and require little equipment other than a microscope and stains for bacteria. Some can be done only in elaborate and specialized laboratories.

A *hemoglobin* should be performed periodically as iron deficiency is common, particularly during pregnancy and in patients with abnormal uterine bleeding. In cases of suspected intraperitoneal bleeding, serial hemoglobin or hematocrit levels can document blood loss. *Leukocyte counts* are helpful if infection is suspected and can assist in the differentiation between a tubal pregnancy and acute salpingo-oophoritis. A *clean voided urine sample* can be tested in the office with a test strip for glucose, protein, blood, acetone, and leukocyte esterase. If any of the tests are positive, appropriate follow-up is required.

Tests for pelvic infections

The physician should try to identify the organisms responsible for the various types of pelvic infections. Delineating between infections of the *lower genital tract* (cervix, vagina, vulva) and *upper genital tract* (endometrium, tubes, ovaries) is helpful; the specific diagnosis and therapy of these entities are covered in later chapters. In some instances diagnosis of the lower genital infections can be made by the physician by examining a *wet smear*. A culture may be taken and sent to a laboratory. Special precautions are necessary when anaerobic infections are suspected.

Wet smear. Obtain a small amount of vaginal discharge, dilute it with about 1 ml of saline, and shake it; place a drop of the suspension on a clean glass slide, cover with a coverslip, and examine under a microscope at 400×. *Trichomonas* may be identified as they are motile and somewhat larger than a leukocyte. If 1 to 2 drops of 10% aqueous potassium hydroxide are added to another slide prep, mycelia with spores signify the presence of *candidiasis*. If the discharge has a strong fishy odor and large, stippled epithelial cells, the "clue cells," the most likely diagnosis is *Gardnerella*.

Cultures. Crusts or exudates should be removed so that material for culture can be obtained directly from the infected area. After culture material is obtained with a sterile cotton swab, it should be placed in a transporting medium and sent to the laboratory as soon as possible.

Bacterial cultures are more informative for diagnosing vulvar or vaginal ulcers and gonorrhea. Besides obtaining a culture, ulcerations, particularly painless ones, should prompt the physician to obtain a dark field examination for syphilis and a serology.

Gonorrhea can be diagnosed more accurately by culture of cervical and urethral secretions than by clinical examination or by stained smear (Chapter 40). The material for culture is best obtained from the cervical crypts rather than purulent exudate in the vaginal canal.

The cervix is exposed and wiped clean, and a dry swab is inserted into the canal and rotated. The applicator should be left in the cervical canal for at least 30 seconds.

Special media and specimen handling are also required to culture *Chlamydia* and *herpes*. In handling all patient bodily secretions, hepatitis B and HIV precautions should be taken.

Stained smears. A Gram stain of cervical or vaginal secretions may provide information necessary to initiate appropriate treatment while awaiting the reports of bacterial cultures. This is particularly important in the treatment of septic abortions and suspected streptococcal, clostridial, and other serious acute infections.

HORMONE ASSAYS

Disturbances in production and metabolism of reproductive hormones may be important as causes of menstrual abnormalities and infertility.

Because, in a sense, the patient presents herself as a bioassay of specific hormone activity, one can determine if the ovary is producing estrogen or if a woman is ovulating through the use of simple, inexpensive tests that can be done in the office.

Specific assays are required when more precise information concerning hormone production is necessary. Examples of conditions for which accurate assay is essential are the follow-up of patients who have been treated for hydatidiform mole; the evaluation of women suspected of having anterior pituitary dysfunction; and the evaluation of women with amenorrhea, infertility, or hirsutism.

Measuring reproductive hormone function is different from measuring activity of other endocrine organs. Thyroid function, for example, varies little from day to day, and one can usually assess thyroid activity reasonably accurately with a set of tests performed on one occasion. This is not true of ovarian function, which changes from day to day throughout the menstrual cycle. It is easy to get a false impression of reproductive endocrine function if one fails to relate the results of the test to the *day of the cycle* or if one accepts a *single study* as representative of a constantly changing production of hormones. The frequency and the pulse amplitude of follicle-stimulating hormone (FSH) and luteinizing hormone (LH) are often more important than a random level of either hormone.

In short, endocrine assays are expensive, and they provide little useful information if they are ordered indiscriminately and unless they are performed in a laboratory in which the techniques are well designed and carefully controlled. Before an assay is ordered, one should have decided whether it will provide the information needed and also whether equally satisfactory information can be obtained by a simpler and less expensive method.

Tests for estrogen

Vaginal cytology. Estrogen stimulates the growth of vaginal epithelial cells. The basal and parabasal cells respond to this hormone by proliferating and becoming *cornified*. During periods of physiologic low estrogen production, before puberty, and after the menopause, the vaginal epithelium is thin and made up almost entirely of basal and parabasal cells. The cells contain little or no glycogen. Estrogen produced by the active ovaries of mature women stimulates epithelial cell growth. These changes can be demonstrated by examining stained spreads of exfoliated cells in vaginal secretions.

The presence of systemic estrogen activity may be assumed when a smear of cellular material collected from the upper vagina and stained by the Papanicolaou technique reveals cornified or precornified cells (Fig. 2-5).

Cervical mucus. Papanicolaou described an interesting pattern of arborization, or *ferning,* in cervical mucus spread on a clean glass slide and allowed to dry. The intensity of ferning is determined by the concentration of sodium chloride and other electrolytes in the cervical secretion; the greater the amount, the more pronounced the ferning. Electrolyte concentration is controlled by estrogen; the higher the concentration of estrogen, the more complete the arborization.

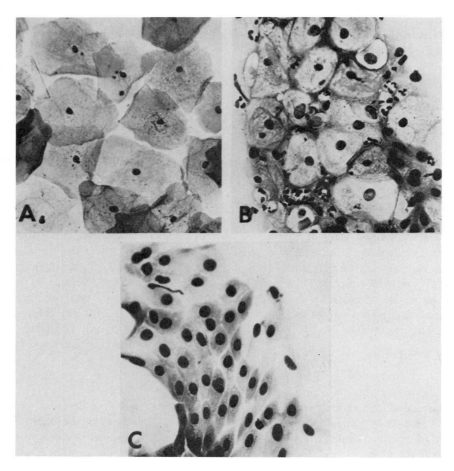

Fig. 2-5 Estrogen-induced changes in vaginal epithelial cells. **A,** Cornified (superficial) cells, a strong estrogen effect. **B,** Intermediate cells and parabasal cells, smaller rounder cells with large nuclei, a progesterone effect. **C,** Clump of basal cells, vaguely outlined with large nuclei, indicating lack of estrogen. (From Riley G: Clin Obstet Gynecol 7:432, 1964.)

Ferning is absent immediately after menstruation when estrogen is low. It increases progressively to the maximum at the time of ovulation when the estrogen concentration peaks (Fig. 2-6). Arborization does not occur in cervical mucus from untreated castrated women and from women after the menopause, but it can be induced in such women by the administration of small amounts of estrogen.

Ferning is inhibited by progesterone; hence the pattern is not present during the postovulatory phase of the normal menstrual cycle and during pregnancy.

To obtain mucus, an unlubricated speculum is inserted into the vagina, exposing the cervix from which the visible discharge is wiped. A cotton-tipped applicator is gently inserted into the cervical canal and rotated. The mucus that adheres to the cotton swab is spread on a clean slide and allowed to dry at room temperature. The dried, unstained spread is scanned under the low power of the microscope. A slightly different technique is used to examine cervical mucus after intercourse for a postcoital exam (Chapter 14).

Bone maturation. Radiograph examination of the hands of peripubertal females can be used to assess *bone age* and, therefore, estrogen activity. Epiphyseal closure is related to the amount and duration of estrogen secretion.

Radioimmunoassay of estrogen. Estrogens can be extracted from plasma, separated from other lipids and steroid hormones, and quantitated.

The technique for the measurement of plasma estrone, estradiol, and estriol enable one to quantitate program quantities of these compounds in serum. The plasma concentrations of estradiol during the early follicular phase of the normal menstrual cycle are in the range of 25 to 75 pg/ml and during the midcycle peak 200 to 400 pg/ml, respectively. During the luteal phase the concentrations fall to a level of 100 to 300 pg/ml for estradiol. In postmenopausal women the concentrations of hormones are as low as 5 to 25 pg/ml for estradiol.

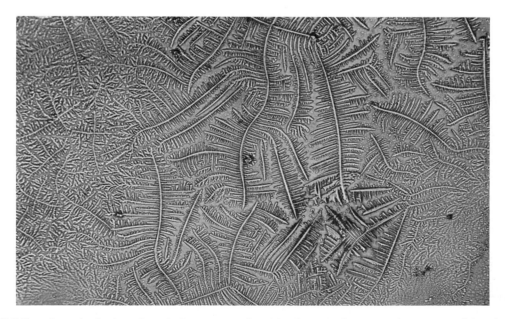

Fig. 2-6 Complete arborization of cervical mucus seen in midcycle peak of unopposed estrogen activity. (×164.)

Tests for progesterone

Progesterone activity can be detected by simple tests; a precise measurement requires a complicated assay.

Basal body temperature charts. Because progesterone has a *thermogenic* property, a sustained rise in the basal body temperature during the latter half of the menstrual cycle is presumptive evidence of progesterone activity. A monophasic curve is suggestive of absent or deficient progesterone secretion. Daily recording by the patient is required to detect the 0.4 to 0.6° F increase at ovulation; the actual event of ovulation probably occurred 1 to 2 days earlier (Fig. 2-7).

Zuspan and Zuspan reported that almost identical temperature curves can be obtained by taking temperatures at 5 PM or at bedtime rather than on awakening. Although the 5 PM temperatures are slightly higher than those in early morning, the late afternoon schedule may be quite appropriate for women whose schedules of arising and retiring are irregular or for those who cannot adjust to the basal temperature regimen.

Progesterone radioimmunoassay. Radioimmunoassay procedures are used for the determination of plasma progesterone levels, which increase from low follicular phase levels (0.4 to 1 ng/ml) to significantly elevated concentrations (3 to 20 ng/ml) during the luteal phase. These luteal phase progesterone levels drop before the onset of the next menstruation or rise sharply in early pregnancy under the stimulus of chorionic gonadotropin upon the corpus luteum. Plasma progesterone concentration increases throughout the course of pregnancy.

Tests for gonadotropins

Concentrations of anterior pituitary gonadotropins in peripheral blood can be determined by radioimmunoassay, which not only distinguishes

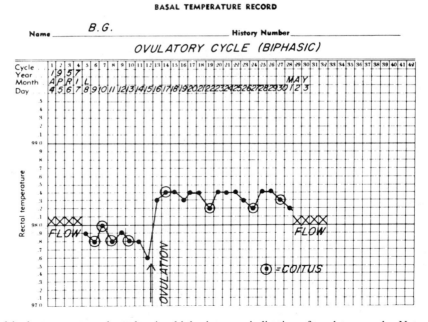

Fig. 2-7 Basal body temperature chart showing biphasic curve indicative of ovulatory cycle. Note drop and sharp rise at time of ovulation. An anovulatory cycle produces a monophasic pattern. If the temperature is elevated for greater than 16 days in the luteal phase, pregnancy should be considered.

between FSH and LH but also measures minute amounts of the hormones in small volumes of serum. The pattern of FSH and LH secretion during a normal menstrual cycle is described in Chapter 7. Follicular phase FSH concentration varies from 5 to 20 mIU/ml, whereas LH concentrations in the serum range from 5 to 25 mIU/ml; the value doubles around the time of the LH surge.

Tests for androgens

Radioimmunoassay procedures are available for the measurement of *testosterone, androstenedione* and *dehydroepiandrosterone sulfate* in serum. During the normal menstrual cycle, the plasma testosterone level is 0.2 to 0.8 ng/ml.

Tests for ovulation

Without ovulation, reproduction is impossible. This makes it important not only to be able to detect ovulation but also to time its occurrence with some degree of accuracy. The only certain methods to document ovulation is to recover an ovum, which, while possible, is clinically impractical, or

by the initiation of pregnancy. However, a number of fairly reliable *indirect* indices that ovulation has occurred may be used to determine and to time this event. The indirect tests depend predominantly upon the presence of progesterone. Some of these tests were discussed earlier.

Endometrial biopsy. Histologic examination of endometrium removed either by curettage or by biopsy 3 to 5 days before the onset of a normal menstrual period should demonstrate a late secretory endometrium. The limitations of this method are that it indicates only what has happened in one isolated cycle and that the expense and discomfort involved make it impractical to repeat the test during several cycles. To obviate the possibility of interfering with an early pregnancy in women who are trying to conceive, some authors have suggested that the endometrial biopsy be obtained during the first few hours of the menstrual flow. This is not always practicable, and, furthermore, the histologic picture of the endometrium during the bleeding phase when it is disintegrating is not nearly so well defined as it is during the

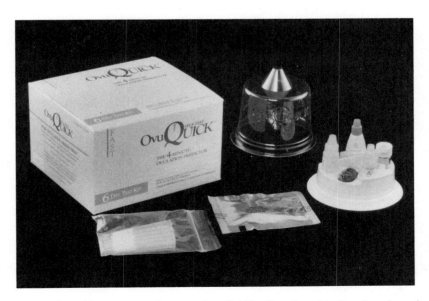

Fig. 2-8 Urinary LH predictor kits are expensive, vary in reliability from brand to brand, and require the patient to perform a simple laboratory test.

premenstruum. Temporary contraception can be used during the study cycle. Current pregnancy tests can detect human chorionic gonadotropin (hCG) at 10 days of gestation.

That the risk of interrupting pregnancy is not great is suggested by the experience of Rosenfeld and Garcia. They obtained endometrial biopsies during the cycles in which 18 infertile patients conceived; 14 delivered normal infants at term, one delivered prematurely, one aborted, and two were lost to follow-up.

Hormone assay. Serum progesterone levels are significantly increased after ovulation. No comparable change occurs during anovulatory cycles.

Examination of temperature curves, endometrial biopsy, and progesterone assay will usually indicate that ovulation has occurred or at least that progesterone is being secreted. None of these tests, however, is of value in determining the exact time of ovulation. It may be possible to anticipate ovulation by the use of *rapid urinary LH assay* to detect the LH surge. Over-the-counter test kits are available for the patient to use at home.

Fertility testing and coital timing can be facilitated if the woman can use the kit (Fig. 2-8).

Ultrasound. Monitoring follicle growth for 2 to 4 days with ultrasound to look for the formation of a *dominant follicle* (DF) is a reliable way of assessing ovulation. A DF in a spontaneous cycle ranges from 18 to 22 mm mean diameter (Fig. 2-9). The collapse of the follicle is thought to correlate with ovum release.

TESTS FOR CHORIONIC GONADOTROPINS

Soon after the ovum is fertilized and implantation occurs, the trophoblast begins to secrete hCG. The detection of this hormone in serum or urine is the basis of all pregnancy tests. It can be detected as early as 7 to 9 days after fertilization by the highly sensitive techniques of beta-subunit radioimmunoassay and radioreceptor assay. The production of hCG increases rapidly; the serum concentration *doubles about every 48 hours* during the early weeks of pregnancy. Serum levels and urinary excretion of hCG rise to a peak at

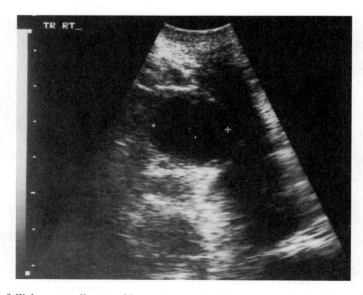

Fig. 2-9 A dominant follicle, mean diameter 20 mm, is seen in this sonogram obtained from the region of the right adnexa by using a 5-MHz endovaginal probe.

about the *sixtieth or seventieth day* after conception and then decline toward a lower plateau, which is maintained throughout the second and third trimesters. Pregnancy tests generally remain positive throughout gestation or as long as viable trophoblastic tissue is in contact with the maternal circulation.

The half-life of hCG is approximately *36 hours.* The rate of disappearance is contingent upon the level of circulating hCG, which can be significantly elevated in patients with gestational trophoblastic disease and those having functioning residual trophoblastic, as occurs following pregnancy termination. Typically, hCG levels return to normal after 10 to 14 days following delivery. Serial hormone levels are often needed in the clinical setting to monitor the disappearance of hCG.

Tests can generally be divided into two groups, *biologic* and *immunologic.* The former category constituted the original pregnancy test and depended upon hCG eliciting a biologic response, the formation of corpora lutea in rabbit ovaries, when present in sufficient quantities. Hence the concept of a *bioassay.* These tests have been replaced with newer assay techniques relying upon an immunologic response, but it is cogent to remember that immunologic and biologic hormone activity are not identical.

Immunologic tests

Immunologic pregnancy tests are based on the reaction of hCG with labeled or "tagged" antibody to hCG to chorionic gonadotropin (rabbit anti-hCG). Many pregnancy tests use the agglutination inhibition principle as an indicator. Either latex particles (slide tests) or sheep erythrocytes (test tube assay) are used.

Although the hemagglutination inhibition test is a 2-hour test as compared with the 2-minute slide tests, it is more accurate and sensitive than currently available slide tests. The hemagglutinin inhibition tests are sensitive enough to detect 500 to 1000 mIU/ml and will usually be positive by about 6 weeks after the first day of the last men-

strual period. The slide tests are even less sensitive, detecting no less than 1500 mIU/ml of urine.

A highly sensitive enzyme-linked immunoabsorbent assay (ELISA) designed to detect concentrations of hCG as low as 25 mIU/ml in urine is available. *Monoclonal antibodies* that react to different areas, the *alpha and beta subunits,* of the hCG molecule can be produced. The first immobilize hCG molecules on a membrane; the second, combined with an enzyme that produces a color change, attach to the captured hCG molecules. If hCG is present, a characteristic color appears on the membrane. If there is no hCG, the color of the membrane is unchanged. The necessary materials are supplied in kit form, and tests can be run in 10 to 20 minutes. Monoclonal antibody tests are far more sensitive than the ordinary immunologic tests and can be used to detect hCG soon after implantation and in women suspected of having ectopic pregnancies. Therefore the test depends on immunologic reaction that results in colorimetric response, thereby eliminating the precautions and equipment required to perform the radioimmunoassay. This test is an example of a *qualitative* pregnancy test.

Radioimmunoassay

Although the alpha subunits of hCG and LH are identical chemically, the beta subunits are different. Thus one can prepare a specific antibody against the beta subunit of hCG that will not react with LH. *Beta-subunit radioimmunoassay* on serum is highly sensitive and quantitative but is not practical for rapid use as a pregnancy test. The assay is more expensive and requires several hours to run. Most large metropolitan hospitals offer this test on a daily basis; it is more difficult to have access to this quantitative assay on a 24-hour basis in smaller institutions. The detection level is 5 mIU/ml.

Clinical utility of pregnancy tests

With the large array and sensitivity of pregnancy tests, it is incumbent upon the practitioner to understand, in detail, what test is being per-

---

**CLINICAL PROBLEMS WARRANTING
hCG MONITORING**

Pregnancy
Spontaneous abortion
Incomplete abortion
Ectopic pregnancy
Gestational trophoblastic disease
Molar pregnancy
Choriocarcinoma
Tumor marker
Ovarian teratoma
Dysgerminoma

---

formed and the extent of its reliability. One should also understand which circumstances can produce *false-negative* or *false-positive* tests; hCG testing is utilized in the management of several clinical problems and usually in conjunction with ultrasound (see box above).

Ordinarily, the diagnosis of pregnancy can be made without the laboratory procedures described. However, there are situations in which the history and physical findings are inconclusive or in which a complication such as threatened abortion or ectopic pregnancy is suspected but cannot be confirmed. Under these circumstances, tests for the beta subunit of hCG may prove to be an invaluable aid in diagnosis.

The standard urine hormone tests for pregnancy are about 98% accurate when carried out by hemagglutination inhibition procedures, when done properly, and when 4 to 6 weeks have elapsed since fertilization. Slide tests are less accurate in early pregnancy. Over-the-counter pregnancy test kits are available. These kits require the patient to follow exact instructions and exercise a degree of objectivity that may be unrealistic for certain patients. Performed at the proper time and in the proper manner, these tests can be reliable.

False-negative tests are encountered more frequently than false positive. The most common reasons for a false-negative test are performing the test too early in pregnancy before there is sufficient circulating hormone, or technical errors either in handling or storing of the test urine occur. Negative standard pregnancy tests are encountered in intrauterine fetal death unless a considerable amount of viable trophoblast tissue is present. A negative qualitative pregnancy test, which occurs in about half of ectopic pregnancies, never excludes the diagnosis.

False-positive tests may be obtained early in the menopause or in other gonadal deficiencies in which there is an overproduction of pituitary LH and because of errors in technique. False-positive tests may be encountered in patients who have been taking tranquilizing drugs, notably phenothiazines.

As the newer monoclonal antibody subunit-specific tests are used, the false positivity and negativity will decline. The quantitative hCG is the most sensitive and most specific and is detectable in 99% of patients with ectopic pregnancy. It is the gold standard!

It must be emphasized that all of these tests demonstrate the production of chorionic gonadotropin and do not necessarily indicate the presence of a normal pregnancy. The only conclusion to draw from a positive pregnancy test is that there is a source of gonadotropin, which may be from a normal pregnancy.

TESTS FOR CANCER

Some of the common benign cervical lesions look much like cancer grossly and can be differentiated only by special tests, all of which require highly trained personnel for their interpretation. The specimens must be properly collected and carefully handled so that they will provide the maximum amount of information. These tests are discussed in detail in Chapter 44.

Cytologic examination. A cytologist can detect abnormal cervical cells in specially prepared and stained spreads from the cervix. The most accurate results are obtained when the material is col-

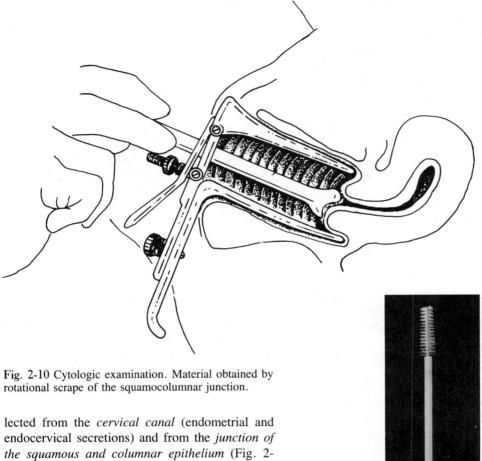

Fig. 2-10 Cytologic examination. Material obtained by rotational scrape of the squamocolumnar junction.

lected from the *cervical canal* (endometrial and endocervical secretions) and from the *junction of the squamous and columnar epithelium* (Fig. 2-10). This is the area at which squamous cell cancer usually originates. The former specimen is best obtained by rotating an endocervical brush within the cervical canal (Fig. 2-11). Material from the squamocolumnar junction is collected by scraping the area with a special spatula and transferring the material to a clean glass slide, which is then stained and read by the cytologist.

Cytologic examination is a screening procedure that indicates patients in whom further study is necessary. Whenever abnormal cells are found in a cytologic spread, more precise investigation, usually by *colposcopy, biopsy,* and *endocervical curettage* is necessary. Cytologic studies should

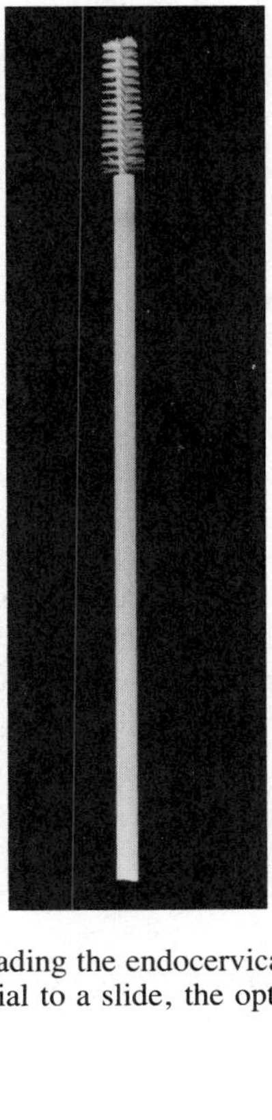

Fig. 2-11 By abrading the endocervical canal and transferring the material to a slide, the optimum sample can be obtained.

be obtained as a part of the periodic examination, even though the cervix appears normal, because the earliest carcinomas are not obvious clinically.

Cytologic examination is of less help in screening for endometrial cancer. Exfoliated endometrial cancer cells can be detected in only a small percentage of women with invasive endometrial lesions.

Cervical biopsy. The use of punch and cone biopsy is discussed in Chapter 44.

Colposcopy. The colposcope is a binocular magnifying instrument through which one can detect epithelial changes that are not visible by gross inspection. Expert colposcopists can identify the early changes in cervical and vaginal epithelium that precede the development of invasive cancer.

Under certain conditions colposcopy can replace cone biopsy in evaluating the cause of abnormal cervical cytologic studies. Tiny areas of dysplasia, carcinoma in situ, and invasive cancer can be seen and biopsied in *colposcopic-directed biopsy*. This is far more accurate than are random punch biopsies.

The requirement for accurate colposcopy is a skillful colposcopist who is able to inspect the portio vaginalis, the *transformation zone* (the squamocolumnar junction) and the endocervical canal. If this is impossible, the examination is inadequate, and additional studies such as cone biopsy are imperative in evaluating the cervix when cytologic analysis suggests the possibility of malignancy.

Endometrial biopsy. Sufficient endometrium can be obtained by office biopsy to determine its histologic pattern, but it is impossible to remove as much tissue as with dilatation and curettage, particularly if uterine polyps or submucosal myomas are present. It may be possible to diagnose carcinoma of the endometrium by office biopsy.

Endometrium can be obtained by *suction curettage*. More tissue can be removed by this technique than with a small biopsy curet. Endometrial biopsy alone cannot be considered an adequate procedure to eliminate suspected endometrial cancer.

A report of hyperplasia, particularly if it is atypical, is usually an indication for more complete curettage or hysteroscopic-directed biopsy.

Vulvar disease. Early carcinoma of the vulva may be multicentric and in its earliest phase presents no characteristic gross appearance. Areas of abnormal tissue can be detected by applying 1% aqueous toluidine blue solution to the vulva, permitting it to dry, and then sponging the vulva with 1% acetic acid. Ulcerated, excoriated, or abraded areas retain a dark blue stain. Although this test is not specific for malignancy, it does indicate areas of abnormal tissue that should be biopsied.

Adequate biopsies can be obtained with a Keyes dermatologic punch. Several specimens can be obtained from various areas of the vulva. If there is a distinct proliferative or ulcerated lesion, the biopsy can be performed with a punch biopsy instrument or by excising a wedge of tissue. These are all outpatient procedures that can be performed with local anesthesia. *Colposcopic evaluation of the vulva* with directed biopsy is the preferred method to detect lesions not discernible without a magnification.

DIAGNOSTIC IMAGING

Diagnostic imaging techniques offer significant potential in the evaluation of the obstetric or gynecologic patient. Table 2-1 presents a list of studies and their applications. With the possible exception of ultrasound, there should always be some reluctance about ordering these procedures during pregnancy. This hesitation is stimulated mostly by our lack of information concerning possible deleterious effects on the embryo or fetus.

X-ray

An important use of x-ray film examination in gynecology is for hysterosalpingography, by which small intracavitary uterine lesions as well

TABLE 2-1 Imaging procedures in obstetrics and gynecology

Study	Assessment
Hysterosalpingography	Uterine cavity contour and tubal patency
Ultrasonography	Pregnancy diagnosis and dating; fetal studies including growth
1. Abdominal	evaluation and to exclude anomalies; pelvic masses
2. Transvaginal	
Mammography	Early detection of malignancy
1. Xeromammography	
2. "Low dose" screen film mammography	
Computerized axial tomography (CT)	Pituitary tumor; adrenal tumor
Bone densitometry*	Osteoporosis
1. Single photon	
2. Dual photon	
3. Quantitative CT	
Magnetic resonance imaging	Abdominal, pelvic, pituitary tumor

*Clinical utility has yet to be determined.

as abnormalities in the tubes can be detected (Chapter 14).

Radiologic studies are used infrequently during pregnancy. X-ray film studies during the first few weeks of pregnancy are more likely to disturb fetal growth than are those during the second and third trimesters, when the organs are reasonably well formed. The tissues are particularly susceptible from the second to the sixth week after conception, when it may be difficult to diagnose pregnancy. After the primary organ systems have developed and the embryonic cells are transformed into those with adult characteristics, it is less likely that ordinary diagnostic procedures will influence fetal development.

One should seldom have to consider the need for therapeutic abortion because of radiation during pregnancy if adequate protective measures are observed consistently. Most of the questions concerning possible fetal damage arise because pregnancy is not eliminated by history or physical examination.

Radiographic studies should be ordered when the patient is in her follicular phase if possible; the newer, more sensitive hCG determination provides greater but not total assurance that an intrauterine gestation is not present when x-rays are needed in the luteal phase.

Ultrasound

This technique is useful in diagnosing both normal and abnormal pregnancy during the early weeks, in identifying multifetal pregnancy and fetal anomalies, in differentiating hydatidiform moles from normal pregnancy, in diagnosing missed abortion and intrauterine fetal death, as an aid in diagnosing ectopic pregnancy, in identifying abnormalities in amniotic fluid volume, in measuring the biparietal diameter of the fetal skull, in assessing fetal size and the rate of fetal growth, for placental localization, and in the differential diagnosis of various uterine and ovarian enlargements. These are discussed in detail in appropriate sections of the book. Diagnostic sound waves appear to have no deleterious effect on maternal or fetal tissues. The recent acquisition of the endovaginal probe has enhanced the diagnostic and therapeutic potential of this modality.

Mammography

Various low-dose techniques improve the detection of nonpalpable lesions. Current equipment allows the examination to be performed with 0.1 to 0.8 rad for a two-view examination. Xeromammography uses selenium-coated aluminum plates with the image being formed by a photoelectric process. Screen film uses special x-ray equipment that enhances soft tissue and reduces exposure time. Additional information can be found in Chapter 12.

Magnetic resonance imaging

Magnetic resonance imaging is based on the principle that nuclei of certain atoms possess the property of angular momentum, or spin, which makes them function as magnets. In a magnetic field the atoms assume positions either parallel to

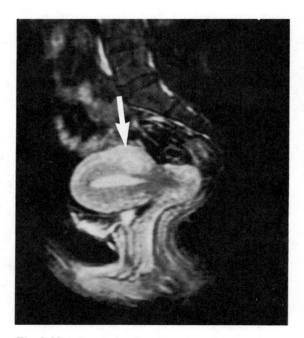

Fig. 2-12 A 2-cm posterior, intramural leiomyoma in a sagittal view obtained with a 1.5 Tesla magnet enhanced with gadolinium.

or opposite from the direction of the field. The tissue images provided by this technique are far superior to those of ultrasound and eliminate the potential dangers from radiation associated with CT scans. Because there are no known ill effects on tissue, magnetic resonance imaging has an important potential for use in obstetrics and gynecology, but it is too early to evaluate its contribution (Fig. 2-12).

Bone densitometry

There is a group of studies that attempt to assess bone density to determine which patients are at greater risk to develop osteoporosis and possible fracture. *Single-photon beam densitometry* evaluates changes predominantly in cortical bone of the distal forearm; *dual-photon beam densitometry* measures bone thickness of the thoracolumbar spine and/or femoral neck. *Quantitative CT* also examines the spine. Currently, there is controversy concerning their clinical utility.

The results from each method relate solely to that technique and cannot be compared with a different technique. Serial studies will prove more useful than one determination as the physician is attempting to detect relatively small losses in bone density, that is, 1.0% to 3.0% annually. The studies should not, at the present time, be utilized as a routine screen in perimenopausal women. Ideally, each institution needs to develop its own normative data with clinical correlation over a period of time.

LAPAROSCOPY

The development of high-intensity, fiberoptic light sources has led to a reevaluation of an old method of examining the peritoneal cavity. With the laparoscope, which is inserted through a subumbilical incision after pneumoperitoneum with CO_2 has been established, it is possible to inspect the contents of both the pelvis and the upper abdomen. The view of the pelvic organs is usually excellent; one looks down from above and can see the bladder, the anterior surface of the uterus, the adnexa, and the posterior cul-de-sac.

The principal *indications* for laparoscopy are the evaluation of pelvic pain, for inspection of small uterine or ovarian masses, infertility, endocrinopathies, amenorrhea, congenital anomalies, and sterilization. The serious *complications* are hemorrhage from punctured blood vessels and perforation of a hollow viscus.

This procedure can be classified as *diagnostic* or *operative*. The latter term applies when electrocautery, laser, or special instruments facilitate the removal of adhesions, biopsy of a pelvic structure, or incision of a fallopian tube with evacuation of an ectopic pregnancy.

HYSTEROSCOPY

The advantages of diagnosing intrauterine disease by direct inspection rather than indirectly by exploring the cavity with a curet are obvious. Hysteroscopy was first described in 1869. Improved optics, lighting sources, and operating instruments have been designed, and hysteroscopy is becoming an important tool.

Lysis of intrauterine adhesions, polyp or IUD removal, and resection of a septum are the major operative procedures. As the cavity must be distended to permit visualization, CO_2 (for diagnostic study) and high-molecular-weight dextran (for operations) are required. In spite of its simplicity, there is potential for serious complications.

AMNIOCENTESIS

A variety of examinations can be performed on amniotic fluid. Almost all tests performed during early pregnancy are to diagnose genetic defects (Chapter 32). The majority performed during the third trimester are to obtain fluid for examination in Rh disease (Chapter 32) and to assess fetal maturity (Chapter 20).

The aim of *genetic amniocentesis* is to detect fetal chromosomal and biochemical abnormalities during early pregnancy so that parents may either obtain an abortion or plan for the care of the child if a defect is present. Fetal cells in amniotic fluid are cultured for karyotyping, identification of certain enzymatic deficiencies, and determination of

fetal sex. The fluid can also be assayed for its *alpha-fetoprotein*, which may indicate open neural tube defects.

The majority of amniocenteses are performed to detect chromosomal abnormalities, which increase with maternal aging. Some abnormalities of carbohydrate, lipid, and protein metabolism can be diagnosed by studying cultured or uncultured cells. The determination of fetal sex is important in considering the possible outcome of sex-linked genetic disorders.

Genetic amniocentesis is usually performed at about 14 to 16 weeks. Before this there may be too little amniotic fluid and too few shed cells to ensure a successful result. If done much later, the pregnancy may be so far advanced when the results are available that the possibility of abortion is eliminated. Genetic amniocentesis is an outpatient procedure performed with local infiltration anesthesia and ultrasound guidance.

The *principal indications* for genetic amniocentesis are:

1. Maternal age of 35 years of more
2. Chromosomal abnormality in a previous child
3. Known chromosomal abnormality in either parent
4. Metabolic disorder in a previous child
5. History of a sex-linked genetic disorder
6. Family history of chromosomal, enzymatic, or metabolic abnormality or of neural tube defects

The *potential complications* are infection of either mother or fetus, injury to the fetus, fetomaternal transfusion with possible Rh alloimmunization if a placental blood vessel is punctured, and abortion. Infection can be kept at a minimum by using meticulous sterile technique. One can usually avoid injuring the placenta by identifying its position with ultrasound and selecting a puncture site beyond its edge. Genetic amniocentesis does not increase the rates of abortion, preterm delivery, fetal or neonatal death, or neonatal complications. It is estimated that fetal death within 3 weeks of midtrimester amniocentesis occurs in about 0.5% of cases when experienced operators perform the procedures.

Occasionally, fetal cells will not grow in the culture, minor chromosomal abnormalities may not be detected, and the techniques for diagnosing many of the metabolic disorders are still in the experimental stages or not even available. There is no way to detect anomalies such as cleft palate, club foot, and other similar defects by studing amniotic fluid.

Because of the importance of accurate diagnosis and the potential complications, amniocentesis should be performed in a perinatal center where the procedures are done regularly and where facilities are available for prompt and accurate evaluation of the cells and fluid.

Amniocentesis during late pregnancy, although easier, is not without danger. Several cases have been recorded of fetal death from hemorrhage after the puncture of an umbilical vessel.

ADDITIONAL PRENATAL DIAGNOSTIC STUDIES

Discussing new prenatal diagnostic developments in detail is beyond the scope of this text. However, a confluence of scientific knowledge has permitted greater study of the intrauterine environment in early pregnancy. Improved optic systems, advances in ultrasound imaging and recognition of anomalies, and molecular genetic techniques form the foundation of this technology.

Chorionic villus sampling (CVS)

This procedure can be performed at about the 8th to 10th week of pregnancy either transabdominally or transvaginally with ultrasound guidance.

Cells can be analyzed for biochemical markers and karyotype, and DNA probes can examine portions of the genome of the fetus. As experience grows, the risk

of infection and spontaneous abortion diminishes; currently, the risk is about 1% to 2%.

Fetoscopy

Fetoscopy, or amnioscopy, is a technique that permits direct inspection of the fetus and placenta through an endoscope, which is introduced through the maternal abdominal and uterine walls. The available instruments have a limited field of vision, and it is not yet possible to inspect the entire fetus and amnionic cavity. Fetal blood samples can be obtained from a placental vein, and the skin can be biopsied.

Percutaneous umbilical blood sampling (PUBS)

Under ultrasound guidance, the blood in the umbilical vessels can be sampled and fetal drug therapy or transfusions can be performed. Although this technique offers enormous potential, there is obvious risk. It is currently being performed in large perinatal centers, and its use will expand as the safety and efficacy improves.

SUGGESTED READING

Batzer FR: Guidelines for choosing a pregnancy test, Contemp Obstet Gynecol: 23:42, 1986.

Crandall BF, Howard J, Lebherz TB, Rubinstein L, Sample WF, and Sarti D: Follow-up of 2000 second-trimester amniocenteses, Obstet Gynecol 56:625, 1980.

De Cherney AH, Romero R, and Polan ML: Ultrasound in reproductive endocrinology, Fertil Steril 37:323, 1982.

Elias S, Simpson JL, Martin AO, Sabbagha RE, Gerbie AB, and Keith LG: Chorionic villus sampling for first-trimester prenatal diagnosis: Northwestern University Program, Am J Obstet Gynecol 152:204, 1985.

Papanicolaou G: General survey of vaginal smear and its use in research and diagnosis, Am J Obstet Gynecol 51:316, 1946.

Siegler AM: Hysterosalpinography, Fertil 40:139, 1983.

Tompkins P: The use of basal temperature graphs in determining the date of ovulation, JAMA 124:698, 1944.

3

John H. Mattox

Pediatric gynecology

Objectives

RATIONALE: Serious gynecologic problems in the pediatric age group requiring physician input are infrequent. However, it is apparent that nearly all of the diseases identified in the adult female population can be found in the very young female. A special approach and knowledge base are important to the successful management of these patients.

The student should be able to:

A. Demonstrate a knowledge of the anatomic and physiologic differences in the genital tract between the prepubertal girl and postpubertal young woman.

B. Outline the management, including a differential diagnosis, of a 6-year-old girl complaining of an odorous, sanguinopurulent discharge.

C. Discuss the assessment of a 7-year-old girl who presents with precocious puberty.

With few exceptions, the gynecologic problems encountered in the adult woman can be manifested in the prepubertal girl. Genital disorders most often encountered in girls from infancy to adolescence include various local infections, injuries, congenital anomalies, and abnormal sexual development. The disorders during the adolescent years are primarily those related to menstrual function. Differences in adult and adolescent anatomy and physiology alter the method of examination and interpretation of findings.

The physician must also tailor an approach to the younger female patient that incorporates a quiet demeanor, greater gentleness, and increased sensitivity. Invariably both the parent and child require the physician's understanding and time.

ANATOMIC AND PHYSIOLOGIC DEVELOPMENT
Neuroendocrine system

Although the ultimate function of the hypothalamic-pituitary-ovarian axis (HPO) is to produce repetitive ovulatory cycles, a defined sequence is initiated in utero and progresses until puberty is complete. The presence of gonadotropins can be identified histochemically *by the tenth week of*

31

gestation. By the second trimester, in vitro studies substantiate that the fetal pituitary will respond to GnRH. The gonadotropins FSH and LH tend to be higher in female fetuses, with a greater concentration of FSH being secreted. Following an initial surge of FSH and LH at birth, these hormones become almost undetectable for several years. The HPO axis is controlled by negative feedback, and this system is extremely sensitive to suppression by small amounts of estrogen. As the maturation of the system occurs, this unique sensitivity disappears, and a greater concentration of estradiol is needed to suppress FSH and LH. The *nocturnal pulses of gonadotropins* occur, and eventually the benchmark of the mature HPO axis, *positive feedback,* can be documented. It can be easily understood how the corresponding fluctuations in gonadotropins would produce similar changes in gonadal steroid production, the latter being responsible for the changes in physiognomy associated with pubescence. A more thorough description of the neuroendocrine relationships can be found in Chapter 7.

Genital tract

Normal variations from adult genitals include a more anterior location of the introitus and a rela-

tive prominence of the clitoris, which may measure 1 to 1.5 cm. During the first few days after birth, the breasts and genitals are swollen, and the latter are moistened by clear secretions from the estrogen-stimulated vagina. The endometrium also is stimulated, and estrogen-withdrawal bleeding may occur within 3 to 5 days of delivery because the placental source of estrogen is no longer present.

All estrogen effects disappear after 2 to 3 weeks and do not return until puberty, when ovarian function is initiated. During this intermediate period, the vaginal epithelium is thin, uncornified, and red. The vaginal smear is made up of basal and parabasal cells, and the vaginal pH is alkaline.

The hymen is redundant and with strain may protrude beyond the surrounding parts. The hymenal opening changes little in size throughout the prepubertal period and is as adequate for passage of the same instruments in the infant as in the girl of 10 years of age. Bartholin's, paraurethral, and cervical glands are rudimentary and virtually functionless.

The vaginal portion of the cervix is flat, and the endocervical epithelium extends for a short distance over the surface. This should not be in-

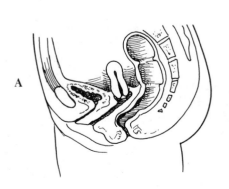
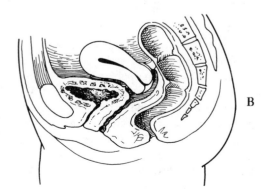

Fig. 3-1 Comparison of immature, **A,** and mature, **B,** pelvic organs. In immature organs the cervix comprises two thirds of the organ, and the vaginal fornices are short.

terpreted or treated as an erosion or cervicitis.

The posterior fornix is short and the cul-de-sac almost nonexistent. The long axis of the uterus is parallel to the long axis of the body in contrast to the anteverted position in the adult (Fig. 3-1). The total length is 2.5 to 3 cm with reversal of the adult cervix-corpus ratio, the *cervix in the immature female comprising two thirds* of the entire organ. Complete reversal of the ratio does not occur until full maturation, which can be within a few months or as long as several years after the menarche.

The ovaries arise embryologically about T10 and are more an abdominal than a pelvic organ during childhood. The greatest number of follicles is present in utero at approximately 20 weeks of gestation and continues to decline (through the poorly understood process of atresia) from birth to adolescence.

The vagina contains the *Lactobacillus* at birth and is acidic; however, during early childhood, the pH is neutral to slightly *alkaline,* and only a few bacteria colonize it. Therefore the usual protective measures, the acidic pH and estrogen-induced vaginal cornification, are absent, making the vulvovaginal area very susceptible to infection and trauma.

APPROACHING THE PREMENARCHAL PATIENT
History

Usually the mother of the patient will want to provide all of the information. It may be relevant to ask about any complications of the mother's pregnancy as well as the growth and development of the child, particularly with suspected anomalies or intersex problems. However, the physician should make significant effort to establish rapport with the girl, first by asking her nonmedical questions perhaps about school or home activities and then inquiring about her thoughts concerning the problem. Eye contact when possible and an unhurried approach are mandatory. The verbal feedback from the pediatric patient will be less than from the adult patient.

Physical examination

The first examination most girls undergo is as infants following birth in the delivery room. Whether that examination has any psychologic ramifications is unclear; certainly the premenarchal examination will be remembered. Customarily the mother is present and perhaps chaperones the examination, but in circumstances such as suspected child abuse having a nurse present will be preferable while performing a general physical examination. Continual assurance concerning what to expect can help minimize any anxiety the child is experiencing. The use of stirrups and a large drape are cumbersome and usually unnecessary and may have an adverse effect upon rapport. The "frog leg" position on the examining table will suffice. As much as possible have all needed instruments, media, and other materials prepared ahead of time. A fine-gauge, lubricated pediatric feeding tube is preferable to a rigid cotton-tipped applicator for assessing vaginal patency and depth. The knee-chest position is particularly useful as the vagina tends to open naturally when the patient is in this position.

The vaginal vault and cervix can be seen through a small, well-lubricated vaginoscope or urethroscope. Makeshift instruments such as a nasal speculum or an otoscope are inadequate be-

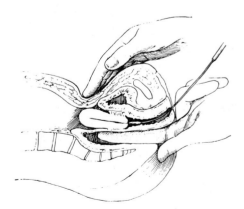

Fig. 3-2 A rectoabdominal exam.

cause they are too short to expose the upper vagina and cervix. If vaginal smears or cultures are to be obtained, a well-lubricated pediatric feeding tube is rolled through the hymenal opening.

A rectoabdominal examination is performed (Fig. 3-2). Copious lubrication is needed, as well as explanations of what to expect to the patient. The uterus may not be palpable to the inexperienced examiner, and no masses should be present under normal circumstances. On occasion some mild sedation in the office may be necessary, and the physician should not hesitate to perform an examination under anesthesia, if necessary, to secure needed information.

GYNECOLOGIC PROBLEMS IN PREADOLESCENTS
Vulvovaginitis

This condition is the most common problem in the premenarchal female. She usually presents with pruritus, discharge, and signs of acute or chronic irritation of the vulva and vaginal introitus. *Poor perineal hygiene* is most frequently the problem. The diagnosis is not usually apparent from the clinical presentation but can be made through a systematic approach. Any bleeding raises the specter of possible neoplasm (see box below).

ABBREVIATED LIST OF CAUSES OF VULVOVAGINITIS

Poor perineal hygiene
Foreign bodies (wads of paper, sand, pieces of crayon)
Pinworms
Chemical agents (soaps, bubble bath, deodorant sprays)
Bacterial infection, nonspecific (from respiratory infections, urinary tract infections, unknown)
Sexually transmitted disease *(Trichomonas,* herpes, gonorrhea, *Chylamydia)*
Allergens
Neoplasm (rare)

Investigation of infections involving the external genitals should include pelvic examination; culture of the discharge; perianal examination, particularly for pinworm ova; and urinalysis to exclude urinary tract infection and diabetes. *Any sexually transmitted disease in a child should suggest the possibility of sexual abuse.*

Acute gonorrheal vulvovaginitis produces an intense inflammatory reaction, edema of the vulva, and a profuse, purulent vaginal discharge. Cervical, paraurethral, and Bartholin's glands are poorly developed and are rarely involved, but an associated proctitis is not uncommon. Upper genital tract infections are extremely rare. Systemic reactions are minimal. The choice of antibiotic can be determined by the cultures.

Chlamydia trachomatis is now considered the most common cause of sexually transmitted diseases in women and of ophthalmia neonatorum in the infant. Cervical erosion and a mucopurulent discharge are usually noted. Smears show characteristic evidence of infection, although both chlamydial and gonorrheal cervicitis are frequently asymptomatic. Mixed infections are common. Culture or an immunofluorescent staining technique is necessary for diagnosis. Chlamydial vaginitis found in a young child can occur by eye-to-vagina transmission but should also raise suspicion of sexual abuse. Therapy with a broad-spectrum tetracycline is usually effective.

Hemolytic streptococcal vaginitis is more often the cause of bloody or serosanguineous discharge than is a foreign body, although the possible presence of the latter should not be overlooked. Evidence of genital infection generally appears 2 to 4 weeks after a streptococcal infection elsewhere, particularly in the throat or the skin. Diagnosis is made by culture.

Nonspecific vaginitis is characterized by a relatively low-grade, often persistent mixed infection. Local irritation by scratching or manipulation is a common cause. Persistent stool secondary to poor wiping technique is responsible. Cultures reveal intestinal flora. *Pinworm infestations* should be suspected in any persistent or recurrent nonspecific vaginitis, and examination should be made for ova and parasites. Nocturnal pruritus sufficient to awaken the child is a key symptom if present.

Treatment consists of local hygiene and removal of irritation. Pinworm infestations, when present, must be eradicated with medication. The use of sitz baths two or three times a day, the application of a 0.5% hydrocortisone ointment, and then local cleansing after defecation will reduce irritation. When inflammation of vulvovaginal tissues is intense, the oral administration of appropriate antibiotics gives more prompt relief than do local measures alone.

Estrogen therapy is indicated for persistent or recurrent vaginitis because cornification of the epithelium and reduction of the vaginal pH increases local tissue resistance. Steroidal estrogen such as Premarin creme, with dosage adjusted to size of the patient, applied to the vulva daily for 21 days, is usually sufficient. Breast stimulation may occur but is reversed when the hormone is discontinued. Loose-fitting clothing and clean cotton panties should be part of the symptomatic care.

Candidiasis is uncommon except in diabetic children and in children following antibiotic administration. A urine or blood glucose determination is indicated in every case.

Trichomonas infections are rare, but, when present, trichomonads are usually found in the urine as well as in the vaginal discharge. Treatment with metronidazole is effective.

Vaginal foreign body. The presence of a persistent vaginal discharge accompanied by pain suggests a foreign body. Endoscopic inspection of the vaginal canal with lavage offers the best means of localization. X-ray or ultrasound examination is necessary if the foreign body has migrated into adjacent tissues. A nonspecific vaginitis occurs secondarily and requires treatment.

Lichen sclerosus. Lichen sclerosus usually is diagnosed in older women, but it sometimes occurs in children. It is discussed in detail in Chapter 43. Surgery, other than biopsy for diagnosis, is contraindicated. In children the lesion will sometimes spontaneously regress.

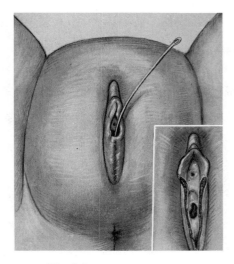

Fig. 3-3 Labial agglutination.

Labial agglutination

Labial agglutination may occur congenitally or as the result of infection or irritation, which denudes the thin membrane and leads to adhesion of the labia minora in the midline (Fig. 3-3). A characteristic livid line, extending vertically down the center of the membrane, distinguishes agglutination from the less commonly encountered imperforate hymen or vaginal atresia.

This condition is self-limiting and disappears as puberty approaches and estrogen levels rise, but it may require therapy before then because the agglutination encourages pocketing of urine, irritation, and infection.

Application of an estrogen cream twice daily induces cornification of the epithelium, and spontaneous separation will usually occur within 2 weeks. Reagglutination can be prevented by regular perineal cleansing.

Prolapsed urethra

Bleeding, the appearance of a mass at the vaginal orifice, and pain, particularly with micturition, suggest prolapse of the urethral mucosa (Fig. 3-4). The congested edematous mass may

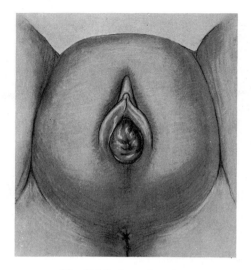

Fig. 3-4 Prolapsed urethra.

occlude the vaginal orifice and is likely to be mis-interpreted as vaginal prolapse or genital tumor. Although no lumen is visible, a lubricated pediatric feeding catheter inserted in the center of the mass will seek the bladder and confirm the diagnosis.

Reduction of the prolapse can be accomplished occasionally; but necrosis often is present, and excision of the redundant tissue at the meatal line of demarcation is necessary.

Trauma

Most injuries to the female genitals produce no permanent damage. A *vulvar hematoma* is the most frequent lesion. Bleeding can usually be controlled by pressure and application of cold compresses. Deep lacerations requiring suturing heal with little scarring. The location of the urethra provides protection against actual injury, but urinary retention as a result of edema and spasm is not uncommon. Reassuring the parents that local genital injuries will not interfere with future functions is one of the most important aspects of treatment.

Trauma caused by *rape* can be a devastating experience for a young child. Team approach, including physician, nurse, psychiatrist, and security officer, is vital to management of the overall problem in order to begin dealing promptly with the potentially long-term psychosocial effects of rape. If trauma is marked or if bleeding persists, examination under anesthesia is necessary to rule out upper genital tears or penetration of the peritoneal cavity.

In the usual case, rape results in circumferential tears, abrasions, and ecchymosis. These evidences or the demonstration of sperm about the genitals are indications for prophylactic antibiotic therapy.

Abuse of the child represents one of the major public health problems in the world. In the United States 4000 children are estimated to die annually from battery or neglect. The physician seeing infants and young girls must be continually vigilant in detecting abuse, which can be physical, sexual, or emotional, the last being the most difficult to detect and substantiate. Estimates of sexual abuse run as high as 200,000 children annually and include a myriad of possible circumstances such as incest, assault, forced witnessing of sexual behavior, fondling of the genitalia, fellatio, cunnilingus, and sodomy. The subject of sexual abuse is covered in greater detail in Chapter 6.

CONGENITAL ANOMALIES

Because of the close embryologic relationship of the genital and urinary tracts, developmental anomalies observed in one system warrant thorough examination of both.

Imperforate hymen. Imperforate hymen is an exception in that it usually occurs as an isolated anomaly. Surgical correction is desirable when the diagnosis is made but is imperative at puberty. Simple puncture of the membrane will heal over and is inadequate. Cruciate incisions across the membrane will maintain patency.

Vaginal agenesis. Complete vaginal agenesis is generally associated with absent or rudimentary development of the uterus and tubes. Ovarian development usually is normal. An expanded dis-

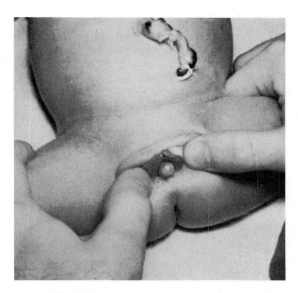

Fig. 3-5 Ectopic ureter with ureterocele.

cussion of congenital anomalies can be found in Chapter 9.

Ectopic ureter with vaginal terminus. Ectopic ureter in the female most often terminates in the vaginal vault or the vestibule; hence there usually is constant loss of urine from the vagina. If the terminus is closed, the *ureterocele* thus formed appears as a cystic mass that protrudes from the vagina (Fig. 3-5). This is the most common "vaginal cyst" in infants. If the ectopic ureter is patent, constant irritation from urine promotes infection, and vaginitis may be the first sign.

Vaginal ectopic anus. Imperforate anus associated with a rectovaginal communication in the female infant is a consequence of erratic migration of the hindgut, occurring by 6 to 8 weeks of embryonic life (Fig. 3-6).

NEOPLASMS

Unfortunately, nearly all of the tumors diagnosed in the adult female patient have been identified in the pediatric age group. Tumors of the genital tract are important not because of their frequency but because of their highly malignant potential. Suspicion should be raised concerning a neoplastic etiology whenever there is a genital ulcer, persistent odorous or bloody discharge, a mass presenting at the introitus, persistent abdominal pain or swelling, and sexual precocity. *Nearly 50% of the genital tumors diagnosed in females under 16 years are premalignant or malignant.*

Benign and malignant lesions of vagina and cervix

Because of the close embryologic origin of the upper vagina and the cervix, both benign and ma-

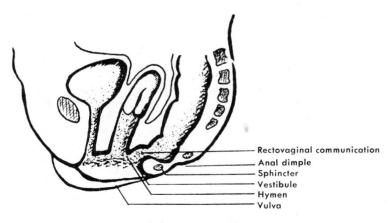

Fig. 3-6 Vaginal ectopic anus.

Rectovaginal communication
Anal dimple
Sphincter
Vestibule
Hymen
Vulva

lignant lesions of similar histologic character can arise from either tissue.

The benign lesions of the vagina are usually remnants of the mesonephric duct, which usually form cystic tumors. They may be small, stable, and asymptomatic; therefore, no therapy is required. Lesions that are large, growing, or otherwise symptomatic should be biopsied.

DES-related lesions. An exception to the low frequency of benign vaginal and cervical lesions was found in young women exposed to diethylstibestrol (DES) during the first 18 weeks of intrauterine life; these involve the unusual but significant occurrence of clear cell adenocarcinoma of the vagina or cervix in DES-exposed women. Characteristic benign lesions identified in at least 80% of women with a history of intrauterine exposure to DES or related synthetic nonsteroidal estrogens, as well as the anatomic deformities recognized in about 20%, give clear evidence of the teratogenic potential of this group of drugs.

Remnants of müllerian anlage persist beneath the vaginal plate of squamous epithelium, where glandular elements are not normally found. Most of the glands are lined by mucin-secreting columnar cells resembling those of the endocervix. In some the lining cells are smaller and resemble tubal or endometrial cells. They may be completely buried beneath the vaginal epithelium, but often ostia of the glands and their secretions are visible on the surface, *adenosis.*

Eversion, or *ectropion,* of the cervix is common. Deformities of the vagina or cervix occur mainly in the form of transverse ridges. The terms *ridges, vaginal hood, cervical collar,* and *cockscomb cervix* are used, depending on the appearance and extent of the deformity.

Upper genital tract abnormalities also occur more frequently in exposed females. These include reduced size and shape of the uterus, synechiae, and constricting bands. The incidence of premature labor and pregnancy failure caused by uterine abnormalities and by incompetence of an anomalous cervical os is increased.

Clear cell adenocarcinoma

More than 90% of the young women exposed to DES in utero who subsequently develop this rare type of lower genital tract malignancy have reached puberty or beyond. Ages at the time of diagnosis range from 7 to 29 years. It is therefore likely that stimulation of the anomalous glandular epithelium plays a key role in

their growth. Studies of women who were exposed to DES in utero indicate that the incidence of cervical dysplasia and carcinoma in situ was 15.7 per 1000 person-years of follow-up in those who had been exposed to DES versus 7.9 cases per 1000 in controls. The risk of adenocarcinoma is between 1.4/1000 and 1.4/10,000 women. Neoplastic lesions arise most commonly in the upper half of the vagina or in the cervix.

Examination and management of DES-exposed women

Every young woman whose mother received DES during pregnancy should be considered at risk of adenosis or adenocarcinoma of the lower genital tract. All should be examined regardless of age if symptoms appear, otherwise beginning about age 12 to 14, before the risk of malignancy becomes significant. Symptoms are vaginal bleeding, discharge, or pain, although about 20% of malignant and benign lesions are asymptomatic.

The screening pelvic examination includes direct visual inspection, which may reveal patchy red areas of adenosis, cervical ectropion or eversion, or marked mucus secretion. Because adenosis may be entirely submucosal, palpation of the entire vagina is necessary to detect small nodular structures.

Cytologic examination is not wholly reliable for diagnosis of this malignancy. False-negative results have been found in approximately 20% of cases.

Colposcopic examination has proved to be of particular value in diagnosis of adenosis, interpretation of findings in the surrounding transformation zone of squamous metaplasia or dysplasia, and selection of suspicious areas for biopsy.

Treatment of adenosis is conservative, with follow-up examinations at regular intervals. Improvement with time or after pregnancy is not uncommon. This is observed particularly in cases with extensive cervical ectopy and apparent deformity of the cervix. Replacement of columnar epithelium by squamous metaplasia and a smoothing of cervical ridges have been observed within a 3- to 5-year period. *Because of the significant decline in DES usage in the late 1960s and early 1970s, the occurrence of carcinoma has been dramatically reduced.*

Mixed mesodermal tumors

Botryoid sarcoma arises from mesenchymal tissue of the cervix or vagina and appears as an edematous grapelike mass of tissue that bleeds readily on touch

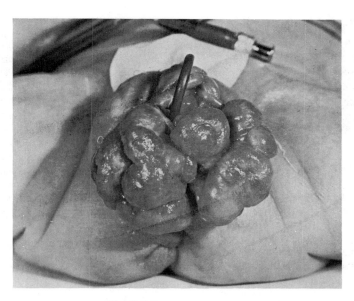

Fig. 3-7 Sarcoma botryoides.

(Fig. 3-7). Extension proceeds locally, involving all pelvic structures. Distant metastasis is not characteristic. The neoplasm is resistant to x-ray or radium therapy and curable only by early radical extirpation.

Ovarian tumors

Ovarian neoplasms are occasionally encountered in preadolescents. Any young female patient presenting with persistent or unexplained abdominal pain or an abdominal mass should be evaluated for an ovarian tumor. Benign cystic teratoma, or *dermoid cyst,* is the most common type and is more likely to cause symptoms as a result of torsion rather than size. The use of pelvic ultrasound and abdominal computerized tomography have facilitated the diagnosis of abdominopelvic lesions. While promising, the utility of magnetic resonance imaging (MRI) has not been firmly established.

In a review of 21 years of experience, Ehren and colleagues reported on 63 children with ovarian neoplasms. More than 75% had a history of chronic abdominal pain; there were 41 benign teratomas; the incidence of torsion in the entire series was 41%.

ABNORMAL SEXUAL DEVELOPMENT

The types of sexual abnormalities encountered can be characterized in terms of the three distinctive stages of sexual development: (1) gonadal, (2) differentiation of the internal genitals, and (3) differentiation of the external genitals.

Clinically, intersex disorders are manifested at birth in infants with *ambiguous genitalia, sexual precocity,* either isosexual or heterosexual, and in patients presenting with *primary amenorrhea.*

Genetic sex is determined at the time of fertilization. The sequence of events leading to gonadal differentiation begins with the appearance of the undifferentiated gonad at the fourth week of embryonic life; the germ cells then migrate from the entoderm to the yolk sac along the hindgut and beyond to enter the primitive gonad; finally, gonadal sex is determined by the sex-controlling genes in the X and Y chromosomes. The Y chromosome, or a specific portion (pericentric), must be present to induce development of the testis. An *H-Y histocompatibility* antigen, the location of which has been recently identified near the testis-determining gene on the Y chromosome, is usually present but is not the major determinant of testes formation. *Testicular-determining factor* (TDF) gene, located on the short arm of the Y chromosome, controls male gonad differentiation.

At about 7 to 8 weeks after conception, the seminiferous tubules and then Leydig cells appear, and the latter begin to produce testosterone, which is essential for any further male development.

Both *wolffian* (mesonephric) and *müllerian* (paramesonephric) ducts are present in the early embryo. Differentiation of the internal genitals is controlled by hormones. Early in embryonic life the testis produces *müllerian-inhibiting hormone* (MIH), which causes regression of the müllerian ducts. Even in the absence of MIH, the female genitalia can develop independently. The early testis also produces *testosterone,* the essential factor in effecting differentiation of the wolffian ducts into vas deferens, epididymis, and seminal vesicles. Through 5-alpha reductase activity, *dihydrotestosterone* is produced. For completely normal male genitalia, internally and externally, both hormones are necessary. If an ovary is present or even in its absence, as in ovarian dysgenesis 45×, the wolffian system, lacking testosterone stimulation, regresses; and the müllerian duct differentiates into uterus, fallopian tubes, and upper vagina.

The last stage, differentiation of the external genitals, involves common primordial structures in both sexes. Androgen stimulation of the genital tubercle, folds, and swellings is essential for differentiation into male external genitals; otherwise, female phenotypia prevails.

Genital ambiguity of the newborn

The proper *recognition of sex of the newborn infant* is one of the first considerations for the obstetrician. Cases of indeterminate sex noted at birth involve abnormalities in development of the external genitals and will require further study before a definitive diagnosis and sex assignment can occur. These fall into three main groups: (1) *congenital adrenal hyperplasia,* (2) *masculinization caused by maternal environmental factors,* and (3) *male pseudohermaphroditism with incomplete development of the external genitals.*

Congenital adrenal hyperplasia (CAH) is the most frequent cause of distinct virilization of the newborn infant. The disorder is an inborn error in metabolism and is an autosomal recessive trait. There is impairment or block of the synthesis of cortisol caused by specific defects in steroid hydroxylating enzyme.

In order of frequency, deficits occur in C-21 hydroxylase, C-11 hydroxylase, and 3-beta-ol dehydrogenase. Impairment of C-21 hydroxylation of 17-alpha-hydroxyprogesterone is followed by diminution in the biosynthesis of deoxycortisol (compound S) and in turn by reduction in cortisol. As the rate of adrenocorticotropic hormone (ACTH) secretion by the pituitary is regulated by cortisol feedback, diminution of this hormone results in excessive ACTH secretion and overstimulation of the adrenal glands, with resultant hyperplasia of the zona reticularis. Overproduction of androgenic hormones ensues in response to ACTH stimulation, as the metabolic pathway for these end products remains unimpaired. The deficit of C-21 hydroxylase can be complete or incomplete. In approximately a third of cases the deficit is so great that virilization is accompanied by the *salt-losing syndrome.*

The clinical characteristics in the newborn are shown in Fig. 3-8. These include relative persistence of the urogenital sinus, accentuation of the labial folds, and enlargement of the clitoris. A small vagina usually communicates with the urethra. The single opening is located at the base of the enlarged clitoris and suggests

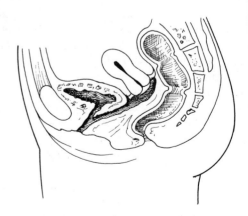

Fig. 3-8 Persistence of urogenital sinus in females with congenital adrenal hyperplasia; there are usually sites of communication between urethra and vagina.

hypospadias. The appearance can be so perplexing that determination of sex on the basis of external examination alone is impossible. Chromosome studies for determination of sex, rectal palpation of the uterus or identification with pelvic ultrasound, and visualization of the cervix by endoscopy or the urinary and genital tracts by x-ray film examination after radiopaque instillation aid in diagnosis. Elevated 17-alpha hydroxyprogesterone levels are diagnostic.

Cortisone will reverse the symptoms. Mineralocorticoids are necessary in the salt-losing type. Early diagnosis of sex and the establishment of a plan for the child's future are of the utmost importance. Surgical revision of the clitoris and reconstruction of the vagina may be required.

Maternal factors. Masculinization of the female fetus can occur when certain progestins, 19 norsteroids, and medroxyprogesterone acetate are administered to the expectant mother during early pregnancy. Except for the importance of accurate diagnosis, this type of masculinization does not pose a serious problem because effects are limited to the external genitals.

The clitoris is enlarged, and the labial folds may be firmly fused in the midline, giving an ambiguous impression of the sex (Fig. 3-9). There is no interference with differentiation of the müllerian and wolffian ducts, and therefore the vagina, uterus, and tubes are normal. The fetal ovary is unaffected.

Diagnosis is made by (1) a history of oral or intramuscular administration of progestins to the expectant mother before the twelfth and through the fifteenth or sixteenth week of gestation, usually for threatened or habitual abortion, (2) normal 17-alpha hydroxyprogesterone secretion, and (3) a 46 XX karyotype.

Treatment begins with reassurance of the parents. In mild cases there is spontaneous regression. Clitoral revision is sometimes necessary.

Male pseudohermaphroditism. Physical characteristics of individuals with male pseudohermaphroditism show gradations of abnormality. The external genitals may appear feminine, doubtful, or masculine. The feminine type *(testicular feminizing syndrome* or *androgen insensitivity)* is most common.

For the types in which feminization is incom-

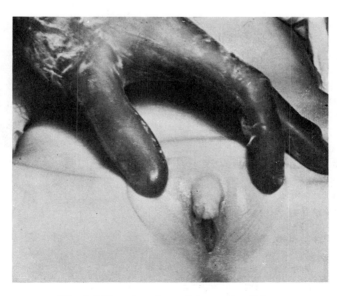

Fig. 3-9 Nonadrenal pseudohermaphroditism.

plete, extreme caution in the assignment of sex is particularly urgent in this condition.

The chromosomal complement is usually 46 XY and one is tempted to make an assignment of male sex on this cursory examination, yet subsequent development tends to proceed along female lines. At birth the absence of a vagina and/or inguinal masses or hernias should call attention to this diagnostic possibility. This problem is discussed in Chapter 9.

SEXUAL PRECOCITY

Manifestations of precocious puberty are either isosexual or heterosexual. *Isosexual types* in the female child are dependent on early or abnormal *estrogen* stimulation that may be hypothalamopituitary (constitutional), a CNS tumor, adrenal, or ovarian in origin. Effects are entirely feminizing. *Heterosexual types,* resulting in virilization, are usually caused by increased adrenocortical activity. The inadvertent administration of estrogen, testosterone, and certain progestins or the presence of a functioning adrenal tumor can produce precocity.

Isosexual

True and pseudoisosexual precocity. The onset of puberty has a wide normal range. Early appearance of secondary sex characteristics usually represents *sensitive end-organ response* to minimal hormone stimulation, but the occurrence of the menarche before the age of 9 years is unusual and deserves investigation.

Premature thelarche, unilateral or bilateral breast enlargement, occurs as an isolated event without other evidence of sexual maturation; the problem is self-limiting and requires only assurance to the patient and parents. *Premature pubarche,* the early development of pubic hair, can also occur as an isolated event. It is prudent to exclude possible problems with androgen secretion or ingestion, and medical therapy is not required.

The most common type (85 to 90%) of isosexual precocious puberty is "constitutional," in

which *idiopathic hypothalamic-pituitary-ovarian activation* occurs. No abnormalities other than early maturity are associated. Hypothalamic, pituitary, ovarian, and adrenal hormones reach normal adult levels; the patient can be ovulatory, and pregnancy is possible. This description defines *true isosexual precocity.* Rarely, *central nervous system lesions* may produce true isosexual precocity.

Social adjustment poses the most serious problem for these children. Sexual awakening and receptivity are far in advance of mental and emotional maturity. Children with idiopathic precocious puberty can be treated with a long-acting GnRH analogue (DepoLupron). It will inhibit gonadotropin secretion, menstruation, and breast development.

Precocious sexual development and uterine bleeding resulting from *feminizing tumors of the ovary, granulosa-theca cell tumors, or functioning follicular cysts* are estrogen induced and anovulatory. Hence pregnancy does not occur, but in other respects clinical features of this type of precocity do not differ from other

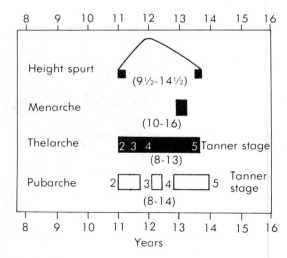

Fig. 3-10 Diagram of sequence of pubarchel events in girls. Range of ages within which some events may occur is given by figures in parentheses. (Redrawn from Tanner JM: Growth at adolescence, ed 2, Oxford, England, 1962, Blackwell Scientific Publications, Ltd.)

isosexual varieties. Pelvic ultrasound can assist in the diagnosis.

Rarer causes for pseudoprecocity include *hypothyroidism, estrogen-producing adrenal tumors,* and *Albright's syndrome* (polyostotic fibrous dysplasia, café au lait spots, and cysts of the skull and long bones).

Heterosexual precocity. Virilization is the striking manifestation of heterosexual precocity and is usually caused by an adrenal lesion. When evident at birth, congenital adrenal hyperplasia is most likely, whereas after the first year of life the onset of an adrenogenital syndrome is usually caused by an adrenal tumor or a mild delayed type of adrenal hyperplasia. Virilization appearing in puberty and in early adulthood is associated with adrenal or ovarian tumors, the incomplete form of male pseudohermaphroditism, and delayed or acquired adrenal hyperplasia. These disorders and their management are discussed earlier in this chapter and in Chapters 9 and 47.

GYNECOLOGIC PROBLEMS IN ADOLESCENT GIRLS

Menarche. The sequence of events leading to the menarche, or first menstrual period, is illustrated in Fig. 3-10. Characteristic body changes precede the menarche by several years. Various

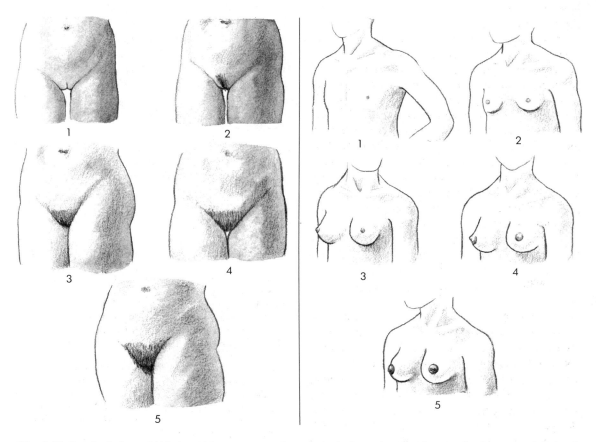

Fig. 3-11 Standards for pubic hair and breast stages. Stage 1 is the least developed; stage 5 represents adult development. (Redrawn from Tanner JM: Growth and endocrinology of the adolescent. In Gardner L, editor: Endocrine and genetic diseases of childhood, ed 2, Philadelphia, 1975, WB Saunders Co.)

factors such as the genetic, socioeconomic, and general health of the individual, climate, and body mass influence the age of onset of menstruation.

Tanner and colleagues observed longitudinal changes in secondary sexual maturation in English schoolchildren. Although nearly four decades old, these guidelines still seem to represent appropriately the progression of the pubertal sequence. The current age of menarche in the United States is approximately 12.3 years. A pictorial representation of the Tanner stages can be seen in Fig. 3-11.

Growth spurt is greatest during this time, the protein requirement being three times that of the adult. Growth continues for another 3 years or so after the onset of menstruation, but the rate is slower and rarely exceeds 5 cm (2 inches). Ossification centers gradually disappear, and growth is complete. Thus girls in whom the menarche occurs at an early age are likely to be shorter as adults than those in whom its appearance is late.

Apparently, there is considerable variation in the sensitivity of breast tissue and the pubic hair follicles to stimulation by estrogen and androgen, respectively. This phenomenon explains the early appearance of breast development and pubic hair growth in many girls in whom endocrine function and onset of menstruation are normal.

PREMATURE MENARCHE. The onset of menstruation before the age of 9 years is precocious and should be investigated. This problem is discussed under abnormal sexual development in this chapter.

DELAYED MENARCHE. Absence of menstruation beyond the sixteenth year, *primary amenorrhea,* should be considered abnormal, and the possibility of a disorder of genetic origin should be given careful consideration in all such cases. Chromosomal abnormalities are found in approximately 40% of phenotypic females in whom menarche is delayed beyond the sixteenth year and no secondary sex characteristics are present. Instances in which the menarche has occurred as late as the twenties are rare. Primary amenorrhea is discussed in detail in Chapter 9.

Adolescent dysfunctional uterine bleeding. Menstrual irregularities, so common at this time of life, are usually the result of fluctuating, unopposed estrogen production by the nonovulating ovary, but even in young girls the possibility of systemic or pelvic lesions must be eliminated before the diagnosis of dysfunctional uterine bleeding is made.

Although a reasonable time must be allowed for the establishment of an ovulatory cycle, adolescent dysfunctional uterine bleeding is not necessarily self-limiting. In a long-range study of 538 adolescents with menstrual disorders conducted by Southam and Richart, 291 cases were diagnosed as dysfunctional uterine bleeding. The follow-up period was as long as 25 years. These authors showed that, if symptoms persist for a period of 4 years or more, there is a 50% chance for future irregularities, a diminution in reproductive potential, and an increased risk of uterine neoplasm.

Abnormal bleeding is discussed in detail in Chapter 8.

Dysmenorrhea. Primary dysmenorrhea, the most common menstrual disorder in adolescent girls, is discussed in detail in Chapter 10.

SUGGESTED READING

Ehren IM, Mahour GH, and Isaacs H: Benign and malignant ovarian tumors in children and adolescents, Am J Surg 147:339, 1984.

Frisch RE: Body fat, menarche, and reproductive ability, Semin Reprod Endocrinol 3:45, 1985.

Herbst AL, Kurman RJ, Scully RE, and Poskanzer DC: Clear-cell adenocarcinoma of the genital tract in young females; registry report, N Engl J Med 287:1259, 1972.

Kemp CH and others: The battered child syndrome, JAMA 181:17, 1962.

Robboy SJ, Noller KL, O'Brien P, Kaufman RH, Townsend D, Gundersen J, Lawrence WD, Bergstral E, McGorray S, Tilley B, Anton J, and Chazen G: Increased risk of cervical and vaginal dysplasia in 3980 diethylstilbestrol-exposed young women: experience of the National Collaborative Diethylstilbestrol Adenosis Project, JAMA 252:2979, 1984.

Southam AL and Richart RM: Prognosis for adolescents with menstrual abnormalities, Am J Obstet Gynecol 94:637, 1966.

Tanner JM: Growth at adolescence, ed 2, Oxford, England, 1962, Blackwell Scientific Publications, Ltd.

4

Lisa M. Fromm and Melissa Schiff

The psychologic aspects of the female life cycle

Objectives

RATIONALE: The responses of a woman to the transitions between childhood, maturity, and senescence may be important determinants in her responses to physiologic reproductive function, to pregnancy, to aging, and to her relationships with others.

The student should be able to:
A. Demonstrate knowledge of the events of the normal life cycle of menarche, pregnancy, menopause, and the postmenopausal phase of life.
B. Understand the psychosocial responses to these changes.

A woman's life is marked by many transitions. From birth to death, various physical events occur that are directly related to her unique reproductive capacity. This chapter highlights some of the important psychosocial aspects of menarche, pregnancy, and menopause.

MENARCHE

Menarche is an important stage in female development. It is one of the few concrete signs of physical maturation. Issues discussed in this section include education and preparation for the onset of menstruation, individual psychologic reactions to menarche, changes in self-perception, and the impact of the event on family dynamics.

Education

Formal education concerning the menarche most often takes place in school health classes. Much of the information provided focuses on basic physiology of sexual maturation, hygienic aspects of menstruation, and the physical discomforts associated with menstruation. Frequently the psychologic aspects of the menarche are overlooked; specifically, how a girl feels about the onset of menstruation and its psychologic impact on her are often not addressed. These issues may not even be addressed in discussions with family members and peers. Because premenarcheal girls who are more knowledgeable about possible physiologic *and* psychologic changes have a more

45

positive reaction to menarche, it is important that they be well informed regarding both aspects.

Psychologic reactions

The onset of menstruation can cause a variety of psychologic reactions. A girl may regard it as a "hygienic crisis," a fearful event, or a natural maturational milestone that is readily accepted. If she views it as a "hygienic crisis," cleanliness and secrecy are emphasized, and the focus is on physical discomforts and limitations. Menstruation is perceived as messy and embarrassing. A fearful reaction often occurs because of a lack of preparation and no knowledge of what to expect. For girls who are informed and who regard this event as a maturational milestone, the reaction is one of acceptance and pride. Menarche confirms that they are developmentally normal and have reached a turning point signifying maturity and the initiation of womanhood.

The timing of menarche in relation to peers can also influence her response. If she begins to menstruate at the same time as the majority of her peers, she perceives the event more positively than if she is either early or late.

Changes in self-perception

With menarche, girls become increasingly aware of their sexual identity and of their ability to bear children. Unlike the physical changes, changes in self-perception can occur suddenly. She has an increased concern with personal appearance, an awareness of sexual differentiation, and the emergence of romantic interests.

Impact on family interactions

Parents view their daughter as more grown-up with the onset of menarche and, as a result, implement changes in their limit setting and increase her responsibilities. The daughter begins the process of separation from her parents as she negotiates the fine balance between closeness with parents and involvement with peers.

In summary, each girl's psychologic reaction to the menarche is unique and is influenced by her knowledge about the process. Questions about the girl's knowledge and her feelings about the onset of menstruation can assist the health provider in guiding her through this time of transition.

PREGNANCY

Each pregnancy is a unique experience for a woman and her family. Whereas the physiologic changes take place in a progressive and orderly fashion, the same is not true of the psychologic changes. This section discusses the psychologic issues that arise during a first successful pregnancy, including the acceptance of pregnancy, the development of the role of mother, the relationship with the partner, changes in body image, concerns and fears, and the relationship to the fetus.

Acceptance of pregnancy

Upon learning that she is pregnant, a woman is immediately faced with the task of deciding whether or not to accept the pregnancy. A common myth is that all women are happy about being pregnant. In fact, approximately 50% of women are ambivalent about or rejecting of pregnancy, whether planned or not. A first pregnancy is the most highly accepted. Subsequent pregnancies are more readily accepted with a longer space between children and fewer number of children. Age, financial status, relationship with the partner, anticipated life-style changes, and interference with career goals also influence acceptance of pregnancy. Sharing the knowledge of the pregnancy with others helps to confirm and accept the fact. During the second trimester, fetal movement causes a vivid awareness of the presence of new life, making the pregnancy real. This sense of reality is enhanced by ultrasonographic technology, which makes possible seeing the fetal image in utero. (Seeing the fetal image may make a woman's grief reaction more intense, should abortion or fetal death occur.) The overwhelming majority of women come to accept their pregnancies by the third trimester. The physical and psychologic changes that occur during the course of the pregnancy facilitate this acceptance. It is not unusual, however, for some ambivalence to persist throughout pregnancy and for that ambivalence to become especially intense during labor and delivery. Ambivalence after delivery is also common.

Development of the role of mother

As pregnancy progresses, preparation occurs in development of the woman's new role of mother. New information is obtained and changes in self-concept occur. Frequently a pregnant woman recalls childhood experiences with her own mother, and she may spend time talking with her mother about pregnancy, labor and delivery, and childrearing practices. She reviews and analyzes the positive and negative characteristics of her own experiences and finally crystallizes her own unique identity as a mother.

Although all pregnant women have to anticipate changes in their life-style, the woman who works outside her home may experience conflicts between her work role and her new role as mother. Decisions on the length of maternity leave, when and if to return to work, and how to arrange for day care are difficult. Many times these issues are not completely resolved until the postpartum period. All pregnant women must adjust to less freedom and more responsibility.

Relationship with the partner

Couples experience a change in their relationship during pregnancy. The majority experience increased emotional closeness and commitment, but others may experience more conflict and strain. For those who have unresolved marital difficulties before the pregnancy, the probability of conflict is greater. Also, women who feel emotionally alone and overburdened by the physical and emotional changes may feel resentment toward the partner. Communication and empathy are especially important at this time. As a couple learns to communicate and nurture each other during the happy and difficult times of pregnancy, they prepare themselves for their new role as parents.

The couple's sexual relationship may undergo change during pregnancy as a result of the numerous physical and psychologic changes. Many women report decreased sexual interest during the first trimester of pregnancy. During the second trimester, sexual desire and responsiveness is improved; as pregnancy approaches term, sexual interest may again decrease. This decrease may be due to the physical changes and limitations occurring late in pregnancy, and couples may need to find new positions or focus on noncoital sexual activities. Many couples worry throughout pregnancy that sexual activity may harm the fetus. Communication, mutual support, and understanding are important in the adaptation to changes in the sexual needs and desires of the individual partners. Sexual activity can enhance a couple's emotional bond to each other and to the pregnancy.

Body image

Women who have a positive body image before pregnancy often continue to have a positive body image during pregnancy. If the individual is happy and accepts the pregnancy, the physical changes may even be desired and welcomed. With increasing abdominal size, some women report a more negative feeling about their body because the pregnant body shape contradicts society's ideal body image, that of a thin woman.

Concerns and fears

Many women experience some fear and anxiety during pregnancy. Common concerns relate to the health and well-being of the unborn child, the changing marital relationship, and the new role as mother. During the third trimester, a woman's fears about labor and delivery increase. Because the physical changes and the process of labor and delivery are out of the pregnant woman's control, she may experience a *general* feeling of loss of control.

Relationship with fetus

During pregnancy a unique relationship develops between the mother and her unborn child. It includes incorporation, differentiation, and separation. During the first trimester, the pregnant woman begins to *incorporate* the idea of being pregnant and her new role as a mother into her concept of herself. Fetal movement helps confirm the reality of the pregnancy and initiates the process of *differentiation,* establishing that another being is within her body. The second trimester is characterized by a turning inward or "binding in" with the unborn child. Many women have vivid dreams and fantasies as they develop a very personal relationship with their unborn baby. As the third trimester progresses and delivery approaches, the process of *separation* begins. The parents choose names for the baby and acquire clothes and furniture in anticipation of the baby's arrival. Although many women are anxious to have the pregnancy over and to see their baby finally, they also experience sadness over this separation and the loss of the special prerogatives pregnancy brings.

In summary, the person caring for the pregnant woman must be aware that each woman reacts in an individual way to the physiologic and psychologic changes that occur during pregnancy. It is important to inquire about her feelings about the pregnancy relating to all these aspects. Many difficulties in coping with changes occurring during pregnancy can be alleviated by education, support, and understanding. A knowledgeable person who is willing to take time can provide this help.

MENOPAUSE

A woman is said to be through the menopause when she has ceased menstruating for 1 year. The average age for this occurrence is about 50 years. The period of time preceding the menopause is the *climacteric* phase of life and is characterized by declining ovarian function and accompanying hormonal changes. In addition to the hormonal and physical changes that occur during the climacteric and menopause, psychosocial changes also take place (see Chapter 47). This section discusses the differing perspectives of the menopause, psychologic reactions to the menopause, and the impact of the menopause on sexuality.

Perspectives on the menopause

As with puberty, menopause is most appropriately viewed as a normal life change. Most women pass through the menopause with no physical or psychologic problems, but, because the menopause involves declining hormone levels that often require medical treatment, some physicians tend to view the menopause as a pathologic condition. Some women experience menstrual irregularities during the climacteric that may require investigation and treatment. Most menopausal women have hot flashes that may vary in frequency and severity, and some have vaginal dryness or atrophy. Hormone replacement alleviates these symptoms.

Psychologic reactions to the menopause

Although some women may experience sadness over loss of reproductive capabilities, they may also feel relief from the physical discomforts of monthly bleeding, dysmenorrhea, or premenstrual tension. Pregnancy and contraception are no longer concerns. Most women experience the menopause as a normal life change and view the physical changes as positive.

The menopause is capable of eliciting a wide range of psychologic responses. The response can be influenced by the experience of a woman's mother, the individual's self-perception, her current role in society, and her present activities. Women who perceived their mothers as having difficulty with menopause may fear that they are destined to have a similar experience. Those who believe menopause signifies the onset of old age may fear loss of personal attractiveness and/or fear that they are no longer useful in society. Women who have focused most of their adult lives on their role as mothers may be more likely to experience depression, and, finally, those who have had difficulty coping with other life transitions may have difficulty during the menopausal transition.

Relationship and the menopause

Sexual interest and activity decrease with age, but no evidence exists for an abrupt change at the time of menopause. The sexual response cycle remains intact, but sexual difficulties may arise for other reasons. The major physical cause for sexual impairment during the menopause is vaginal dryness, which is alleviated by hormone replacement. Marital status is important in how a woman copes with menopausal changes. Women who are separated, divorced, or widowed tend to have a higher incidence of depression. Married women in a poor relationship may also have difficulties in adjusting, whereas women in a good relationship report increased marital satisfaction.

In summary, the health provider who understands the variety of physical and psychologic changes that may occur during menopause can provide anticipatory guidance during this normal life event. Hormone replacement is helpful for physical changes. In order to understand a woman's psychologic adjustment to the menopause, the health provider should investigate her life situation and attitude toward the menopause.

SUGGESTED READING

Menarche

Golub S: Menarche: the transition from girl to woman, Lexington, Mass, 1983, Lexington Books.

Greif EB and Ulman KJ: The psychological impact of menarche in early adolescent females: a review of the literature, Child Dev 53:1413, 1982.

Koff E, Rierdan J, and Jacobson S: The personal and interpersonal significance of menarche, J Am Acad Child Psychiatry 20:148, 1981.

Morse JM and Doan HM: Adolescents' response to menarche, J Sch Health 57:385, 1987.

Swensen I and Havens B: Menarche and menstruation: a review of the literature, J Community Health Nurs 4:199, 1987.

Pregnancy

Colman AD and Colman LE: Pregnancy: the psychological experience, New York, 1971, Seabury Press.

King HE, Calhoun LG, and Selby JW: Psychological changes in pregnancy. In Selby JW, Calhoun LG, Vogel AV, and King HE, editors: Psychology and human reproduction, New York, 1980, The Free Press.

Lederman RP: Psychosocial adaptation in pregnancy: assessment of seven dimensions of maternal development, Englewood Cliffs, NJ, 1984, Prentice-Hall, Inc.

Rubin R: Maternal tasks in pregnancy, MCN 4:143, 1975.

Menopause

Frey KA: Middle-aged women's experience and perceptions of menopause, Women and Health 6:25, 1981.

Greene JG: The social and psychological origins of the climacteric syndrome, Brookfield, Vt, 1984, Gower Publishing Company.

McKinlay JB, McKinlay SM, and Brambilla D: The relative contribution of endocrine changes and social circumstances to depression in mid-aged women, J Health Soc Behav 28:345, 1987.

Notman MT: Midlife concerns of women: implications of the menopause. In Nadelson CC and Notman MT, editors: The woman patient: concepts of femininity and the life cycle, New York, 1982, Plenum Press.

5

Lisa M. Fromm and Teresita A. McCarty

Female sexual physiology: normal and dysfunctional

Objectives

RATIONALE: Sexual dysfunction is common and often undiscovered because physicians do not regularly take sexual histories and do not encourage women to talk about sexual problems.

The student should be able to:

A. Describe the phases of the physiologic responses to sexual stimulation in women.

B. Be comfortable in discussing sexuality and in obtaining information concerning sexual function, both normal and abnormal.

C. List the disorders of sexual dysfunction and indicate those that warrant referral.

Most of what we know about female sexual physiology can be attributed to the research of Masters and Johnson, which took place in the early 1960s. They were the first to treat the female sexual response as a natural biologic function and to observe it under the same kinds of laboratory conditions used to study other biologic functions. Their work resulted in the description of the four sequential phases of the female response cycle: *excitement, plateau, orgasmic, and resolution.* Two basic physiologic changes during the sexual response cycle were observed: vasocongestion and increased neuro-muscular tension or myotonia. Vasocongestion occurs in the body tissues in the internal and external genitalia and in the female breasts, whereas myotonia occurs throughout the body in response to sexual arousal and not simply in the genital region. Because most of the physiologic changes occur in the external genitalia and breasts; those changes are described in greater detail. Table 5-1 shows how these changes are integrated and which changes occur simultaneously. The physiology of the female sexual response is the same for all women, whether heterosexual or homosexual.

TABLE 5-1 Peripheral manifestations of the female sexual response cycle

	I. Excitement phase (several minutes to hours)	II. Plateau phase (30 sec to 3 min)	III. Orgasmic phase (3-15 sec)	IV. Resolution phase (10-15 min; if no orgasm, ½-1 day)
Skin	No change	Sexual flush; inconstant; may appear on abdomen, breasts, neck, face, thighs. May resemble measles rash	No change	Flush disappears in reverse order
Breasts	1. Nipple erection 2. Venous congestion 3. Areolar enlargement	Venous pattern prominent. Size may increase one fourth over resting state. Areolae enlarge; impinge on nipples so they seem to disappear	No change	Return to normal
Clitoris	Glans: glans diameter increased Shaft: variable increase in diameter. Elongation occurs in only 10% of subjects	Retraction: shaft withdraws deep into swollen prepuce	No change (Shaft movements continue throughout if thrusting maintained)	Shaft returns to normal position in 5-10 sec Full detumescence in 5-10 min
Labia majora	Nullipara: thin down, flatten against perineum Multipara: rapid congestion and edema. Increase to 2-3 times normal size	Nullipara: may swell if phase II unduly prolonged Multipara: become enlarged and edematous	No change	Nullipara: *increase* to normal size in 1-2 min or less Multipara: *decrease* to normal size in 10-15 min
Labia minora	Color change: bright pink in nullipara and red in multipara. Size: increase 2-3 times over normal	Color change: bright red in nullipara, burgundy red in multipara. Size: enlarged labia form a funnel into vaginal orifice	Proximal areas contract with contractions of lower third	Return to resting state in 5 min

Modified from Sherfey MJ: The nature and evolution of female sexuality, New York, Random House, 1972.

Continued.

TABLE 5-1 Peripheral manifestations of the female sexual response cycle—cont'd

	I. Excitement phase (several minutes to hours)	II. Plateau phase (30 sec to 3 min)	III. Orgasmic phase (3-15 sec)	IV. Resolution phase (10-15 min; if no orgasm, ½-1 day)
Vagina	Vagina: transudate appears 10-30 sec after onset of arousal. Drops of clear fluid coalesce to form a well lubricated vaginal barrel. (Aids in buffering acidity of vagina to neutral pH required by sperm.)	Copious transudate can continue to form. Quantity of transudate generally increased by prolonging preorgasm stimulation	No change	Some transudate collects on floor of the upper two thirds formed by its posterior wall (in supine position)
Upper two thirds	Balloons: dilates as uterus moves up pulling anterior vaginal wall with it. Fornices lengthen; rugae flatten	Further ballooning occurs, then wall relaxes in a slow, tensionless manner	No change; fully ballooned out and motionless	Cervix descends to seminal pool in 3-4 min
Lower third	Dilation of vaginal lumen occurs. Congestion of walls proceeds gradually	Maximum distension reached rapidly; contracts lumen of lower third. Contraction around penis aids thrusting traction on clitoral shaft via labia and prepuce	3-15 contractions of lower third and proximal labia minora at ¾ -sec intervals	Congestion disappears in seconds. (If no orgasm, congestion persists for 20-30 min)
Uterus	Ascends into false pelvis in phase I	Contractions: strong sustained contractions begin late in phase II	Contractions strong throughout orgasm. Strongest with pregnancy and masturbation	Slowly returns to normal position
Rectum			Inconstant rhythmical contractions	All reactions cease within a few seconds

THE BREAST

In the breast, the first signal of increased sexual excitement is erection of the nipple. During this phase the length of the nipple may increase from 0.5 to 1.0 cm, and the base diameter may increase by 0.25 cm over unstimulated measurements. Erection of the nipple is caused by involuntary contraction of the muscle fibers within the structure of the nipple. The nipples may not become erect simultaneously and the amount of nipple erection varies (Figs. 5-1 and 5-2).

Another physiologic reaction in the breast during the excitement phase is that of increased blood flow. The resultant venous engorgement causes an increase in the size of the breast, although the amount of the increase varies among women.

During the plateau phase, venous engorgement continues and becomes evident in the areolae. As a result of the increased tension, the areolae enlarge, and an illusion of loss of nipple erection is created. Before orgasm breast size may increase by as much as 20 to 25% over baseline measurements. As sexual tension increases during this phase, a pink mottling or "measleslike rash" often appears over the abdomen and then the breasts. This vasocongestive reaction of the breast is known as the *sex flush*.

After orgasm a rapid disappearance of the sex flush and the simultaneous detumescence of the areolae occur. The nipples return to the prearousal state more slowly, and this difference in timing between the areolae and the nipples gives the appearance that the nipples are becoming erect again. The venous engorgement of the breasts may take 5 to 10 minutes or more to return to the prearousal state. The speed with which this return occurs is related to the size of the venous drainage system.

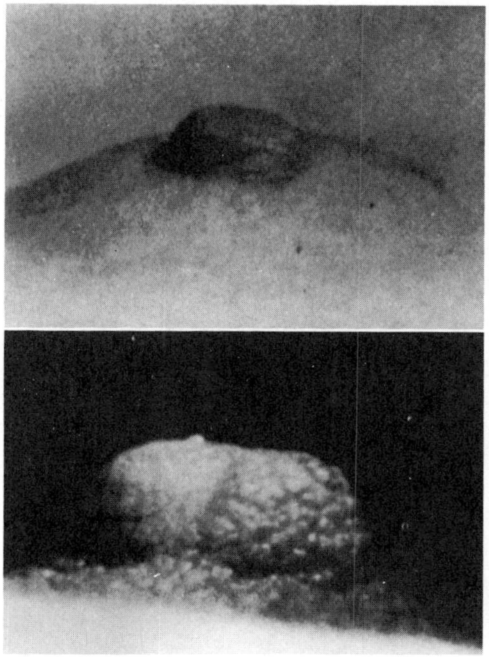

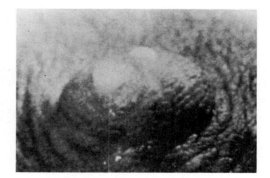

Fig. 5-1 **A,** Nipple erection in early excitement phase. **B,** Close-up of nipple erection (side view) in later excitement phase. (From Wagner G: Physiological responses of the sexually stimulated female in the laboratory, Institute of Medical Physiology, University of Copenhagen, and Focus International, New York City [film].)

Fig. 5-2 Following genital stimulation, both the nipple and the areola are erected. A milk drop is seen exuding from the top of the nipple. (From Wagner G: Physiological responses of the sexually stimulated female in the laboratory, Institute of Medical Physiology, University of Copenhagen, and Focus International, New York City [film].)

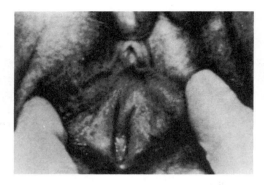

Fig. 5-3 Soft, unstimulated head of the clitoris visible under the prepuce upon spreading of the labia. (From Wagner G: Physiological responses of the sexually stimulated female in the laboratory, Institute of Medical Physiology, University of Copenhagen, and Focus International, New York City [film].)

THE CLITORIS

During the excitement phase, the clitoris becomes hard and increases in size. Stimulation of the mons area close to the clitoris quickens this response. As plateau levels of excitement are reached, the clitoris elevates and retracts behind the clitoral hood (Figs. 5-3 and 5-4).

This retraction does not interfere with the orgasmic response because the clitoris is contiguous with the labia minora, and the traction exerted on the labia minora by penile thrusting is usually sufficient to stimulate orgasm. Mons contact with the male pelvis enhances the probability of orgasm. Following orgasm is a rapid return to the pre-arousal state. If orgasm does not occur, resolution may take 2 to 6 hours and may be associated with irritation and discomfort.

THE VULVA: LABIA MAJORA

The major labia normally meet in the midline and protect the underlying structures, that is, the minor labia, the vaginal outlet, and the urinary meatus. Changes in the normal anatomic relationship secondary to obstetric trauma affect the sexual response pattern of the major labia. Thus, the response patterns for women who have not borne

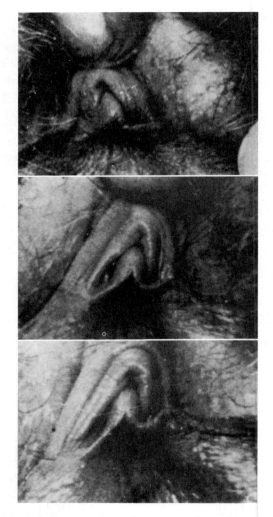

Fig. 5-4 Close-up views of the progressive enlargement of the clitoris and surrounding tissues with stimulation. (From Wagner G: Physiological responses of the sexually stimulated female in the laboratory, Institute of Medical Physiology, University of Copenhagen, and Focus International, New York City [film].)

children (nulliparous) are different from those who have borne more than one child (multiparous).

For nulliparous women, the excitement phase is characterized by thinning and flattening of the labia majora against the perineum. The labia also move in an upward and outward direction away from the vaginal outlet. This movement is thought to be secondary to engorgement of the labia minora and vasocongestion of the external one third of the vagina. The labia majora remain in this position through the plateau and orgasm phases and return rapidly to the midline position during resolution. If orgasm does not occur or if stimulation is prolonged, the result may be marked engorgement and edema that may take several hours to abate.

For multiparous women, the labia majora, instead of thinning in the excitement phase, become markedly distended as a result of vasocongestion. The movement away from the midline position may occur, albeit to a lesser degree than for nulliparous women.

THE VULVA: LABIA MINORA

During the excitement phase, the labia minora of both nulliparous and multiparous women expand markedly and may increase two or three times in thickness by the time the plateau stage is reached. The minor labia may then actually protrude through the labia major adding about 1 cm to the length of the vaginal barrel. In the plateau phase, the minor labia and the clitoral hood undergo vivid color changes secondary to vasocongestion. For nulliparous women the color change may range from pink to bright red and for multiparous women, from a bright red to a deep wine color. Women do not attain orgasm without first demonstrating these color changes. After orgasm, the loss of color is rapid.

THE VAGINA

Vaginal response to sexual stimulation occurs in a pattern and is the same whether the stimulation is physical or psychologic in origin.

Vaginal lubrication, the first physiologic evidence of sexual responsiveness, begins within 10 to 20 seconds after initiation of effective sexual stimulation. The vaginal secretion is a transudate that occurs secondary to dilation of the venous plexus that encircles the vaginal barrel. Initially, it appears on the vaginal walls as droplets, which then coalesce to form a smooth, slippery surface over the entire vaginal wall. The production of vaginal lubrication is greatest during the excitement phase and actually slows during the plateau phase, particularly if the level of sexual tension is extended for a long time (Figs. 5-5 to 5-7).

As sexual tension mounts, the inner two thirds of the vagina lengthens and distends. The cervix and the body of the uterus are slowly pulled backward and upward into the pelvis to create a tenting effect. The total vaginal length may increase by as much as 3 cm and the width by as much as 4 cm.

In the excitement phase, the vaginal walls undergo a distinct color change because of vasocongestion. The normal pink-red coloring of the unstimulated vagina changes to a darker purplish hue. When pelvic congestion becomes intense during the plateau phase, the entire vaginal mucosa shows a perceptible further darkening. The outer third of the vagina demonstrates minimal change during the excitement phase, but, as the plateau phase is reached, the outer third of the vagina also becomes distended with venous blood.

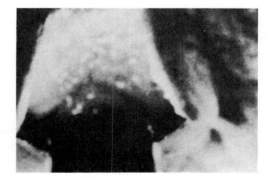

Fig. 5-5 Individual droplets of a lubricating transudate appearing on the vaginal walls in the early excitement stage. (From Wagner G: Physiological responses of the sexually stimulated female in the laboratory, Institute of Medical Physiology, University of Copenhagen, and Focus International, New York City [film].)

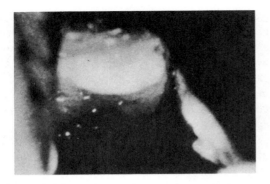

Fig. 5-6 Tenting effect in the excitement phase, producing considerable expansion of the inner portion of the vagina. (From Wagner G: Physiological responses of the sexually stimulated female in the laboratory, Institute of Medical Physiology, University of Copenhagen, and Focus International, New York City [film].)

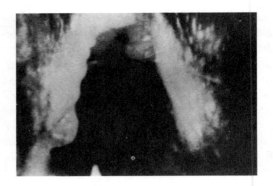

Fig. 5-7 Vagina during orgasm. Considerable increase in volume is seen. A large droplet of lubrication can be seen in the lower left corner of the vaginal outlet. (From Wagner G: Physiological responses of the sexually stimulated female in the laboratory, Institute of Medical Physiology, University of Copenhagen, and Focus International, New York City [film].)

The degree of vasocongestion in this phase is such that the central lumen of the outer third of the vaginal barrel may be reduced by as much as one third from the distension that was established during the excitement phase. The anatomic change associated with the vasocongestion that encompasses the outer third of the vagina and labia minora is termed the *orgasmic platform*. The response of the vaginal barrel during orgasm is confined to the outer one third of the vagina or the orgasmic platform. Reflex muscular contractions occur during orgasm at 0.8-second intervals. The number ranges from a minimum of 3 to 5 to a maximum of 10 to 15 contractions per orgasm. There are no other physiologic responses of the vagina during the orgastic phase.

The resolution phase is characterized by a rapid dispersion of the localized vasocongestion established during the plateau phase. As a consequence of this loss of vasocongestion, the central lumen of the outer third of the vagina increases in diameter. Gradually the expanded inner two thirds of the vaginal barrel return to the collapsed, unstimulated state. The cervix also returns to its normal position from its elevated position in the pelvis.

These changes take place over 3 to 4 minutes. The color of the vaginal mucosa also returns to normal but more slowly, frequently requiring as long as 10 to 15 minutes for completion.

THE UTERUS

During the plateau phase, the uterus and cervix rise in the pelvis as the vaginal walls expand. This expansion creates a tenting effect and an anatomic basin for a seminal pool. Full uterine elevation is not achieved until the plateau phase is complete. Late in the plateau phase, the uterus undergoes strong, sustained contractions that last 2 or more minutes. The cervix shows slight swelling at this time and changes in color to a patchy purple. The contractions continue throughout the orgasm phase. Following orgasm, during the resolution phase, the elevated uterus descends to its normal resting position. The size and color of the cervix return to normal in 4 minutes, and it is patulous for 10 minutes.

SEXUAL DYSFUNCTION

Sexual dysfunction can cause embarrassment and unhappiness in an otherwise satisfactory life.

Sexual problems often used to be ignored because they were considered unmentionable. Patients feared that sexual dysfunctions indicated underlying psychopathology, perversion, or immorality. Physicians believed that sexual dysfunctions required treatment that was lengthy, costly, and usually ineffective. In spite of such prohibitive attitudes, 10% of patients presenting for medical evaluation spontaneously report sexual problems, and physicians who ask patients about their sexual functioning as part of a sexual history find that 50% have a sexual problem. Evidently, the prevalence of sexual dysfunction is high. Health care providers should routinely ask their patients about sexual functioning to facilitate discussion, diagnosis, and treatment.

Patients need information about the stages of normal sexual development, and they need permission to enjoy healthy sexual play as part of adult life. Accurate sexual information can prevent unwanted pregnancy and the spread of sexually transmitted diseases. Knowledge of a patient's sexual functioning might unearth problems caused by medications, illness, or injury. Taking a sex history facilitates communication, education, prevention, and treatment.

Sexual history

Health care providers hesitate to ask questions about sexual functioning for many reasons, including lack of knowledge about sexual topics; embarrassment regarding sexual issues; judgmental beliefs; a wish to ignore their own sexual worries; a lack of comfort with homosexuals, heterosexuals, or bisexuals; a desire to avoid unpleasant realities of sexual abuse or violence, and unwillingness to investigate sexual symptoms. They may worry that the patient will be embarrassed or angered by sexual questions, misinterpret professional inquiries as personal sexual interest, or discover that the physician does have sexual feelings in response to the patient. (Actual sexual feelings between patient and physician are a very serious matter and require immediate professional ethics consultation.)

Because human sexuality is now taught in most medical schools and reference texts are widely available, physicians no longer have a reason to be uneducated about sexual issues. The primary impediment to patient-physician dialogue about sexual issues is the personal attitude of the physician. Considering how one's own sexual attitudes were formed is important before beginning to ask patients about their attitudes.

Remembering the freedom of child's play is another avenue to understanding one's own and the patient's sexual behavior. Children pretend, imagine, and imitate. Infants put everything into their mouths, and no one thinks they are strange. Children skip, run, and jump just to enjoy their bodies. Adult sexual activity is often reminiscent of childhood play. It should be a time to retreat from adult responsibilities and dust off the fantasy, games, and physical sensations children enjoy.

After having sorted out one's own sexual attitudes, one must decide how to bring up sexual issues with patients. Almost all patients think that discussion of sexual issues is appropriate for physicians. The specific questions, of course, vary with the patient's presentation and needs. New patients need to have a complete sexual history taken sometime during the initial evaluation (see box on p. 58). At the first visit of those coming for ongoing care, straightforward questions can be asked about the age of menarche, age and nature of first sexual experience, and present sexual activity and interest. However, some patients require more care in the approach to sexual questions than others. For example, an adolescent may need a more subtle approach. Volunteering developmentally appropriate sexual information lets adolescents know sexual issues can be discussed freely and they are more likely to answer sexual questions honestly.

Taking a sexual history does not end with the first visit. Established patients need an alert physician who remembers to ask sexual questions again as conditions change. When a level of comfort has been established with patients, the physician can ask open-ended questions about sexual

SEXUAL HISTORY

General information

Patient: age, occupation, education, ethnic/cultural/religious background, gender identity, marital status

Childhood sexuality

Family attitudes about sex: modesty, nudity, religion, siblings

Learning about sex: information sources, too soon, too late?

Childhood sexual beliefs: conception, birth, body parts

Childhood sexual activity: genital self-stimulation, pleasure, guilt, consequences, peer sexual play, sexual abuse or exploitation by same sex or opposite sex

Adolescent and adult sexuality

Masturbation: frequency, guilt, orgasm

Necking and petting: age started, partners, type of activity

Body image: body habits, gender identity, peer acceptance, self-esteem

Sex practices: type, frequency, partners, contraception, enjoyment, pain, orgasm

Sex in relationship/marriage: sexual compatibility, mutual and reciprocal satisfaction, enjoyment, masturbation

Pregnancies: number, result, effect on sex life

Extramarital sex: partners, attachment, frequency, emotional results, relationship effects

Sexual illnesses: Genital trauma or surgery, mastectomy, hysterectomy, sexually transmitted diseases

Sex after loss (widowhood, separation, divorce): sex outlets, family attitudes, personal attitudes, fantasies

Sex trauma: violence, rape, resultant fears

Sexual variations: bestiality, pedophilia, voyeurism, exhibitionism, fetishism, transsexualism, transvestism

enjoyment and specific questions about how a new medication or illness has affected their sexual activity.

Some sexual questions have to be asked specifically; patients often will not disclose this information in response to open-ended questions. Examples of such sensitive areas are experiences of childhood sexual abuse, rape, violence as a prelude to sex, or any sexual activity that makes the patient physically or psychologically uncomfortable. Patients assume their physician will be uncomfortable discussing these issues and thus avoid them until asked directly. The approach to these sensitive areas is illustrated here, using childhood sexual abuse as an example.

Sexual trauma like childhood sexual abuse and rape are such violations of a person's sense of self that the event(s) and emotional reaction may be partitioned off in memory. Victims of childhood sexual abuse are often threatened with harm if they tell anyone. If a child reports the assault and is not believed and not protected, injury to a child's self-concept and ability to trust grows and lasts into adulthood. This repression of memory, together with the perpetrator's or caretaker's injunction against telling and the unwillingness of many to "hear" about sexual violence, often prevents patients from volunteering this information. To overcome these barriers, one can ask if anything physically or sexually frightening ever happened to them when they were young. One can then ask about uncomfortable touches, molestation, and rape. If the patient affirms these events, one can ask who they told and what the response was. If the patient has never discussed the events and if they remain very upsetting, the patient should be referred for treatment of the psychologic sequelae of sexual trauma.

With a basic understanding of a patient's sexual history, one can fill in information gaps, correct misinformation, and anticipate new phases in their sexual activity. For instance, telling a menopausal woman about vaginal lubricants helps her avoid unnecessary discomfort and indirectly gives permission to continue having intercourse. A sexual history can take many forms, but the goal is to understand the patient's unique emotional and experiential sexual development.

Sexual effects of illness

Most physical and psychologic illnesses have some effect on sexual functioning. These consequences may be part of a general malaise or may be a specific effect of the disease. Illnesses can alter any or all of the phases of sexual desire, excitement, and orgasm. Illness can also lead to or mask a psychologic sexual dysfunction that persists when the precipitating illness or injury is gone. Telling a patient about the sexual effects of the medical illness or injury can prevent the development of a subsequent sexual dysfunction.

Very sick patients often have a decrease in or total absence of sexual desire. Examples of such illnesses are severe infections, advancing malignancies, and degenerative diseases. The sexual effects of brief illnesses are usually transient, and no intervention is required.

Chronic illnesses can have many sexual effects that, in turn, can have a severe impact on intimate relationships. *A physician cannot assume that patients who seem to have adapted to their chronic illness have adapted to the associated sexual dysfunction.* In fact, the sexual adaptations may be maladaptive, unnecessary, or suboptimal.

Other illnesses have a more direct effect on sexual functioning because they affect the brain centers necessary for sexual activity. Illnesses of the peripheral nervous system and disorders of the hypothalamic-pituitary-gonadal axis such as Addison's disease, endogenous depression, and hypopituitarism also have many direct effects on sexual functioning. The major illness categories with specific sexual consequences are neurologic, neuromuscular, and endocrine diseases.

General information about illnesses that affect sexual desire is listed in the box at right. Most illnesses have some impact on sexual functioning, and it is helpful to pinpoint whether the change has occurred in the desire for sexual activity, in the ability to become aroused, or in the ability to

---

ILLNESSES CAUSING CHANGES IN SEXUAL DRIVE

Decreased sexual drive
Epilepsy
Hypothalamic lesions
Drug-induced changes
Medical illnesses
    Liver disease
    Kidney disease
    Carcinoid syndrome
    Addison's disease
    Hypothyroidism
Depression
Schizophrenia (chronic)
Increased sexual drive
Neurologic disorders
    Epilepsy
    Diencephalic lesions
    Kleine-Levin syndrome
    Bilateral temporal lobe injury (Klüver-Bucy syndrome)
    Frontal lobe syndromes (tumors, head trauma)
Medical conditions and pharmacologic agents
    Hyperthyroidism
    Cushing's disease and steroid administration
    Androgen administration
    Levodopa administration
Psychiatric disorders
    Mania
    Schizophrenia (early stages)

Modified from Cummings J: Clinical neuropsychiatry, New York, 1985, Allyn and Bacon.

---

reach orgasm. Treating the illness that is causing the sexual symptoms is the best way to eliminate the offending symptoms. This applies to primary endogenous depression as well as hypothyroidism. Unfortunately, some of the medications used to treat these illnesses also cause sexual dysfunction.

Sexual side effects of drugs

Most of what we know about the sexual effects of medications comes from clinical reports or

TABLE 5-2 Effects of commonly used drugs on sexual function

Drug	Libido	Effect on sexual function	
		Arousal or erection	Orgasm or ejaculation
Antihypertensive agents			
Reserpine, A-methyldopa	Decreased	Decreased (common)	May be impaired
Diuretics	—	May be impaired	—
Clonidine	—	—	May block emission in males, orgasm in women
Propranolol	May be decreased	May be decreased	—
ACE inhibitors	—	—	—
Calcium channel blockers	—	—	—
Hormonal agents			
Androgens	Increased	Increased (men)	Increased (men)
Estrogens	Decreased in men; variable in women	May cause impotence in men	Delay
Thyroxine	Increased	—	—
Adrenal steroids	Decreased in high doses	—	—
Histamine (H₂) antagonists			
Cimetidine	May be decreased	May be impaired	—
Ranitidine	May be decreased	May be impaired	—
Famotidine	—	—	—
Alcohol/drugs of abuse			
Alcohol	Initially increased	Reduced	Impaired; correlates with blood level
Barbiturates	Reduced	Reduced	—
Narcotics	Impaired in high doses	Impaired in high doses	Impaired in high doses
Amphetamines/cocaine	Enhanced with low doses; reduced with high doses	Decreased with chronic use	Increased with low doses; diminished with high doses
Marijuana	Variable	Decreased in chronic hashish users	—
Psychotropic agents			
MAO-inhibiting antidepressants	May be increased	—	Impaired
Tricyclic antidepressants	May be impaired	May be impaired	May be impaired; may cause spontaneous seminal emission
Trazodone	—	May cause priapism	May be impaired, rarely spontaneous orgasms

Modified from Cummings J: Clinical neuropsychiatry, New York, 1985, Allyn and Bacon.

TABLE 5-2 Effects of commonly used drugs on sexual function—cont'd

Drug	Libido	Effect on sexual function	
		Arousal or erection	Orgasm or ejaculation
Fluoxetine	—	May be impaired	May be impaired, rarely spontaneous orgasms
Lithium carbonate	Impaired	Impaired	—
Neuroleptic agents	May be decreased	Impaired (rare priapism)	Retrograde ejaculation rarely
Antianxiety agents	Variable	Impaired with chronic usage	—
Anticholinergic agents	—	May be impaired	—
Miscellaneous			
Levodopa	May be increased	—	—
Disulfiram	—	Occasional impotence	Delayed

studies of men. Changes in sexual functioning are more obvious and therefore more easily studied in men but are thought to be similar in women. In general, medications that cause impotence in men can impair excitement or prevent orgasm in women, but specific verification of this assumption is not available for most medications. As with illnesses, most medications cause a decrease in sexual interest, excitement, or orgasm, although a few medications can cause increased sexual interest or tendency to orgasm.

Three major classes of medications cause most of the sexual functioning problems (Table 5-2). They are the antihypertensive agents, the histamine H_2-receptor antagonists, and the psychotropic medicines, especially antidepressants. Some medications have secondary effects that cause sexual problems. Examples are a vaginal yeast infection precipitated by antibiotics or decreased vaginal lubrication because of the drying effects of anticholinergic agents.

Drugs of abuse are often rumored to increase sexual desire. Although alcohol and marijuana may have such an effect at low doses, overall these and other central nervous system (CNS) depressants impair desire and sexual functioning.

Several treatment options are available for drug-induced sexual dysfunction. If the sexual problem is dosage related, try decreasing the dose to a level that is medically effective but does not cause the undesirable sexual effects. Timing sexual activity to coincide with the lowest possible blood level and having intercourse just *before* taking the next dose of medication can minimize the dysfunction. If decreasing the dosage or changing the time when the medication is given does not help, try changing to a medication with a different mechanism of action. Patients who must stay on the same medication at the same dose sometimes find the sexual effects ameliorate with time. Patients can also be instructed in methods of increasing stimulation to maximize the remaining sexual response. These techniques are outlined under treatment of sexual dysfunctions.

Dyspareunia (painful intercourse)

Patients often report painful intercourse as a specific symptom, although it has many causes. The etiologies of painful intercourse are divided into those that cause pain in the lower portion of the vagina and those that cause pain high in the vagina, as experienced with deep thrusting.

Congenital malformations, scarring, bladder infections, and vaginitis with discomfort near the introitus can cause painful intercourse. Vaginal irritation is sometimes caused by allergies to deodorants in tampons, laundry or hand soaps, spermicides, or the materials used in artificial barriers like condoms or diaphragms. Inadequate lubrication, a frequent cause of dyspareunia, can be caused by anxiety and premature vaginal entry or by a decrease in estrogen after menopause. An intact hymen or an episiotomy scar can cause pain. Patients and their partners sometimes need to change their sexual activity or use additional lubrication if direct clitoral stimulation is causing the pain. *Vaginismus* or spasm of the vaginal muscles can cause painful entry or actually prevent vaginal entry. Vaginismus often has a psychologic origin but is not under voluntary control and is considered one of the disorders of sexual desire. Anatomically, the unstimulated vagina is a potential rather than an actual space. In other words, unless menstruation or sexual stimulation is occurring, the anterior and posterior walls of the vagina are contiguous.

When the pain occurs high in the vagina or is felt as pelvic pain known as *deep dyspareunia,* a thorough physical evaluation is required. Such pain can be caused by active pelvic inflammatory disease or its residual scarring effects. Tumors, cysts, endometriosis, and inflammatory bowel disease can also cause dyspareunia and pelvic pain. Pelvic pain can also be associated with childhood sexual abuse as a somatic or body memory of previously experienced pains. Patients with a history of childhood sexual abuse who also have pelvic pain should have a psychiatric evaluation and psychologic treatment as well as continuing gynecologic care.

Treatment of sexual dysfunction

Kaplan reconceptualized the sexual response cycle of Masters and Johnson into three phases beginning with sexual desire. Kaplan's *triphasic model of sexuality* is based on the basic physiologic changes namely vasocongestion and reflex muscle contractions, that occur. *Sexual desire* is the first phase, and Masters and Johnson's phases of excitement and plateau are condensed into the second phase, *excitement,* because they both involve vasocongestion. The third phase, the *orgasmic* phase, involves reflex muscular contraction of pelvic muscles. Kaplan dropped the resolution phase because it involves a return to the normal prearousal state and no disorders are associated with it. Kaplan's triphasic model of sexuality is clinically useful and is used here to discuss sexual dysfunction and treatment. Disorders of sexual desire, excitement, and orgasm are discussed, along with appropriate treatment.

Sex therapy overview. The contribution of organic factors to the sexual dysfunction should be determined as much as possible. This judgment is often more difficult than it seems. Consider a patient with diabetes mellitus. She may have altered sexual sensation and responsiveness because of circulatory changes and neuropathy. More prone to bladder and vaginal infections because of the diabetes, she will have intermittent dyspareunia. When these organic factors are combined with a possibly ambivalent desire for pregnancy, the increased attention to body malfunction caused by any illness, and the possibility of a premature death, separating the relative contribution of the organic and psychologic factors becomes difficult. Sex therapy is usually prescribed for psychologic sexual dysfunction, but it can be helpful even when the sexual dysfunction is almost entirely organic. Psychotherapy for organic dysfunction should be secondary, adjunctive to the principal medical management.

Sex therapy involves a combination of education, behavioral therapy (including densensitization), and psychotherapy. Sex therapy can be done with individuals, but partners are treated together whenever possible. The relative emphasis on behavioral therapy over psychotherapy may depend on the severity of the psychologic dysfunction. Dysfunctional psychologic reactions to sexual experience can be caused by immediate emotions and/or deeper conflicts. Reactions caused by immediate emotions are often very responsive to brief behavioral or supportive therapy; reactions arising from deeper conflicts may require longer-term psychotherapy.

Immediate emotions. The immediate emotional response to the initiation of sexual activity has an impact on the outcome. Morning people living with night people, compatible in other ways, may have trouble coordinating their sexual desire cycles. Even enjoyable sexual activity can end in rancor if the partner "just turns over and goes right to sleep."

Ignorance, distaste, anger, fear, and anxiety can all interfere with any stage of sexual activity. Some women lack fundamental knowledge of their own or their partner's anatomy and patterns of normal sexual functioning. They have never explored their own bodies to discover what sensations cause pleasure. Budding sexual interest is easily squelched by distaste, poor timing, or an inconsiderate partner. An unwashed partner or one who smells of alcohol or is in an altered state from drug abuse is not sexually attractive. A crying baby quickly puts a damper on sexual activity, as do worries about work, finances, or undone household chores. Anger or fear are rarely sexy. To "kiss and make up" soon after an argument or a violent episode is often difficult. Sexual actions that take place in the midst of anger and fear are closer to rape than to intimacy. Anxiety commonly interferes with sexual enjoyment, but it can have many forms. The anxiety that interferes with sexual activity can be spectating, performance anxiety, fear of loss of control, or unrelated intrapsychic anxiety.

Now and then most people watch themselves perform and act as their own spectators instead of remaining absorbed in their activity. This self-consciousness is frequently dramatized in movies. Woody Allen has a famous sports announcer doing a play-by-play of a couple's sexual activity in one of his films. Paying too much attention to the details or method of the sexual experience robs it of its excitement.

Some people overvalue the idea of sexual per-

formance. The ability to perform defines their worth as men or women. They compete mentally with the imagined sexual skills of their rivals. Of course, this overconcern with performance causes anxiety, which makes failure more serious and more likely.

Some anxious people worry that they will not be able to recover normal control over their bodies and emotions if they fully experience sexual feelings. Such a fear may diminish with increased sexual experience. If this anxiety does not diminish, this fear of loss of control may be a deeper problem requiring more extensive treatment.

Finally, anxiety not directly related to the immediate sexual activity can cause sexual dysfunction. For example, a patient with claustrophobia could become fearful when the partner is on top. Nonspecific panic attacks can be triggered by improper breathing during sex. In some cases how a more general fear like claustrophobia is triggered during sexual activity is easy to see. Other patients have never identified the larger cause of their anxiety and may need psychiatric evaluation to help define the problem.

Deeper factors. Some sexual dysfunctions are caused by deeper, intrapsychic conflicts. These intrapsychic conflicts can be impossible for the patient to express because they are not available to the conscious mind, nor are they understood by the patient. When the physician has trouble conceptualizing the patient's problem, or when appropriate treatment of the apparent sexual problem does not relieve the symptoms, a deeper underlying conflict may be present.

Intrapsychic conflicts originate in the patient's thinking as it has been influenced by upbringing. Culture and religion have a tremendous impact on sexuality and, at least in most of North America, the effect is repressive. For example, sexual issues are not widely discussed. Family traditions may not allow a mother to be sexual. Some intrapsychic conflicts are actually conditioned fears. A rape victim may develop a specific fear of the sexual act that was forced upon her. An angry partner who unconsciously feels the woman provoked the rape can activate dormant fears of inadequacy and intensify the victim's reaction to the rape. For reactions based on intrapsychic conflicts, one's partner can either exacerbate the problem or play a therapeutic role, depending on the quality of the interaction between the two.

Most patients who suffer from intrapsychic conflicts resulting in sexual dysfunction need to be referred for psychotherapy or a combination of sex therapy and psychotherapy. Reactions caused by deeper factors take longer to define and to treat than reactions caused by immediate emotions.

The sexual variations or *paraphilias* require special mention. Patients may be distressed by their less common sexual practices. The amount of distress often reflects the acceptance and accommodation of their partners. A physician has to find out if the activity creates a problem, causes pain, or is illegal. If patients say they like younger partners and further questioning reveals that *younger* means prepubertal children, a report to a child protection agency and referral for psychologic treatment is necessary. Alternatively, a woman who feels guilty about being excited when her husband wants to wear her underwear is relieved to hear this described as retained childhood play. The deeper factors do not have to be uncovered when they are part of consensual adult sexual activity.

Disorders of sexual desire

A persistent indifference to sexual activity is a disorder of sexual desire. This disorder may be primary, as in a woman who has never had any interest in sex, or secondary, which occurs when previous sexual interest is lost. Secondary losses of desire may be organic, as previously discussed, situational, or the result of hidden inhibitions. Many situations such as bereavement, stress, anxiety, or loss of erotic attraction to a partner may cause loss of sexual interest.

Treatment of a primary disorder of sexual desire requires psychotherapy and specific sex therapy. A secondary disorder of desire is best treated by identifying and treating the underlying cause.

Disorders of sexual excitement

When vasocongestion fails to cause or maintain adequate lubrication and swelling during sexual activity, a disorder of sexual excitement occurs. Disorders of excitement are often associated with orgasm problems. Many psychologic causes have to be considered once physical causes have been evaluated. For example, a woman may not be able to tell her partner what is stimulating and what is not. Conversely, the partner may object or react personally to being told. Fear of pregnancy, marital strife, or fear that either partner will be judged as inadequate may exist.

Sex and behavior therapy is useful in disorders of excitement and orgasm. In sex therapy both partners are treated whenever possible so that neither is identified as "sick." The therapist begins by interviewing the partners separately and then together to gather the history and understand the difficulties. Sexual activity is usually prohibited except as prescribed by the therapist.

Only after the partners are comfortable with nonsexual touching and able to tell one another what feels good do they progress to exploring the bodies' erotic regions. When comfortable with touch, sexual stimulation or masturbation is prescribed. Reassured that their bodies function normally, the couple is usually ready to resume full sexual activity. The overall goals of sex therapy are to provide accurate information, decrease performance fears, and increase communication. These goals can often be reached in a few weeks.

Vaginismus is the inhibition of vaginal relaxation. A disorder of desire, the symptoms appear during the excitement phase. This involuntary constriction of the vaginal muscles can completely prevent penile insertion. Vaginismus can be secondary to an illness that has made intercourse painful, or it can be the result of unconscious conflicts or sexual trauma. A newly married woman with a strict religious upbringing may have difficulty reconciling marital sexual relations with previous sexual prohibitions. This conflict is nonverbally represented by vaginismus, which can even prevent introduction of the speculum.

Vaginismus treatment is usually very successful and involves gradual dilation of the vaginal opening. Using a lubricant, the patient inserts one finger into the vagina. Graduated dilators may be substituted for fingers. When comfortable with the largest dilator (which is larger then a penis), the patient is ready for insertion of the penis.

Inhibition of orgasm (preorgasmia or anorgasmia)

Peripherally, orgasm consists of the reflex contractions of genital muscles. Inhibitions of orgasm range from mild to total. A stimulation threshold must be reached to trigger this reflex, so anxiety or other inhibiting emotions should be minimized. Such inhibitions can be under voluntary control or unconscious. Primary preorgasmia, in which a woman has never had an orgasm either as a result of coitus or masturbation, is relatively uncommon and may be serious. Secondary inhibition of orgasm, or anorgasmia, in which a woman has previously experienced orgasm, is a common complaint. The complaint may be of discomfort from the extended vasocongestion of prolonged excitement. Some women fear that they may become uncontrollably aggressive, that their orgasm will not meet their own or their partner's standards, or that they do not deserve pleasure.

Primary preorgasmia is treated by prescribing masturbation and practicing contracting genital muscles. Kegel exercises—contracting muscles as if to stop urination—strengthen the pubococcygeal muscles. Secondary inhibitions of orgasm often respond to sex therapy. Longer-term psychotherapy may be indicated when deeper factors or unconscious conflicts are the causes of inhibition.

SUMMARY

Medical schools have included human sexuality courses in their curriculum since the 1970s. Physicians now should have the information necessary to *educate* their patients about sexuality, to *evaluate* their concerns, and to *refer* them for sex therapy when appropriate. Many sexual dysfunctions can be treated relatively simply and effectively.

SUGGESTED READING

Abramowicz M, editor: Drugs that cause sexual dysfunction, The Medical Letter 29:65, 1987.

Buffum J, Smith DE, Moser C, Apter M, Buston M, and Davison J: Drugs and sexual function. In Lief HI, editor: Sexual problems in medical practice, Chicago, 1981, American Medical Association.

Cole JO, and Bodkin JA: Antidepressant drug side effects, J Clin Psychiatry 51:21, 1990.

Ende J, Rockwell S, and Glasgow M: The sexual history in general medical practice, Arch Intern Med 144:558, 1984.

Harrison WM, Rabkin JG, Ehrhardt AA, Stewart JW, McGrath PJ, Ross D, and Ouitkin FM: Effects of antidepressant medication on sexual function: a controlled study, J Clin Psychopharmacol 6:144, 1986.

Kaplan HS: Disorders of sexual desire, New York, 1969, Brunner/Mazel.

Kaplan HS: The new sex therapy, vol 1, New York, 1974, Brunner/Mazel.

Kolodney RC, Masters WH, and Johnson VE: Textbook of sexual medicine, Boston, 1979, Little, Brown and Co.

Masters WH and Johnson V: Human sexual response, Boston, 1970, Little, Brown, and Co.

Modell JG: Repeated observations of yawning, clitoral engorgement, and orgasm associated with fluoxetine administration, J Clin Psychopharmacol 9:63, 1989.

Pauly IB and Goldstein SG: Prevalence of significant sexual problems in medical practice, Med Aspects Hum Sexuality 4(11):48, 1970.

Simons RC: Understanding human behavior in health and illness, ed 3, Baltimore, 1985, Williams & Wilkins.

Sherfey MJ: The nature and evolution of female sexuality, New York, 1972, Random House.

6

Kate Moffitt Musello

Sexual assault

Objectives

RATIONALE: As many as half of all women will be threatened with rape during their lifetime. Because the sequelae of rape may have long-term effects, physicians should learn how to assist the patient in overcoming the emotional and physical effects of sexual assault.

The student should be able to:
A. Demonstrate knowledge of the effects of sexual assault on women.
B. Conduct an appropriate evaluation of an alleged victim of rape.
C. Demonstrate knowledge of the legal aspects of sexual assault.

Rape is a crime of anger and aggression expressed as a sexual act without consent of the victim. Physicians, especially gynecologists and family practitioners, too often come unprepared to the examination of the alleged rape victim. The purpose of this chapter is to provide background information on rape and specific guidelines for those physicians involved in the care of rape victims. Let us emphasize in the beginning that, although the proof of rape must be left to the courts, competent care of the victim may provide the data with which a recovering victim and the district attorney can pursue the legal process.

It has been estimated that as many as one of every two women will be threatened with rape in her lifetime. As many as one half of all rape victims know their assailant. Although the majority of reported rapes involve one assailant, in one study approximately 30% resulted from group rape. Group rape is usually premeditated, involves street drugs and/or alcohol, and generally elicits more brutality and sexual humiliation of the victim. According to Nadelson, Notman, and Hilberman, approximately 25% of victims sustain extragenital as well as genital injury.

A significant psychologic injury to the victim's sense of self-determination should also be taken into account. Self-recrimination and guilt over one's powerlessness to avoid or deflect the attack are common reactions to rape. Appetite, sleep, and concentration disruption may be profound during the healing process. Many victims suffer from disabling fear, nightmares, intrusive recollection of the event, and even panic triggered by violence in the media. Some victims probably develop full-blown anxiety and depressive states, perhaps even psychosis, as a result of rape.

Sexual assault is an umbrella term that includes manual, oral, or genital contact by the assailant. This contact occurs without the victim's consent. Rape specifically refers to genital contact perpetrated by the assailant through some element of force. *Force* may be defined as anything from threats made against the victim or the victim's family now or in the future to actual display of a deadly weapon. Although resistance on the part of the victim is no longer required in most states to prove rape, evidence of force and/or resistance is very persuasive in court. A psychiatrically (for example, schizophrenic) or otherwise mentally handicapped person, including someone under the influence of drugs, is considered legally unable to offer consent.

An overview of the examination explained in lay language will help prepare the patient for its more uncomfortable aspects. During this initial contact, the physician can observe the patient's emotional state; that is, if it is one of anger, agitation, or inordinate calm. Some victims may find catharsis in recounting the rape, whereas others will relive the most terrifying and humiliating aspects of the assault. The presence of someone from a rape victim support group, as well as a friend or family member, can be an invaluable stabilizing influence on the patient in this situation. The names and affiliations of those present should be recorded on the medical record (for example, Jenny Moore present from Rape Crisis Center).

Victims of sexual assault often experience significant trauma in the form of fear of death, fear of loss of a loved one, physical injury, isolation, confusion, or mental torture. It is important that the treatment offered does not incur further trauma. Describing the available diagnostic and therapeutic techniques so that the patient can make choices for herself should be the physician's goal. Facilitating the reestablishment of the patient's sense of safety and control is a priority and yet is made difficult in the emergency room setting where other priorities and/or values dominate.

The following is a list of five goals (not necessarily listed in order of importance) of the rape examination:

1. Promotion of emotional healing
2. Evaluation and treatment of physical injury
3. Evaluation and treatment to prevent treatable sexually transmitted diseases
4. Evaluation and treatment to prevent pregnancy
5. Collection of evidence

In the first four tasks, the physician acts as the patient's advocate. In the fifth task, the physician must be a careful, impartial collector of data to be presented at a later time under the auspices of the court. All five tasks are accomplished in the usual familiar process of history taking, physical examination, laboratory testing, and treatment.

It is important to allow the patient to choose whether or not to be treated as a step in regaining control over her life and body. One way to accomplish this is through an informed consent for both the examination and the collection of evidence (see box below).

I authorize Dr. _____ to perform a complete medical examination, including a pelvic (internal) examination on my person and to record for the proper law enforcement agency the findings as related to the prosecution of my assailant(s).

Signed_____ Date/Time_____

Witness_____ Guardian_____

If the victim is under the age of consent in a given state, social services need to be informed; however, parental permission is not required in a sexual assault case when a law enforcement agent presents the child for medical care. Because trace evidence is considered to be "fleeting," no search warrant is necessary. Obstruction of the exam by a parent or guardian may be grounds for charges of coconspiracy.

HISTORY AND PHYSICAL EXAMINATION

The physician carries the responsibility of detecting both genital and nongenital trauma. The ACOG technical bulletin "Alleged Sexual Assault" provides a standardized sexual assault history and physical that can be used instead of the usual emergency room log sheet. States such as New Mexico also include a standardized sexual assault history form in their rape evidence collection kits (see *Sexual Assault History Form*). By standardizing the sexual assault medical record, important information will not be inadvertently omitted. If at all possible, the report of the history and physical should be dictated, because dictation facilitates recording a more detailed description. Including nonmedical explanations of medical terminology can be useful, should interpretation come into question later in court. As with any legal scrutiny, the physician's and the victim's strongest ally is a comprehensive medical record.

History

Gently ask the patient to tell you what happened. Make every attempt to ask nonleading questions (such as, "What happened?") rather than "Tell me how you were raped." She does not need to tell you all the details because a sex crimes detective will go over the attack with the patient. The minimum information that the physician needs to know includes the following:

1. The sequence of accosting and assault to determine jurisdiction and to assess evidence;

where the crime began so that evidence may be collected and given to the appropriate authorities (the timing is important for assessing the likelihood of a viable specimen being present as well).
2. The types of threat and injury (what the assailant actually said may be painful to recount but may give a clearer picture of the threat and the emotional/psychologic trauma).

Documentation of the history should be in the patient's own words with as little additional opinion or interpretation from the physician as possible. Many people have difficulty describing aspects of the assault that were bizarre or unusual. Clearer descriptions of the assault may be prompted by everyday language (for example, "oral sex" may not be as clear as "Did he force you to put his penis in your mouth?"). Although it is important that the physician not contribute to the victim's tendency toward self-blame by implying that she should not have performed such tasks as washing, the patient should be asked if she has showered, urinated, defecated, brushed her teeth, douched, or changed her appearance since the assault. A description of the assailant's behavior, the use of drugs by either the victim or the assailant, the use of foreign objects in the attack, the use of a condom, or the assailant's achievement of orgasm should be included in the history. Some conditions shown to correlate with a higher risk of sexual assault include mental retardation, alcoholism, mental illness, indigency, and transiency.

A general brief medical history should be included after the above questions have been answered. This should include a history of past or current medical conditions as well as a gynecologic history (date of last menstrual period, character of last period, gravidity, parity, cycle length, flow, previous history of infections such as herpes, syphilis, gonorrhea, condylomata, method of birth control, and the time of the patient's most recent consenting intercourse).

Physical examination

The physical examination has a dual purpose. The first is to evaluate for injury. The second is to collect evidence for future prosecution of the assailant. Because the patient is essentially the crime scene, the evidence being collected is trace evidence. Hairs and seminal fluid, along with standards from both the victim and suspect, are commonly the two most important types of trace evidence in sexual assault cases. Most states have standardized rape evidence collection kits that should be available in the emergency room at all times. The collection of evidence and its untampered transfer to the court is extremely important. Unless there is a verifiably unbroken chain of custody and transfer of the collected evidence (that is, evidence can be accounted for from the time of collection until it is turned over to the police), the evidence may be ruled inadmissable in court. All specimens should be signed by the person who collected them, and the amassed evidence should be labeled and locked in a police box by those who collected the evidence if it is not transferred directly to the officer in charge.

The victim should be asked to undress over a paper or cloth floor sheet. This sheet should be carefully folded and submitted as evidence.

Clothing that demonstrates struggle or contains specimens from the assailant such as blood or semen should be described in the medical report and submitted with the other evidence. Foreign matter on the patient's body should also be collected and submitted. Debris beneath the nails or nail clippings may be included. If semen stains are identified, these can be collected. Some hospitals have Wood's ultraviolet lamp, which can be used to examine for semen. Because of the high histone content of semen, it will fluoresce under a Wood's lamp in a dark room.

The physical examination itself offers a healing touch to the assault victim. Doing an overall examination permits evaluation and treatment of the patient rather than of an invaded orifice alone. A good first step is to visualize the entire skin surface, the scalp, and the mucosal membranes.

Nongenital injury may be important evidence. Document injuries by careful descriptions with the help of diagrams or burn sheets. Although photographs sound promising, they often do not show up well and can diminish rather than verify injury. Nongenital injuries may include choke marks, bites, scratch marks, abrasions, fractures, and hematomas. Besides possibly requiring medical attention, these injuries are objective evidence of lack of consent or resistance on the part of the victim. If the victim is examined soon after the assault, the physician may detect only tenderness. The victim should be reassured about the healing process and instructed to return if these areas of tenderness manifest visual signs of injury. If a patient returns several days after the initial examination, new evidence of injury should be documented.

After an examination of the skin, a general physical examination should be done. When this is completed, pausing to ask the patient for permission to perform the pelvic exam can give the victim a sense of control that may help her negotiate this difficult aspect of the examination. The pelvic examination should begin with the external genitalia; the physician should look for lacerations, abrasions, blood, ecchymoses, secretions, and dried semen, which looks like a whitish yellow flaking stain. Some authors recommend applying toluidine blue to the mucosa to visualize lacerations not visible to the unaided eye.

The condition of the hymen should be described without offering an opinion as to the cause of its appearance. Hymens vary. Hymenal rupture or the lack of it is not required to prove or disprove rape. A speculum moistened with water (not lubricant, which interferes with the acid phosphatase and Papanicolaou test) is then gently introduced into the vagina. If a plastic speculum is used, warn the patient about the clicking sound it makes as it is opened. (In our experience, one patient responded hysterically when the physician opened the speculum because it sounded like the gun that had been placed in her vagina to play Russian roulette.) Examination of the cervix and vaginal mucosa should include a description of any trauma observed. With preadolescent children or severe injury, general anesthesia may be required to perform an adequate examination.

Two types of specimens are collected. Certain specimens fall under the category of evidence, whereas other specimens are used to identify the presence of disease. Swabs of the vaginal pool, anus, and oral cavities along with a wet mount should be obtained for evidence. When describing the wet mount, the physician needs to note the presence or absence of sperm and whether or not they are motile. The presence of motile sperm in the vagina has been studied and found to decrease rapidly after coitus (Soules and associates), probably because of the pH of the vagina. Motile sperm were identified in only 50% of the women studied after 3 hours. In this group of women, however, whole sperm were identifiable for up to 18 hours, and sperm heads were identifiable for up to 24 hours. Other studies have shown that motile sperm can be seen for as long as 28 hours after coitus, and, according to Findley, nonmotile sperm may remain for up to 48 hours. Spermatozoa may be seen later upon examination of the other specimens after special staining, even if the examining physician did not identify sperm on the wet mount. Because rape is not a crime of passion, it is not surprising to discover that some rapists suffer from sexual dysfunction and often fail to ejaculate. Other rapists will be azospermic because of any number of conditions such as inherent infertility or vasectomy. The use of condoms or coitus interruptus are other possible explanations for the absence of motile sperm on wet mount.

The vaginal swabs are used to prepare air-dried slides, which are submitted for future examinations by the forensic laboratory. After the identification of a fluid as semen with the use of either an acid phosphatase screening test or direct identification of sperm, the forensic laboratory in Albuquerque, New Mexico, can subject the specimen to screening for four genetic markers. These markers are phosphoglucomutase, glyoxalase I, esterase-D, and peptidase-A. Prostatic Ag can be used to identify semen from vasectomized males. All of these markers are identified with electrophoretic methods. The ABO and secretor status are also determined. If ejaculation has occurred, acid phosphate will be identifiable (Wertheimer). Significant concentrations of this prostatic enzyme were seen in 50% of women 9 hours after intercourse. No acid phosphatase was seen 36 hours later. Dried acid phosphatase as found in clothing or gathered from skin may be detectable for months after an assault. The Johnson Rape Kit contains a colorimetric test strip that changes from blue to dark purple when exposed to acid phosphatase. Acid phosphatase is present in a concentration of from 400 to 8000 King-Armstrong U/ml in fresh ejaculate.

Secretor or ABO status of the victim is obtained as another means of discriminating between the victim and the assailant. Approximately 80% of the population secrete blood group antigens in saliva, sweat, semen, and vaginal secretions. As of this writing, DNA typing remains too controversial to be utilized widely.

Under the category of laboratory specimens, a culture for gonorrhea and a Papanicolaou smear are collected and submitted, although the Papanicolaou test is done mostly as a courtesy to the patient and may be eliminated from the exam.

Blood may be drawn at any time that seems appropriate during the examination and should be analyzed for complete blood count, serum pregnancy test, syphilis, and alcohol/drug screening as indicated. A urine specimen should be obtained for urinalysis and toxicologic screening, if necessary.

Examination of the child victim

As described in Sgroi's *Handbook of Clinical Intervention in Child Sexual Abuse,* determination of sexual abuse in children may be more difficult than in adults for various reasons. Children usually do not come to the attention of authorities because of an acute episode of rape but after a long episode of repeated abuse. To validate sexual abuse, where physical evidence is often lacking, investigative interviewing is much more important.

Special skills are required to establish enough rapport with the child to obtain the child's consent. Sometimes in-depth interviewing of a child is best done by others involved with the alleged sexual abuse, such as a social worker or a physician the child already knows. Family members should not be present when a child is being questioned, as the child may be unable to discuss details in front of a family member. If an in-depth history has already been taken from a child, the examining physician should elect to defer from repetitive questioning.

The progression from history to physical exam should be made clear to the child. The examination should be complete, with as much deemphasis of the genital/rectal exam as possible. Questions such as "Did anything happen here?" or "Were you touched here?" may be helpful during the exam.

Although most child victims do not have physical evidence of trauma, if force has been employed, there may be soft tissue trauma to the urethral, vaginal, or rectal orifices. As with adult patients, examination for the presence of sperm and pregnancy should be performed. Pregnancy can occur even without vaginal penetration. Girls age 10 or older should be evaluated for pregnancy. The throat, urethra, and vagina in prepubertal girls along with the cervix in postpubertal girls should be cultured for gonorrhea. A moistened swab inserted into the rectal opening for approximately 10 seconds provides a sample. Blood testing for syphilis should be included in STD testing.

The absence of physical evidence in child sexual abuse does not negate the child's allegations. Finally, the child and family need to be reassured many times from various professionals that the child will be all right, and not necessarily damaged for life.

EXAMINATION FOLLOW-UP

The victim should be offered protection against pregnancy. The pregnancy status of a patient should be assessed before she is given protection. The patient should be counseled that efforts to prevent pregnancy after coitus must be initiated within 72 hours of the assault and are not uniformly successful. If contraception is not successful, the patient may want to consider abortion, should she become pregnant as a result of a rape. One method of contraception is the administration of two Ovral birth control pills at the time of the examination if the monoclonal urine pregnancy test is negative, to be followed 12 hours later by two more Ovral birth control pills. The theory behind this therapy is that the birth control pill renders the endometrial lining relatively resistant to implantation. As nausea can be a side effect of this method, the patient may be offered an antiemetic.

The prevention of sexually transmitted disease is offered to all victims of sexual assault. This includes prevention of syphilis, gonorrhea, and chlamydia. Unfortunately, we have no preventive methods for herpetic or human papilloma virus infections. Other infections such as trichomoniasis or bacterial vaginitis should be treated when they are diagnosed. Gonorrhea is transmitted in 3% to 4% of all reported rapes, whereas syphilis develops in approximately 0.1% of all reported rapes. The patient must be counseled on the importance of follow-up syphilis serology because of potential inadequacy of prophylactic antibiotics.

The CDC recommendations for prophylaxis after rape is to give the patient tetracycline, 500 mg four times daily by mouth for a total of 7 days. Pregnant women or patients allergic to tetracycline should receive amoxicillin, 3.0 g, or ampicillin, 3.5 g, each given with probenecid, 1.0 g, as a single oral dose. A final alternative is erythromycin base, 500 mg four times daily for 7 days, or 250 mg four times daily for 14 days. The dosage of ampicillin to be given to a child is calculated as 50 mg/kg, which is also given with probenecid, 25 mg/kg orally as a single dose.

CONSEQUENCES

Each victim will respond to such an assault variously depending on coping mechanisms developed during previous events in her life and on the circumstances of the assault. During the acute reaction, which may last from a few days to several weeks, the victim experiences a grief response expressed as shock, disbelief, or even emotional disintegration. The normal integrity of her life may be totally disrupted. The victim may become absorbed in self-recrimination or guilt. The phase resolves if the victim is able to construct an outward adjustment to being victimized, even though she has further to go in reintegrating her anger and sense of loss of control. The long-term effects of the assault may be denied or repressed. At this time the victim may withdraw from counseling or discontinue previous contact with the rape victim support group. The third phase is characterized by integration of the assault into the victim's self-image, which may be preceded by a period of depression. Evidence of the rape trauma syndrome or posttraumatic stress disorder may be admissible in court. Successful prosecution of the assailant can be a constructive force in resolving the victim's loss of control over her life.

LEGAL CONSIDERATIONS

A physician subpoenaed to testify in a rape case should take several preparatory steps. Obtain and review records. Discuss the case at length with the district attorney. Ask what tack the defendant's lawyer is considering to discredit the victim's charge (defamation of character, attempting to prove consent, discrediting the examiner, invalidating the evidence). Unfortunately, sexual assault cases may all too frequently be determined by whose story the jury finds more convincing. A few caveats to keep in mind are: (1) rape is a legal, not a medical, definition; (2) although the physician can offer a medical opinion concerning the presence/absence of trauma, it is not his or her responsibility to prove rape or to say what caused any trauma; (3) it is admissible to state that the victim appeared to have had traumatic intercourse; (4) the words *rape* or *sexual assault* should always be preceded by the word *alleged;* (5) the physician should avoid being cornered by a defendant's lawyer into answering yes and no questions, especially those concerning situations about which no medical research exists to support the answer (for example, "Doctor, is it not true that a woman could develop a reddened vaginal opening if she had prolonged consenting intercourse?"). It is perfectly acceptable to answer, "There is no medical information with which to answer such a question," or "That question cannot be answered with an unconditional yes or no." It is important that the physician remember that he or she is not on trial and thus that he or she must remain as calm and unemotional as possible. Insults made by the defendant's lawyer are the lawyer's way of trying to unhinge the physician's reason and thereby elicit a particular response. By listening carefully, the physician can often predict and thus avoid that answer.

Cooperative efforts between medical personnel and law enforcement agencies can greatly improve a community's ability to deal effectively and compassionately with rape. There is much left to do in the way of informing both physicians and their communities that will greatly improve their response as a medical team to rape. Furthermore, rape is a crime associated with a high rate of recidivism of the rapist if untreated and a high percentage of recovery if treatment is completed; thus it behooves physicians to provide the best care of victims and most accurate collection of evidence so that a successful court outcome can be obtained.

SUGGESTED READING

American College of Obstetricians and Gynecologists: Alleged sexual assault, Technical Bulletin no 52, Chicago, 1978, American College of Obstetricians and Gynecologists.

Breen JL and Greenwald E: Rape. In Glass RH, editor: Office gynecology, ed 2, Baltimore, 1981, The Williams & Wilkins Co.

Findley TP: Quantitation of vaginal acid phosphatase and its relationship to time of coitus, Am J Clin Pathol 68:238, 1977.

Hilberman E: The rape victim, Baltimore, 1976, Garmond Pridemark Press.

Nadelson CC, Notman MT, and Hilberman E: The rape experience. In Curran WJ, McGarry AL, and Petty CS, editors: Modern legal medicine, psychiatry, and forensic science, Philadelphia, 1980, FA Davis Co.

Porter E: Treating the young male victim of sexual assault: issues and intervention strategies, Safer Society Press, 1986.

Sgroi SM: Handbook of clinical intervention in child sexual abuse, Lexington, Mass, 1987, DC Heath & Co.

Soules MR, Pollard AA, Brown KM, and Verma M: The forensic laboratory evaluation of evidence in alleged rape, Am J Obstet Gynecol 130:142, 1978.

STD treatment guideline, 1985, US Department of Health and Human Services.

Wertheimer AJ: Examination of the rape victim, Postgrad Med 71:173, 1982.

7

John H. Mattox

The menstrual cycle

Objectives

RATIONALE: The hallmark of female health, particularly in the reproductive years, is the event of ovulation. This event is the result of the integrated and coordinated function of the hypothalamic-pituitary-ovarian axis. In order to comprehend the onset, normalcy and decline of menses, as well as the endocrinopathies and therapies involving the menstrual cycle, a thorough understanding of this axis is required.

The student should be able to:

A. Understand thoroughly the hypothalamic, pituitary, and ovarian hormones involved in the menstrual cycle and their interrelationship.

B. Draw a graph depicting the patterns of FSH, LH, E_2, and P_4 secretion and the relationship to ovulation.

C. Define the parameters that characterize a normal menstrual cycle in terms of periodicity, duration of flow, and amount of flow.

Menstruation is the periodic discharge of blood and disintegrating endometrium after a normal ovulatory cycle. Normal menstrual cycles are comprised of two phases depending upon the point of reference: *follicular* (ovary) or *proliferative* (endometrium) *phase*, beginning with the first day of menstrual flow and culminating in ovulation; and a *luteal* (ovary) or *secretory* (endometrium) *phase*, which ends with the onset of menstruation.

OVERVIEW OF THE MENSTRUAL CYCLE

Normal menstruation depends mainly on the functional integrity of three endocrine sites: the *hypothalamus*, the *anterior pituitary gland*, and the *granulosa-theca cells of the ovary*. They are often referred to as the *hypothalamic-pituitary-ovarian axis*. The process is precisely coordinated, but stimuli from the cerebral cortex mediated through the hypothalamus can influence menstrual function. Examples are cessation of periods or irregular menstruation associated with fear of pregnancy, emotional crises, exercise, or rapid weight loss.

A neurochemical transmitter known as *gonadotropin-releasing hormone* (GnRH), which is produced in the hypothalamus, is liberated in a pulsatile fashion into the capillary plexus from the median eminence *(arcuate nucleus)* and is carried through the portal vessels to the anterior lobe of the pituitary gland, the *adenohypophysis.* The result of its neurohormonal action is the production and release of the gonadotropins *FSH* and *LH* from the anterior pituitary cells. These hormones are transmitted to the ovary, where they stimulate follicle development and ovulation. The hypothalamus becomes active before puberty as the first step in the maturation process.

The production of FSH and LH by anterior pituitary cells is not steady; rather, the hormones are secreted in pulsatile discharges. The characteristic cyclic pattern of FSH and LH secretion during the normal menstrual cycle is governed by cyclic changes in ovarian estrogen and progesterone secretion (Fig. 7-1).

The principal modulator of hypothalamic-pituitary activity is *estrogen.* Estradiol (E_2) has a strong negative feedback relationship with FSH. Ovarian steroidogenesis is at a minimum during the first few days of a menstrual cycle (Fig. 7-2). The initial growth of the follicle is stimulated by specific *growth factor(s).* Then the low concentration of estrogen triggers secretion of GnRH with a consequent release of FSH and LH. These hormones stimulate follicle growth and an increase in E_2 production, which in itself plays an essential role in follicle growth and maturation. The increase in E_2 in conjunction with a rising concentration of FSH increases the number of *FSH receptors* and also results in granulosa cell proliferation. Intraovarian and circulating E_2 rises more steeply during the latter part of the follicular phase, reaching a maximum just before ovulation. The rising estrogen concentration inhibits FSH secretion; then a sharp peak acts on the hypothalamic-pituitary system and stimulates LH and, to a lesser extent, FSH release. *E_2 triggers the midcycle surge of LH, which must be precisely timed to induce ovulation.* The secretion of LH continues at a lower level. Its principal function is to support the growth of the corpus luteum.

The secretion of *progesterone* (P_4) increases rapidly after ovulation, and there is a concurrent but lesser increase in estrogen production. High levels of P_4 are maintained until about day 23 or 24 of the cycle, when the corpus luteum begins to regress if the ovum has not been fertilized. The withdrawal of hormone support of E_2 and P_4 to the endometrium is followed by its disintegration and menstruation. The low concentration of ovarian hormones permits the cycle to be reinitiated.

Hormones of menstruation

Hormones of the hypothalamus. *GnRH is a decapeptide* that is produced and secreted in the hypothalamus by special neuronal tissue in the region of the median eminence. It is secreted in a pulsatile fashion becoming *circhoral* (about every 60 minutes) around the time of ovulation but less frequently during the luteal phase. The half-life of GnRH is several minutes. Although exact control mechanisms have not yet been fully elucidated, there are certain neuromodulators that are known to affect the secretory patterns of GnRH.

Endogenous opioids suppress LH secretion presumably because of the direct effect upon the GnRH neurons. *Catecholamines* play a major role in the control of GnRH secretion. *Dopamine* generally *inhibits* LH secretion, whereas *norepinephrine* via alpha receptors *facilitates* LH secretion. The exact interrelationship of the centrally located aminergic, opioidergic, and petidergic neurons and their control is unclear.

The pulsatile release of GnRH is also subject to feedback from the ovarian sex steroids E_2 and P_4.

Hormones of the anterior pituitary. The exquisite timing of gonadotropin secretion is of paramount importance to a normal menstrual cycle. The *gonadotrope* is a pituitary cell that is responsible for the synthesis, storage, and release of

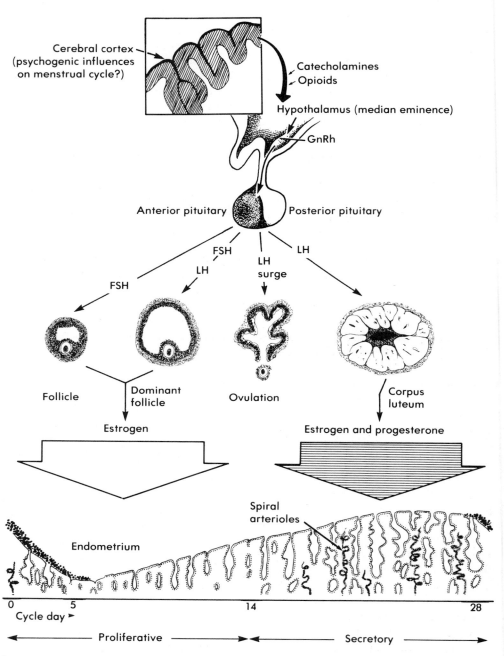

Fig. 7-1 Hormone and anatomic relationships during a menstrual cycle. There is also feedback from the ovarian hormones E_2 and P_4 to the pituitary and the hypothalamus.

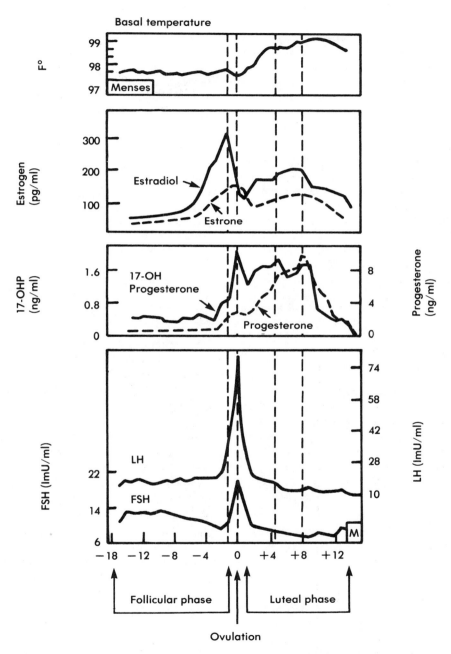

Fig. 7-2 Means of serum FSH, LH, estrone, E_2, P_4, and 17-hydroxyprogesterone during a normal menstrual cycle.

FSH and LH. Most of the pituitary gonadotropes produce both hormones. However, the cell population is heterogeneous, and some cells predominantly release one hormone or the other. The anterior pituitary is part of an endocrine unit called the *hypothalamic-hypophyseal complex,* which is subjected to numerous "messages" that result in secretion of gonadotropin hormones. The amplitude and the frequency of hormone release is determined by altering the sensitivity of this complex by making it more sensitive or less sensitive to incoming stimuli. The *negative feedback response* (E_2-inhibiting FSH and LH secretion) predominates during most of the menstrual cycle. At the time of ovulation, the *positive feedback response* (E_2-stimulating LH and FSH secretion) is the key event that ultimately results in ovum release. This stimulatory response is unique to the hypothalamic-pituitary-ovarian axis.

FSH and LH are glycoproteins that have similar alpha and different beta subunits and a somewhat similar molecular weight, 33,000 and 28,000, respectively. The half-life of these hormones is contingent upon the amount of sialic acid in the molecule and is approximately 4 hours for FSH and 1 hour for LH.

Hormones of the ovary. Estradiol (E_2) and estrone (E_1) are elaborated by the ovary, and there is an ongoing dynamic interconversion of estrone to estradiol and vice versa; during the reproductive years the net result favors E_2 secretion. E_2 has the greater biologic potency and plays a more significant role in modulating and effecting the normal menstrual cycle. Estrogens are *18-carbon compounds* that circulate bound to *sex steroid–binding globulin.* They are inactivated at a relatively rapid rate by the liver and excreted in conjugated forms as glucuronates and sulfates by the way of the urine predominantly and the feces to a lesser extent. Estrogens are secreted as a result of the interaction of the *ovarian theca and granulosa cells;* the latter aromatize the androgens, androstenedione, and testosterone to E_2. The positive-feedback response requires that E_2 concentration be at least 200 pg/ml for 48 hours in order to

trigger the LH surge. During the second half of the cycle, the *luteinized granulosa cells* that comprise the corpus luteum secrete estrogen and P_4.

The biologically active estrogens have an important maturational effect on the genital tissues; they also bring about the feminine habitus and stimulate growth of the ductal system of the breasts. Estrogens also play a role in long-bone growth and epiphyseal closure. The absence of estrogen after the menopause predisposes women to osteoporosis and genital and breast atrophy.

Knowledge of the role of intraovarian hormones in controlling events of the menstrual cycle continues to expand. Several protein hormones have been identified. *Inhibin,* a peptide synthesized by the granulosa cells, is secreted into the follicular fluid and ultimately can be measured in the peripheral circulation. FSH stimulates the production of inhibin, which in turn feeds back to reduce FSH levels. The secretion of inhibin also appears to be under paracrine control. A major role of inhibin is postulated to be ensuring that a dominant follicle is formed by reducing the available FSH to the cohort of follicles in that cycle.

Progesterone (P_4) is a 21-carbon compound that is secreted by the luteinized granulosa cells of the corpus luteum and is found predominantly in the latter half of the cycle. Serum concentration of at least 3 ng/ml is found in an ovulatory cycle. The plateau of its secretory pattern is reached about 7 days after ovulation. Just before ovulation, there is a small increase in P_4 that enhances pituitary sensitivity and is necessary for an optimal LH surge. P_4 circulates bound to *cortisol-binding globulin.* For tissues to be sensitive to the action of P_4, they must first have been exposed to estrogen, which induces P_4 receptors.

The primary reproductive function of P_4 is to induce secretory activity in the endometrial glands, thereby preparing the endometrium to receive a fertilized ovum. Its other biologic effects include desensitizing the myometrium to oxytocic activity, altering the histologic appearance of the vagina, inhibiting the secretory activity of the cervical glands, stimulating development of the alveolor system of the breasts, and, because of its thermogenic property, being responsible for the increase in basal body temperature following ovulation.

Changes in the genital tract

The ovary. At the time menstruation is taking place, *recruitment* of a number of primordial ovarian follicles, stimulated primarily by FSH, is initiated and continues for 5 days; LH stimulation also is required. The *dominant follicle* is then *selected,* although it cannot be easily identified for 2 to 3 more days. The increased production of E_2 resulting from the increase of both FSH receptors and granulosa cells is responsible for the process of selection. The ova that are excluded regress under the influence of intraovarian androgen production to undergo atresia. As the dominant follicle evolves, its lining granulosa cells become more cuboidal and multilayered; and a central cavity, the *antrum,* becomes filled with a transudate, *liquor folliculli.* The oocyte surrounded by its own granulosa cells awaits release.

Follicle growth and volume can be determined by ultrasound. The maximum mean diameter before rupture is 19.5 mm with a range between 18 and 25 mm. However, there may be variation from cycle to cycle in the same woman (Fig. 7-2).

E_2 secretion in the follicular phase is thought to occur because of the interaction between the *theca* and the *granulosa* cells. LH receptors are present in the thecal cells, and small amounts of that pituitary hormone stimulate thecal cell androgen production via the second messenger c-AMP. Receptors on the granulosa cell are predominantly FSH; these cells, when stimulated by FSH, increase aromatase enzyme activity, which enables the granulosa cells to convert androgens to E_2. Hence the interaction of both cells is required for normal estrogen production.

As a result of positive feedback, E_2 produces the onset of the LH surge, which is followed in 28 to 36 hours by ovulation. The LH spike also facilitates the resumption of meiosis in the oocyte, the luteinization of the granulosa cells, and the synthesis of prostaglandins required for the rhexis of the follicular wall and extrusion of the oocyte.

Oocyte maturation inhibitor (OMI) and *luteinization inhibitor* (LI) are nonsteroidal intrafollicular hormones that facilitate the entire series of events, preventing the premature release of an egg and early luteinization of the granulosa cells, respectively.

The rupture of the follicle is attended by capillary bleeding. The blood replaces the spilled follicular fluid, and a *corpus hemorrhagicum* is formed. Through the continued action of LH, the granulosa cells become luteinized, and a corpus luteum results. The corpus luteum continues to grow and function, aided by the pulsatile secretion of LH, until about day 23 or 24 of the cycle, when it begins to regress. If the ovum, which was discharged at the time of ovulation, is fertilized, this regression does not take place; the corpus luteum continues to function as the corpus luteum of pregnancy being maintained by the LH effect of hCG.

In the absence of pregnancy the corpus luteum becomes progressively less sensitive to LH stimulation. As the corpus luteum regresses, it becomes hyalinized and has a characteristic convoluted structure that can be seen histologically, the *corpus albicans.*

Luteal cells become less efficient at synthesizing P_4 if the ovum is not fertilized. The luteal tissue has also been found to contain a nonsteroidal substance that prevents LH from binding to the receptor on the granulosa cells. The *LH receptor-binding inhibitor* (LHRBI) increases in concentration during the luteal phase.

The uterus. The cervical mucosa, the myometrium, and the blood vessels of the uterus are all influenced by the cyclic changes in the levels of the hormones of ovary, but the endometrium shows the most dramatic effect of the influence of estrogen and progesterone. The changes are divided into three phases.

PROLIFERATIVE PHASE. Immediately after menstruation the endometrium is thin, the epithelium is cuboidal, and the glands are straight and nar-

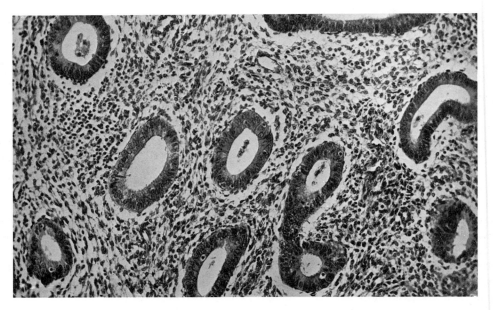

Fig. 7-3 Proliferative endometrium. Increase in number and size of glands and compact stroma. Although some glands are elongated, they are not tortuous. (×197.)

row. The stroma is compact. This stage lasts until the ninth day of the cycle.

The continued stimulatory effect of estrogen brings about an increased thickness of the mucosa during the late proliferative phase. The epithelium becomes columnar. As the phase progresses, the stroma becomes looser, more abundant, and more vascular. This phase lasts until about day 14 of the menstrual cycle (Fig. 7-3).

SECRETORY PHASE. During the postovulatory premenstrual stage, the progesterone from the corpus luteum stimulates the proliferative endometrium to exhibit secretory activity. The mucosa becomes thick and velvety. The glands become widened and assume a corkscrew pattern, and the stroma becomes edematous and loose. Early in the secretory phase the nuclei appear to move away from the basement membrane, leaving a characteristic area of *subnuclear vacuolization*. Secretion within the lumen of the glands is maximal by day 25 (Fig. 7-4). Special staining techniques reveal that secretions are rich in glycogen. There is an increasing coiling of arterioles.

By carefully examining the endometrial architecture with the use of well-defined criteria developed by Noyes, Hertig, and Rock, it is possible to monitor the progressive maturation. It is these dating criteria that are used to assist with the diagnosis of the luteal phase defect.

If the ovum is fertilized during the cycle and the corpus luteum persists, this phase progresses to the formation of the *decidua,* the endometrium of pregnancy.

MENSTRUAL (BLEEDING) PHASE. The decline in E_2 and P_4 initiates the process of menstruation. Although the structural changes in endometrial shedding have been observed directly in the elegant investigation of Markee, who transplanted endometrium into the anterior chamber of the eye of the rhesus monkey, the precipitating cause is unknown.

Following ovarian steroid decline, the height of

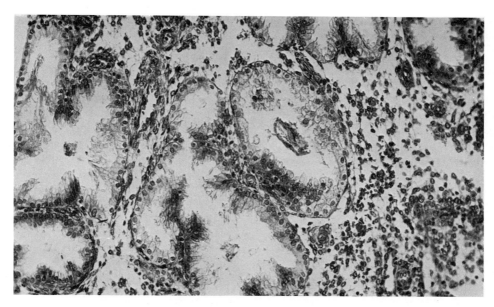

Fig. 7-4 Secretory endometrium. Stroma is scanty and loose, and dilated tortuous glands show intraluminal tufting and secretory activity. (×220.)

the endometrium diminishes, with a subsequent reduction in blood flow and vascular stasis. The *spiral arterioles* play a special role in menstruation by undergoing rhythmic vasoconstriction and relaxation. Ischemia is followed by tissue breakdown with cellular migration from the vascular bed; subsequently, enzymatic destruction of the endometrium occurs. The separation along the endometrial surface occurs between the layers *basalis* and the *spongiosa* and *compacta,* the latter two being discarded. Concomitantly, small vessels are being "plugged" with thrombin, and the growth of a new endometrial surface is being stimulated by estrogen. The entire event is relatively precise and uniform, occurring over the entire endometrial surface.

Christiaens, Sixma, and Haspel noted that the endometrial surface diminishes from 4 mm to 1.25 mm during this phase in a course of several hours.

Concentration of prostaglandin F_2alpha increases throughout the menstrual cycle; the highest amounts are measured at the time of menstrual flow. This potent vasoconstrictor probably plays a key role in initiating spiral arteriolar spasm.

THE CERVICAL MUCUS. In the immediate postmenstrual phase, the cervical mucus is scant, viscid, and opaque. During the follicular phase the columnar cells become taller, and the cervical glands begin to secrete increasing quantities of thin, clear, watery mucus that exhibits the physical properties of *spinnbarkeit* (the ability to form long, thin threads) and *arborization* (Chapter 2). These changes are a result of *estrogen stimulation.*

In the normal menstrual cycle the peak of estrogen activity is reached in the immediate preovulatory phase. The cervical mucus at this point is greatly increased in amount, is watery, and exhibits maximal spinnbarkheit and arborization. This remarkable change in the amount and character of the mucus favors sperm motility and survival and enhances its penetrability. These changes in the quality and amount of cervical mucus are a major source of information for those women wishing to practice natural family planning (Chapter 15).

After ovulation, under the influence of increasing *progesterone* production, the cervical mucus gradually decreases in amount and becomes viscid and tenacious; the arborization phenomenon disappears.

The vagina. The adult vaginal epithelium is composed of three stratified layers of squamous cells that shed representative cells reflecting the state of hormonal stimulation (Fig. 7-5). In a hematoxylin and eosin–prepared vaginal smear, cells from these layers can be identified. The *superficial cell,* the most mature cell, is large and flattened and is usually an eosinophilic staining cell with a small pyknotic nucleus. The layer below the superficial cells, the *intermediate cell* layer, is made up of medium-sized basophilic

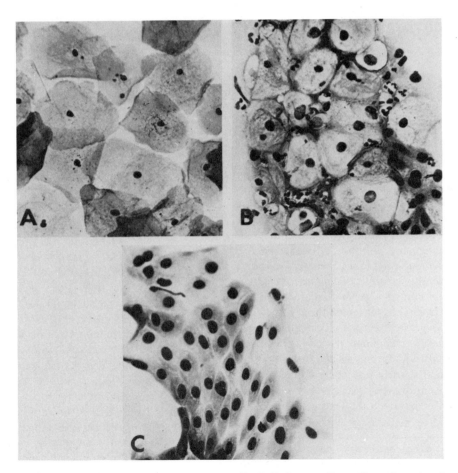

Fig. 7-5 **A,** Cornified (superficial cells, a strong estrogen effect). **B,** Intermediate cells and parabasal cells, smaller rounder cells with large nuclei, associated with progesterone influence. **C,** Clump of basal cells, vaguely outlined with large nuclei, indicating lack of estrogen. (From Riley G: Clin Obstet Gynecol 7:432, 1964.)

staining cells with vesicular nuclei. These are transitional cells. In an unstimulated vaginal epithelial surface that has been recently exposed to estrogen or if estrogen concentration is relatively low (for example, during the early proliferative phase of the cycle), this cell type predominates. Also, women who are in the progestational phase of their cycle have a preponderance of these cells. The *parabasal cell* is a more immature cell and has a larger nucleus-to-cytoplasm ratio. These cells are not usually seen in the vaginal epithelial profile of a female in the reproductive age range unless infection has aided in the denudation of the surface. The predominance of basal cells is seen in the absence of estrogen stimulation.

The fallopian tube. Although the physiology of the fallopian tube is not completely understood, it is more than a simple conduit through which gametes pass. The tubal epithelium, consisting of at least three cell types, ciliated, nonciliated or secretory, and peg cells, varies in height and activity throughout the menstrual cycle. The cells are at their smallest immediately following menses. Cellular changes can also be documented during pregnancy and when women take hormone therapy.

CLINICAL ASPECTS OF NORMAL MENSTRUATION

The length of the menstrual cycle and the duration and amount of flow vary considerably among normal women, but pronounced deviations from the accepted norms should suggest the possibility of functional or anatomic abnormality. Clinically significant characteristics of the menses are the *age at onset, periodicity, duration, amount of flow, character of flow,* and *associated symptoms.*

Age at onset. The first period usually occurs at about 12 years of age, but the menses may appear at age 9 or may be delayed until age 16 without being considered abnormal. Many factors are responsible for this wide variation. The most significant are race, heredity, the general health, nutritional status, and body mass of the individual girl. If the periods start before the age of 9 years, it is spoken of as *precocious menstruation;* if they

are delayed past the age of 16 years, it is spoken of as *primary amenorrhea.*

Periodicity. The theoretic normal interval from the beginning of one period to the onset of the next is 28 days, but few women menstruate that predictably. However, most women establish a somewhat reproducible pattern in the absence of pelvic disease or hormone therapy. Ranges between *25 and 34* days may be considered normal. The postovulatory phase is constant at 14 ± 2 days, whereas the preovulatory interval may be as short as 3 or 4 days or as long as 21 days. Cycles shorter than 3 weeks or longer than 5 weeks may indicate some disturbance of ovulation. Patients with short cycles are said to have *polymenorrhea.* If the cycle intervals are unusually long (45 to 60 days), the condition is designated as *oligomenorrhea.*

Duration. The usual length of flow is *5 ± 2 days,* but periods may last as long as 8 days or stop after 2 days and yet be within normal limits. Extremely short or scant periods are designated as *hypomenorrhea,* whereas unusually long or profuse menses are referred to as *hypermenorrhea.*

Amount of flow. The amount of blood lost at each period varies greatly. The average is about *40 ± 20 ml* and may be less than 20 ml; a loss of more than 80 ml is considered abnormal but may not be reflective of an ovulatory disorder.

Character of flow. The menstrual discharge consists of blood, mucus, and desquamated particles of endometrium. It is usually dark red and has a characteristic, musty odor. An interesting feature of menstrual blood is its failure to clot under normal circumstances.

Associated symptoms. A characteristic group of symptoms may appear several days before the menstrual flow. These symptoms, which include weight gain, edema, breast fullness and discomfort, heaviness of the legs, and irritability or depression, are referred to as *molimina.* An exaggeration of these symptoms is usually termed *premenstrual syndrome* (Chapter 10).

Even though menstruation is a normal function and should be free from disturbing symptoms, most women experience some degree of discomfort during the period of bleeding. A sense of weight in the pelvic region, mild backache, and cramping are such common complaints that they may be considered as normal accompaniments of the menses. When the pain become more severe, the patient is said to be suffering from *dysmenorrhea* (Chapter 10).

HYGIENE OF MENSTRUATION

Women need not restrict their usual daily routine in any way during the menstrual flow; this includes work, social, and athletic activities. Many couples abstain from sexual intercourse during menstruation because of aesthetic reasons or because of the concern of uncleanliness.

A daily bath or shower is not only permissible but most helpful in eliminating the characteristic odor that is sometimes present during the menstrual period.

External pads have been used for many years to absorb the menstrual discharge, but currently the majority of women use intravaginal tampons. Their safety is not entirely absolute or universal. A relatively rare acute infection, *toxic shock syndrome* (TSS), although limited to neither females nor the menses, occurs far more often in women specifically at the time of the menstrual period or shortly thereafter. TSS has also been reported in women utilizing a diaphragm and the contraceptive sponge. The risk is higher for women between ages 15 and 24 and during the postpartum period. The organism involved is *Staphylococcus aureus;* an *endotoxin* produced by this bacterium is believed to be responsible for the clinical problem. The illness is characterized by fever, rash, myalgia, fatigue, nausea, and emesis; TSS can progress into shock, coma, and death.

Tampon use has been identified as one of the risk factors. Although the incidence, estimated at 3 to 14 cases per 100,000 menstruating women per year with mortality rate at 2.3%, is low, certain precautions have been advised. Tampons should be changed at least every 4 to 6 hours, and intermittent rather than regular use appears advantageous; for example, they may be used during the day, but external pads should replace them at night. Also, external minipads can be used when the flow is scant. Handwashing is advised before inserting anything, including a tampon, sponge, or diaphragm, into the vagina.

Some women prefer to douche after menses if they perceive an odor to be present. Although this practice is reasonable, there is no medical information that it is necessary to cleanse the vagina.

SUGGESTED READING

Christiaens, Sixma JJ, and Haspel AA: Hemostasis in menstrual endometrium: a review, Obstet Gynecol Surv 37:281, 1982.

Fritz MA and Speroff L: The endocrinology of the menstrual cycle: the interaction of folliculogenesis and neuroendocrine mechanisms, Fertil Steril 38:509, 1982.

Knobil E: The neuroendocrine control of the menstrual cycle, Recent Prog Horm Res 36:53, 1980.

McLachlan RI and others: Circulating immunoreactive inhibin levels during the normal human menstrual cycle, J Clin Endocrinol Metab 65:954, 1987.

Markee JE: Menstruation in intraocular endometrial transplants in the rhesus monkey, Contrib Embryol 28:219, 1940.

Noyes RW, Hertig AT, and Rock J: Dating the endometrial biopsy, Fertil Steril 1:3, 1950.

Treloar AE, Boynton RE, Behm BG, and Brown BW: Variation of the human menstrual cycle through reproductive life, Int J Fertil 12:77, 1967.

Wager GP: Toxic shock syndrome: a review, Am J Obstet Gynecol 146:93, 1983.

8

John H. Mattox

Abnormal uterine bleeding

Objectives

RATIONALE: Abnormal uterine bleeding is one of the most common complaints of females and one of the most frequent indications for hysterectomy. Whereas effective medical therapy is available, its usage requires a thorough understanding of the pathogenesis of abnormal uterine bleeding and the need to tailor the evaluation and the therapy to the age of the patient and her specific problem.

The student should be able to:
A. Define dysfunctional uterine bleeding.
B. List at least five causes of abnormal uterine bleeding.
C. Outline an evaluation and differential diagnosis of abnormal uterine bleeding during adolescence, the reproductive age, and the premenopausal period.

Excessive or inappropriately timed bleeding through the vagina is one of the most common symptoms encountered by the practitioner providing health care for women. Abnormal bleeding can be the harbinger of serious pelvic disease or denote a relatively minor problem. The source of the bleeding can be any of several sites along the menstrual outflow tract. Therefore, a thorough and systematic examination is required in every patient presenting with this complaint. Blood loss of more than 80 ml during a period is called *hypermenorrhea,* whereas too frequent bleeding episodes (cycles less than 21 days) is *polymenorrhea.* Abnormal uterine bleeding be-

tween periods is called *metrorrhagia.* Another common word that denotes excessive uterine bleeding is *menorrhagia.* These descriptive terms characterize the patient's symptomatology and should not be used as the diagnosis. To understand abnormal uterine bleeding, the reader should be familiar with normal menstruation, which was discussed in Chapter 7.

ETIOLOGIC FACTORS

Most abnormal uterine bleeding is caused by a *complication of pregnancy,* a *tumor,* or *hormonal dysfunction.* The last term is used to characterize a disorder of the hypothalamic-pituitary-ovarian axis, which impacts on the endometrium to produce abnormal bleeding. Women receiving exogenous hormone therapy for contraception, estrogen-progestin replacement, or as treatment for certain endocrine disorders may experience abnormal endometrial shedding as a bothersome side effect. Less commonly, a serious constitutional illness such as chronic hepatitis is associated with abnormal bleeding. The following classification provides an overview of the causes of abnormal uterine bleeding:

I. Complications of pregnancy
II. Organic lesions
   A. Endocervical or endometrial polyp
   B. Cervical malignancy
   C. Benign leiomyoma or malignant uterine tumors
   D. Chronic endometritis
   E. Adenomyosis
   F. Endometriosis
   G. Salpingo-oophoritis
   H. Ovarian tumors
      1. Nonneoplastic cysts
         a. Follicular
         b. Corpus luteum
      2. Functioning stromal tumors (granulosa-thecal cell type)
   I. Trauma (intrauterine device)
III. Hormonal disorders
   A. Menstrual cycle
      1. Anovulatory
      2. Ovulatory
   B. Exogenous
      1. Hormone replacement therapy
      2. Contraceptive therapy
IV. Constitutional diseases
   A. Disorders of coagulation
   B. Liver disease
   C. Leukemia
   D. Anticoagulant therapy
   E. Thyroid disorders
   F. Adrenal disorders

Complications of pregnancy

Women of reproductive age should be suspected of being pregnant when presenting with abnormal bleeding. *Threatened, complete,* or *incomplete abortions* are by far the most common complications of pregnancy associated with bleeding. Other less common causes are *ectopic pregnancy* and *gestational trophoblastic disease.* All of these topics are discussed in other chapters.

Organic lesions

Uterine leiomyomas, particularly those of the *submucous* variety, are the genital tract lesions that most often cause abnormal bleeding in women who are not pregnant. Other entities include *carcinoma of the vagina, cervix, uterus,* and *ovaries; adenomyosis; endometriosis;* and *chronic salpingo-oophoritis* with extensive ovarian destruction. These are discussed in other chapters.

Endometrial polyps may cause intermenstrual staining and postmenopausal bleeding, as well as menorrhagia and hypermenorrhea. Because polyps generally do not cause an appreciable enlargement of the uterus, they are frequently overlooked. *Endocervical polyps* protruding from the os may cause spotting following coitus.

Dysfunctional uterine bleeding

Definition. *Dysfunctional uterine bleeding is abnormal endometrial bleeding caused by an endocrine dysfunction of the ovarian steroid hormones, estrogen and progesterone.* The clinical manifestation is bleeding that is abnormal in amount, duration, or timing in a female of reproductive age. When this diagnosis is entertained, it is understood that the physician has ruled out organic causes of abnormal uterine bleeding.

Incidence. Dysfunctional uterine bleeding may occur at any age between menarche and menopause. It is encountered most frequently at the two extremes of menstrual life, when disturbances of ovarian function are most common. More than 50% of dysfunctional bleeding occurs in premenopausal women 40 to 50 years of age, about 20% occurs during adolescence, and the remaining 30% is distributed among the other women in the reproductive period. About 85% of cases are associated with *anovulation*.

Pathophysiology. Dysfunctional uterine bleeding reflects a disturbance in the critical sequential hypothalamic-pituitary-ovarian interaction that is essential for ovulation, normal corpus luteum function, and normal endometrial growth and development. Bleeding associated with anovulation is caused by unopposed estrogen effects on the endometrium that results in "breakthrough bleeding" or by relative declines in circulating estrogens, causing "estrogen withdrawal bleeding."

If there is a deficiency of progesterone following ovulation, there may be abnormal bleeding, a *luteal phase defect*. If the corpus luteum fails to regress appropriately and progesterone continues to be secreted (Halban's syndrome), *"progesterone breakthrough bleeding"* occurs. Somewhat related is the chronic administration of a long-acting progestin, *medroxyprogesterone acetate. Abnormal endometrial bleeding occurs in the ab-*sence of sufficient estrogen to maintain a structurally sound endometrium. An atrophic endometrium is formed that is subject to breakdown resulting in bleeding.

Ovarian dysfunction may be caused by a primary defect or pathologic lesion within the ovary itself, or it may be a result of malfunction of other endocrine glands, notably the hypothalamus, pituitary, and thyroid. Anovulatory cycles tend to be self-perpetuating. They are discussed in Chapter 9.

When the ovary is unresponsive, as is the case in the aging gland of the perimenopausal woman, follicles fail to develop and become luteinized, despite increased gonadotropic stimulation. Conversely, if the ovaries are healthy and responsive, the defect in ovulation may be a result of inadequate gonadotropin secretion secondary to hypothalamic-pituitary dysfunction. In either case the result is the same—absence of progesterone secretion. The granulosa-theca cell complex contin-

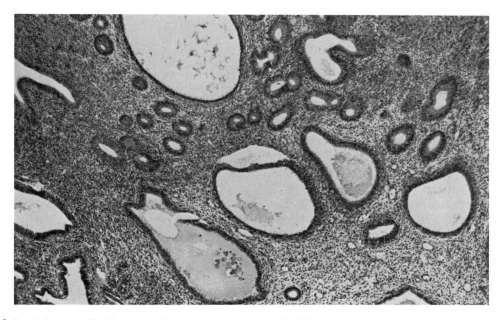

Fig. 8-1 Cystic hyperplasia. Note nonsecretory character of glands and great variation in their size, resembling holes in Swiss cheese. (×60.)

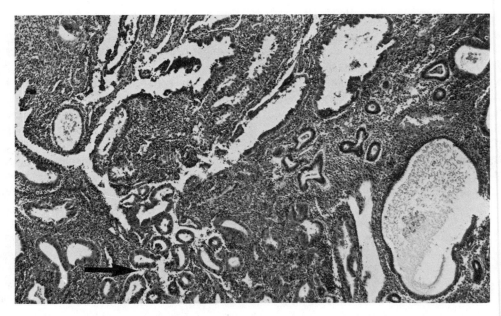

Fig. 8-2 Adenomatous hyperplasia. Glands are closely packed and back to back as a result of extraluminal budding. (×60.)

ues to secrete variable quantities of estrogen. This continued secretion causes a *relative excess* of estrogen that results in bleeding from the endometrium.

Pathologic findings of the endometrium. Dysfunctional bleeding is often associated with hyperplastic endometrium, a result of long-standing, unopposed estrogen stimulation. It may also occur with normal-appearing proliferative endometrium.

Hyperplastic endometrium with dysfunctional bleeding is characteristically thickened and may be polypoid, but in some cases it may be normal in appearance. Microscopically, the typical picture is that of benign cystic (Swiss cheese) hyperplasia (Fig. 8-1). There is great disparity in the size and shape of the glands, the epithelium is cuboid or cylindric with deeply stained nuclei, and usually there is no evidence of secretion. The stroma is dense and hyperplastic. In a small percentage of patients an adenomatous pattern is seen (Fig. 8-2).

Rarely, dysfunctional bleeding occurs with "mixed" endometrium, showing estrogen and progestational changes. In these instances the cycle is regular, but the bleeding period is prolonged, and the flow is irregular. This is called *irregular shedding,* a term that denotes asynchronous prolongation of shrinking, shedding, and involution of the endometrium rather than the rapid disintegrative process during the normal cycle.

The concentration of *estrogen and progesterone receptors* in endometrial cytosol varies during the menstrual cycle and is influenced by the circulating levels of the female sex steroids. Estrogen receptors and progesterone receptors reach maximum concentration during the late proliferative phase. Diamond, Aksel, and Speir measured receptor concentration in endometrial cytosol preparations in 36 women with dysfunctional uterine bleeding. Although their findings were of interest, they concluded that the *endometrial histology* rather than the concentration of receptors provided the most reliable information to determine the course of management.

Psychogenic uterine bleeding

There have been reports of irregular uterine bleeding with no evident cause other than emotional factors. The exact mechanism for the production of this type of bleeding is poorly understood.

The most likely explanation is that neurotransmitters are altered by emotional changes and adversely affect GnRH secretion upon the pituitary-ovarian axis, *thereby interfering with ovulation.* Markee, Everett, and Sawyer have shown that fright causes bleeding in endometrial transplants in the eye of the monkey. This suggests that the vasoactive substances released during acute stress could affect the endometrial arterioles and result in tissue breakdown. Even when confronted with a patient having acute psychologic distress, a thorough systematic evaluation must still be conducted by the physician.

Constitutional disease

Although these causes are uncommon, they must be considered, particularly in the female with continued, recurrent episodes of abnormal uterine bleeding. Constitutional diseases most likely to cause uterine bleeding such as thrombocytopenia, factor VIII deficiency, and leukemia interfere with the blood-clotting mechanism. Hypothyroidism has been shown to induce a secondary factor VIII deficiency, which may be responsible for the bleeding problem.

MANAGEMENT

An accurate diagnosis must be made before one can treat abnormal bleeding effectively. This implies that the physician is thoroughly aware of what constitutes normal bleeding and acceptable variations from the norm. The ultimate goal is to determine the cause of all cases of prolonged, excessive, or irregular flow. A general approach that can be applied to the assessment of most women with abnormal bleeding is found in the box at right.

DIAGNOSIS OF ABNORMAL UTERINE BLEEDING

Problem-oriented history
General physical and pelvic examination
Papanicolaou smear
Complete blood count
Serum hCG
Assessment of the endometrium
Other hormone studies as indicated

When this outline is followed, several factors such as the age of the patient, the chronicity or recurrence of the problem, and the patient's risk of genital tract malignancy must be considered. Also, some specialized studies such as *hysteroscopy* or *hysterosalpingography* may be helpful in diagnosing certain problems that might otherwise have been overlooked.

Adolescence

Diagnosis. In adolescent females, abnormal bleeding is almost always caused by a disturbance of ovarian function that results in anovulation. It occurs because of immaturity of the hypothalamic-pituitary axis with a lack of appropriate ovarian stimulation and positive estradiol feedback. However, clinical observations suggest that fewer than 20% of postpubertal females remain anovulatory for more than 5 years after menarche.

The possibility of pregnancy, blood dyscrasia, or malignancy must be kept in mind. Adenocarcinoma of the vagina or cervix has been described in young women who were exposed to diethylstilbestrol in utero. If an acute hemorrhage occurs in the adolescent, particularly with the first menstrual flow, a blood dyscrasia or more serious illness would be suspected. Usually, a careful history will rule out the more serious conditions.

Classens and Cowell found that 28% of 79 adolescents hospitalized at the Toronto's Hospital for Sick Children from 1971 through 1980 had an underlying coagulation disorder; 10% had other pathologic conditions.

In the young female, a gentle rectal examination may suffice to evaluate pelvic structures. The use of *pelvic sonography* can also be considered. If the uterus and adnexa cannot be assessed readily, the physician should consider examining the patient under general anesthesia.

When ordering a *complete blood count,* interpretation of the red blood cell indices should not be overlooked. A *serum ferritin* level may be helpful in diagnosing iron deficiency anemia. If a *clotting disorder* is seriously considered, a platelet count, partial thromboplastin time, prothrombin time and bleeding time will assist in making the diagnosis.

As the risk of malignancy is remote in the adolescent female, endometrial curettage is rarely necessary. It may be required and can be useful in temporarily controlling acute hemorrhage in selected cases.

Therapy. Because most dysfunctional uterine bleeding in this age group occurs because of abnormal hormonal stimulation of the endometrium, it can usually be effectively controlled by endocrine therapy. The underlying issue with which to deal in the anovulatory patient is unopposed estrogen. This effect on the endometrium can be combated by a combined progestin-estrogen contraceptive agent or cyclic progestin therapy. Oral administration of one of the *progestin-dominant oral contraceptive steroids* for 3 to 6 months will usually regularize uterine bleeding. Periodic administration of progesterone such as *oral medroxyprogesterone acetate,* 10 mg daily for 13 days/month, will eliminate the endometrial hyperplasia caused by unopposed estrogen stimulation and regulate uterine bleeding; *this is not an effective contraceptive agent.*

On occasion it will be necessary to control an acute episode of bleeding; *conjugated estrogens* administered intravenously, 25 mg every 4 hours for 24 hours, or a *progestin-dominant oral contraceptive steroid* such as Lo Ovral, one tablet every 6 hours for 3 to 4 days, will usually control the acute bleeding. After the acute episode is controlled, combined estrogen-progestin oral contra-

ceptives should be continued cyclically for 3 to 6 months. *Progesterone therapy alone, orally, or intramuscularly, is not useful in controlling acute bleeding.*

Bed rest, increasing oral fluid intake if a curettage is not contemplated, and iron replacement therapy are additional measures that should be instituted. In those adolescents who have a particularly heavy flow, it is prudent to continue iron therapy. If significant blood volume depletion occurs as a result of the heavy bleeding that cannot be controlled by hormone therapy and the patient is developing shock, a dilation and curettage should be performed.

Childbearing period

Diagnosis. In women in the reproductive age range, complications of pregnancy, pelvic infections, endometriosis, leiomyomata, and neoplasia are the most likely causes of irregular bleeding. Particularly appropriate questions to be asked are: Is there intermenstrual bleeding or staining? (Suspect endometrial polyp or malignancy.) Does bleeding occur after coitus? (Suspect cervical neoplasia.) Have there been any recent periods of amenorrhea? (Suspect pregnancy or oligoovulation.) Is the patient taking any hormones? (Suspect endometrial hyperplasia.)

Women in this age range are less likely to have an unrecognized coagulopathy than are adolescents. However, *hypothyroidism* is likely, and a serum thyroid-stimulating hormone (TSH) level may be helpful. Also, for any woman with a disorder of ovulation, a *serum prolactin* should be ordered. Because uterine malignancy is uncommon before the age of 30, an endometrial sampling is not required routinely. If the physician has any reason to be suspicious of malignancy or a precursor, an in-office or outpatient endometrial sampling using an aspiration curet will usually be sufficient (Fig. 8-3). In dealing with recalcitrant or recurrent dysfunctional bleeding, a *hysterogram* can be a valuable aid. Endometrial polyps and submucous myomas can be diagnosed by this procedure (Figs. 8-4 and 8-5). *Hysteroscopy* can

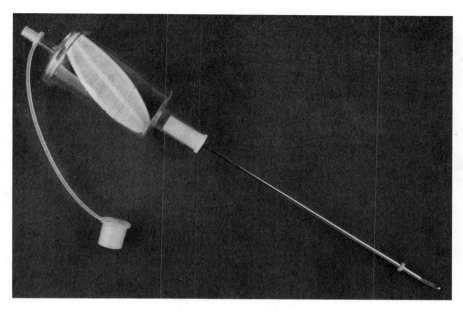

Fig. 8-3 Endometrial biopsy suction curet; there are several types available. Curet is attached to pump producing negative suction. Uterine cavity depth is determined, since curet is calibrated in centimeters. Sample obtained is collected in tissue trap. Preprocedure tranquilizer or paracervical block can reduce the discomfort and should be used as necessary.

often provide additional diagnostic information. The advantages of hysteroscopy include being able to perform a directed biopsy, identification and removal of endometrial polyps, and perform lysis of intrauterine adhesions. In a patient who has not responded to initial therapy, *dilation and curettage* with exploration of the uterine cavity by hysteroscopy or with forceps should be carried out. *Uterine curettage should generally be viewed as a diagnostic and not as a therapeutic procedure; it does not in itself correct the factors that are responsible for anovulation.* Curettage is best performed premenstrually or at the time of bleeding if it is acylic; this will indicate whether or not there is a progesterone effect.

Therapy. In the patient with dysfunctional bleeding, if no contraindications exist, *cyclic hormone therapy* with a combination estrogen-progestin medication may be tried for 3 to 6 months.

In the patient who has a long-standing history of oligoovulation or anovulation, *cyclic progesterone therapy,* medroxyprogesterone acetate (MPA), 10 mg; or norethindrone acetate, 5 mg, for 13 days each month, should eliminate estrogen-induced endometrial hyperplasia and should produce regular withdrawal bleeding episodes. MPA also has a more favorable effect upon serum lipids than the 19 nonsteroids. Patients with prolonged anovulation may need additional medical evaluation as discussed in Chapter 9. It is *seldom necessary to remove the uterus* because of dysfunctional bleeding. However, hysterectomy may be indicated if the bleeding cannot be controlled by hormone therapy or if there is a contraindication to its use. Some patients are unable to tolerate endocrine treatment because of side effects related to the medication; other women prefer hysterectomy to many years of hormonal therapy.

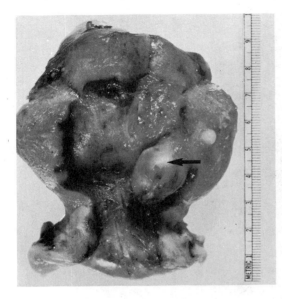

Nonsteroidal antiinflammatory medication has been shown to be effective in reducing uterine menstrual flow in women who have regular, ovulatory, but excessive menses. It is ineffective in controlling anovulatory bleeding. An *oral iron preparation* should be administered if the patient gives a history of heavy flow; her iron stores may be depleted, but her hemoglobin may not yet have decreased enough to permit a diagnosis of anemia.

Greenberg noted that menorrhagia may be accompanied by *depression*. He diagnosed mild-to-moderate depression in 31 of 50 women being considered for hysterectomy because of excessive uterine flow.

Fig. 8-4 Pedunculated submucous myoma. Uterus is normal size. Diagnosis is made by hysterogram (see Fig. 8-5).

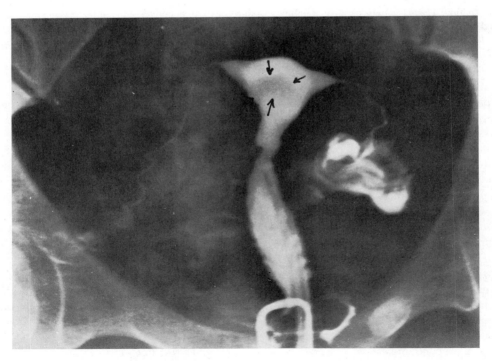

Fig. 8-5 Hysterogram showing submucous myoma. Uterine cavity is normal but has filling defect. Two previous curettages failed to disclose tumor.

The severity of blood loss with excessive, but regular uterine bleeding correlates poorly with the patient's history of how many tampons or maxipads are required to contain the flow.

Chimbira, Anderson, and Turnbull also found that endometrial surface area did not prognosticate the severity of flow: the larger uterine cavity, 46 cm^2, produced a mean loss of 85 ml; however, the largest mean loss, 525 ml, was found with a uterine surface area of 26 cm^2.

Endometrial ablation with laser or a resectoscope has been utilized as a procedure to reduce uterine bleeding in the absence of uterine pathology.

The role of GnRh agonists to treat this disorder has yet to be determined.

Perimenopausal period

The assessment of women with abnormal bleeding during the *climacteric* (perimenopausal period) is similar to that of women in the child-bearing years. However, *sampling the endometrium* should be part of the routine evaluation in this group. If the bleeding cannot be controlled easily with cyclic progestin therapy or if the patient cannot tolerate the medication, hysterectomy should be considered. The risks and benefits of estrogen replacement therapy in women over the age of 40 must be considered when discussing any surgical treatment with the patient (Chapter 47).

The patient with *postmenopausal bleeding* should be considered to have precancerous or malignant disease until proven otherwise. However, benign lesions such as atrophic endometritis and cervical polyps are a more frequent cause of postmenopausal bleeding. *Fractional dilation and curettage* is essential in the study of patients in this age group. Although endometrial hyperplasia may be the result of unopposed endogenous estrogen production, particularly in the obese female because of the conversion of androstenedione to estrone, the patient should still be thoroughly questioned as to whether or not she is taking estrogen. *Digoxin* has also been reported as having estrogenic activity and has been associated with endometrial hyperplasia. The possibility of an *ovarian estrogen-producing tumor* must also be considered. It is particularly important in this age group for the physician to search for an explanation of why there is excessive estrogen production at a time when it should be waning.

If anemia is diagnosed, other sources of blood loss such as *colon cancer* should be considered, and appropriate screening advised. *Hypothyroidism* is more common in this age group, and the evaluation of thyroid function should be considered a routine measure.

Therapy. The treatment of irregular bleeding in the postmenopausal age group consists mainly of treating pathologic conditions of the uterus and ovaries. Endocrine therapy is less likely to be appropriate; however, *cyclic progestin therapy* (medroxyprogesterone, 10 mg daily for at least 13 days/month) may be tried after malignancy has been excluded.

Progesterone prevents the replenishment of estrogen receptors in the endometrial cells and thereby reduces the growth effect of estrogen. It also facilitates the intracellular conversion of estradiol to estrione, a weaker estrogen. This cellular effect is related more to the length of time progesterone is administered.

SUGGESTED READING

Chimbira TH, Anderson ABM, and Turnbull AC: Relation between measured menstrual blood loss and patients' subjective assessment of loss, duration of bleeding, number of sanitary towels used, uterine weight and endometrial surface, Br J Obstet Gynaecol 87:603, 1980.

Classens EA and Cowell CL: Acute adolescent menorrhagia, Am J Obstet Gynecol 139:277, 1981.

Diamond E, Aksel S, and Speir BR: Endometrial estrogen and progesterone receptors in patients with dysfunctional uterine bleeding, Semin Reprod Endocrinol 2:351, 1984.

Greenberg M: The meaning of menorrhagia: an investigation into the association between the complaint of menorrhagia and depression, J Psychosom Res 27:209, 1983.

Markee JE, Everett JW, and Sawyer CH: The relationship of the nervous system to the release of gonadotropin and the regulation of the sex cycle, Recent Prog Horm Res 7:139, 1952.

9

John H. Mattox

Amenorrhea

Objectives

RATIONALE: The absence of menses at an unexpected time is always a cause for concern. The explanation may be physiologic but it is also a symptom of malfunction of the hypothalmic-pituitary-ovarian axis. Amenorrhea may be associated with serious systemic illness. The appropriate management requires not only a thorough understanding of menstruation but a systematic approach to insure a serious endocrinopathy or other illness is not overlooked.

The student should be able to:
A. Define primary and secondary amenorrhea.
B. List three etiologies of amenorrhea by using the hypothalamic-pituitary-ovarian-utero-vaginal compartment model.
C. Outline an approach to evaluate a patient with amenorrhea.
D. Outline an evaluation of a patient with polycystic ovary syndrome.

The term *amenorrhea* indicates the absence of menstruation. It is a symptom, not a disease entity, and may be caused by a variety of physiologic and pathologic processes.

Oligomenorrhea customarily refers to the occurrence of infrequent menstruation when the interval is usually 45 days or more. The term can also refer to short episodes of amenorrhea.

Amenorrhea is considered to be *primary* if a normal, spontaneous period has not occurred by age 16 years. *Secondary amenorrhea* indicates

cessation of menstruation after a variable period of normal function, usually three consecutive cycles.

Although a distinction concerning the evaluation of women with primary and secondary amenorrhea is no longer diagnostically relevant, some observations about these two groups of patients presenting with the symptom of amenorrhea may be clinically useful. Women with primary amenorrhea are more likely to have a uterovaginal anomaly, a genetic disorder, or a defective gonad;

those with secondary amenorrhea are more likely to have a disorder of the hypothalamic-hypophyseal complex or a prolactinoma.

ETIOLOGIC FACTORS

Amenorrhea can be induced by physiologic, anatomic, pathologic, or constitutional factors. Although the underlying problem may be physiologic or perhaps caused by a minor and negligible systemic or psychologic disturbance, it also may be an early symptom of a serious constitutional disease or endocrinopathy for which prompt treatment may be critical.

The following classification of the possible etiologic factors involved in amenorrhea is offered as a guide to the diagnostic study of this problem.

Causes of amenorrhea

I. Physiologic
  A. Periods during which amenorrhea occurs
    1. Adolescence
    2. Pregnancy
    3. Lactation
    4. Menopause
II. Anatomic
  A. Uterovaginal
    1. Imperforate hymen
    2. Absence of vagina/uterus
      a. Atresia
      b. Androgen insensitivity (testicular feminization)
      c. Müllerian agenesis (Mayer-Rokitansky-Kuster-Hauser syndrome)
      d. Hysterectomy
    3. Destruction of endometrium
      a. Uterine synechiae (Asherman's syndrome)
      b. Atrophy caused by irradiation or medication
      c. Severe infection (tuberculosis, schistosomiasis)
  B. Ovarian (gonadal)
    1. Gonadal dysgenesis
      a. 45 X (Turner's syndrome)
      b. Mosaicism, isochromosome formation

      c. "Pure" 46 XX or 46 XY (Swyer's syndrome)
    2. Premature ovarian failure
    3. Destruction
      a. Mumps
      b. Irradiation
      c. Surgery
    4. Tumors
      a. Hormone-secreting neoplasms
        (1) Androgen (arrhenoblastoma, hilus cell)
        (2) Estrogen (granulosa-thecal cell)
        (3) hCG (dysgerminoma)
      b. Persistent corpus luteum (Halban's syndrome)
    5. Polycystic ovarian syndrome
  C. Pituitary
    1. Infarction following delivery (Sheehan's syndrome)
    2. Tumor
      a. Prolactinoma
      b. Craniopharyngioma
      c. Acromegaly
    3. Irradiation
    4. Surgery
  D. Hypothalamic/CNS
    1. GnRH deficiency (Kallmann's syndrome)
    2. Eating disorders
      a. Weight loss (with or without bulimia)
      b. Anorexia nervosa
    3. Stress-induced
    4. Exercise-associated
    5. Tumor
    6. Psychotropic medication
    7. Drug addiction
  E. Miscellaneous
    1. Thyroid disease (usually hypothyroidism)
    2. Adrenal disease
      a. Congenital adrenal hyperplasia
      b. Cushing's syndrome
      c. Hormone-secreting tumor
      d. Adrenal insufficiency (Addison's disease)

Physiologic causes

Amenorrhea during adolescence. The average healthy American girl usually experiences her first menstrual period at about the age of 12.3 years, but it is not at all unusual for the menarche to be delayed until 15 or 16 years of age, particularly if the young female is athletic. Similarly, although some girls menstruate regularly after the onset of the first period, many exhibit considerable irregularity with periods of amenorrhea during the first three years. This variation during adolescence is so common that it may be considered normal.

Failure to menstruate by age 16 warrants investigation. *Delayed menarche* is sometimes a biologic variant of normal maturation, but it may result from anatomic causes or serious endocrine or genetic abnormalities. The complaint of primary amenorrhea in a young woman will occasionally provide the first opportunity to uncover one of these conditions.

In women who have never menstruated, particular attention should be paid to whether or not secondary sex characteristics are present, a pivotal observation that aids in the evaluation. If no *breast budding* occurs by 14 years of age, it is neither desirable nor necessary to wait until age 16 because this female is not undergoing the normal physiologic progression seen in puberty.

Pregnancy. Pregnancy is the most common cause for amenorrhea during the reproductive years and should *always* be considered as a possible cause in all patients in the childbearing period. Instances of uterine bleeding during pregnancy are caused by a disturbance of pregnancy or by an organic lesion and not by menstrual periods.

Lactation. The first menstrual period after delivery usually occurs within 8 weeks unless the infant is breast-fed, in which event menstruation may be delayed until nursing is discontinued because of the persistence of increased levels of serum prolactin. Further discussion of this entity can be found in Chapter 42.

Climacteric. Variable periods of oligomenorrhea may occur for a number of years preceding the final cessation of menopause. This is frequently a source of considerable anxiety to the middle-aged woman, who may consider the amenorrhea to be a symptom of pregnancy. Vaginal bleeding that occurs after 5 to 6 months of amenorrhea should be investigated carefully as the risk of neoplasia increases at this time. Ovulatory cycles are uncommon after age 50.

Anatomic causes

Amenorrhea may be caused by congenital malformations that preclude the possibility of menstruation. These abnormalities account for about 2% of all amenorrhea not caused by pregnancy.

Atresia of the vagina and imperforate hymen (Fig. 9-1). These anatomic causes for primary amenorrhea, although not common, underscore the importance of complete examination of girls at birth and during subsequent examinations.

Absence of menstruation can result from an obstruction at some point in the vagina or cervix. An *imperforate hymen* is one of the possible congenital malformations. Because the ovaries and endometrium in these patients are perfectly normal, a discharge of blood from the uterus occurs at the time of menstruation, but it is retained and hidden in the vagina. This process is repeated from month to month and leads to *hematocolpos*, a progressive distension of the vagina with blood (Fig. 9-2). If the situation is unrecognized, the uterus and even the fallopian tubes may become filled with this material, resulting in *hematometra* and *hematosalpinx*. Periodic episodes of lower abdominal pain and backache are characteristic. Inspection of the vulva and rectal examination will readily confirm the diagnosis. A simple cruciate incision of the hymen is corrective of these disorders. In the course of the evaluation, laparoscopy should be carried out, as these young women may have developed endometriosis.

Absence of the uterus and vagina. Abnormal development of the müllerian system can result in partial or complete absence of the vagina, uterine hypoplasia, or only rudimentary muscular cords. Rarely, a small functional uterine cavity may be

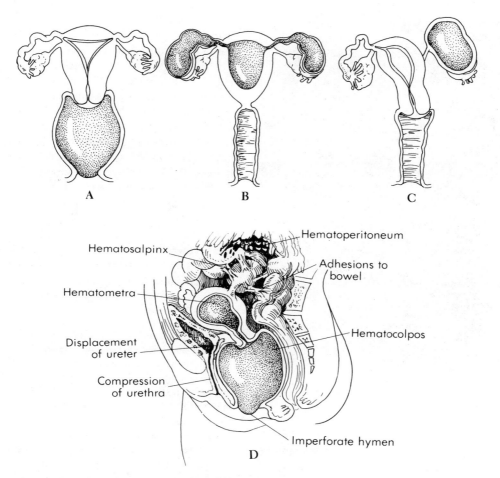

Fig. 9-1 **A**, Imperforate hymen, hematocolpos. **B**, Congenital atresia of cervix, hematometra, bilateral hematosalpinx. **C**, Uterus bicornis unicollis, lateral hematometra in blind, rudimentary form.

present. Menstrual flow can be retained, resulting in periodic pelvic pain. Complete aplasia of the vagina associated with a poorly defined uterine anlage, *Mayer-Rokitansky-Kuster-Hauser syndrome,* is a relatively common cause of primary amenorrhea; about one third of these women have a renal anomaly, and 12% have skeletal defects. This diagnosis should be entertained when young women with secondary sex characteristics fail to menstruate. A careful examination of the genitalia

should be performed and will usually disclose a diagnosis.

Androgen insensitivity, testicular feminization syndrome, should be included in the differential diagnosis. Testicular feminizing syndrome (male pseudohermaphroditism) is truly a misnomer. The clinical picture occurs because the male tissues are partially or totally *unable to respond to androgen hormone messages* because of the lack of intracellular receptors and is not caused by the

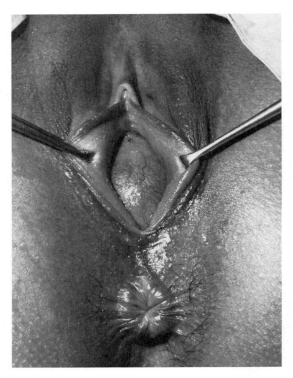

Fig. 9-2 Imperforate hymen distended by hematocolpos.

testis secreting estrogens as the wording implies. A strong familial tendency transmitted probably by an X-linked recessive mode is responsible. These individuals are chromatin negative, with a karyotype of 46 XY and thus genotypic males; however, most are completely feminine in appearance but variations do occur. Breasts are distinctively developed; height is normal; and axillary, pubic, and facial hair is absent or sparse. A vaginal indentation, less deep than usual is present, but other internal female genitals are absent. The male gonads are usually found as swellings in the inguinal canal or within the abdominal cavity.

The gonad produces both estrogen and androgen. Estrogen values are higher than those found in normal males. LH levels are elevated. Inability of end-organ response to androgen is further demonstrated by the fact that serum testosterone and dehydroepiandrosterone sulfate (DHEAS) levels are in the range for normal males.

These individuals are psychologically and morphologically female and function normally in this role except that they are amenorrheic and infertile. The gonads containing a Y chromosome should be removed because of their propensity to become malignant; extirpation can be deferred until the endogenous estrogen effects of puberty are gained. Gonadal malignancy is rare before the age of 20. This condition should be strongly suspected in female infants with inguinal hernias or labial masses.

Counseling of these patients and their parents and partners is a delicate matter. Artless emphasis on the genetic and chromosomal sex can be unduly traumatic. They should be considered to be and spoken of as women. The term *gonad* is obviously preferable to *testis*.

After they studied 17 families in Santo Domingo, Peterson and co-workers demonstrated the necessity of 5-alpha reductase, the enzyme required to convert testerone to dihydrotestosterone (DHT) for the formation of normal male genitalia. At birth the affected genetic males had labial-scrotal or inguinal testes, a small phallus, and a single perineal opening; they were raised as females in the society until puberty. Partial virilization with testicular descent and some penile enlargement occur, but prostatic enlargement, facial hair growth, temporal recession, and acne are absent; those biologic phenomena require dihydrotestosterone. These males undergo psychosexual reassignment and assume the role of young men after puberty.

Endometrial abnormalities. Prolonged *endometrial suppression* following the use of injectable medroxyprogesterone acetate can result in endometrial atrophy. Although the condition is self-limiting, the uterine lining may be partially resistant to exogenous or endogenous estrogen stimulation, giving the impression that there is endometrial obliteration.

Secondary amenorrhea as a result of *endometrial cavity obliteration* with adhesions may develop after repeated or too strenuous curettage,

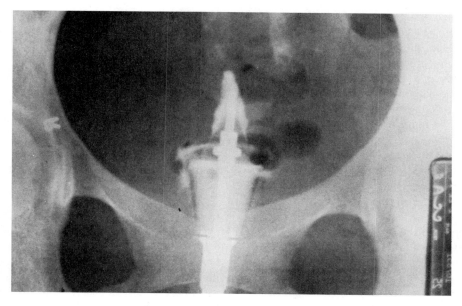

Fig. 9-3 Attempted hysterogram. Endometrial cavity obliterated following postpartum curettage. Cannula tip at cervicouterine junction, and no endometrial cavity is visualized.

particularly in the postpartum and postabortal uterus, *Asherman's syndrome* (Fig. 9-3). *Endometritis* may be responsible for the development of synechiae that may partially or almost completely obliterate the endometrial cavity. The hypoestrogenic state seen in the early period following pregnancy is also believed to be contributory, as endometrial proliferation is less active.

The recent use of *hysteroscopy* has greatly improved both diagnosis and management of this problem. Although a hysterogram will demonstrate a filling defect, the precise location and extent of the adhesions are far more accurately determined under direct vision. Symptoms in patients with a moderate number of adhesions are hypomenorrhea and a tendency to abort if implantation occurs.

Irradiation of the pelvis to treat pelvic malignancy can result in either temporary or permanent amenorrhea, depending on the dose employed. This effect is produced by the destructive action on the endometrium or ovaries. If periods recur after a long period of irradiation-induced amenorrhea, an intrauterine malignancy must be ruled out as a cause of bleeding.

Ovarian causes

Gonadal dysgenesis (Turner's syndrome). Classic features of Turner's syndrome include congenital webbed neck, low-set ears, cubitus valgus, short stature, shield chest, high-arched palate, increased pigmented nevi, and sexual infantilism. Other anomalies such as congenital heart disease, particularly *coarctation of the aorta* and *renal malformation,* often are present. The complete picture of this syndrome, including all the foregoing anomalies, is relatively rare, whereas sexual infantilism and short stature are consistent findings. About 30% of infants have lymphedema of the lower extremities at birth; this finding should alert the clinician to the possibility of this diagnosis.

It is not unusual for the patient to have amenorrhea as the first complaint. About 80% to 90% of these patients are chromatin negative and have a chromosome constitution of 45X. The chromosomal patterns in others may show *mosaicism* such as X/XX or X/XXX. Thus the chromosomal number of the majority is 45, whereas some have chromosomal counts of 46. An X/XY form occurs and tends to be familial.

Turner's syndrome represents primary and complete ovarian failure. The ovaries are represented by elongated, whitish ridges or streaks on the broad ligament. They contain neither primordial follicles nor germ cells, but the stromal tissue is similar to that of the ovary. The absence of estrogen secretion is reflected by a lack of breast development, genital hypoplasia, amenorrhea, and high serum concentrations of FSH and LH.

Diagnosis is confirmed by examination of the buccal smear for nuclear sex evaluation, determination of chromosomal constitution, and detection of high gonadotropin excretion.

Premature ovarian failure, a clinical problem presenting with secondary amenorrhea afflicts about 5% of the female population. The condition is usually permanent but can be transient. Although there are some known causal agents such as irradiation, cytotoxic drugs, genetic factors, and specific viral infection such as mumps oophoritis, the cause frequently remains a mystery. There is a significant association between premature ovarian failure and reduced function of other endocrine systems, specifically the pancreatic beta cells and the thyroid, adrenal, and parathyroid glands, suggesting that the ovarian failure is part of an autoimmune disease. A high incidence of ovarian failure has also been identified in women with abnormal galactose metabolism.

Nonneoplastic ovarian cysts such as a *follicular cyst* of the ovary may on occasion cause a short period of amenorrhea. As a rule, this type of ovarian cyst produces no menstrual disturbance, nor is it associated with dysfunctional uterine bleeding. A *corpus luteum cyst* (larger than 5 cm) that persists may induce a short period of amenorrhea followed by irregular bleeding. The problem

is self-limiting. The symptoms and presentation of an adnexal mass may lead the physician to suspect ectopic pregnancy. With a careful history, pelvic examination, appropriate use of serum hCG levels, and ultrasound, the correct diagnosis can be reached.

POLYCYSTIC OVARIAN SYNDROME (PCO). Although PCO patients are more likely to present with oligomenorrhea or abnormal uterine bleeding, primary or secondary amenorrhea can be seen. The classic features of the clinical symptom complex originally described by Stein and Leventhal in 1935 were amenorrhea, infertility, obesity, and facial hirsutism. The ovaries were described as oysterlike in appearance with a thick grayish capsule, numerous tiny cysts beneath the thickened tunica, and an enlargement amounting to approximately two to three times their normal size. Typical microscopic findings in PCO are hyperplasia and luteinization of the theca interna.

It became evident later that neither ovarian enlargement nor theca luteinization was an invariable finding. Stein and Leventhal recognized that some of the symptoms were inconstant; hirsutism occurred in only about 50% of the cases, and instead of amenorrhea, menstrual irregularities with episodes of menometrorrhagia were not uncommon. The amenorrhea tends to develop gradually over a period of years. Obesity is not always present. However, ovaries with thick fibrous tunica reflecting anovulation and infertility are consistent findings.

There has been great confusion and controversy regarding the etiologic factors in PCO. It is apparent that it represents the end result of long, uninterrupted periods of anovulation. A wide spectrum of disorders causing anovulation is associated with malfunction of the hypothalamic-pituitary-gonadal axis. Many are temporary derangements. Polycystic ovarian syndrome reflects prolonged, persistent anovulation—the development of a "steady state" in the feedback effects of estrogen on gonadotropin secretion. FSH levels fall in the low normal range with absence of the midcycle peak (negative feedback effect);

LH secretion is sustained at an elevated level (positive feedback effect) with lack of an appropriate midcycle surge. In addition, there is increased LH secretion in response to testing with GnRH. The polycystic ovary produces an excess of androgens, mainly androstenedione and testosterone.

Persistent gonadotropin stimulation causes growth of follicles and an increase in estradiol and estrone at first, but ova are not released. The follicles arrest and become cystic or atretic, and stromal tissue is increased. The amount of estradiol produced is diminished, but estrogen precursors, androstenedione and testosterone, are significantly increased. Androstenedione can undergo conversion to testosterone within the ovary and peripherally. It also undergoes conversion to estrone by fatty tissue, and this contributes to the circulating estrogen pool. These derangements, characteristic of PCO, are thus self-perpetuating. The persistent LH excess causes some increase in adrenal and ovarian androgen secretions. However, the ovary is the major source of androgens in the majority of hirsute women with polycystic ovaries.

Diagnosis. Clinical features, including menstrual irregularities, may begin in the teens or early twenties. Infertility is caused by anovulation. Obesity and hirsutism may or may not be associated. Enlargement of the ovaries on pelvic examination is a common but not essential feature. The size is within normal limits in about a third of cases. The smooth, gray, sclerotic capsule is characteristic of persistent anovulation (Fig. 9-4).

The basal body temperature is monophasic, cervical mucus displays arborization with no significant change during the cycle, and the endometrium is proliferative or hyperplastic. The secretion of estrogen is within normal limits but unopposed by progesterone.

Gonadotropin secretion assumes a relatively steady state, although the actual values vary. As a rule, FSH is in a low normal range, and LH is elevated. The LH:FSH ratio is usually greater than 2:1. The urinary 17-ketosteroid level is normal or

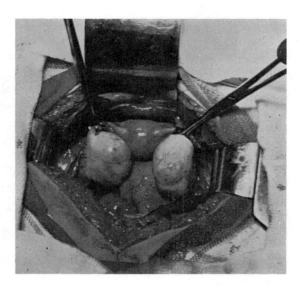

Fig. 9-4 Polycystic ovaries in young woman with polycystic ovarian syndrome.

slightly elevated. The serum DHEAS is normal or mildly elevated. Plasma testosterone is usually elevated when hirsutism is associated but is usually less than 200 ng/ml.

About 4% of PCO patients have an underlying adrenal disorder, *late onset congenital adrenal hyperplasia,* an autosomal recessive disorder that results from a 21-hydroxylase deficiency (the most common enzyme deficiency). A baseline 17-α hydroxyprogesterone level will be elevated above 300 ng/mL or an exaggerated response occurs after ACTH stimulation testing measuring the changes from baseline of 17-α hydroxyprogesterone level.

Dihydrotestosterone, the 5-α reduced form of testosterone, is responsible for stimulating growth of the hair follicle. The major circulating metabolite of DHT is 3-α androstanediol glucuronide, *3-AG;* therefore, one can measure indirectly 5-α reductase activity. This information may assist with understanding why some women have greater or lesser amounts of hirsutism.

If the patient is hirsute and hypertensive, primary adrenal disorders must be excluded. The abbreviated adrenal suppression test is the administration of dexamethasone, 1.0 mg, at 11 PM. A se-

TABLE 9-1 Summary of hormone abnormalities in PCO

Hormone	Status
Testosterone	Mildly elevated; <200 ng/mL
DHEAS	Normal to mildly elevated; <700 mcg/dL
LH:FSH	Follicular phase level 2:1
E_2	Normal to slightly elevated
PRL	Mildly elevated in 10-15% of patients; <50 ng/mL

rum cortisol drawn at 8 AM the next morning should be less than 6 μg/dl. If mild adrenal hyperplasia is suspected, prednisone therapy may be useful. A summary of the hormone abnormalities in PCO is seen in Table 9-1.

Polycystic ovarian syndrome patients often have associated medical problems such as diabetes mellitus, essential hypertension, and hyperlipidemia.

HYPERTHECOSIS. This condition is closely related to the polycystic ovary syndrome, but hirsutism is more pronounced, temporal recession of hair is characteristic, and hypertension is usual. Hyperthecosis is not confined to the theca interna in these cases. Instead, nests of luteinized cells are found throughout the ovarian stroma. Plasma testosterone levels are higher than in patients with PCO. This condition undoubtedly accounts for some failures of wedge resection performed in patients in whom an adrenal disturbance was excluded and a diagnosis of polycystic ovary syndrome was entertained.

OVARIAN NEOPLASMS. Hormone-secreting ovarian tumors are rare but may cause amenorrhea and must be considered in the differential diagnosis.

Because of its malignant potential, the masculinizing Sertoli-Leydig stromal cell tumor, *arrhenoblastoma,* is the most important of the virilizing tumors of the ovary, all of which can cause amenorrhea. The serum testosterone is usually greater than 200 ng/dl.

Masculinizing hilus cell tumor is an exceedingly rare growth arising from the hilus cells of the ovary, which are probably the homologs of the Leydig cells of the testis. Therefore these tumors, although rather small in size, produce distinct virilization.

The *granulosa-thecal cell* stromal tumors can secrete estrogen and result in amenorrhea.

Pituitary gland causes. The finding of abnormally low gonadotropin values associated with either primary or secondary amenorrhea points to an anterior pituitary or hypothalamic disorder. Differential diagnosis between the two can be extremely difficult. Major advances in diagnostic radiographic techniques, including *magnetic resonance imaging,* MRI, and new methods for dynamic testing using hypothalamic-releasing hormones have made possible greater accuracy of diagnosis.

Primary hypopituitarism with resultant amenorrhea may result from destruction of the pituitary (the anterior lobe more frequently than the posterior lobe) by tumor, irradiation, surgery, or infarction. It is estimated that 70% of the adenohypophysis can be destroyed before clinical manifestations occur. Some recovery of pituitary function following an insult can occur, and only a partial deficiency of tropic hormones may result. Following gland destruction, defective growth hormone secretion occurs in virtually 100% of patients; alteration in gonadotropin secretion is next.

Pituitary adenomas are much more common than once appreciated in the past. Three adenomas were recognized because of their dramatic clinical presentation: (1) *acromegaly* as a result of excess growth hormone, (2) hypercortisolism with sequelae caused by increased ACTH secretion *(Cushing's disease),* and (3) amenorrhea-galactorrhea secondary to a prolactin-secreting adenoma. It has now been documented that in clinically reported cases that pituitary adenomas may produce many protein hormones completely or in fragments; pituitary tumors secreting TSH, LH, FSH, and beta endorphins have been reported. Immunohistologic staining of tumor material identifies the tumor cells more appropriately.

Amenorrhea-galactorrhea represents a marked disturbance of the hypothalamic-pituitary function and often is the first clinical evidence of a small pituitary prolactinoma. The tumors are usually, but not invariably, benign. Hyperprolactinemia is found in a high proportion of these cases, and high levels tend to correlate with the tumor and its size. Normal serum prolactin values range from 3 to 22 ng/ml in women. When both amenorrhea and galactorrhea are present, prolactin values over 100 ng/ml should lead to suspicion of a functioning macroadenoma. Growth of microadenomas (below 1 cm in size) may be so insidious that hyperprolactinemia, amenorrhea, and/or galactorrhea may be present for years before an abnormality in the sella turcica is evident by x-ray film study.

Recently developed techniques in diagnostic radiology using high-resolution computerized tomography (CT) and contrast material make it possible to detect microadenomas of 4 to 10 mm with surprising accuracy. Availability of these diagnostic aids makes it apparent that pituitary adenomas are far more common than previous reports indicate. The accuracy of MRI has proven more beneficial in certain cases. This technique may supplant CT scanning to diagnose pituitary tumors.

When hyperprolactinemia in women is assessed, it should be remembered that tranquilizers and antihypertensives (phenothiazines, tricyclic antidepressants, and reserpine), oral contraceptives, and even stress situations can inhibit prolactin-inhibiting factor, *dopamine,* through hypothalamic suppression with consequent release of prolactin. Amenorrhea-galactorrhea is also found in some cases of *hypothyroidism.*

Diagnostic workup of patients with amenorrhea-galactorrhea should include determination of the serum prolactin level as a screening test, as high levels tend to correlate with a tumor. Early pregnancy should be excluded. A careful drug history and examinations for evidence of other endocrinopathies, particularly hypothyroidism, are obviously important, as these disorders can be easily treated. Visual field measurements and a CT scan should be included.

Prolactin-secreting adenomas, particularly microadenomas, do not mandate therapy. Other variables to be considered are other findings or symptomatology such as headaches, visual field deficit, a desire for pregnancy, risk of osteoporosis, and the patient's anxiety about the tumor or hyperprolactinemia-associated depression. March and colleagues studied a group of 43 patients with radiographic evidence of tumor-associated hyperprolactinemia from 3 to 20 years. Only two patients underwent transsphenoidal surgery for tumor growth; three patients became eumenorrheic and euprolactinemic, suggesting spontaneous resolution. The remainder of the patients demonstrated no significant change in their tumor.

EMPTY-SELLA SYNDROME. Empty-sella syndrome, with similar clinical symptomatologic findings, must be differentiated from pituitary adenoma. The sellar abnormality is believed to be developmental in that the sellar diaphragm is incomplete.

The sella is filled with cerebrospinal fluid, which compresses and flattens the pituitary gland against the sellar floor. Because of the sensitivity of gonadotropin secretion, amenorrhea is likely to be the dominant symptom. Galactorrhea is occasionally associated with this syndrome, but other endocrine functions are usually normal. The main importance of this abnormality is that it must be distinguished from other more common causes of enlarged sella, such as degenerated pituitary tumors or cysts. Prolactin-secreting adenomas have been described in women with "empty sella syndrome."

PITUITARY ADENOMA AND PREGNANCY. The pituitary gland normally increases in size primarily as a result of changes in the lactotropes during pregnancy. A preexisting pituitary adenoma likewise enlarges and may become symptomatic. Headaches occur first, and visual disturbances may follow. Magyar and Marshall studied 73 women with previously untreated pituitary microadenomas and macroadenomas during 91 pregnancies. Most experienced no complications and could be managed expectantly.

PITUITARY HYPOFUNCTION (SHEEHAN'S SYNDROME). Pituitary hypofunction is usually related to a preceding severe postpartum hemorrhage or a serious puerperal infection. The lactotropes undergo hypertrophy and hyperplasia during pregnancy and are more susceptible to hemorrhage, thrombosis, infarction, and resultant necrosis in the immediate period following delivery. If a considerable portion of the anterior lobe is destroyed, gonadotropic, adrenal, and thyroid functions are severely depressed, cachexia develops, and lactation is inhibited. Hormone replacement is essential to protect against adrenal insufficiency, hypothyroidism, and estrogen deficiency.

There are other causes of anterior hypopituitarism, such as surgery, irradiation, and nonfunctioning tumors.

Hypothalamic causes. Because higher centers in the brain exert control over pituitary activity by affecting neurotransmitters that impact ultimately on the hypothalamus, it is not difficult to understand that "psychogenic factors" can cause disturbances in ovarian physiology. Lesions that cause destruction of or impinge on the hypothalamus can result in diminished or poorly coordinated pulsatile secretion of GnRH. Tumors such as craniopharyngioma, glioma, endodermal sinus tumor, or histiocytosis along with head trauma and external therapeutic irradiation have all been associated with an absence of menses.

The concept of *hypothalamic amenorrhea* should be defined in its broadest sense as the absence of menses secondary to an alteration in psychoneuroendocrine events characterized by alterations in pulse amplitude, frequency, or amount of GnRH released. Currently, not all of the biochemical pathways or interactions are clearly understood, but that should not detract from the concept.

A striking example of the intimate relationship between the psychic and the soma is *pseudocyesis*. The condition usually occurs in emotionally unstable women who are infertile and have an intense desire for pregnancy. Current evidence indicates that there is a hypersecretion of prolactin and LH with circulating estradiol and progesterone levels comparable to those found in the early luteal phase.

Anorexia nervosa is a condition in which amenorrhea is an early and common symptom. Although the exact incidence is unknown, it was found in one of 150 adolescent girls in Sweden. It is seen in those who are obsessed by the necessity to remain thin. Their objective is fulfilled either by restricting food or becoming *bulimic;* that is,

they periodically go on eating binges, usually associated with catharsis or self-induced emesis.

These individuals are very intense and hyperactive and frequently are hyperachievers. They are usually members of an upper-middle-class family whose parents are dominating. There may also be a history of sexual molestation. Hormonally, there is a significant inhibition of GnRH secretion similar to prepubertal state. There is also a significant effect involving the hypothalamic-pituitary-adrenal axis in that there is a hypersecretion of cortisol but diminution in adrenal androgen secretion. Although there is a wide clinical spectrum, most cases are not severe; however, death can result. Treatment centers around psychotherapy, hormone replacement therapy, and eventually regaining weight.

Miscellaneous causes

WEIGHT. *Exercise amenorrhea* varies with different athletic endeavors. The incidence is higher in long-distance runners and ballet dancers than it is in swimmers. Although there has been some attempt to relate this to body weight, amenorrhea associated with athletic competitiveness can occur without weight loss. In a large number of women, *a 15% loss* of total body weight from ideal body weight will result in oligoamenorrhea. It is clear that, although the cause of the hormonal problem is mediated through deficient secretion of GnRH, it is multifactorial.

Frisch and MacArthur noted that menarche depended on the acquisition of 22% body fat. This percentage is required to maintain normal menses, and therefore diminution of percentage of body fat or an increased lean-to-fat ratio would be associated with a menstrual abnormality. Women who are obese may also have a menstrual abnormality; although the mechanism is not well understood, it is known that severely obese women ($>100\%$ over ideal body weight) have *decreased sex steroid–binding globulin* levels and therefore more free circulating hormone, specifically testosterone.

THYROID GLAND. Ovarian function often is disturbed in women with hypothyroidism or hyperthyroidism. Amenorrhea may be associated with either mild or severe hypothyroidism and occasionally may be a symptom of Graves' disease.

Primary hypothyroidism is one of many causes for amenorrhea-galactorrhea syndrome. TRH, which is increased in this condition, induces release not only of pituitary TSH but also of prolactin. Thyroid substitution therapy alone is corrective of this disorder.

ADRENAL GLAND. Amenorrhea and signs of masculinization may be produced by hyperplasia, benign adenomas, or malignant tumors of the adrenal cortex. Apart from amenorrhea, which is common to each, more specific clinical syndromes and laboratory findings reflect involvement of different components of the adrenal cortex.

Cushing's syndrome is characterized by excessive production of the major glucocorticoid, cortisol, whereas congenital adrenal hyperplasia is characterized by excessive production of adrenal androgens. Adrenal neoplasms may produce either substance, or the typical features of each may overlap. Furthermore, adrenal hyperactivity may be secondary to excessive pituitary adrenocorticotropic hormone (ACTH) secretion.

Menstrual abnormalities, including amenorrhea, can be found in 25% of patients with primary adrenal cortical insufficiency, Addison's disease, or in a higher percentage of women with secondary deficiency related to destructive or infiltrative lesions of the pituitary or hypothalamus.

DIAGNOSIS

Often the physician can establish the cause of amenorrhea after taking a complete history, performing a pelvic examination, or ordering a simple laboratory test. However, the etiologic factors of the symptom may require extensive investigation of genetic, systemic, psychic, and endocrine factors. The same algorithm can be followed for women who fail to initiate menstrual function or who develop secondary amenorrhea.

A thorough physical examination, including inspection of the genitals and palpation of the pelvic organs, will enable the physician to detect gross anatomic abnormalities as well as deviations in somatic growth and genital development. Endocrine stigmas such as hirsutism, body fat pattern, absence of breast development, and enlargement of the clitoris are significant physical findings in the clinical evaluation of amenorrhea. Pregnancy must be excluded as part of the initial evaluation.

When the general examination does not provide specific clues, a practical approach as outlined in Fig. 9-5 can be followed. A baseline *serum prolactin level, a TSH level and total T_4 determination,* along with the *progesterone challenge* constitutes the initial assessment. If hyperprolactinemia is encountered (23 ng/ml is the upper range of normal for the nonpregnant woman in most laboratories), other causes of this problem should be investigated. If a prolactinoma is strongly suspected, high-resolution computerized tomography with dye enhancement will aid in the diagnosis. If androgen excess is clinically apparent, a serum testosterone and DHEAS should be ordered. If the testosterone is above 200 ng/dl, an ovarian or adrenal testosterone-producing tumor should be sought. A DHEAS above 700 µg/dl should make one suspicious of severe disease originating from the adrenal gland.

The progesterone challenge consists of attempting to induce uterine bleeding by administering 100 mg of progesterone-in-oil or oral medroxyprogesterone acetate, 20 mg daily for 5 days; if bleeding occurs, it may be assumed that the amenorrhea is probably not caused by any serious derangement of the pituitary, ovary, or uterus because enough estrogen is being produced to stimulate the endometrium. This result would indicate a functional derangement of gonadotropic release with anovulation.

If no bleeding occurs following the progestin challenge test, either there may be failure of the ovary to secrete an appropriate amount of estrogen to prime the endometrium, or the surface may have been destroyed by surgery, medication, or irradiation. To rule out *endometrial failure,* estrogen stimulation in the form of 2.5 mg/day of conjugated estrogens for 25 days, immediately followed by 7 days of medroxyprogesterone acetate,

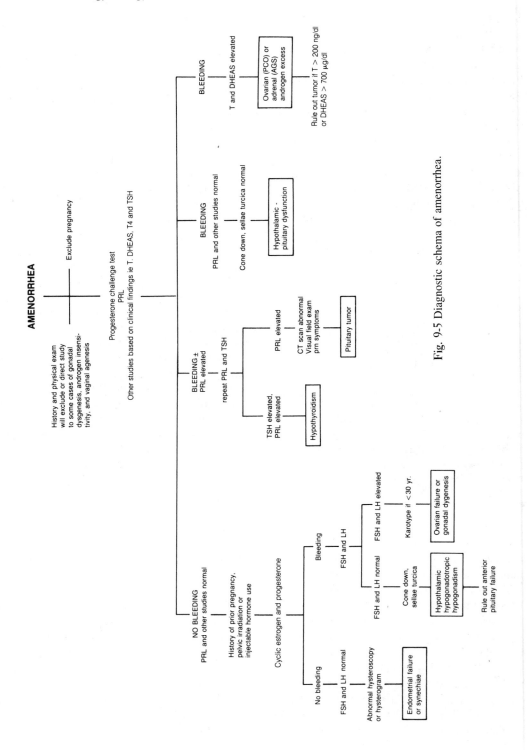

Fig. 9-5 Diagnostic schema of amenorrhea.

10 mg, will assist in the differential diagnosis. If bleeding does occur, one can assume that the endometrial surface is only atrophic, perhaps because of prolonged use of medication or inactivity of the ovary. If bleeding does not occur, hysterosalpingography or hysteroscopy will provide the necessary information to diagnosis intrauterine scarring, *synechiae*.

To differentiate these two causes for the amenorrhea, it is necessary to perform an immunoassay of gonadotropins. When serum gonadotropin levels, FSH, and LH are above 50 ImU/ml, *ovarian failure* is likely. A buccal smear determining the presence or absence of a Barr body and a fluorescent Y chromosome can be helpful, but a serum karyotype is often needed to ensure the accuracy of the diagnosis. Absence or low levels of gonadotropins indicate hypothalamic or pituitary failure.

TREATMENT
General principles

Appropriate therapy depends on an accurate diagnosis. With that information the physician can decide whether effective treatment is feasible or necessary. Even if no medical or surgical intervention is required, it is important that the patient be given sufficient information to ensure that she understands the problem.

Because the range of disorders found in patients with amenorrhea is extensive, an overview of therapy will be approached under four categories. Any one patient may require several treatment modalities. The physician should be continually aware of the need to address all facets of treatment, including how the patient perceives the problem, how her diagnosis may alter her relationships with friends and family, and the effect on an intimate interpersonal relationship.

Constitutional therapy

Most patients with amenorrhea will benefit from measures directed toward the improvement of their general health and well-being. One of the major considerations is *adequate nutrition*. Normal menstruation is contingent upon an appropriate body mass. When obesity is associated with amenorrhea and no other abnormalities are found, weight reduction may be corrective. It may also be desirable for a patient to regain her ideal body weight to enable her hypothalamic-pituitary-ovarian axis to resume normal function. An increase in the amount of *exercise* may be a very important adjunct to an individual who is overweight; young females who participate in competitive sports or extremes of exercise such as long-distance running may need to curtail these activities in order to resume menstruation. Substance abuse, including nicotine and excess caffeine, should be eliminated.

Psychotherapy

Psychotherapy plays an important role in the management of all patients with amenorrhea. A variable amount of anxiety and emotional distress is present in most women whose menstruation is delayed or absent. Under certain circumstances the psychologic distress may actually be the cause of the amenorrhea. Listening in a sensitive manner, providing sympathetic encouragement and a factual explanation of the mechanism of menstruation, and, at the same time, being willing to approach the patient's sexual problems are basic elements in physician counseling. Many patients will readily respond to this type of therapy. However, patients with severe eating disorders like anorexia nervosa with or without bulimia, vaginal agenesis, intersex disorders, and premature ovarian failure may require more in-depth and long-range psychotherapy.

In patients with gonadal dysgenesis and müllerian dysgenesis, other anomalies should be sought, and a thorough family history should be obtained. As part of the counseling procedure, a geneticist may be included to ascertain what, if any, risk is present for other members of the family.

Hormone therapy

The use of hormones should be reserved to treat specific problems: *reestablish periodic endometrial shedding with the hope of preventing endometrial hyperplasia, induce ovulation, combat the adverse cosmetic effects of androgen excess,* or *reduce the size of a pituitary tumor.* When the amenorrhea is associated with infertility, ovulation-induction therapy is the obvious treatment. The administration of estrogen-progesterone combination will result in regular uterine flow, but such bleeding is unaccompanied by ovulation. The uterine response occurs only in relationship to the repeated courses of hormone therapy. Emotionally, women often feel relief by the reappearance of flow, even though the basic problem of anovulation is not being solved. Whether hormone replacement therapy has an intrinsic salutary effect on improving the state of emotional well-being remains to be answered. Estrogen-progesterone replacement is of particular value in cases of primary or secondary ovarian failure to protect the relatively young woman from developing atrophy of the genital pelvic structures, prevent osteoporosis, and reduce the incidence of cardiovascular disease.

Hypothyroidism is an uncommon cause of amenorrhea. It is often associated with hyperprolactinemia. The response to thyroid hormone replacement is dramatic and corrects the menstrual abnormality quickly. The empiric use of thyroid medication is not beneficial.

Adrenal insufficiency is an unusual cause of amenorrhea and responds promptly to corticosteroid therapy in replacement doses. Adrenal hyperfunction is usually secondary to a congenital adrenal hyperplasia secondary to a 21-hydroxylase deficiency. Suppressive therapy with prednisone or dexamethasone is in order; the patient should be apprised of the benefits and risks of this medication and the need for additional replacement if she is involved in a serious accident or requires a major surgical operation.

Estrogen replacement therapy. Conjugated estrogens (CE), 0.625 to 1.25 mg or equivalent daily, with the addition of a progestational agent such as medroxyprogesterone acetate, 5 to 10 mg on the fifteenth through the twenty-ninth day, will induce regular withdrawal bleeding episodes without encouraging endometrial hyperplasia. Osteoporosis can probably be prevented with as little

as 0.3 mg of CE if the patient has a regular program of weight-bearing exercises (walking 30 minutes three times per week) and uses calcium supplementation. Larger dosages are necessary to meet the hormone needs of younger women. Patients on this regimen should be monitored carefully by examining their weight, blood pressure, and serum lipids, as well as the patient's tolerance to the medication. FSH and LH levels are not a clinically useful parameter to assess the adequacy of treatment. It must be remembered that 19-nonsteroid progestins have a greater adverse effect on HDL-cholesterol than the substituted C21 progesterones.

It is beneficial to induce withdrawal bleeding on a monthly basis by the use of oral progestins alone administered for at least 13 days of the cycle in those who are secreting enough estrogen to stimulate endometrial proliferation. Even though oral contraceptive steroid therapy is convenient because of its packaging, it is not the preferred hormone regimen for replacement therapy. With oral contraceptive therapy, the patient will be taking a greater amount of hormone than is necessary for her physiologic needs.

Oral contraceptives. Birth-control pills, containing a minimally active androgen as the progestin component, can be extremely beneficial in treating PCO patients. This medication has the advantage of *reducing LH levels* (decreasing thecal cell stimulation), *increasing sex hormone–binding globulin* production (making less free testosterone available), and *producing regular bleeding episodes* (reduces hyperplasia of the endometrium and amenorrhea).

Spironolactone. Spironolactone, an aldosterone antagonist, has also been shown to be an androgen receptor antagonist that interferes to some extent with androgen steroidogenesis. This medication is somewhat useful in treating hirsutism; as a PCO patient may ovulate periodically, contraception must be used when taking this medication.

Clomiphene citrate. Clomiphene citrate is a nonsteroid estrogen antagonist that is used to induce ovulation. To be effective, it does require functioning ovaries and production of gonadotropins. The drug acts on hypothalamic estrogen receptors, and there is a resultant secretion of GnRH with ensuing FSH and LH secretion that stimulate follicular growth resulting in ovulation. Clomiphene citrate (Clomid or Serophene) is ineffectual in the absence of endogenous estrogen, particularly when the cause is ovarian failure, anterior pituitary obliteration, or congenital absence of GnRH. Although clomiphene therapy in properly treated patients results in ovulation in a high percentage of cases, the achievement of pregnancy is only about half as successful.

Menotropins. Human menopausal gonadotropins (Pergonal) has been successful in inducing ovulation in women who have estrogen deficiency but ovaries that are capable of ovulating with the proper stimulus. Most appropriate candidates are usually women who have been unresponsive to clomiphene or who have a GnRH deficiency. Dosage of menotropin is required daily until a dominant follicle(s) is produced. The latter is determined by monitoring serial serum estradiol concentrations and follicular growth by ultrasound. When a dominant follicle is identified, an "LH surge" is produced by an intramuscular dose of hCG (Profasi, A.P.L.), 5000 to 10,000 U. Both clomiphene and menotropins can overstimulate the ovaries, give rise to multiple births, and result in severe ovarian enlargement and ascites in a small percentage of cases. These effects occur more readily with menotropins.

GnRH. Synthetic GnRH is currently available, is approved by the FDA for diagnostic testing, and it can be used to induce ovulation. The medicine is administered in a pulsatile fashion either subcutaneously or intravenously by pump every 1 to 2 hours. Serum estrogen levels and ultrasound monitoring of the ovarian follicles are helpful to adjust the dosage to the proper level. The most suitable patients for this medication are those women who are GnRH deficient. Ovarian hyperstimulation and multiple pregnancies are still a possibility but are less likely with this medication.

Bromocriptine. Bromocriptine mesylate (Parlodel) is a dopamine agonist. This medication can be used to treat both tumor- and nontumor-related hyperprolactinemia. It is the most effective agent to treat prolactinomas; ovulatory cycles and fertility are usually established within 2 to 3 months after therapy, but permanent remission is not possible unless the medicine is continued.

The surgical treatment (transsphenoidal adenomectomy) of prolactin-secreting tumors as well as irradiation with external beam therapy or implantation of yttrium-90 seeds have been used less frequently since the introduction of bromocriptine.

It is extremely effective in inducing ovulation in those individuals with hyperprolactinemia with or without documented prolactinoma. If the patient achieves euprolactinemia, restoration of ovulatory cycles returns. During early therapy it is not unusual for the patient to have one or two cycles with an inadequate luteal phase. When pregnancy does occur, the medicine should be discontinued, although there is no information at the current time that it acts as a teratogen or is embryotoxic.

Surgery

Surgery is essential and generally curative in cases of obstruction to menstrual flow such as imperforate hymen, vaginal or cervical stenosis, and uterine synechiae. In those individuals with vaginal agenesis, self-induced pressure with vaginal dilators of increasing size can result in a pouch that is sufficient for coitus. If this method of treatment fails, an artificial vagina can be created with the use of a skin graft, the *McIndoe procedure*.

When there is definite evidence of pathologic changes in the ovary such as an androgen- or estrogen-secreting tumor, oophorectomy may remove the cause of the amenorrhea. Because of the risk of malignancy, any Y-bearing gonad such as would be found in a patient with Swyer's syndrome or androgen insensitivity should be removed.

Gonadal neoplasms, the gonadoblastoma or dysgerminoma, are rare before age 20.

In selected patients, ovarian wedge resection or utilizing the CO_2 laser to produce multiple sites of damage results in a reduction of ovarian androgen secretion and permits ovulation to return temporarily.

SUGGESTED READING

Frisch RE and MacArthur JW: Menstrual cycles: fatness as a determinant of minimum weight for height necessary for their maintenance or onset, Science 185:949, 1974.

Griffin JE and Wilson JD: The syndrome of androgen resistance, N Engl J Med 302:198, 1980.

Keettel WC and Bradbury JT: Premature ovarian failure: permanent and temporary, Am J Obstet Gynecol 89:83, 1964.

Kleinberg DL, Noel GL, and Frantz AG: Galactorrhea: a study of 235 cases including 48 with pituitary tumors, N Engl J Med 296:589, 1977.

March CM, Kletzky OA, Davajan V, Teal J, Weiss M, Apuzzo MLJ, Marrs RP, and Mishell DR: Longitudinal evaluation of patients with untreated prolactin-secreting pituitary adenomas, Am J Obstet Gynecol 139:835, 1981.

Peterson RE, Imperato-McGinley, Gautier T, and Sturla E: Male pseudohermaphroditism due to steroid 5α-reductase deficiency, Am J Med 62:170, 1977.

Speroff L, editor: Polycystic ovary disease, Chang RJ, guest editor, Semin Reprod Endocrinol 2:3, 1984.

Stein IF and Leventhal ML: Amenorrhea associated with bilateral polycystic ovaries, Am J Obstet Gynecol 29:181, 1935.

Toaff R and Ballas S: Traumatic hypomenorrhea-amenorrhea (Asherman's syndrome), Fertil Steril 30:379, 1978.

Tulandi T and Kinch RAH: Premature ovarian failure, Obstet Gynecol Surv 36(suppl):521, 1981.

10

John H. Mattox

Dysmenorrhea and the premenstrual syndrome

Objectives

RATIONALE: Dysmenorrhea and premenstrual syndrome in their severest form cause major incapacitation. Pain with menstruation is a common reason for teenagers especially to seek medical care. As many as 10% of high school females are thought to be absent from classes monthly because of dysmenorrhea. PMS with all of its protean manifestations must be differentiated from other affective disorders. With proper management the majority of women with these problems can be kept comfortable and functional.

The student should be able to:

A. Define *primary* and *secondary dysmenorrhea*.
B. Enumerate four causes of dysmenorrhea.
C. Outline the management of a 16-year-old woman with disabling primary dysmenorrhea and a 37-year-old woman who has had increasingly severe menstrual pain for 3 years.
D. Give a definition of premenstrual syndrome (PMS).
E. Outline a management plan for patient with PMS.

The past decade has brought to the gynecologist a greater demand from women to participate in their health care and for increased sensitivity. Increasing physician awareness and medical knowledge have served to reduce stereotypic attitudes concerning the discomfort associated with menstruation. *Dysmenorrhea,* crampy pain that accompanies menstruation, often with a constellation of other troublesome symptoms, not only carries significant dread for about a fifth of the female population in the United States who are moderately to severely compromised each month but also produces far-reaching economic and societal ramifications. Dysmenorrhea is the primary cause of absenteeism in school and the workplace, with an estimated loss of over 2 million hours of work annually. Dysmenorrhea is associated with ovulatory cycles in the majority of cases and has been classified as primary and secondary, based somewhat upon age of onset and the pathogenesis.

Primary dysmenorrhea usually begins in women under 20 years and is probably the result of excessive uterine prostaglandin production; no other pelvic disease should be identified.

Secondary dysmenorrhea, sometimes referred to as *acquired,* occurs after 20 years of age in women with pelvic pathology such as endometriosis, adenomyosis, submucous myomas, severe cervical stenosis, and chronic pelvic infections. In addition, either in times of severe anxiety or stress, it has been postulated that pain tolerance is reduced thereby exaggerating what may have been tolerable uterine cramping, or that pelvic somatization occurs. These theories are difficult to prove or disapprove; formulating clinical studies to answer the questions they pose is also difficult.

PRIMARY DYSMENORRHEA

Primary dysmenorrhea usually appears shortly after the onset of ovulatory cycles after the menarche. It is not caused by pelvic disease. Dysmenorrhea, which is not associated with ovulatory cycles or which begins more than 3 years after the menarche, is probably secondary rather than primary. The pain is usually crampy in nature, emanates from the lower abdomen, and may radiate to the back and the thighs. Of women suffering from primary dysmenorrhea, 50% also have other symptoms such as nausea, vomiting, headache, diarrhea, or fatigue. These symptoms usually begin before or shortly after the onset of the menstrual flow and persist for 12 to 36 hours. In rare instances, syncopy and collapse may occur. Childbirth and advancing age may lessen the severity of the symptoms of primary dysmenorrhea.

Dysmenorrhea is thought to be more common in women whose mothers were symptomatic.

Anderson and Milsom surveyed by questionnaire 586 Swedish female 19-year-olds, of whom 72.4% replied that they suffered from primary dysmenorrhea and 15.4% reported that they experienced severe pain that could not be adequately controlled with medication. The pain was more severe in women with early menarche, heavy flow, and a longer duration of menstruation.

Etiology

In the early 1970s infusions of dilute solutions of prostaglandins (PG) into women to terminate pregnancy resulted in a cluster of symptoms similar to what some women experienced with dysmenorrhea: uterine cramping, nausea, headache, diarrhea, and emesis. The association between PG release and dysmenorrhea became evident. Although the precise cause of pain is unknown, the role of PG as a causal agent in primary dysmenorrhea appears to be significant (see box below).

The presence of an excess amount of prostaglandin increases myometrial contractions, which cause a reduction of uterine blood flow and ischemia of the uterine muscle. This in turn results in an increased stimulation of the autonomic pain fibers from the uterus.

Women who suffer from primary dysmenorrhea have been shown to have an elevated uterine basal tone, greater than 10 mm Hg. They also demonstrate an increased frequency of contractions and an incoordinate contractile pattern caused by prostaglandin stimulation.

As with other forms of pain, there may be associated anxiety, fear, or guilt. In addition, stress

---

THE ROLE OF PG IN PRIMARY DYSMENORRHEA

- Infusions of $PGF_{2\alpha}$ result in similar symptoms.
- PG levels in menstrual fluid are higher in women with primary dysmenorrhea than in controls.
- $PGF_{2\alpha}$ metabolites are higher in symptomatic women.
- PG synthetase inhibitors are effective therapy.

of either external or internal origin may affect the pain threshold.

Therefore, the biochemical stimulation of pain fibers from the pelvis and the interpretation of this stimulation by the central nervous system are important factors in the cause of primary dysmenorrhea. Both may be affected by the emotions or may bring about an emotional response. Both physiologic and emotional responses are important considerations in patients with severe menstrual cramps.

Diagnosis

The patient's history should indicate that the onset of the menstrual pains began shortly after the menarche. The pain coincides with the onset of menstruation and lasts from 48 to 72 hours. The pain is cramplike in nature.

The physician should ascertain what relieves and what exacerbates the pain. How much analgesia is being taken? A pelvic examination and a rectovaginal examination should reveal no pelvic masses or uterine fixation. The uterine corpus may be tender during menstruation. For patients for whom the diagnosis is uncertain or for those who do not respond to standard treatment, endometriosis and chronic pelvic infection particularly should be excluded.

Management

The physician should listen carefully to the patient's account of her symptoms. A sympathetic and understanding approach should be taken.

The patient should be advised about the need for increasing physical activity; moderate exercise can help to alleviate her symptoms. Careful attention to diet (such as eating more whole grains, beans, vegetables, and fruit, and less or no salt, caffeine, and sugar) have also been helpful to some women. Relaxation, massage, and biofeedback techniques have been effective in reducing pain.

If the patient is sexually active, low-estrogen-containing *oral contraceptives* offer effective therapy for primary dysmenorrhea for 90% of the women who take them. Oral contraceptives suppress ovulation, cause a reduction of endometrium and a corresponding reduction in menstrual flow. This reduction results in a decreased production of prostaglandin.

Women who should not or will not use oral contraceptives can be placed on *prostaglandin synthetase inhibitors* (PGSI). There are many types of PGSI such as aspirin, indomethacin, mefenamic acid, and ibuprofen. All bring about a reduction in endometrial prostaglandin release.

Clinical trials conducted by Dawood suggest that aspirin is not much better than a placebo. Of the several types of PGSI, the fenamates may prove to be more effective. Mefenamic acid (Ponstel), 250 to 500 mg three to four times a day, has resulted in excellent relief. Ibuprofen (Motrin) was one of the first agents available and has the advantage now of being available over the counter (Advil, Nuprin). Using the latter preparation requires an adjustment in dosage.

Pretreatment with PGSI is not necessary. They should be given at the onset of symptoms and may be used for the first 3 days of the menstrual flow. Contraindications for the use of PGSI include gastrointestinal ulcers and hypersensitivity to aspirin.

If the patient does not respond to either oral contraceptives or PGSI, secondary causes must again be considered, and a laparoscopy is indicated. If pelvic disease is discovered, appropriate treatment should be carried out. If significant emotional stress seems to be present, a *psychiatric consultation* should be suggested.

SECONDARY DYSMENORRHEA

Although women presenting with this symptom have been presumed to have pelvic disease, that is not always true. However, a thorough evaluation including a hysterosalpingogram or hysteroscopy and laparoscopy may be required to make an accurate diagnosis. A list of possibilities can be seen in the box on p. 114.

**DIAGNOSTIC POSSIBILITIES IN
SECONDARY DYSMENORRHEA**

Endometriosis
Adenomyosis
Chronic pelvic infection
Submucous leiomyoma
Pelvic adhesions
Cervical stenosis
Hypermenorrhea
Pelvic congestion syndrome
Stress

Etiology

Most of the disease entities listed in the box above are discussed in greater detail in other chapters. How each of these diagnoses produces secondary dysmenorrhea is unclear. In addition, many women with pelvic disease have chronic low-grade pain that becomes aggravated by menses; the distinction between the patient with chronic pelvic pain and secondary dysmenorrhea may become blurred. Surprisingly, cancer in the pelvis, the most serious disease, does not often present with pain unless the disease is quite advanced.

Pedunculated submucous myomas or *large endometrial polyps* usually present with abnormal uterine bleeding. However, these lesions, depending on their location, can "irritate" the uterus, which contracts excessively in an attempt to expel the tumor.

Normally, the menstrual effluent liquefies before it is expulsed. When menstrual flow is excessive in amount but normal in duration *(hypermenorrhea),* clots form inside the uterine cavity that require excessive contractions to be expelled.

Cervical stenosis can be a congenital anomaly or the result of therapy such as overzealous cryotherapy or conization. This condition is much less common than was originally believed. To be a significant etiology of dysmenorrhea, the external os is nearly obliterated and the canal will admit only a fine wire probe.

Pelvic congestion syndrome, the existence of

which is debated among gynecologists, is purportedly seen in parous females; the pelvic vasculature, particularly the veins in the broad ligament, are dilated and engorged. Patients present with pelvic "fullness," mild to moderate pelvic pain, and dysmenorrhea. Although visualizing the pelvic congestion at laparoscopy is simple, the relationship between the findings and pelvic pain remains problematic.

Management

Detailed management of the diagnoses listed can be found in other chapters. However, some management principles can be outlined.

1. Listen to the patient.
2. Perform a meticulous assessment to identify the cause of the pain.
3. Surgical measures such as laparoscopy may facilitate the diagnosis.
4. Dilatation and curettage as an empiric therapy is not effective; it may be required for diagnosis.
5. Significant stress or anxiety may be integrated into the problem, and the patient is exercising denial.
6. A precise diagnosis to explain the dysmenorrhea is not always attainable.
7. General health measures such as increasing exercise, appropriate weight loss, and caffeine and salt reduction may make the patient more comfortable.

Errors in differentiating primary and secondary dysmenorrhea have frequently been made. Some patients have been diagnosed as having primary dysmenorrhea when they suffered from such forms of secondary dysmenorrhea as nonpalpable endometriosis. Other patients have been diagnosed as having adenomyosis, another etiology of secondary dysmenorrhea, when indeed they suffered from primary dysmenorrhea. The distinction may be difficult, but it is critical because the treatment of secondary dysmenorrhea requires eradication of the particular pelvic disease that is producing the pain.

In summary, in managing patients with severe menstrual pain, the physician should rule out a secondary pathologic condition within or about the pelvis. Primary dysmenorrhea, in which there is no definable pelvic pathology, will usually respond to medical treatment. Oral contraceptives are generally effective in treating primary dysmenorrhea, particularly if contraception is desired. Patients who do not wish oral contraceptives or for whom there are contraindications to their use will usually respond to PGSI. Laparoscopic examination should be done on those patients who do not respond to either oral contraceptives or PGSI. The patient's emotional response to dysmenorrhea should be evaluated. A psychiatric consultation should be suggested for those few patients who manifest a great deal of anxiety or depression. A surgical procedure is helpful only in rare cases.

PREMENSTRUAL SYNDROME

The manifestations of premenstrual syndrome (PMS) were first described by Frank in 1931. He suggested that women who demonstrated edema, weight gain, and emotional disturbances before the onset of menstruation had a premenstrual disease due to excess estrogen. In 1953 Dalton and other investigators suggested that women with these symptoms should be categorized under the heading PMS. The symptoms now attributed to this condition number well over 40 and are outlined in Moos' Menstrual Distress questionnaire. This questionnaire is divided into eight categories with symptoms related to (1) pain, (2) concentration, (3) behavioral change, (4) autonomic reactions, (5) water retention, (6) negative affect, (7) arousal, and (8) control.

Although premenstrual tension has been recognized for over 50 years, only recently has there been concentrated interest in the whole group of symptoms because women have become more involved in jobs outside the home and are assuming many responsible positions in the work force. Premenstrual symptoms sometimes prevent women from attaining their best level of performance. In addition, PMS has occasionally been used as a legal defense in criminal cases involving charges such as murder. A great deal has been written in both the lay and professional press because of the renewed interest in this area.

Most women experience some changes in bodily sensation and mood before the onset of menstrual flow *(molimina)*. For some women, the number and the severity of the symptoms are so extreme that they are classified as a medical disorder. Otherwise healthy women experience one or more of these symptoms in a mild-to-moderate form. The incidence of PMS has been reported from 5% to 95% of population studied; 2% to 3% of women in the childbearing age have severe PMS. It has been suggested that about 5 to 6 million women experience severe symptoms each month in the United States. Fortunately, threatening symptoms such as homicidal or suicidal ideation occur only in a very small percentage of women. More frequently, the life of the woman and significant others is disrupted, which may lead to feelings of guilt on the part of the woman.

Etiologic factors

The postulated etiologic factors involved in this syndrome are *insufficient progesterone, fluid retention, nutritional problems, glucose metabolism,* and *estrogen.* The exact cause of premenstrual tension is unknown, but its cyclic nature and timing suggest that there is a progesterone insufficiency or withdrawal in women who experience the symptoms. This insufficiency results in a relative estrogen imbalance. It has also been shown that PMS is more apt to occur in women with endometriosis or luteal phase defect, which may explain why the symptoms appear as long as a week before the onset of the menstruation, when progesterone levels are usually high.

Fluid retention. In the past fluid retention was believed to precipitate the various manifestations of PMS, and diuretics were used as part of the clinical management. Studies assessing weight change, sodium exchange, and total body water have failed to uncover a pattern of fluid retention in most women with PMS. Aldosterone levels are not significantly elevated. Progesterone does, however, affect the renin-angiotension-aldosterone mechanism and water metabolism by inducing a temporary natriuresis followed by fluid retention.

Nutrition. A great deal of emphasis has been placed on proper nutrition and the importance of exercise in reducing PMS. Deficiencies in vitamin B_6 (pyridoxine), vitamin D, and calcium have been suggested as a cause of PMS, although the supporting data are questionable. It has also been suggested that pyridoxine affects the biosynthesis of brain catecholamines that regulate mood behavior. Hypoglycemia may also invoke symptoms of PMS. The relationship between the amount of carbohydrates and protein in the diet may be important. Some studies have suggested that the reduction of carbohydrates and the increase of protein may be beneficial.

Hyperprolactinemia. Hyperprolactinemia has been cited by some as another possible cause. However, some studies do not indicate that women with PMS have elevated prolactin levels. In addition, women with hyperprolactinemia rarely have symptoms of PMS.

Endogenous opioids. More recently, Reid and Yen have suggested that an endogenous opiate peptide may be responsible for the symptom in some women, especially those with the depressive symptoms. Opiate peptides do affect the amount of gonadotropin secretion and produce changes in the concentration of LH. Direct measurement of beta-endorphin concentrations in the portal-hypophyseal blood of the rhesus monkey has revealed that levels of opiate peptides are high during the midluteal phase and undetectable at the onset of menstruation. These authors postulate that progesterone, acting either alone or in combination with estrogen, can increase central endogenous opiate peptide activity. They further suggest that this may trigger the subsequent neuroendocrine manifestations of PMS.

Symptomatology

Headache, nervous irritability, insomnia, and crying spells are the most common manifestations of premenstrual tension. Many women complain of backache, lower abdominal pain, and tender or painful breasts as well. These symptoms usually appear about a week to 10 days before the period is due, and they gradually increase in intensity. Usually, they disappear once the menstrual flow is well established. A weight gain of 1 to 3 kg (2 to 6½ lb) during the premenstrual phase is common. Generalized edema and diminished urine output occur frequently. Rapid loss of weight gained and marked diuresis usually follow the onset of menstruation, along with regression of the other symptoms. The doctor should also consider other possible diagnoses, including chronic depression, which may become aggravated before menstruation, and manic depressive illness. Schizophrenia should also be excluded as a possible cause of the symptoms.

Management

Women who suffer from PMS may experience irritability, depression, fatigue, edema, breast discomfort, and the other symptoms associated with this syndrome for quite some time before they consult a physician. Frequently, when they first seek medical help, they inform the doctor that they have the feeling they are "going crazy." *It would be helpful for physicians to inquire about the symptoms of PMS every time they take a menstrual history.* Such information provides a more complete picture of the patient. Frequently, the early diagnosis of patients with PMS can prevent many emotional difficulties within the home and on the job.

Once symptoms characterizing PMS are identified, the patient should be reassured that she is not becoming psychotic and that measures can be taken to help her. Early in the management of the patient, it is usually helpful to bring any immediate family members into a discussion concerning the symptoms.

It is essential to have the patient keep a daily diary about her symptoms and behavior. She should be told that PMS is a common hormonal disorder of women in their childbearing years, that the symptoms usually disappear at menopause, and that there are a number of things that can be done to alleviate them. With treatment, the patient will learn to cope with her symptoms in a more effective manner. She should be taught the importance of a *good exercise program* such as walking regularly, and she should be put on an *appropriate diet*. The *elimination of tobacco and caffeine* has been beneficial to some patients. A diet that is low in carbohydrates but contains a reasonable amount of protein, vegetables, and fruit will help other women. Protein should be obtained primarily from fish rather than from red meat. *Pyridoxine* in doses of 100 to 400 mg/day may also be helpful.

Progesterone in pharmacologic amounts administered by suppository or intramuscularly has been recommended by Dalton. In large doses progesterone does inhibit smooth muscle contractions and is a CNS depressant. Substituted progesterone, medroxyprogesterone acetate, and the 19-norsteroids, the progestins in oral contraceptives, are not "pure" progesterones according to aficionados. Unfortunately, prospective, placebo-controlled studies have not been promising; progesterone is no more effective than a placebo.

In women with severe breast pain *(cyclic mastodynia)* and swelling, *bromocriptine* or *danazol* has proven to be helpful. However, these medications should not be necessary for most patients.

Some patients report improvement of their symptoms with *oral contraceptives*. This form of therapy should probably be restricted to patients under the age of 35 who need contraception or who have associated dysmenorrhea. In addition, *prostaglandin inhibitors* such as mefenamic acid (250 mg) and naproxen sodium (275 mg) taken orally every 4 to 6 hours may relieve not only dysmenorrhea but symptoms of PMS as well.

Unfortunately, diuretics are probably the most frequently used medication in the treatment of PMS. Although there is very little evidence of the contribution of fluid retention to this syndrome, 25 mg of spironolactone, to be taken orally four times a day, may be prescribed the week before menstruation when edema is severe. *GnRH analogs* are currently being evaluated and may prove effective.

Certainly, patients showing marked alteration in mood swings with manic and/or severe depressive symptoms, as well as those exhibiting psychotic behavior, should have a psychiatric evaluation before treatment. Tricyclic antidepressants have not been effective in treating this syndrome. Lithium carbonate, in dosages of 600 to 1800 mg/day taken orally, is sometimes effective in the control of manic depressive symptoms and psychotic behavior. If the patient is placed on lithium therapy, the physician needs to monitor serum lithium levels carefully because of the possibility of serious side effects from this medication.

In summary, PMS encompasses a number of symptoms that women experience before their menstrual period; control of these symptoms is clearly important. Patients who are prone to the syndrome should first be evaluated carefully. They should maintain a diary, itemizing their symptoms for a number of cycles. They should be reassured that they are not psychotic and that their symptoms are brought about by hormonal changes affecting their body chemistry. It is helpful to educate not only the patient but the family as well about the effects of PMS, so that the family can provide strong emotional support. With appropriate changes in life-style, which might include the start of an exercise program, a balanced diet, certain drug therapies, and the support of an understanding physician, most women with PMS can be helped significantly.

SUGGESTED READING

Abraham GE, Elsner CW, and Lucas LA: Hormone and behavioral changes during the menstrual cycle, Senogolia 3:33, 1978.

Andersch B and Milsom I: An epidemiologic study of young women with dysmenorrhea, Am J Obstet Gynecol 144:655, 1982.

Chan WY and Dawood MY: Prostaglandin levels in menstrual fluid of nondysmenorrhea subjects with and without oral contraceptive or ibuprofen therapy, Adv Prostaglandin Thromboxane Res 8:1443, 1980.

Dalton K: Cyclical criminal acts in premenstrual syndrome, Lancet 2:1970, 1980.

Dawood MY: Dysmenorrhea, Clin Obstet Gynecol 26:3, 1983.

Frank RP: The hormonal causes of premenstrual tension, Arch Neurol Psych 26:1052, 1931.

Reid RL and Yen SSC: The premenstrual syndrome, Clin Obstet Gynecol 26:3, 1983.

11

John H. Mattox

Endometriosis and adenomyosis

Objectives

RATIONALE: Whereas endometriosis is a benign disease, it progresses and can be responsible for major morbidity in terms of pelvic pain or infertility. The pathogenesis is incompletely understood. Still, it is important to understand how to formulate an early diagnosis and which therapeutic modalities are appropriate.

The student should be able to:
A. List three theories of pathogenesis for endometriosis.
B. Identify three symptoms and physical findings.
C. Discuss the rationale for medical versus surgical therapy.
D. Describe three differences between endometriosis and adenomyosis.

Endometriosis is the abnormal growth of endometrial tissue outside the uterine cavity. The disease was first mentioned in the medical literature in 1860 by the reknowned Viennese pathologist, von Rokitansky. The observations of Sampson in the 1920s focused on one of the current major theories of the origin of the disease and documented its histologic variability. Whether aberrant endometrium is located on the serosal surface of the peritoneal structures, on the ovary, *external endometriosis,* or in the tissues contiguous with the uterine mucosa, *internal en-*dometriosis* (adenomyosis), functioning endometrial tissue that responds to ovarian hormones, predominantly estrogen, is the prerequisite for the genesis and maintenance of this condition. Therefore, it is rarely encountered before menarche and usually becomes quiescent after the menopause. *Adenomyosis* can be considered as endometriosis involving the myometrium, whereas *endosalpingiosis* is located in the fallopian tube.

It is estimated that between 1% and 2% of the female population has endometriosis, and many physicians believe that the incidence is increasing. Characteristic lesions can be recognized during at least 5% of pelvic operations and in 30% of women with infertility, and frequently it is an unexpected finding. Some women may have asymptomatic endometriosis; it is more likely to be problematic in the third and fourth decades of life.

PATHOGENESIS

No single hypothesis can explain all of the varied clinical presentations seen with endometriosis. The possible explanations include theories of coelomic metaplasia, retrograde menstruation, blood or lymph dissemination, immunologic induction, and combinations of the above.

According to the *metaplasia theory,* undifferentiated coelomic epithelial cells, like those from which the paramesonephric ducts are formed, remain dormant on the peritoneal surface until the ovaries begin to function. They respond to cyclic stimulation by ovarian estrogen and progesterone in a manner similar to that of normal endometrial cells and eventually can be identified as definite lesions on the peritoneal surface. The longer cyclic stimulation and withdrawal persist without a break, such as that provided by pregnancy, the larger the lesions can become.

Sampson's investigations indicate that endometriosis can be caused by *retrograde transport of menstrual fluid from the uterus through the tubes during menstruation.* Blood often can be seen in the cul-de-sac, and endometrial tissue can be identified in the tubal lumen in women who undergo surgery during menstruation. The typical lesions of endometriosis can be produced in monkeys by diverting the menstrual flow into the peritoneal cavity. Endometriosis also occurs in young women with congenital obstructing defects in the cervix or vagina, which are associated with reflux menstruation into the peritoneal cavity.

A tenable etiologic theory is a combination of *metaplasia* and *retrograde tubal transmission.* An irritating substance in the menstrual fluid entering the peritoneal cavity may induce the formation of endometrial glands and stroma in undifferentiated mesenchyme. This would explain the location of the lesions in the ovary and the cul-de-sac, the areas first affected by reflux menstruation.

The theory that a *substance, perhaps an immune complex,* in menstrual fluid *induces* a change in certain susceptible individuals resulting in endometriosis is more tenable than is the single hypothesis of the growth of transplanted endometrial cells. Endometrial cells from menstrual discharge usually do not grow in tissue culture, so it is difficult to accept cell transplantation as the most important factor in the development of a condition as common as endometriosis.

Heredity may be a factor in the development of endometriosis. Simpson and colleagues conducted genetic interviews with 123 women who had been treated for endometriosis. The incidence of the condition in female siblings over age 18 years (5.8%), mothers (8.1%), and first-degree relatives (6.9%) was considerably higher than that in the husbands' female relatives (1.0%) and mothers (0.9%). The precise genetic mechanism is not known.

GROSS PATHOLOGIC FINDINGS

The gross appearance of endometriosis is variable, depending on the stage of the disease and the length of time it has existed. Minimal lesions appear as bluish red spots, each surrounded by a ring of puckered scar tissue, scattered over the pelvic peritoneal surfaces. Each of these small foci may grow as a result of repeated cyclic stimulation; the larger lesions are known as *endometriomas* (Fig. 11-1). As the endometriomas continue to grow, they coalesce and with scar tissue may completely obliterate the cul-de-sac. The tubes and ovaries become densely adherent to the posterior surfaces of the broad ligaments, and in more advanced cases the rectosigmoid adheres to the posterior surface of the uterus, further immobilizing the adnexal structures (Fig. 11-2). "Windowlike" defects in the peritoneum can be a result of endometriosis. Eventually, the entire pelvis

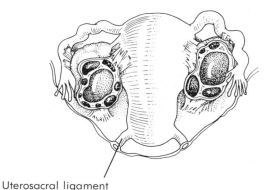

Uterosacral ligament

Fig. 11-1 Cross-section showing uterus in center with bilateral ovarian endometriomas adherent to uterus, posterior leaves of broad ligament, and tubes.

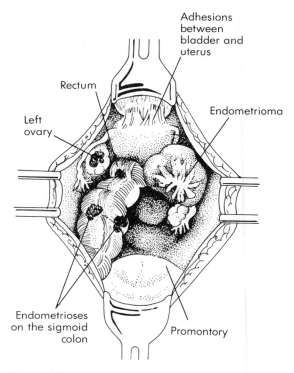

Fig. 11-2 Advanced endometriosis with lesions and adhesions on various pelvic structures.

may be filled with a solid mass of agglutinated structures that may be completely obscured by adherent small bowel and omentum.

The adhesions produced in response to the lesions are dense and firm and can be separated only by sharp dissection. As the planes are opened, thick brown fluid escapes. This fluid consists of old blood and cellular debris formed within the endometrioma. The blood may be the irritant that initiates the peritoneal reaction, which is eventually responsible for the dense scarring.

Ovarian involvement varies from small cystic collections to a single loculated structure, which may measure as much as 10 cm in diameter *(ovarian endometrioma)*. Other lesions such as hemorrhage into an ovarian cyst or a corpus luteum cyst can form the "chocolate cyst" and be confused with ovarian endometriomas. Whenever possible, an exact diagnosis should be made before a definitive operative procedure is performed because the treatment of each of these lesions is different.

The rectosigmoid and urinary tract may be involved. The lesions are on the peritoneal surface and rarely penetrate the entire thickness of the wall. Occasionally, the vagina, cervix, episiotomy scars, laparotomy scars, umbilicus, round

ligaments, lungs, and extremities are sites of endometrial implants. Wherever the lesion is found, its behavior is essentially the same.

A typical lesion of endometriosis contains glands and stroma like those of endometrium in its normal location (Fig. 11-3). Repeated episodes of bleeding within a lesion may produce enough pressure atrophy to destroy the glandular epithelium, leaving only the stroma and hemosiderin-containing macrophages. Usually a considerable amount of fibrous tissue surrounds the older lesions. During pregnancy the lesions usually exhibit a typical decidual reaction.

A classification system developed by a committee of the American Fertility Society is simple and informative. Points are awarded for each of several aspects of the lesions as they are seen through the laparoscope or at laparotomy. The total number accumulated is an indication of the severity of the process (Fig. 11-4).

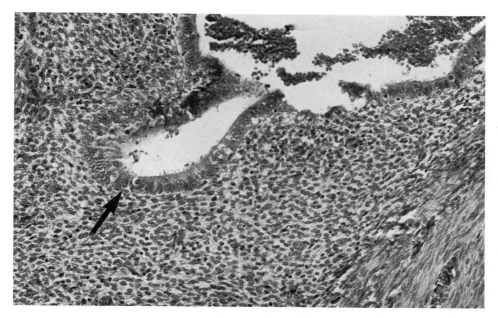

Fig. 11-3 Internal endometriosis or adenomyosis. Endometrial gland *(center)* with myometrium identified in lower right corner.

SYMPTOMS

Pain. Lower abdominal and pelvic pain in some form is the most common symptom of endometriosis. The cycling ectopic endometrium bleeds in conjunction with the normal menstrual flow, but the blood is contained within the involved organ or affected tissue, distending it and the surrounding peritoneum. Pain is most severe in areas of peritoneal scarring, which are put under tension as the lesions expand during the bleeding phase.

Dysmenorrhea is a common symptom, but dysmenorrhea in women is not always a result of endometriosis. Most women who have had painful periods since the menarche *(primary dysmenorrhea)* do not often have endometriosis; the pain caused by endometriosis appears at a later time *(secondary dysmenorrhea)*.

The pain associated with endometriosis is generally severe and steady rather than cramplike. Whenever pain is caused by endometriosis, there usually is considerable involvement of the uterosacral ligaments and the cul-de-sac.

Pelvic pain that increases in severity with the onset of menses is postulated to be indicative of endometriosis, whereas the dysmenorrhea that is relieved as menses progress is less likely to be caused by endometriosis. Although it is interesting to try to establish this clinical correlation, the character of the menstrual pain is not sufficiently discriminatory to exclude the diagnosis of endometriosis. The discomfort associated with endometriosis is usually described as deep, constant, grinding pressure in contrast to the colicky pain of primary dysmenorrhea. It often radiates to the back and down the legs. *Rectal tenesmus* and *dyspareunia* are common and severe before and during menstruation if there is considerable involvement in the cul-de-sac and uterosacral ligaments. Most women are free from pain during the first half of the cycle.

Disturbing features of endometriosis are that

THE AMERICAN FERTILITY SOCIETY
REVISED CLASSIFICATION OF ENDOMETRIOSIS

Patient's Name _____ Date _____

Stage I   (Minimal)   - 1-5
Stage II (Mild)   - 6-15
Stage III (Moderate) - 16-40
Stage IV (Severe)   - >40
Total _____

Laparoscopy _____ Laparotomy _____ Photography _____
Recommended Treatment _____
_____
Prognosis _____

PERITONEUM	**ENDOMETRIOSIS**	<1cm	1-3cm	>3cm
	Superficial	1	2	4
	Deep	2	4	6
OVARY	R Superficial	1	2	4
	Deep	4	16	20
	L Superficial	1	2	4
	Deep	4	16	20

	POSTERIOR CULDESAC OBLITERATION	Partial		Complete
		4		40

	ADHESIONS	<1/3 Enclosure	1/3-2/3 Enclosure	>2/3 Enclosure
OVARY	R Filmy	1	2	4
	Dense	4	8	16
	L Filmy	1	2	4
	Dense	4	8	16
TUBE	R Filmy	1	2	4
	Dense	4*	8*	16
	L Filmy	1	2	4
	Dense	4*	8*	16

*If the fimbriated end of the fallopian tube is completely enclosed, change the point assignment to 16.

Additional Endometriosis: _____
_____
_____

Associated Pathology: _____
_____
_____

To Be Used with Normal
Tubes and Ovaries

L   R

To Be Used with Abnormal
Tubes and/or Ovaries

L   R

Fig. 11-4 Classification of endometriosis. (From The American Fertility Society: Revised American Fertility Society classification of endometriosis, Fertil Steril 43:351, 1984. Reproduced with the permission of the publisher, The American Fertility Society.)

all degrees of involvement are encountered without a single symptom and that severe pelvic pain occurs in women with minimal endometriosis.

Abnormal bleeding. Abnormal uterine bleeding may occur in women with endometriosis. It most often results from a considerable amount of ovarian destruction by advanced lesions.

Infertility. Many women with endometriosis are infertile. It is easy to understand why this occurs when the lesions are so extensive that the tubes and ovaries are immobilized by or even buried within the masses of endometriosis. The mechanism of infertility is not obvious when there are only scattered lesions that do not appear to disturb tubal or ovarian function.

Several theories based on experimental findings have been proposed to explain infertility coexisting with endometriosis in the absence of a mechanical factor. It has been postulated that an *autoimmune response* is triggered in some women when endometriotic tissue is phagocytized and absorbed by the host; this results in the rejection of the embryo or disrupted sperm transport. Another theory involves the existence of the *luteinized unruptured follicle syndrome.* It is postulated that the ovarian follicle fails to release the ovum despite the occurrence of the biochemical changes that are associated with ovulation. *Increased prostanoids* have been identified in some women with endometriosis, and their presence might alter tubal smooth muscle activity, thus compromising ovum transport. Another possibility is that *increased numbers of macrophages* in the peritoneal cavity phagocytize spermatozoa.

Ruptured ovarian endometrioma. As an ovarian endometrioma increases in size because of repeated hemorrhages, its walls become progressively thinner; eventually it may rupture. The sudden prostrating pain associated with dissemination of the old blood throughout the peritoneal cavity as the cyst ruptures may be preceded by gradually increasing pain as the tumor enlarges. The treatment is prompt operation. It may be necessary to remove the ovary as well as the cyst, but ovarian tissue can often be saved even though the endometrioma is large.

Risk of cancer. Although it is rare, malignant transformation in endometriosis does occur.

Sampson carefully described the qualifying criteria. These endometrioid cancers are usually adenocarcinoma and are more likely to be observed in an ovarian endometrioma. Therapy is similar to that for other ovarian malignancy.

PHYSICAL FINDINGS

There may be historic information suggesting the presence of endometriosis such as pelvic pain, dysmenorrhea, or infertility. There are also certain findings on pelvic examination that should raise suspicion. A fixed retroflexed uterine corpus, extreme uterosacral ligament tenderness with nodularity, bilateral fixed tender masses in the adnexa, and tender thickening of the rectal-vaginal septum are findings that have a significant association with pelvic endometriosis.

Endometriosis can be diagnosed with certainty only by direct inspection, and optimally by microscopic examination of the lesions. In some instances, histologic confirmation is impossible because both glands and stroma have been destroyed as the lesions enlarge. In this event the only remaining suggestion of endometriosis may be deposits of hemosiderin.

Laparoscopy with the use of the dual-puncture technique should be performed to confirm the diagnosis in women suspected of having endometriosis because of the presumed characteristic history and physical findings. This is particularly true in women who cannot conceive; the extent to which the reproductive organs, particularly the tubes and ovaries, are involved can be determined only by direct inspection.

DIFFERENTIAL DIAGNOSIS

It is difficult to accurately diagnose endometriosis by history and physical examination alone. Small lesions, particularly those involving the tubes and ovaries, cannot be felt, and even those in the cul-de-sac may be missed. Endometriosis can also be confused with other conditions.

Pelvic infection. The lesions that most often simulate endometriosis are those that follow repeated attacks of salpingo-oophoritis. Both conditions may cause pain before and during menstruation and deep dyspareunia. The tubes and ovaries adhere to the posterior leaves of the broad ligaments and in the cul-de-sac in both. The residua of recurrent salpingitis are smoother as compared with a fixed nodular mass of endometriosis involving the uterosacral ligaments and the cul-de-sac. Both may be tender, but old quiescent salpingo-oophoritis is usually less so than endometriosis, except during recurring acute attacks or in conjunction with menstruation.

The history often is helpful. There is nothing in the history of a patient with endometriosis that is similar to that of recurrent attacks of acute salpingo-oophoritis; the latter is often associated with fever.

Ovarian carcinoma. Cul-de-sac nodularity may on occasion resemble ovarian carcinoma. Endometriosis usually is associated with dysmenorrhea, and pelvic examination is painful. Women with ovarian cancer usually are older, there is no associated increase in dysmenorrhea, symptoms usually are minimal and may consist only of vague gastrointestinal discomfort, and pelvic examination often produces no pain.

Benign ovarian neoplasms. An endometrioma of the ovary cannot be distinguished from a primary benign ovarian neoplasm by pelvic examination alone. Direct inspection of the enlarged ovary is necessary.

Urinary tract lesions. Urinary tract endometriosis is suggested in women with cyclic or intermittent hematuria. This is an unusual symptom and occurs only if an endometrial lesion penetrates the bladder wall. The ureters usually are involved in extrinsic lesions, which constrict rather than penetrate. These may eventually constrict the ureter completely. Intrinsic bladder lesions can be seen and biopsied. Ureteral involvement can be suspected by pyelography.

Bowel lesions. Cyclic dyschezia or hematochezia is an uncommon symptom of endometriosis and usually reflects bowel mucosal involvement. Any lesion visualized at sigmoidoscopy should be biopsied. On barium enema extraluminal disfiguration or annular constriction can be seen when pelvic endometriosis involves the colon.

Other lesions. Cyclic hemoptysis has been ascribed to *bronchial endometriosis;* a well-timed bronchoscopy and directed biopsy will usually confirm the diagnosis.

LABORATORY TESTS

It would be of enormous benefit to be able to diagnose, as well as monitor, women with serologic testing. Unfortunately, no such assay exists. CA-125, a cell surface antigen, can be detected by radioimmunoassay in the serum in many patients with endometriosis; however, it does not have any clinical utility at this time. Although the erythrocyte sedimentation rate or leukocyte count may be slightly elevated, particulary with an acute painful episode, these tests are not particularly helpful in the management of women with endometriosis.

TREATMENT
General principles

The symptoms associated with endometriosis can be relieved by surgery or a variety of hormone regimens. The treatment one chooses for a specific patient is determined by her age, the severity of symptoms, the extent of the disease, whether she wishes to become pregnant, and, if so, now or in the future. Teenagers may acquire endometriosis; therefore reproduction might be postponed for many years. An overview of the potential therapies can be seen in the box on p. 125.

1. Not every women needs therapy. *Expectant management* is a term that has been used to characterize the female who is not interested in conceiving, whose minimal endometriosis is causing no menstrual disturbance, and who has little or no discomfort.
2. Whether or not infertile patients with minimal endometriosis (American Fertility Society stage I) require therapy is currently debatable.
3. Conservative surgery is definitely more suc-

POTENTIAL THERAPY FOR
ENDOMETRIOSIS

I. Surgical
   A. Conservative
      1. Laparoscopy with electrocautery or laser vaporization of lesions
      2. Removal of specific lesions and possible uterine suspension with presacral neurectomy
   B. Definitive
      1. Abdominal hysterectomy
      2. Salpingo-oophorectomy if diseased
      3. Bowel resection rarely
II. Hormonal
   A. Progestin-dominant with control pills: norgestrel (Lo-Ovral)
      1. Cyclically
      2. Continuous
   B. Progestin (medroxyprogesterone acetate)
      1. Intramuscular (Depo-Provera)
      2. Oral
   C. Androgen (Danazol)
   D. GnRH analog (Synarel, Lupron)
III. Combined medical and surgical

cessful for moderate and severe endometriosis when improving fertility is the major objective.

4. Hormonal therapy is usually administered for at least 6 months.

5. Ovarian endometriomas larger than 2 cm in diameter are not permanently responsive to medical therapy.

6. In spite of appropriate hormonal or conservative surgical therapy, a conservative estimate of recurrence over 7 years is approximately 15%.

Specific therapy

Conservative operations are those in which the most important goals are to reduce the severity of the symptoms and to retain or improve fertility. A conservative approach includes resection, or destruction by cautery or laser, of most or all visible endometriosis; freeing tubes and ovaries that are immobilized by disease or adhesions; removing an extensively damaged tube and ovary if the other is reasonably normal; freeing and suspending a retrodisplaced uterus that is bound down in the posterior cul-de-sac; and presacral neurectomy to relieve dysmenorrhea.

Definitive operations are those in which the major goal is to relieve symptoms. They are appropriate for women who have no desire for pregnancy or when the endometriosis is so extensive that preservation or restoration of fertility is impossible. Frequently, these patients have been unsuccessfully treated with medicine or surgery. The operation most often performed is hysterectomy, bilateral salpingo-oophrectomy, and resection of as much disease as possible.

Hormone therapy eliminates the repeated cyclic variations in ovarian estrogen and progesterone that stimulate periodic growth and disintegration of the ectopic endometrium. Hormone therapy includes the following: *cyclic low-dose combined oral contraceptives,* which produce minimal endometrial growth and scant withdrawal bleeding; *continuous high-dose estrogen-progestogen combinations* to produce a pseudopregnancy state in which uterine and ectopic endometrium is converted to decidua, which eventually undergoes necrosis; *long-acting progestogens,* which also produce decidualization, necrosis of the endometrium, and amenorrhea.

Danazol, an attenuated androgen, can produce a pseudomenopausal state by interfering with gonadotropin secretion and steroidogenesis. By inhibiting the secretion of estrogen and progesterone, the reproductive tissues and the endometriosis undergo atrophic change. The side effects—weight gain, hot flashes, and oily complexion—can be disagreeable, albeit temporary. The dosage varies from 600 to 800 mg daily, and the medication is expensive.

The use of a *GnRH agonist* (Lupron, Synarel) may be an important adjunct to treat this disease. By *down-regulating* (see Chapter 7) the gonadotrope, FSH and LH are inhibited. In the absence of ovarian stimulation, E_2 declines to postmenopausal levels, a milieu that cannot sustain endometriosis. GnRH agonists are gradually becoming primary therapy and are usually prescribed in the more difficult cases. Daily self-administration is required for some agonists but a monthly depot preparation is available. Osteoporosis has been reported in women using these analogs for 6 months or longer.

Specific indications

Patients for whom treatment must most often be planned are (1) young women who want to delay pregnancy for several years, (2) women who are infertile, and (3) those who are seeking only symptomatic relief. Each is treated differently. Laparoscopy should usually be performed to confirm the diagnosis and to determine the extent of the disease before a treatment plan is developed. This procedure can be repeated if necessary to assess the effectiveness of therapy.

Delay of pregnancy. The major concern for *young women who want to delay pregnancy* is to preserve fertility by limiting further growth of the lesions.

Creation of a pseudopregnancy state with *continuous estrogen-progestogen combination* controls the growth of endometriosis, although probably less effectively than with danazol. A product containing norgestrel can be given daily although other progestin-dominant preparations are also effective. This produces a decidual change and eventually necrosis in the ectopic endometrium and presumably limits its growth. Breakthrough bleeding is controlled by increasing the daily dosage when spotting occurs.

A possible approach is to use *cyclic low-dose oral contraceptives.* Endometrial stimulation is minimal, and bleeding is scant; this may serve to inhibit the growth of ectopic endometrium.

Low-dose oral contraceptives also may be considered for young women with family histories of endometriosis and as a treatment of dysmenorrhea. The development and growth of the lesions may be inhibited or at least retarded by these preparations. The risks involved in using these substances by women in this age group are minimal.

Infertility. *Women with endometriosis who are also infertile* require special consideration. The major goal in treatment is to improve fertility; hence oral contraceptives and the production of pseudopregnancy states usually should not be considered. These regimens are less effective in destroying lesions already present and in preventing the spread of endometriosis than is surgery.

These women benefit most from *conservative surgical procedures* designed to remove as much endometriosis as possible and to correct endometriosis-induced scarring that reduces fertility. *Uterine suspension* may be performed if the uterus is adherent in cul-de-sac endometriosis, and *presacral neurectomy* to relieve dysmenorrhea. Pregnancy rates from 30% to 90% have been reported after surgical procedures. The major factors that affect the result are the extent of the disease and the skill of the surgeon. Buttram reported that 73% of his patients with mild, 56% with moderate, and 40% with severe endometriosis became pregnant within 15 months after their operations.

Ordinarily, hormone therapy should not be used after surgery, even though a few small areas of endometriosis are left. Because most conceptions occur during the first 12 to 15 months after surgery, the patient should be given an opportunity to use this time without suppressing ovulation. Medication may be prescribed later for patients who do not conceive or for those whose lesions recur after operation.

Danazol may prove to be as effective as conservative surgery in establishing fertility; its major disadvantage is the delay while it is being given. It may also serve an important role in preparing patients with extensive lesions for operation. If such women are pretreated for 3 to 6 months, many of the lesions will have disappeared, and those that remain will be smaller and more easily removed.

Relief of symptoms. When the only concern is the *relief of symptoms,* the most logical treatment is surgical, and the most appropriate operation is *hysterectomy and resection of major masses of endometriosis.* Small areas may be left in place. In women over the age of 40 the tubes and ovaries should usually be removed, but normal adnexa may be left in young women. Replacement estrogen should be prescribed for those who are castrated.

The remaining endometriosis will be troublesome in only a few women whose ovaries are left in place or who are receiving estrogen. Danazol will relieve the symptoms in the former, and the latter can be relieved by stopping the estrogen.

A long-acting progestogen, such as medroxyprogesterone (Depo-Provera) in doses sufficient to produce and maintain amenorrhea, is effective in relieving pain. Because anovulation and amenorrhea sometimes persist for many months after it is discontinued, this drug should not be used in women who may want to become pregnant.

Other indications. Surgery is indicated for reasons other than relieving symptoms or improving fertility. An operation is indicated whenever one or both ovaries are larger than 5 cm in diameter, regardless of the age of the patient and even though she is known to have endometriosis. *Ovarian endometriomas* rarely produce symptoms, and it is impossible to differentiate them from ovarian neoplasms by pelvic examination alone. *Oophorectomy is not often necessary, even for large ovarian endometriomas.* Individual cysts can be dissected out of the normal stroma. One can usually preserve enough ovarian tissue for normal hormone secretion and even pregnancy. A conservative approach is particularly important in young women.

Endometriosis of the rectosigmoid can cause partial or complete bowel obstruction. Bowel resection is appropriate if the lesion cannot be differentiated from cancer or whenever there is significant narrowing of the bowel lumen.

ADENOMYOSIS

Adenomyosis, a benign uterine condition in which endometrial glands and stroma are found deep in the myometrium, is often considered to be a form of endometriosis; they probably are not related disorders but only share histologic similarity. The frequency with which adenomyosis is diagnosed depends largely on how many sections of uterine wall are studied. By definition, the ectopic endometrium is located 2.5 mm (a single low power) below the basal layer of endometrium. The reported incidence varies from about 10% to about 90% of all hysterectomies. It is diagnosed most often in women between the ages of 40 and 50 (Table 11-1).

The pathogenesis is not entirely clear, but adenomyosis is related in some way to estrogen simulation. The cells in the basal portions of the endometrial glands grow downward between the myometrial muscle bundles and may lose their connection to the uterine cavity. The lesions are usually diffuse with patches of endometrial tissue scattered throughout the entire thickness of the uterine wall. The process may be extensive enough to enlarge the uterus but not often beyond a size comparable to a pregnancy of 8 to 10 weeks. Occasionally, the process may be more circumscribed with the formation of a distinct nodule, an *adenomyoma,* but this formation is much less common than is diffuse involvement. Adenomyosis is often associated with uterine fi-

TABLE 11-1 Clinical differentiation

	Endometriosis	Adenomyosis
Approximate age when symptomatic	25-35 years	35-50 years
Parous	Sometimes	Usually
Symptoms	Usually	Sometimes
Abnormal uterine bleeding	Yes	Yes
Dysmenorrhea	Yes	Yes
Infertility	Yes	No
Pelvic pain	Yes	Yes
Responsive to hormone therapy	Yes	No
Responsive to conservative surgery	Yes	No
Requires hysterectomy	Sometimes	Sometimes

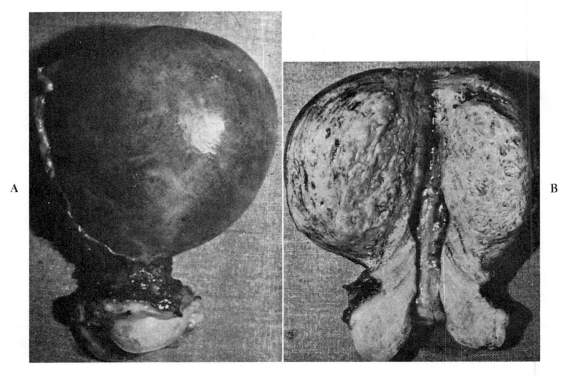

Fig. 11-5 **A,** Hysterectomy specimen from a 37-year-old woman. Note globular appearance of uterus. **B,** Bisection of posterior wall of uterus. (From Emge LA: Am J Obstet Gynecol 83:1551, 1962.)

broids. The most frequently reported symptoms are *colicky secondary dysmenorrhea* and *abnormal bleeding,* but many women with adenomyosis have no symptoms.

The pain is caused first by swelling and then by hemorrhage in the uterine wall as the confined patches of endometrium grow under the stimulus of a rising estrogen concentration and subsequently disintegrate and bleed as the stimulus is withdrawn. Excessive bleeding may reflect the expanding endometrial surface as the uterus enlarges or abnormal prostaglandin production. Increased and irregular bleeding may also occur because of ovulatory failure (dysfunctional bleeding).

The diagnosis is suspected in a woman over 40 who complains of increasingly severe dysmenorrhea and excessive bleeding if the uterus is enlarged and tender, particularly during menstrual flow.

Hormone therapy relieves the pain of ordinary dysmenorrhea and that associated with endometriosis, but these preparations have little effect on the pain associated with adenomyosis.

The only uniformly successful treatment for adenomyosis is hysterectomy. However, operation will not be necessary if the menopause can be expected to occur soon and if the dysmenorrhea can be controlled. The symptoms will disappear after ovarian hormone secretion ceases. Replacement estrogen therapy is not contraindicated (Fig. 11-5).

SUGGESTED READING

Barbieri RL and Ryan KJ: Danazol: endocrine pharmacology and therapeutic applications, Am J Obstet Gynecol 141:453, 1981.

Buttram VC Jr: Conservative surgery for endometriosis in the infertile female: a study of 206 patients with implications for both medical and surgical therapy, Fertil Steril 31:117, 1979.

Meldrum DR, Chang RJ, Lu J, Vale W, and Judd HL: Medical oophorectomy using a long-acting GnRH agonist. A possible new approach to the treatment of endometriosis, J Clin Endocrinol Metab 54:1081, 1982.

Ranney B: The prevention, inhibition, palliation, and treatment of endometriosis, Am J Obstet Gynecol 123:778, 1975.

Sampson JA: Cysts of the ovary, Arch Surg 3:245, 1921.

Simpson JL, Elias S, Malinak LR, and Buttram VC Jr: Heritable aspects of endometriosis. I. Genetic studies, Am J Obstet Gynecol 137:327, 1980.

Von Rokitansky K: Uber uterusdausen—neubildung in uterus und ovarial-sarcomen, Ztscghr d, k k Gesellsch d aerette du Wien 37:577, 1860.

Elsie Reid Carrington

12

The breast

Objectives

RATIONALE: Breast cancer is among the leading causes of death in women. Moreover, women with breast symptoms often exhibit anxiety as a result of their fear of breast cancer. Every physician should understand the basic approach to evaluating the common symptoms associated with the breast.

The student should be able to:

A. Demonstrate knowledge of the standards of surveillance of an adult woman including breast self-examination, physical examination, and mammography.

B. Demonstrate knowledge of the diagnostic approach to a woman with the chief complaint of breast mass, nipple discharge, or breast pain.

C. Demonstrate knowledge of the history and physical findings that might suggest the following abnormalities:
   1. Intraductal papilloma
   2. Fibrocystic changes
   3. Fibroadenoma
   4. Carcinoma

D. Teach a woman how to perform breast self-examination.

Carcinoma of the breast is among the leading causes of death in women. For 1989, the American Cancer Society projected that 142,000 women in the United States would develop breast cancer and 43,000 would die from this disease. Approximately 85% of cancers are detected after the age of 40, whereas occurrence in women under age 30 is only 1.5%. The death rate for breast cancer in the United States is 22.1 per 100,000 women per year. Knowledge and understanding of the nature of the various disorders of the mammary gland are essential parts of the obstetrician-gynecologist's role in providing primary health care for women of all ages.

DEVELOPMENT

The mammary glands develop from specialized skin stimulated by an induction mechanism inherent in the mammary mesenchyme underlying the epidermis. Bands of tissue gradually thicken to form the "milk line" extending from the midclavicular line to the groin. This epithelial mammary ridge is visible in the human embryo at the end of the fourth week of gestation. Regression of the caudal end and thickening of the bands limited to the region of the permanent gland become evident in the embryo of about 6 weeks. Ductal development begins at about the fifth month, and the mammary gland is fully differentiated at birth.

The normal breast hypertrophy of the newborn and secretion from the nipple, if present, regress with the decline in the levels of estrogen-progesterone of placental origin and fetal pituitary prolactin. Breast tissues are dormant until the onset of puberty when estrogen levels begin to rise. Other hormones, including growth hormone, insulin, cortisone, thyroxine, and prolactin, are involved to a lesser degree in adolescent mammary gland growth. Under these influences, differentiation and budding of ducts and an increase in fatty and connective tissues take place and are reflected in breast growth characteristic of the thelarche. The addition of progesterone accompanying ovulatory cycles is essential for optimal acinar growth.

METHODS OF EXAMINATION

Because breast cancers are so prone to metastasize while still small, early detection is essential for control. Significant strides have been made in screening techniques and in therapeutic approaches, but methodical physical examination at regular intervals remains a key factor in early detection. In a majority of cases, the patient first discovers a mass in the breast, usually by accident and often late in the course of its development. Education of the patient in technique, timing, and reasons for self-examination should be a standard part of primary health care.

Breast self-examination. Self-examination should be carried out at monthly intervals, preferably just after the menstrual period when hormonal stimulation is at lowest ebb if the woman is premenopausal. Starting the examination during bathing is advantageous because the soapy water reduces friction and facilitates deeper palpation. With one arm raised, glide the flats of the opposite fingers over every part of the breast, axilla, and supraclavicular areas. Next, with a good light, the breasts are examined in a mirror, first with the arms at the sides and then raised high overhead. Attention is directed to any bulging areas, skin changes such as discoloration, edema, dimpling, or retraction, and any abnormalities of the nipples.

The remainder of the examination is done in the supine position using a rolled-up towel under the back to elevate the side of the chest to be examined. This flattens the breast against the chest wall. Systematic palpation with the flat of the fingers is carried out in concentric circles beginning at the outer margins until every part of each breast is examined (Fig. 12-1). The areolar areas are similarly palpated, and the nipple base compressed and stripped for evidence of secretion. The physician's sensitivity to individual patient needs during instruction encourages self-motivation and helps allay anxieties.

Mammography. Techniques for breast x-ray film examination have improved in quality, and radiation dosage necessary for identification of various breast disorders has been reduced significantly.

The sensitivity rate for these films is about 90%. The type of breast examined influences the accuracy of interpretation. The denser, more glandular breasts of young women make it more difficult to recognize early stages of the disease. Nevertheless, mammography has the capability of detecting many cancers smaller than 1 cm, or 1 to 2 years before they would be clinically palpable. Data from the large national screening project reported by Strax revealed that a total of 2379 early cancers were found among approximately 280,000 screened women who had both clinical and mammographic examinations. Of these, 44% were detected by mammogram alone; in this group, 77% had no nodal involvement. However,

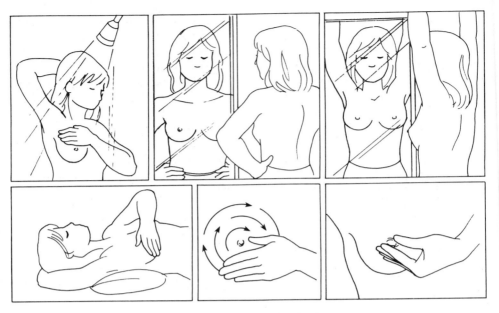

Fig. 12-1 Breast self-examination.

mammography is not infallible. It is an important complement to, but not a substitute for, clinical examination. A negative mammogram, for example, should not induce one to defer aspiration biopsy or excision of a suspicious palpable mass. Films are particularly useful for evaluating intraductile papillary lesions in which microcalcifications highly suggestive of carcinoma can be seen before a mass is palpable.

Xeroradiography. Xeroradiography, a variation of mammography, uses a selenium plate that produces the breast image on paper instead of film. Some radiologists prefer this technique, but results show no real advantage of one method over the other.

Breast aspiration biopsy. Fine needle breast aspiration biopsy is a simple, safe, and cost-effective test. It is particularly useful in the management of fibrocystic disorders so commonly found in young women. If the mass is cystic and the fluid is not grossly sanguinous, aspiration frequently obviates the need for radiologic procedures or surgery. A 21- or 22-gauge needle is preferable to one of larger gauge for both fluid aspirates and tissue samples to minimize both trauma and retrieval of bloody samples. Blood-stained fluids and aspirates from solid tumors require cytologic examination or cell block histology.

Other particular indications include aspiration of masses in the superficial tissues or incisional areas following mastectomy and in suspicious breast masses in pregnant women, in whom delays in diagnosis are far too frequent. Complications are rare. Because even small hematomas and edema may present diagnostic difficulties in interpretation of mammography, the procedure should be deferred for 2 to 3 weeks if findings on the aspirate are inconclusive.

With the use of breast aspiration biopsy in experienced hands, indications are that false-positive results occur in less than 1% of reported cases and that false-negative results range between 10% and 20%.

Other techniques. *Ultrasonography* has its greatest use in evaluating breast masses in young women in whom density of the parenchyma presents difficulty for mammography and xerography because of ultrasound's ability to accurately differentiate cystic and solid masses. Cystic masses should be sharply marginated and contain no internal echos. Early cancers are far more accurately detected by mammography. *Radioisotope scans* have not proved very practical.

The practical use of available methods of examination in relationship to the earliest possible detection of breast cancer is summarized in the American Cancer Society recommendations for breast cancer screening:

Breast self-examination monthly after age 20
Annual physician examination after age 40
Baseline mammogram between ages 35 and 40
Mammogram every 1 to 2 years, depending on physical or film findings, between ages 40 and 49
Annual mammogram after age 50

DEVELOPMENTAL ABNORMALITIES

Supernumerary breasts or *accessory nipples* are remnants of the mammary ridge. The most common locations are just below the normal breast and in the axillary region. These are usually of no clinical significance except during pregnancy, when stimulation of the glandular elements, if present, causes enlargement, sometimes discomfort, and even secretion of milk.

Amastia, or failure of breast development, is extremely rare; when this condition exists, it is usually associated with deformity of the chest wall.

Minor degrees of *asymmetrical growth of the breasts* are exceedingly common. The concerned adolescent girl and her parents usually need only reassurance. Occasionally, either excessive growth or hypoplasia of one breast can be of such magnitude that cosmetic surgery is warranted. Augmentation or reduction mammoplasty should be deferred until maturation is assuredly complete.

Massive hypertrophy of the breasts, although not a common condition, is most likely to occur during puberty. Endocrine studies are within normal limits; hence enhanced end-organ sensitivity is the apparent cause. The condition is psychologically traumatic and can also be physically debilitating. Reduction mammoplasty is indicated when full maturation is attained.

ABNORMALITIES OF SECRETION

Inappropriate lactation, or *galactorrhea,* is caused by a great variety of conditions, including mechanical factors that act through neural reflexes such as vigorous nipple stimulation and reactions to chest or breast surgery or disease. Certain pharmacologic agents, particularly the psychotropic drugs, tend to deplete central nervous system catecholamines and thus reduce secretion of prolactin-inhibiting factor. Occasionally, galactorrhea follows withdrawal of oral contraceptives. Thyroid and, to a lesser extent, adrenal disorders may be associated with abnormal lactation. These and the more common central nervous system and hypothalamic-pituitary disorders associated with galactorrhea are discussed in Chapter 9.

ACUTE INFECTIONS

Localized infections. *Sebaceous cysts* arising from glands normally located in the skin of the areola frequently become infected. Similarly, *periareolar abscesses* may arise in one or more of the lactiferous ducts in association with inversion of the nipple, chronic maceration, ductal obstruction, and secondary infection. Incision and drainage may not be curative, particularly for periareolar abscess, which is prone to recur. Excision of the involved duct is advisable as a final step when the acute infection has subsided.

Puerperal mastitis. In most areas of the United States, postpartum breast infections are relatively rare, usually not exceeding 1%. Puerperal mastitis is discussed in Chapter 41.

Epidemic puerperal mastitis. Epidemic puerperal mastitis is an altogether different type of infection. The responsible agent is almost invariably a penicillin-resistant *S. aureus,* and the infection is most frequently hospital acquired. When the microorganism is present in the nursery, colonization of the nasopharynx occurs in an alarmingly high percentage of infants in 24 to 48 hours. Treatment is like that for sporadic mastitis.

Mammary duct ectasia. Mammary duct ectasia (comedomastitis or plasma cell mastitis) is a benign process usually occurring at about the age of 40. The primary changes occur in the dilated subareolar ducts that become filled with inspissated breast secretions and debris. Chronic inflammation and marked periductal fibrosis develop later. Signs and symptoms include nipple discharge, recurrent pain, and often nipple retraction. The ducts, filled with thick, pastelike material and surrounded by fibrosis, are readily palpable, and the axillary glands may be enlarged. The findings during examination are, in fact, indistinguishable from breast cancer; hence excision biopsy is mandatory. No further treatment is necessary if duct ectasia is found.

Mammary fat necrosis

This condition presents as a localized area of fat necrosis followed by the development of a firm, readily palpable mass located just below the skin. Ecchymosis may or may not be associated. It is more common in women with pendulous breasts. A history of trauma is expected, but in about half the cases the woman recalls no specific injury. Pain and tenderness are early signs. Later fibrosis and scarring occur; the mass then has a firm consistency and an irregular outline closely resembling carcinoma. Excision biopsy is necessary for diagnosis and treatment.

Mondor's disease. Mondor's disease, or *superficial thrombophlebitis of the veins of the breast and anterior chest wall,* does not occur often; however, familiarity with this condition is important because it often is overtreated. The cause is unknown. It is not necessarily associated with trauma, surgery, or oversized breasts. As a rule the first symptom is pain, although acute symptoms may not be a dominant complaint. Next, a hard, usually tender, cord appears in the superficial tissues following the course of one of the superficial veins, particularly the lateral thoracic or the superior epigastric. Retraction of the skin occurs where the vein crosses the breast and can be mistaken as evidence of infiltrating cancer. The course of the thrombophlebitis is self-limiting, although the time required for resolution varies from a few weeks to 6 months. Treatment is symptomatic during the period of pain and tenderness and includes reassurance that neither underlying breast lesions nor complications such as embolism are associated with this condition.

BENIGN DISORDERS
Fibrocystic disorders

Fibrocystic changes are the most common cause of breast "lumps." Typically, these are bilateral and multiple. They can be found in women throughout the reproductive years, most frequently in the thirties, and they regress after the menopause, implying hormonal dependence. Variation in response to estrogen and progesterone with estrogen dominance is believed to cause the ductal and stromal proliferations that characterize this condition. Premenstrual pain and tenderness are relatively common complaints, but the condition often is asymptomatic. Palpation of the breast may reveal a diffuse increase in consistency, shottiness, nodularity, or a fluctuant or rubbery mass. Most of the cysts are thin walled, filled with a turbid fluid, and often bluish in color. The stromal tissues show varying degrees of fibrosis. Although lymphocytic infiltration is common, it does not indicate mastitis.

Treatment depends on the age of the patient and on the nature of the breast changes. Patients over 25 years of age should have mammography studies. Readily palpable cystic masses can be aspirated. If cystic fluid is obtained and the mass disappears completely, no further treatment is needed. If the fluid is bloody, or if no fluid is obtained, excision biopsy is indicated.

Medical treatment for mastodynia associated with diffuse breast involvement is mainly supportive. Oral contraceptives with low estrogen content or a progesterone preparation can reduce pain and tenderness in about 60% to 80% of cases of severe mastodynia, but there is little effect on nodularity. Symptoms recur on cessation of treatment. The antigonadotropin danazol, given in 200- to 400-mg dosages daily, relieves pain in about three fourths of cases. However, the side effects of menstrual irregularities, amenorrhea, acne, weight gain, and the fact that symptoms recur after the course of treatment seriously limit its use.

Adenosis. Adenosis is frequently associated with fibrocystic changes and may be the dominant feature. Proliferation of ducts and acini and marked interlobular fibrosis create a firm irregular mass clinically suggestive of carcinoma. Preoperative mammography and excision biopsy are indicated.

Fibroadenomas. Fibroadenomas may occur at any age, but they are most frequently seen in women under the age of 30. They are usually solitary and asymptomatic. The tumor is firm and mobile, and the margins are well defined. When they arise in the teenage or pregnant patient, they may enlarge remarkably, presumably because of the rapid increase in hormone stimulation. Solid masses should be excised for definitive diagnosis and treatment.

Intraductile papilloma. Intraductile papilloma produces a serous or bloody discharge from the nipple, most often during the perimenopausal years. The growth is small, often less than 1 cm, and difficult to locate. Application of pressure at different points around the areola usually elicits discharge when the involved duct is pressed. In most cases a benign, friable, villous growth is found, but the possibility of papillary carcinoma must always be considered. Treatment is complete excision biopsy of the involved duct.

Galactocele. A galactocele is a cystic mass that develops in women who have recently lactated. The mass is smooth walled, movable, and filled with a thick inspissated milky fluid. Needle aspiration is curative if the fluid obtained is typical and the mass disappears thereafter. If a mass remains, excision biopsy is indicated.

MALIGNANT LESIONS

The incidence and the number of deaths caused by breast cancer have increased during the past 25 years, in part because of increased aging of the population. Currently, one in 10 women will de-

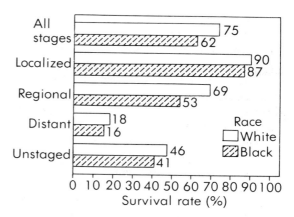

Fig. 12-2 Breast cancer (females) 5-year survival rates, 1979-1984. (From National Cancer Institute, Division of Cancer Prevention and Control, 1987.)

velop breast cancer in her lifetime. Certain features of the disease and identifiable risk factors of importance to the clinician are now well established. Mammary cancer tends to be multicentric and may metastasize at a relatively early stage. Five-year survival rates approach 90% in the early localized stage of the disease. The rate drops to about 60% with involvement of the axillary nodes; if the supraclavicular nodes are involved, the prognosis is extremely grave (Fig. 12-2). Multiple foci are frequently found with the primary lesion; the overall incidence of bilateral breast involvement is between 7.5% and 10%.

Types

Mammary carcinoma is usually classified according to the site of origin in the ducts or lobules:

Intraductile carcinoma
    Scirrhous carcinoma
    Papillary carcinoma
    Colloid carcinoma
    Comedocarcinoma
    Lobular carcinoma
Special types
    Paget's disease

Inflammatory carcinoma

Phyllodes tumors

Approximately 90% of cases arise in the ducts. *Lobular carcinoma* is sometimes found in an in situ stage with small, round, malignant cells filling the acini without stromal invasion. This tumor is frequently multicentric, and in about a third of cases involvement is bilateral.

Paget's disease is different because of the epidermal involvement and because delays in diagnosis are unfortunately so common. Although this is an intraductal lesion, involvement of the nipple epidermis occurs early. Itching, burning, and the gradual development of an eczematoid lesion are the first signs. The lesion may remain indolent for some time and then spread to the areola and deeper into the ducts as an in situ or infiltrating carcinoma. In the absence of a palpable mass, surgical treatment is usually curative. If a mass or axillary nodes are palpable, the prognosis decreases significantly. The 5-year survival rate is only about 50%.

Inflammatory carcinoma comprises 1% to 4% and has the poorest prognosis of all breast cancers. Pain and diffuse enlargement of the breast are first evidences. The superficial tissues become indurated and pitted in appearance. A mass may or may not be palpable. Biopsy reveals dermal lymphatics plugged with neoplastic cells in most, but not all cases. This finding is sufficiently unique that controversy has arisen as to whether this disease should be considered a distinct entity. Despite the fact that fever, leukocytosis, and other systemic components of breast abscess are minimal or absent, infection is often the initial diagnosis made and appropriate therapy may be delayed for weeks or months. Delay is critical because the course of the disease is so virulent that metastases are almost invariably present at the time of diagnosis. Survivals rarely exceed 1 to 2 years.

Phyllodes tumors, often termed *cystosarcoma phyllodes,* is a relatively rare tumor originally thought to be entirely benign. Like a fibroadenoma, from which it must be differentiated, the tumor contains both epithelial and mesenchymal elements, but the stromal cells in phyllodes tumors are far more prominent and may vary in size and shape. Although the tumor seldom undergoes neoplastic changes and rarely metastasizes, it does have a tendency to recur locally. Benign types and most malignant phyllodes tumors may be treated successfully by local incision allowing a wide margin of tumor-free tissue.

Risk factors

Age. Breast cancer is a rarity below age 25, but its frequency increases steadily after age 35. About 85% of the total cases are in women over age 40.

Family history. The risk is doubled with a positive family history and increased eightfold if the mother or sister has had bilateral breast cancer during her premenopausal years.

History of previous benign breast disease. Risk is increased twofold to fourfold, *but only if previously excised tissues showed atypia;* the risk rises with increasing degree of dysplasia.

Previous cancer in one breast. Risk of cancer in the remaining breast is five times greater than the risk of a primary lesion in the general population.

Parity. Nulliparous women and those over age 34 at the time of their first pregnancy are twice as prone to breast cancer as are women who bore children earlier in life. Lactation presumably offers some protection against the development of breast cancer.

Other factors. Exposure to radiation or chemical agents, the use of estrogens, and prolonged exposure to estrogens including oral contraceptives through early menarche and late menopause are less clear-cut risk factors that nevertheless belong in the patient's history.

Diagnosis. The *primary complaints* leading to suspicion of breast cancer are (1) discovery of a lump; (2) serous or bloody discharge from the nipple; (3) nipple retraction, eczema, or ulceration; and (4) skin redness, dimpling, or ulceration. Pain is not a common initial complaint for malignant breast lesions, but it does occur in some cases, mainly if the initial symptom is related to axillary or vertebral metastasis.

Details concerning these symptoms—date of onset, duration, and change in size or other features—and inquiry concerning each of the risk factors mentioned previously should be included in the history.

Physical examination of the breast should be performed systematically as previously described. If the patient is under 25 years of age and the mass is smooth and freely movable or obviously cystic, management as outlined for benign lesions may be most appropriate, but mammographic studies should be obtained on any woman, regardless of age, with suggestive clinical signs or symptoms or dubious findings. Mammography can identify many lesions that are not palpable because of their small size or their location in fatty tissues or within the duct. Intraductal papillary cancers, which are relatively soft and friable and may cause bloody discharge early, are frequently nonpalpable but often produce microcalcifications that are visible on film.

Aspiration biopsies may be examined on frozen section, as well as on permanent sections. The possibility of detecting multifocal lesions, not uncommonly within the same breast and often in the opposite breast, is further reason for mammographic evaluation before biopsy. A tissue diagnosis is essential before any form of therapy is instituted.

Trends in management of breast cancer

Bilateral breast cancer. At least 15% of women with one breast cancer will develop or may already have cancer in the other breast. About 75% of these will be primary rather than metastatic tumors. The risk for the second breast tumor is particularly high in the premenopausal patient with a strong family history or with an initial multicentric or lobular carcinoma. Preoperative mammography is advantageous to rule out suspicious densities or microcalcifications in the opposite breast and to localize the area for bi-

opsy. Management of the contralateral breast is controversial, especially in the high-risk patient, and ranges from close follow-up examinations to prophylactic mastectomy.

Radical mastectomy with or without postoperative radiation remained unchallenged as optimal treatment for cancer of the breast for at least six decades. Failure to alter survival rates significantly during this period, new knowledge of the biology of breast cancers, and the larger number of cases with early occurrence of lesions of less than 2 cm were important factors in the growing trend toward conservatism and individualization. The changing concept of tumor spread is the basis for recent therapeutic approaches. There is good evidence that some mammary cancers have already metastasized by the time the tumor is clinically detectable. In patients with small breast lesions and negative axillary nodes, 75% reach a 10-year survival period without recurrence, but about 25% experience recurrence. Of those with positive axillary nodes and no evidence of distant metastasis, only 25% survive for 10 years without recurrence. These results suggest differences in mammary tumor behavior and host resistance and have stimulated current studies of their interaction.

SURGICAL TREATMENT. A two-stage approach to primary surgical management is usually preferable to biopsy, frozen section evaluation, and immediate operation. The short delay has no deleterious effects, and it permits more precise pathologic assessment and participation of the patient in decisions concerning the overall therapeutic program.

The *modified radical mastectomy,* which involves total (simple) mastectomy and axillary dissection but preserves the pectoralis muscle and nerves, has practically replaced the radical procedure. The trend toward more conservative surgery for early breast cancers with better functional and cosmetic results led to a long-term study formulated by the National Surgical Adjuvant Breast Project in 1971. A total of 1665 women with a primary tumor confined to the breast or breast and

TABLE 12-1 Comparison of total mastectomy with lumpectomy and with lumpectomy and radiation therapy, according to nodal status*

Nodal status and treatment group	Number	Disease-free survival		Distant-disease–free survival		Overall survival	
		5 years	8 years	5 years	8 years	5 years	8 years
Negative nodes							
Total mastectomy	366	75.1±2.3	65.5±3.3	81.5±2.1	73.8±3.2	87.7±1.8	78.7±3.2
Lumpectomy	392	67.6±2.4	60.7±2.8	74.5±2.2	69.6±2.6	87.1±1.8	76.6±2.8
Overall P value		0.05		0.03		0.5	
Lumpectomy and irradia-tion	399	77.3±2.2	65.6±3.3	80.9±2.0	70.7±3.2	88.3±1.7	82.9±2.3
Overall P value		0.7		0.6		0.8	
Positive nodes†							
Total mastectomy	224	53.5±3.4	44.5±4.0	60.8±3.3	50.7±4.2	72.2±3.1	59.9±4.1
Lumpectomy	244	55.4±3.3	41.6±4.1	63.9±3.2	49.1±4.6	75.6±2.9	60.3±4.5
Overall P value		0.6		0.4		0.7	
Lumpectomy and irradia-tion	230	59.0±3.3	46.6±4.1	62.8±3.3	53.1±3.9	77.2±2.9	68.3±3.9
Overall P value		0.2		0.6		0.3	

*The values are life-table estimates of the results 5 and 8 years after surgery and are expressed as mean (±SE) percentages. The P values are for comparisons with the total mastectomy group.
†The values have been adjusted for the number of positive nodes (1 to 3, 4 to 9, or ≥10).
From Fisher B, Redmond C, Poisson R, and others: N Engl J Med 320:822, 1989.

axilla and movable over the underlying muscle were treated by radical mastectomy, total mastectomy without axillary dissection but with irradiation, and total mastectomy alone with axillary dissection only if nodes were subsequently positive. There were no significant differences in the 10-year survival rates related to the procedure used. In patients with clinically negative nodes, overall survival in each group was about 57%. Patients with positive nodes had a 10-year survival rate of about 38% with either modified management or radical surgery.

Other more conservative procedures are now utilized more frequently for small breast cancers in stages I and II, notably lumpectomy with and without radiation therapy (Table 12-1).

Although no one procedure is superior to another, lesser procedures have a greater incidence of local recurrences. Survival time does not differ significantly.

Breast reconstruction is feasible in properly selected cases. It can be done immediately but in most cases it is performed about 6 months after mastectomy when decisions regarding radiation or chemotherapy have been made and the wound is healed.

The estrogen receptor (ER) and progesterone receptor (PgR) status of a portion of the tumor tissue removed should be determined, as results obtained have a bearing on prognosis and also provide guidelines for subsequent therapy, should recurrence arise.

PRIMARY RADIATION THERAPY. Interest in the use of radiation therapy as an alternative to mastectomy has gained impetus following reports showing 5-year survival rates comparable to those with surgical management. Clinical trials of longer duration are necessary and are in progress. Results from the Harvard Joint Center for Radiation Therapy reported in the 1980 National Institutes of Health Summary reveal a 5-year survival rate of 91% for stage I and 66% for stage II lesions. In most centers excision biopsy and axillary node sampling are performed for pretherapy diagnosis, but in some cases needle biopsies are used.

ENDOCRINE THERAPY. Hormone treatment has an important role in palliation of metastatic breast cancer. Availability of reliable methods for assay of estrogen and progesterone receptors within the tumor tissue has aided substantially in selecting therapy for individual patients. About 60% to 70% of patients with tumors that are ER positive will respond to hormonal manipulation, but only about 8% to 10% of those with ER-negative tumors will respond. Progesterone represents a critical end-step in estrogen action, and the presence of progesterone receptors appears to be more predictive of response. Numerous clinical trials have shown that women with tumors possessing both estrogen and progesterone receptors have the most favorable response to endocrine therapy.

Antiestrogens such as tamoxifen have proved effective in approximately 50% of ER-positive cases; this response can be used as a predictor of patients who are likely to respond similarly to oophorectomy, should drug effectiveness fail. Tamoxifen has the advantage of almost complete absence of side effects. It is particularly applicable for the postmenopausal patient with ER-positive breast tumor.

Aminoglutethimide (AG), a derivative of glutethimide (Doriden) has antitumor activity in metastatic breast cancer similar to adrenalectomy and is as effective as adrenal surgery. Glucocorticoid replacement is given with the drug to prevent Addison's disease. Although response rates as high as 43% have been reported, side effects limit its use.

Ablative procedures of adrenalectomy or hypophysectomy and to a lesser extent the adrenal suppressant AG also have response rates of about 30%.

Patients with ER-negative tumors and those unresponsive to hormonal manipulation can still be given palliative chemotherapy.

CHEMOTHERAPY. The most recent approach to treatment of mammary cancer involves the sequential use of chemotherapy after mastectomy, axillary node dissection, and determination of the estrogen-receptor status of the tumor. The rationale for this approach is based on the concept that micrometastases will already have occurred when positive axillary nodes are found.

Numerous clinical trials have been conducted using various drugs and their combinations since such studies were initiated by the National Surgical Adjuvant Breast and Bowel Project 32 years ago. Their reports in 1988 and 1989 indicate that chemotherapy is effective in the management of estrogen-receptor-negative tumors, particularly in reduction of local, regional, and distant metastases, but not in overall survival. The most recent randomized study focused on premenopausal women with ER-negative breast tumors but with no nodal involvement. Relapse-free survival in the chemotherapy group was 80% versus 71% in the group receiving no adjuvant therapy. The overall survival rate was not significantly improved. The use of chemotherapy in this group is controversial, but it provides an option for patients at greatest risk.

Carcinoma of the breast during pregnancy. Pregnancy does not predispose to mammary cancer; but growth, extension, and metastasis may be accelerated by the physiologic expansion of vascular and lymphatic channels.

DIAGNOSIS. Diagnosis during pregnancy or lactation is frequently delayed because a small mass in the hypertrophied breast may be difficult to detect or may be misinterpreted. Regular prenatal examinations of the breast and prompt biopsy of palpable nodes are mandatory if early lesions are to be discovered.

PROGNOSIS. The outlook for the patient with concurrent mammary cancer and pregnancy is not hopeless. The pessimistic view of inoperability of these lesions in gravid women is no longer tenable. Treatment, particularly when initiated in the early stage, is almost as effective as in the nonpregnant patient. In a series of 63 cases treated between 1950 and 1980, King and associates reported a survival rate of 82% in patients with zero to three positive nodes. In patients with more than three positive nodes, the 5-year survival rate was only 27%. In a smaller series of 19 cases, Nugent and O'Connell determined that 10 of the 14 tumors tested for estrogen-receptor status proved to be ER-negative, for which response to endocrine therapy is effective in only about 10%.

MANAGEMENT. The criteria of operability should be the same for pregnant as for nonpregnant patients. The value of terminating pregnancy in the first and second trimesters after radical mastectomy is still a moot question except for patients for whom chemotherapy is indicated. White found little to recommend the procedure in 78 women in whom therapeutic abortion was performed. Obviously, the management of this problem must be individualized. No benefit is derived from interference with the pregnancy in late-stage inoperable carcinoma of the breast.

Subsequent pregnancies usually cause no complications if the patient is well and without evidence of recurrence after 3 to 4 years.

SUGGESTED READING

American Cancer Society: Cancer Facts and Figures, New York, 1989, American Cancer Society, Inc.

Bottles K and Taylor RN: Diagnosis of breast masses in pregnant women by aspiration biopsy, Obstet Gynecol 66:763, 1985.

Clark GM, McGuire WL, Hubay CA, Pearson OH, and Marshall JS: Progesterone receptors as a prognostic factor in stage II breast cancer, N Engl J Med 309:1343, 1983.

Donovan WL: Breast cancer and pregnancy, Obstet Gynecol 50:244, 1977.

Donovan WL and Perz-Mesa CM: Lobular carcinoma: an indication for biopsy of the second breast, Ann Surg 176:178, 1972.

Early Breast Cancer Trialists' Collaborative Group: Effects of adjuvant tamoxifen and of cytotoxic therapy on mortality in early breast cancer: an overview of 61 randomized trials among 28,896 women, N Engl J Med 319:1681, 1988.

Fisher B, Bauer M, Margolese R, Redmond C, Fisher ER, Bauer M, Wolmark N, Wickerham L, Deutch M, Montague E, Margolese R, and Foster R: Ten-year results of a randomized clinical trial comparing radical mastectomy and total mastectomy with or without radiation, N Engl J Med 312:674, 1985.

Fisher B, Redmond C, Dimitrov NV, Bowman D, Legault-Poisson S, Wickerham DL, Wolmark N, Fisher ER, Margolese R, Sutherland C, Glass A, Foster R, and Caplan R: A randomized clinical trial evaluating sequential methotrexate and fluorouracil in the treatment of patients with node-negative breast cancer who have estrogen-receptor-negative tumors, N Engl J Med 320:473, 1989.

Foster RS Jr and Costanza MC: Breast self-examination practices and breast cancer survival, Cancer 53:999, 1984.

Grace WR and Cooperman AV: Inflammatory breast cancer, Surg Clin North Am 65:151, 1985.

Harper P and Kelly-Frye E: Ultrasound visualization of the breast in symptomatic patients, Radiology 137:465, 1980.

Harris JR, Hellman S, Henderson IC, and Kinne DW: Breast diseases, Philadelphia, 1987, JB Lippincott Co.

Hart J, Layfield LJ, Trumbull WE, and others: Practical aspects in the diagnosis and management of cystosarcoma phyllodes, Arch Surg 123:1079, 1988.

Henderson ID, and Canellos GP: Cancer of the breast: the past decade (part I), N Engl J Med 302:17, 1980.

Henderson IC, and Canellos GP: Cancer of the breast: the past decade (part II), N Engl J Med 302:78, 1980.

King RM, Welch JB, Martin JK, and Coulam CB: Cancer of the breast associated with pregnancy, Surg Gynecol Obstet 160:228, 1985.

Manni A: Hormone receptors and breast cancer, N Engl J Med 309:138, 1983.

Marchant DJ and Myirjesy I, editors: Breast disease: proceedings of an international symposium, May 13-17, 1978, New York, 1979, Grune & Stratton, Inc.

Meuller CB: Options in surgical treatment of "curable" breast cancer: results of controlled clinical trials. In Grunfest-Broniatowski and Esselstyn CB, editors: Controversies in breast cancer diagnosis and management, New York, 1988, Marcel Dekker, Inc.

Moxley JH, Allegra JC, Henney J, and Muggia F: Treatment of primary breast cancer: summary of NIH consensus development conference, JAMA 244:797, 1980.

National Cancer Institute, Division of Cancer Prevention and Control 1987: Annual Cancer Statistics Review, Bethesda, 1987, National Cancer Institute.

Nugent P and O'Connell TX: Breast cancer and pregnancy, Arch Surg 120:1221, 1985.

Pressman PI: Selective biopsy of the opposite breast, Cancer 57:577, 1986.

Recht A, Connolly JL, Schnitt SS, Cady B, Love S, Ostein RT, Patterson WB, Shirley B, Silen W, Come S, Henderson IC, Silver B, and Harris JR: Conservative surgery and primary radiation therapy for early breast cancer: results, controversies and unsolved problems, Semin Oncol 13:434, 1986.

Sickles EA, Filly RA, and Callen PW: Benign breast lesions: ultrasound detection and diagnosis, Radiology 151:467, 1984.

Silverberg E: Cancer statistics 1984, Cancer 7:23, 1984.

Strax P: Evaluation of screening programs for early diagnosis of breast cancer, Surg Clin North Am 58:669, 1978.

Wenebo HJ, Senofsky GM, Fechner RE, Kaiser D, Lynn S, and Paradies J: Bilateral breast cancer: risk reduction by contralateral biopsy, Ann Surg 201:667, 1985.

13

Russell K. Laros, Jr.

Fertilization; development, physiology, and disorders of the placenta; fetal development

Objectives

RATIONALE: An understanding of the physiology of reproduction enables the student to understand the abnormalities that may occur during the antepartum, intrapartum, and postpartum periods.

The student should be able to:

A. Demonstrate a knowledge of the process of human fertilization.

B. Explain the development, physiology, and disorders of the placenta.

C. Describe the development of the fetus.

Successful human reproduction is dependent on an integrated sequence of physiologic mechanisms that first of all ensures normal maturation, fertilization, and growth of the ovum and then, as pregnancy advances, permits normal differentiation and adequate nutrition for the fetus.

FERTILIZATION

Union of male and female elements of procreation must be preceded by *maturation* of the germ cells. In the sexually adult male, spermatogenesis occurs continuously, whereas in the female, oogenesis is cyclic. Under the influence of hypothalamic-releasing factors and, in turn, secretion of pituitary FSH, many follicles are stimulated during the first 10 days of the cycle. Generally, only the dominant follicle is destined to reach ma-

turity at each cycle. Its rate of growth is greatly accelerated as the ripening follicle migrates to the surface of the ovary. At present the mechanism that determines which follicle will be singled out to play a leading role in the cycle is not understood. At approximately the fourteenth day, the wall of the follicle ruptures, and the ovum with some of the surrounding granulosa cells and follicular fluid is discharged into the fallopian tube. Release of pressure allows the walls of the follicle to collapse, and blood from the congested vessels of the theca fills the cavity. The point of rupture *(blutpunkt)* seals off. Theca cells and especially granulosa cells undergo luteinization, producing a yellow, lipid-laden body, the *mature corpus luteum.*

Final preparation of the ovum for fertilization

142

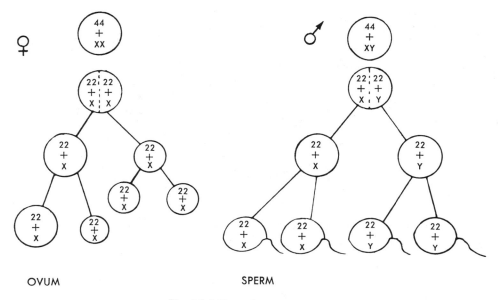

Fig. 13-1 Normal gametogenesis.

involves the unique process of *meiosis* (Fig. 13-1). In contrast to somatic cell division, or mitosis—wherein a complete diploid chromosomal set, each chromosome an exact replica of itself, is passed to the daughter cell—gametogenesis results in reduction of the nuclear chromosomes to half the number characteristic of the species. This is accomplished by two maturation divisions, the steps involved being of utmost importance to an understanding of human chromosomal abnormalities.

Homologous chromosomes arrange themselves in pairs, and in the first *meiotic (reduction) division,* which occurs before ovulation, they separate *(dysjunction)* to form the first two daughter cells. Each daughter cell contains a haploid complement of chromosomes (23 X). Although the chromosomal material is equally divided, the oocyte retains the bulk of the cytoplasm. The other cell is the *first polar body.* The second division may begin before ovulation, but it is not completed until the oocyte is penetrated by a spermatozoon. At this time the *second polar body* is released.

Union of the ovum and the spermatozoon restores the normal diploid number with formation of the zygote, containing 44 autosomal chromosomes and two sex chromosomes; the zygote is female if the sex chromosomes are XX and male if they are XY (Fig. 13-2). Thus the genetic or nuclear sex is determined and fixed at fertilization.

The sex genes direct and control differentiation of the gonad and accessory structures, beginning about the sixth week of embryonic life (Chapter 3). However, the external sex is not clearly apparent until about the sixteenth week. The physical appearance of sex may be influenced by a nonphysiologic hormonal environment to which the fetus is exposed. If gonadogenesis is normal, if the fetal hormonal environment is appropriate, and if there is no interference from harmful physical factors or from exogenous hormonal influences, the physical appearance of sex (phenotype) will be appropriate for the chromosomal sex (genotype).

The genetic constitution may be altered in the

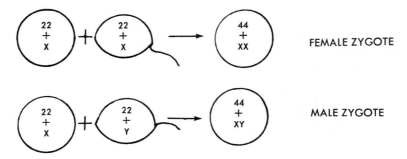

Fig. 13-2 Male and female zygotes.

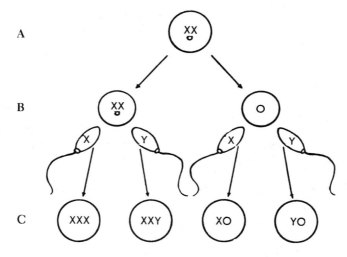

Fig. 13-3 Effects of nondisjunction during gametogenesis. **A,** Haploid daughter cell with two chromatids united by centromere. **B,** Meiosis I, nondisjunction. **C,** Meiosis II, four types of zygotes may be produced during fertilization.

process of gonadogenesis by *nonassociation* or by *nondisjunction of chromosomes,* resulting in defects that are often lethal if autosomes are involved; however, there are exceptions. Nonlethal consequences are seen in developmental abnormalities that result from the number of chromosomes either exceeding or being less than normal (Fig. 13-3).

The normal chromosomal number of 46 is shown in the diagram in Fig. 13-4. The 22 autosomal pairs are similar in the female and the

male, whereas the sex chromosomes differ in the two sexes (XX or XY, respectively).

The true genetic sex can be determined by cytologic examination of various somatic cells. The morphologic difference in the resting cell nuclei of the two sexes was first described in 1950. A dense mass of chromatin known as the *sex chromatin mass* or *Barr body* (Fig. 13-5) situated at the periphery of the nucleus just within the nuclear membrane is found in up to 90% of the somatic cell nuclei of normal females (chromatin

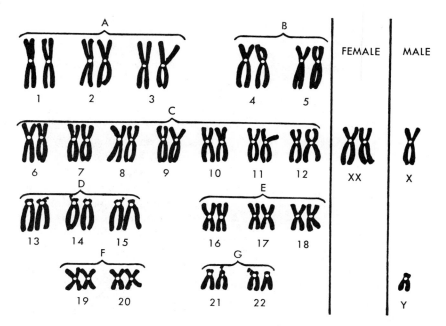

Fig. 13-4 Idiogram of human chromosomes—International System of Nomenclature (Denver).

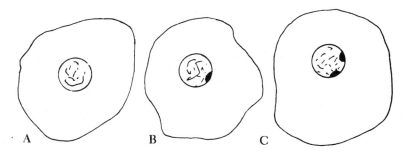

Fig. 13-5 Sex chromatic mass (Barr body) and examples. **A,** Chromatin negative XY, XO. **B,** Chromatin-one positive XX, XXY. **C,** Chromatin-two positive XXX, XXXY.

positive) but is absent or is found in only about 1% to 3% of the nuclei of normal males (chromatin negative). The chromatin mass is derived from the female X chromosome.

The number of Barr bodies found in each nucleus equals the number of X chromosomes minus one. Thus in normal females with an XX constitution, one Barr body is seen. In females with Turner's syndrome bearing the most characteristic XO pattern and in normal males with an XY constitution, the nuclear sex is chromatin negative. In Klinefelter's syndrome, individuals with an XXY or an XXXY constitution display a chromatin-one or a chromatin-two positive nuclear sex pattern, in spite of the fact that the phenotype is male.

Cells obtained by buccal smear are most commonly used for examination; occasionally, skin or vaginal smears are taken. Polymorphonuclear leukocytes can also be used; a characteristic mass, or "drumstick," is found in normal females in about 3% of the neutrophils. However, this may appear as an accessory lobule, and differentiation is therefore more difficult.

The *Y chromatin* of the male interphase nucleus can be identified by the characteristic fluorescent spot seen by ultraviolet microscopy after staining with quinacrine dyes.

Migration of the ovum. After release from the follicle, the ovum is surrounded by sticky cumulus cells. One long projection of the fimbria that contains muscular elements, *fimbria ovarica,* is attached to the ovary, usually at the upper pole. (1) Contraction of these and muscular elements of the parovarium approximate the fallopian tube and ruptured follicle site. (2) Motion of the *epithelial cilia* lining the fimbria promotes migration into the ostium, and, aided by *tubal peristalsis,* which is maximal at this time, the ovum is carried rapidly into the ampulla of the tube. (3) The ovum is retained for about 2½ days at the ampullary-isthmic junction. The luminal fluid provides metabolic substrates and conditions suitable for survival of sperm, ovum, and zygote. (4) Cell division and cleavage continue during transport to the uterus, where implantation during the blastocyst stage occurs at 6 to 8 days after fertilization.

Using culdoscopy for 4- to 5-hour periods, Doyle reported direct observation of ovulation in three patients. He noted elongation, edema, and congestion of the tube and spread of the fimbria over the supermedial aspect of the ovary. The ovum probably is expelled directly into the ampulla of the tube. Trumpet-shaped cones of contraction developed at the fimbria at the rate of six per minute. Peristalsis continued to the isthmus, followed by a to-and-fro motion, and again peristalsis to the cornu. After about 2 hours the fimbria slid down the ovary to the cul-de-sac. Suction developed in this location may provide a means by which the tube on one side may pick up ova ruptured from either ovary.

Fertilization. The ovum is fertilized in the outer third of the tube within a short time after ovulation, probably less than 24 hours. Viability of the ovum is somewhat less than that of spermatozoa.

The seminal fluid vehicle for transport is slightly alkaline, with a pH of 7.5. When the spermatozoa are deposited in the vagina, they are placed in an environment with a pH of 4.5. Although the buffering action of semen is to some extent capable of offsetting this difference, prompt entrance into the cervical canal is important to the continued viability of the spermatozoa. The normal pH of cervical mucus is 7.5. Tyler suggests that the difference in vaginal and cervical pH is one of the factors that favor migration of spermatozoa into the cervical canal; cyclic variations in cervical secretion further enhance their passage. At the time of ovulation the mucus is thin, abundant, rich in glycogen, and most conducive for penetration.

Active spermatozoa reach the fallopian tube within as little as 5 minutes, but the spermatozoa require a period of time within the female reproductive tract to gain the capability of fertilizing the ovum. This process, *capacitation,* is not well understood; however, it seems to involve enzymatic activity and structural alteration termed *acrosomal reaction.*

On penetration of the ovum's vitelline membrane, male and female pronuclei, each with 23 chromosomes, unite to form the segmentation nucleus and restore the original 46 chromosomes.

Repeated cell divisions result in the formation of a mulberry mass, the *morula.* The outer layer of cells secretes fluid that accumulates, forming the segmentation cavity. The mass at this time is called the blastodermic vesicle or *blastocyst.*

Implantation occurs at the blastocyst stage 6 to 8 days after ovulation. Formative cells crowded to one side represent the embryonic pole or inner cell mass. The single layer of cells surrounding the vesicle is the primitive *trophoblast.*

There is much unresolved speculation regarding possible mechanisms in operation during implantation that may account for control of invasion on the one hand and prevention of immunologic rejection on the other. Just before attachment on the uterine endometrium, an aggregate of cells, the *syncytial knob,* appears in the trophoblastic syncytium. These knobs are the portions of the trophoblast that penetrate the decidua. At the implantation site, fusion of maternal and fetal cells occurs temporarily. Behrman and Koren have speculated that such fusion of cytoplasmic and nuclear material may change the immunologic characteristics of maternal tissues and induce tolerance to fetal antigens rather than sensitization.

The pregravid endometrium is prepared to provide for nidation and nutrition of the fertilized ovum. The *decidua* develops under the influence of increasing amounts of ovarian hormones, principally progesterone. The stroma is made up of characteristic large, polyhedral decidual cells; glands become thick and tortuous; and glycogen content is high. Vascularity is greatly increased.

The trophoblast secretes proteolytic and cytolytic enzymes, which permit these cells to invade the prepared endometrium, destroying vessels, glands, and stroma locally. *Implantation bleeding* may occur. This is small in amount, is not associated with pain, and disappears within 1 to 2 days, when the aperture in the endometrium is sealed over. Decidua covering this portion of

the ovum is the *decidua capsularis,* and that beneath the ovum is the *decidua basalis.* The remainder of the uterine cavity is lined by the *decidua vera.* During nidation, trophoblastic cells provide nutrition for the embryo, first by destruction and absorption of decidua and later by absorption of substances from maternal blood (Figs. 13-6 and 13-7).

DEVELOPMENTAL ANOMALIES

Normal growth and development of the fetus may be altered by a great variety of hereditary and environmental factors. These are outlined here and discussed elsewhere in the text. For a detailed description the reader may wish to refer to the work of Thompson and Thompson; Gerbie, Nadler, and Platt; or Simpson and co-workers.

It is important to realize the fact emphasized by Fraser that a minority of congenital malformations have either major environmental or genetic causes. Instead, complicated interactions between genetic predispositions and subtle factors in intrauterine environment form the basis for most malformations. Furthermore, abnormal embryogenesis can produce both gross structural alterations in any of the systems undergoing sequential interrelated actions during development of the fetus and functional derangements such as those re-

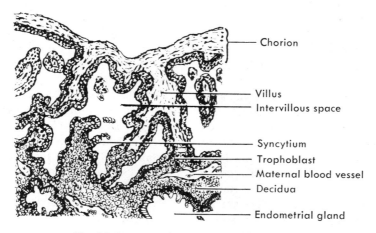

Fig. 13-6 Placental formation at 3 to 4 weeks.

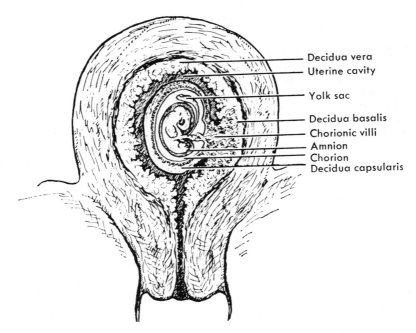

Fig. 13-7 Decidual, chorionic, and fetal growth at approximately 5 weeks.

flected in inborn errors of metabolism or mental retardation.

Congenital defects may be classified on the basis of intrinsic factors (that is, genetic defects) and extrinsic factors. The latter may have a temporary effect on development or may cause genetic alterations of a hereditary nature.

Intrinsic factors (genetic disorders)

Human genetic disorders are generally classified as follows.

Chromosomal aberrations. Chromosomal aberrations include deviations from the normal *chromosomal number* of 46 and abnormalities in the *chromosomal structure*. Numerical aberration involving an individual chromosome is termed *aneuploidy*, which results from *nondisjunction* as shown in Fig. 13-3. Nondisjunction aberrations are related to advanced maternal age. The striking autosomal example of this phenomenon is seen in Down's syndrome (trisomy 21). A second type

Down's syndrome (D/G) involves a structural abnormality, *translocation,* with the G chromosome translocated to the D group. This condition carries a greater risk for the offspring of a maternal carrier, and it is not age dependent.

Sex chromosomal aberrations also include both numerical and structural deviations. Klinefelter's syndrome (47 XXY) is one of the most common of those containing extra genetic material. Turner's syndrome (45 XO) represents a *deletion.* Autosomal deletions are generally lethal, and the conceptus is usually aborted.

Mosaicism is found in many syndromes associated with an abnormal chromosomal number. Adjacent cells from a given individual show different chromosomal counts; for example, patients with gonadal dysgenesis do not always show a chromosomal constitution of 45 XO. A variety of mosaics are now recognized in patients with this disorder, and these findings may modify the classic clinical picture to some degree, for example, 45

XO/46 XX or 45 XO/46 XX/47 XXX. Mosaicism involving autosomal abnormalities is seen in some cases of mongolism (46/47—trisomy 21).

Aberrations in chromosome morphology include the following: *Isochromosomes* represent genetic material that is split horizontally instead of vertically. The arms on either side of the centromere therefore are identical. If the short arm is lost, the functions carried on by the genes on the short arm are also lost. Certain cases of amenorrhea are believed to result from this abnormality.

X-linked disorders. There are now more than 150 recognized X-linked disorders, most of which occur in an *X-linked recessive inheritance* pattern with the male offspring of a female carrier being affected. Examples are hemophilia, Duchenne's muscular dystrophy, and X-linked agammaglobulinemia. *X-linked dominant inheritance* is rare because the male who has a single X chromosome is "hemizygous" rather than homozygous or heterozygous with respect to X-linked traits. Vitamin D–resistant rickets with hypophosphatemia is an example.

Single-gene disorders. There exist more than 930 autosomal dominant and 580 autosomal recessive single-gene disorders that represent a genetically determined biochemical disorder that results in a specific enzymatic block. These conditions are designated *inborn errors of metabolism.* Prenatal diagnosis can be made for a number of recognized disorders of this type that affect carbohydrate, lipid, amino acid, mucopolysaccharide, and other metabolic activities. Glycogen storage disease, Tay-Sachs disease, cystinuria, Hurler's disease, thalassemia, and sickle cell anemia are examples.

Multifactorial disorders. Multifactorial or polygenic disorders affect approximately 1% of neonates who have a normal complement of chromosomes and no apparent single-gene abnormality. These disorders are assumed to represent polygenic inheritance. Examples include disorders limited to a single organ system such as cardiac defects, neural tube defects (hydrocephaly, anencephaly, and spina bifida), cleft lip and palate,

omphalocele, pyloric stenosis, club foot, uterine fusion defects, and hip dislocation. The recurrence risk in subsequent offspring is 1% to 5%, which is far less than would be seen in a single gene defect but much greater than for the general population.

Extrinsic factors

The classic teratogenic period is from 17 to 57 days after conception. The exact time of exposure to a teratogen determines which organ system is affected. Although by 8 weeks after conception all major organ systems have been established, significant damage can still be done by continued exposure of the fetus during the second and third trimesters of pregnancy. Table 13-1 lists agents known to be noxious to the developing fetus. Chemicals such as lead, mercury compounds, biphenyls, and ionizing radiation are also teratogenic.

Antenatal diagnosis

The growing number of developmental disorders that can be diagnosed in utero has had a dramatic impact on genetic counseling. The obstetrician needs to be knowledgeable regarding the general spectrum of these conditions, the testing methods available for diagnosis, their risks, and the fact that there are options for treatment that must be fully and fairly presented by the counselor and decided on by the patient. Accuracy of diagnosis is so critical a matter that referral to a perinatal or genetic center should be advised. Methods used in diagnosis include the following.

Amniocentesis. Ultrasound-directed amniocentesis has proved to be a relatively safe procedure with a complication rate of less than 0.5%. Genetic amniocentesis is discussed in Chapter 2.

Chorionic villus biopsy. Chorionic villi are collected by transcervical aspiration under ultrasonic guidance. The procedure is carried out at 8 weeks of gestation and has the advantage of sampling rapidly growing trophoblast cells rather than slow-growing fibroblasts. Thus results of both chromosomal analysis and DNA probe studies are available in days rather than weeks.

TABLE 13-1 Drugs and environmental agents known to have adverse effects on the human fetus

Extrinsic factors	Effects
Infectious agents	
Cytomegalovirus	
Rubella	
Toxoplasma gondii	
Treponema pallidum	
Varicella	
Drugs	
Sex hormones	
Estrogens (synthetic)	Abnormalities of uterus, cervix, and vagina
Androgens	Masculinization of female fetus
Anticonvulsants	
Dilantin	Hydantoin syndrome (flat nasal bridge, epicanthic folds, hypertelorism, wide mouth and prominent upper lip, mental retardation, growth deficiency)
Trimethadione	Hydantoin syndrome
Valproic acid	Neural tube defects
Retinoids	
Isotretinoin	Abortion and multiple defects (hydrocephalus, microtia, and cardiac)
Anticoagulants	
Warfarin	Warfarin syndrome (nasal hypoplasia, bone stippling on radiologic examination, microophthalmia, optic atrophy, microcephaly, and mental retardation)
Antithyroid agents	
Methimazole	Scalp abnormalities
Antineoplastic agents	
Methotrexate	Multiple congenital anomalies
Alkylating agents	Limited data
Antibiotics	
Tetracyclines	Staining of teeth; inhibition of bone growth
Aminoglycosides	VIII nerve injury
Environmental agents	
Alcohol	Growth retardation, mental retardation, microcephaly, abnormal facies
Smoking	Increased low-birth-weight and premature infants
Cocaine	Prematurity, intrauterine growth retardation, abnormal neonatal behavior
Narcotics	Prematurity, intrauterine growth retardation, neonatal withdrawal

This technique is currently available in only selected centers and its safety is being evaluated by a national collaborative study. It is anticipated that the risk of abortion secondary to the procedure will be no greater than 1.5%.

Ultrasonography. Technologic advances in ultrasonography have minimized the need for x-ray film examinations. An increasing number of gross anomalies have been identified by this method, including anencephaly, limb defects, and omphalocele. Conditions such as fetal ascites and polyhydramnios that lead to suspicion of a fetal abnormality are usually readily detected with ultrasound visualization.

Fetal blood sampling. *Fetal blood sampling* can be accomplished safely under ultrasonic guidance. The umbilical vein or artery is punctured with a 25-gauge needle at its insertion into the placenta. Fetal blood is differentiated from maternal by the size of the red cells by utilizing flow cytometry.

Fetoscopy. Studies evaluating the use of endoscopy in examination of the fetus, umbilical cord, and placenta and its safety are only now beginning to emerge. The small area of vision provided by an endoscope is a limiting factor, but several fetal deformities have been accurately detected. Fetoscopy's unique capability of obtaining skin biopsy from the fetal flank or scalp for culture and analysis and cord or placental blood samples for diagnosis of hemoglobinopathies and other disorders has generated considerable interest.

DEVELOPMENT AND PHYSIOLOGY OF THE PLACENTA

The primitive *trophoblast* proliferates rapidly after implantation. Three layers appear, all of which are believed to be derived from this structure, which first develops as typical Langhans's s cells. These in turn undergo differentiation into an outer syncytial layer, the *syncytiotrophoblast,* and the proliferating Langhans's inner cell layer, the *cytotrophoblast,* underneath which is a thin layer of connective tissue, the *mesoblast.* The mesoblast provides, in effect, a supporting structure or central core of the villus and the site in which villous blood-forming elements and vascular structures make their appearance.

The outer syncytial layer is far more complex than was formerly recognized. Detailed study by electron microscopy reveals the so-called brush border to be a profusion of microvilli projecting from the free surface of the syncytium and of abundant highly developed structures—pinocytotic vesicles, lipoid droplets, and mitochondria—all providing structural evidence of secretory activity. This tissue is like a continuously streaming *ameboid mass* that is capable of actively engulfing substances, including maternal plasma, into the substance of the syncytium.

The fact that syncytial cells are rich in cytoplasmic ribonucleoproteins suggests that synthesis of proteins required by the growing embryo is one of the early functions of the trophoblast. Villee demonstrated that the early trophoblast has the *ability to synthesize glucose.* This function begins to decrease at about 12 weeks, when the fetal liver becomes capable of secreting glucose; in late pregnancy, placental synthesis disappears entirely. *Secretion of hormones* by the syncytiotrophoblast begins shortly after implantation, when chorionic gonadotropin appears; placental steroid hormones are secreted by cells of the syncytium.

During the first 2 to 3 weeks the chorionic villi are devoid of blood vessels. The villi project into the surrounding decidua and become filled with a core of mesoderm from the embryonal side. Islands of red blood cells develop in situ, and vascular channels appear. The villi in contact with the decidua basalis are exposed to a rich blood supply and multiply rapidly, becoming the *chorion frondosum,* or future placenta. Those in contact with the decidua capsularis become the *chorion laeve;* these eventually atrophy.

Formation of the amnion occurs while the chorion develops. Two small cavities appear in the embryonic pole. The dorsal amniotic cavity is derived from ectoderm, and the ventral yolk sac from entoderm. The amnion enlarges rapidly, causing disappearance of the extraembryonic coelom, and forces the body stalk, rudimentary blind allantois, vessels, and vitelline duct into a single pedicle, the beginning of the *umbilical cord.* The outer surface of the amnion applies itself to the inner aspect of the chorion. The two membranes are adherent but not fused (see Figs. 13-6 and 13-7).

Immunologic properties

The placenta corresponds to a natural homograft in that it is a transplant of living tissue within the same species, yet it does not normally evoke the usual immune response reaction to homografts, resulting in destruction and rejection of the graft.

The explanation for the apparent immunologic privileged status of the placenta is most related to the fact that all major class II histocompatibility antigens (HLA) are absent from trophoblastic tissue at all stages of gestation. However, the type I HLA antigens are expressed and may in fact be beneficial to the pregnancy. This expression may stimulate production of various tissue growth factors. Finally, there is a blunting of maternal lymphocyte function during pregnancy. Both decidua and trophoblast produce substances that affect lymphocyte function.

Circulation

By the fourteenth week the placenta is a discrete organ. Most of the villi lie free in maternal blood sinuses; anchoring villi are attached to the decidua basalis. At the points of anchorage, a band of fibrin is deposited as a result of degeneration of fetal and decidual cells. This "fibrinous layer of Nitabuch" is presumed to resist overinvasion of maternal tissues by chorionic epithelium. It is absent in placenta accreta.

Circulation of the blood through the intervillous spaces (choriodecidual spaces) is dependent on (1) maternal blood pressure, with resultant gradient between arterial and venous channels, and (2) uterine contractions. Ramsey's work on placental circulation has clarified certain problems hitherto unexplained. These problems are concerned with (1) delivery of oxygenated arterial blood with suitable mixing throughout the organ, (2) an allowance of sufficient time for metabolic exchange, and (3) venous drainage through multiple channels, which Ramsey demonstrated in the various areas at the base of the placenta, rather than through a single "marginal sinus." Ramsey contends that "marginal lakes" are actually the peripheral portion of the intervillous space lying within the placenta and that the course of the marginal lakes is discontinuous. This arrangement permits segmental "trapping" of blood when intervillous pressure is higher than that in endometrial veins and permits drainage when pressure is lower.

According to Ramsey, arterial blood enters the placenta from the endometrial arteries under a head of pressure. The incoming stream is driven up in fountainlike jet toward the chorionic plate. The villi act as baffles, mixing and slowing the stream. The force is gradually spent, and eventu-

ally the blood that has dispersed laterally falls back on multiple orifices in the basal plate, which connects with maternal veins. Further fall in pressure in the intervillous space results in drainage through the endometrial veins. The circulatory process is enhanced by myometrial contractions. Ramsey demonstrated these events convincingly by x-ray film study of the circulation in the placenta of the rhesus monkey (Fig. 13-8).

Transfer mechanisms

Oxygen and substances for nutrition of the fetus must pass from the intervillous spaces through the surface epithelium of the villus, the thin stroma, and the endothelium of its capillary. Carbon dioxide and waste products from the fetus are transferred in reverse order.

Normally, there is no direct connection between maternal and fetal circulations, but damaged villi occasionally break off into the maternal lakes and allow the escape of small amounts of fetal blood into the maternal circulation. Certain cases of Rh sensitization in which incompatible blood has never been given the mother and instances of ABO isoimmunization are related to this phenomenon.

Fetal growth is considerably greater than that of the placenta from the twelfth or fourteenth week to term. The placenta accommodates to greater demands (1) by increasing the surface area of the villi through arborization and (2) by thinning of the villus covering. Langhans's cells become thinned out but do not disappear. Many of these cells persist and continue to function throughout pregnancy; however, reduction in their number and in the size of the cells that persist leaves, in effect, a single layer of syncytial cells, thus increasing permeability.

Numerous factors, many of which are yet unknown, influence the *rate* of transfer of substances across the placental barrier. Materials of small molecular size such as electrolytes, water, uric acid, creatine, and creatinine can but do not always pass by simple diffusion. Many drugs, notably narcotics, barbiturates, general anesthetics, sulfonamides, and antibiotics, pass readily. How-

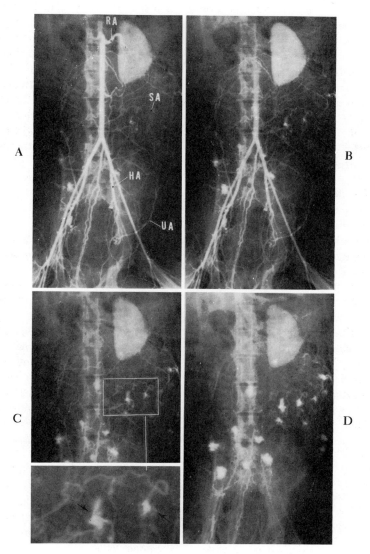

Fig. 13-8 Photographs of four of series of radiographs made at 3½ **(A)**, 4 **(B)**, 5 **(C)**, and 6 seconds **(D)**, respectively, after injection of radiopaque dye into right femoral artery of monkey 111 days pregnant. *Inset* in **C** is magnification (×4) of area enclosed in box. *Arrows* indicate spurts of dye into intervillous space. *RA,* Renal artery; *SA,* spiral artery of endometrium; *HA,* hypogastric artery; *UA,* uterine artery. (From Ramsey EM, Corner GW Jr, Donne MW, and Stran HM: Proc Natl Acad Sci USA 46:1003, 1960.)

ever, despite its obvious influence, the *size of the molecule* is not necessarily the determining factor in movement of materials in either direction. For example, the aldohexoses (glucose, mannose, and galactose) cross the placenta more readily than the ketohexoses (fructose and sorbose).

Facilitated diffusion is the process of speeding up the transfer of certain molecules, such as glucose. This is a form of *active transfer,* carried out by carrier molecules oscillating between the boundaries of the cell. In addition, the placenta achieves active transfer of a far more complex nature by the use of *enzymatic processes* requiring expenditure of energy. In some instances large molecules are broken down by enzymatic action before passage to the fetus, and in others enzyme transport is accomplished against the concentration gradient without alteration of the molecule. Histidine is an example of rapid active transfer of amino acid to the fetus. Fats, on the contrary, do not normally cross the placenta as such. Fats are broken down into fatty acids before passage and are resynthesized by the fetal liver. The passage without structural change of certain antibodies of higher molecular weight and diphtheria or tetanus antitoxin is not readily explained by any of the mechanisms mentioned. Visualization of the ameboid motion of syncytial cells has made tenable the concept of "droplet transfer," or *pinocytosis.* By this means, intact macromolecules may be transferred slowly across the membrane.

A great deal remains to be learned in regard to *selective activity* in placental transfer. It is evident that the various mechanisms operate in accordance with the particular demands of the fetus, but the placenta may act as governor. For example, after removal of the fetus, the intact placenta continues to extract iron from the maternal circulation at approximately the same rate as it did beforehand. Furthermore, in the absence of the normal fetal destination, the placenta is capable of storing iron. Normally, certain substances essential for fetal growth occur in higher concentration in the fetal than in the maternal circulation. These include calcium, inorganic phosphorus, free amino acid, nucleic acid, and ascorbic acid.

Bacteria do not normally cross the placenta. Thus the danger to the fetus of pneumonia in the mother is generally related to the degree of maternal anoxia rather than infection. Tuberculosis does not endanger the fetus in utero except when complicated by placenta tuberculoma that erodes into the fetal circulation. *Spirochaeta pallida* cross the placenta, but, fortunately, penicillin administered to the mother for treatment will also pass the barrier and provide fetal protection or treatment, depending on whether the fetus is already infected. Placental transmission of certain *viruses* has engendered justifiable cause for concern. Virus diseases are considered in Chapter 40.

Placental hormones

In addition to its function as an intrauterine organ of *respiration, nutrition,* and *excretion* for the growing fetus, the placenta functions as an *endocrine gland.* Maternal endocrine functions capable of providing a balance in the hypothalamic-pituitary-ovarian-endometrial axis to ensure ovulation and implantation are all-important in conception, but early in pregnancy endocrine regulation is taken over by the fetus and its accessory endocrine organ—the placenta. The interrelationships of fetal, placental, and maternal compartments are extremely complex, but under normal conditions the conceptus maintains regulatory control of its own private hormonal environment. Abnormal conditions arising in any of the three compartments may jeopardize the fetus. The obstetrician encounters many situations in which assessment of the fetus at risk is mandatory. Under these circumstances, a clear understanding of the physiologic and metabolic activities involved is of exceptional value.

The chief purpose of the dramatic changes in endocrine function during pregnancy is to maintain the pregnancy and to support the fetus in utero until the termination of the gestation period. Modern hormone assay techniques and methods for study of biosynthetic pathways and transfer mechanisms have evoked new concepts of endo-

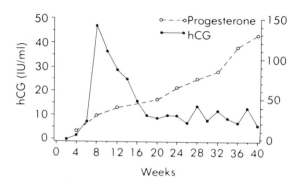

Fig. 13-9 Average values for hCG and progesterone during normal pregnancy. It is important to remember that there is a wide standard deviation at each gestational age and that the trend is clinically more important than the absolute value.

crine activity. Several of these are of practical significance.

The classic hormone excretion curves (Fig. 13-9) provide a valid overall view of alterations during normal pregnancy, although the excretion curves accepted as normal standards are oversimplified. Normal ranges are variable, and day-to-day changes in excretion rates are found for all measurable hormones; some of them show more pronounced deviations than do others. Means of assessing the actual amounts of the various hormones secreted by (1) maternal endocrine glands, (2) placenta, and (3) fetal endocrine glands are limited. Degradation, inactivation, and other metabolic changes are carried out in maternal, placental, and fetal organs. Thus excretion rates of the steroids, for instance, represent the end result of many complex actions. Furthermore, increases in one hormone may cause changes in production and metabolism of another.

From a practical point of view, the fetus and placenta should be regarded as a single functional unit, with the uterus as an integral part of this unit.

Human chorionic gonadotropin. Human chorionic gonadotropin (hCG) provides the basis for biologic tests for pregnancy. Like other glycoprotein hormones, hCG consists of two nonidentical subunits. The alpha subunit is similar to the alpha subunits of LH, FSH, and TSH. The larger beta subunit is hormone specific.

The precise site of production of hCG has been identified as the syncytiotrophoblast. It is found only there; none can be identified in cytotrophoblasts. It is likely that the syncytium, which is derived by differentiation from the cytotrophoblast, plays an active role in production rather than simply storage and transport of this material.

By about the eighth to tenth day after conception (1 to 2 days after implantation), hCG is present in detectable amounts; it reaches a peak 50 to 60 days thereafter. During this time the hormone augments and prolongs corpus luteum function and thus maintains the endometrial bed.

A glycoprotein, hCG in highly purified form exhibits an activity of 12,000 IU/mg. One international unit represents the reaction produced by 0.1 mg of a pure standard preparation. Ideally, sensitivity of laboratory test animals (immature rats) is attained when 1 IU just induces hyperemia in the rat ovaries. Then 1 IU equals 1 hyperemia unit.

The hormone is found in all maternal tissues, blood, urine, cerebrospinal fluid, saliva, and vaginal secretions as well as in placental tissue. Appreciable amounts are found in the amniotic fluid, but only trivial amounts in cord blood. The amount transferred to the fetus directly is not known; however, as the fetus swallows amniotic fluid, differences in concentration suggest that the fetus is able to metabolize hCG and convert the hormone to compounds with little or no biologic activity.

QUALITATIVE AND QUANTITATIVE ASSAYS. The immunnoassay is exceedingly accurate in diagnosis of pregnancy and has all but replaced the less sensitive bioassay as a straightforward pregnancy test. Immunoassays are often positive by the eighth day after conception and may remain positive for 8 days or longer after delivery, although most undiluted samples are negative within 2 to 3 days.

All of the simple immunoassay methods performed with urine samples on slide or in tube tests cross-react with LH. Elevated LH levels associated with the preovulatory LH surge or with the hormonal changes of the premenopausal period may produce false-positive results if the test is sufficiently sensitive. To prevent this problem, these tests are adjusted to reliably detect levels of hCG for normal pregnancy at 2 to 3 weeks after the first missed period. The desirability of earlier, more accurate diagnosis in the management of problems in both infertility and fertility has resulted in recent development of a number of new hormone-specific tests. (See tests for pregnancy, Chapter 2.)

Progesterone. Progesterone can be formed by all steroid-producing endocrine tissues: a small amount by the adrenal, much larger amounts by the corpus luteum, the major production by the placental syncytial cells, and an undetermined amount by the fetal adrenals. In the human adrenal gland, progesterone is an intermediary in the biosynthesis of cortisone and aldosterone. It can also be converted to androgens by adrenal glands and testes. In the ovary, progesterone can be converted to estrogens.

FUNCTIONS. The functions of progesterone are mainly the development and maintenance of the decidual bed.

METABOLISM. In late pregnancy the placenta produces about 250 to 300 mg of progesterone per day. Blood progesterone is metabolized rapidly primarily in the liver but also in the tissue at its site of action, and a considerable amount disappears into depot fat. The turnover time is approximately 3 minutes. Thus the excretion of the metabolic end product, pregnanediol, excreted in the urine as a glucuronide conjugate, averages only about 10% to 20% of the progesterone produced. On an individual basis, excretion rates of pregnanediol show a wide normal range. The mean value is about 50 mg/24 hours near term.

Although assays of progesterone or its end products are useful in certain gynecologic conditions, they have little, if any, use during pregnancy.

Estrogens. The amount of estrogens secreted in the third trimester is enormously increased over nonpregnant levels. The gestational increase in estrone and in estradiol is approximately one hundredfold, whereas the increase in estriol is one thousandfold as compared with individual nonpregnant values. Pregnancy levels drop precipitously after delivery or after intrauterine death of the fetus.

BIOSYNTHETIC PATHWAYS. In normally menstruat-

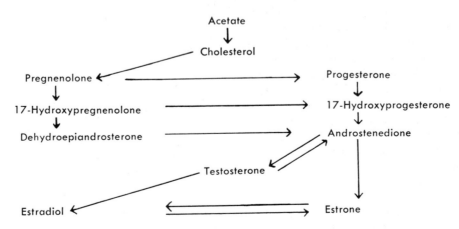

Fig. 13-10 Ovarian estrogen biosynthesis.

ing women the ovary produces estrogens de novo principally, if not entirely, in the biologically active forms of estradiol and estrone. Most of the estriol in nongravid women is derived from the peripheral metabolism of estrone and estradiol.

The diagram of ovarian estrogen biosynthesis (Fig. 13-10) is based on the results of ovarian tissue incubation experiments. With the use of radioactive substrates, these investigators obtained a yield of estrone plus estradiol amounting to 0.03% from acetate, 0.1% from cholesterol, 5.5% from progesterone, and 15% from androstenedione. (Note the increasing yield from intermediates closer on the pathway to the end product.)

The finding of these compounds in the incubation experiments indicates that any one or all of the biosynthetic pathways shown could be operative in human ovaries. Estradiol can be converted to estrone and vice versa, but estriol cannot be reconverted to either. Estradiol is by far the most biologically active, whereas estriol is biologically weak. The biologic activity of estriol is approximately $\frac{1}{100}$ that of estrone and $\frac{1}{500}$ that of estradiol.

The placenta does not synthesize estrogen de novo to any significant degree. If placental tissues were capable of producing estrogens, high excretion might be expected in cases of hydatidiform mole; however, such is not the case. Clearly, the placenta is not autonomous in this regard. Instead, a viable placenta, a healthy fetus, and an intact fetal circulation are necessary for continuous production of this steroid. When these three prerequisites exist, the placenta is highly efficient in conversion of steroid precursors to estrogens, mainly estriol. A much lower percentage of estriol is formed from conversion of estrone and estradiol in pregnant than in nonpregnant women.

Most of the estriol of late pregnancy is derived from primitive steroids such as pregnenolone and dehydroepiandroesterone. These precursors are produced by the maternal and the fetal organisms, the fetal adrenal playing a major role. This concept is supported by studies of pregnancies associated with an anencephalic fetus. Anencephaly is commonly associated with atrophy of the characteristically large fetal zone in the adrenal cortex,

which may be almost absent. Frandsen and Stakemann studied 15 cases of pregnancy associated with an anencephalic fetus and found critically low levels of estriol excretion in all but one. In the only exception the infant adrenals were of normal size and contained a well-developed fetal zone. Excretion of 17-ketosteroids, 17-ketogenic steroids, pregnanediol, and hCG was normal. All fetuses were alive at the time of urine collection for assay. The placentas were normal, and there were no signs of a disturbed fetal circulation.

These investigators further demonstrated the important role played by the fetal adrenals by simultaneous injection of fetal adrenal tissue and placental tissue in castrated mice. Vaginal smears for estrogen effect were obtained daily after injection of fetal adrenal tissue alone. Smears were negative in all tests. Negative results were also obtained after injection of placental tissue alone. But when both tissues were injected intraperitoneally or subcutaneously at the same time, estrogen-positive vaginal smears were obtained in 12 of 15 cases. It was necessary to use living fetal adrenal and living placental tissues to obtain a positive response. The foregoing clinical and laboratory data point to fetal adrenals as the source of precursors and to the placenta as the organ for their metabolism to estrogens.

The importance of an intact fetal circulation in estrogen production is illustrated by the experiments of Cassmer. Therapeutic interruptions carried out by the vaginal route at approximately 20 weeks' gestation were studied as follows: The umbilical cord was brought through the cervix, ligated, and sectioned. Fetus and placenta were allowed to remain in situ for 3 days. Within 24 hours, estriol values dropped more than 70% below previous levels. Progesterone values dropped only 20%, and hCG titers remained the same.

The fetus actively conjugates estrogens, mainly as sulfates and, to a far lesser extent, as glucosiduronates. This ability is acquired at an early stage—usually by 16 weeks' gestation. Sulfurylation can be performed by fetal liver, lungs, gastrointestinal tract, and skin. By means of conjugation, biologically active compounds are converted to relatively weak compounds. The efficiency of this action suggests that it may be an important step for fetal defense against excessive estrogenization.

Results of in situ perfusion studies with various radioisotopes may be summarized as follows: The primitive steroids are produced mainly by the fetus, principally the fetal adrenal glands. The main precursor is dehydroepiandrosterone sulfate (DHAS). In the nonpregnant state, most of the urinary estradiol is derived from estrone and estradiol. During pregnancy the pathway exists within the fetoplacental unit for direct conversion of DHAS to estriol without estradiol as an intermediate. This involves the formation of 16-hydroxy-DHAS, which takes place in the fetal liver. The placenta shows little 16-hydroxylating activity but strong enzymatic activity in the final conversion to estriol, the aromatization of ring A of the steroid nucleus. The conjugates are returned to the placenta and transferred to the maternal circulation, mainly as estriol. The estrogen is metabolized and conjugated in the maternal liver mainly as a glucosiduronate and is excreted largely in this form in the urine. The 24-hour urinary estriol values therefore can serve as an indication of fetoplacental function in the gravid woman whose hepatic and renal functions are within normal limits.

One other aspect of estriol metabolism of clinical importance is the amount found in amniotic fluid in late pregnancy. Most of the free estriol returned to the fetus from the placenta is sulfurylated by various fetal organs, but a small amount is conjugated as the glucosiduronate, presumably by the fetal liver. Both the free and the sulfate forms clear the amniotic membrane rapidly, but the glucosiduronate accumulates. Compromise of fetal hepatic function, which occurs in erythroblastosis, for example, before fetal adrenal activity is affected, may be reflected in low amniotic fluid estriol values, whereas maternal urinary estriol is still in the normal range.

The range of normal urinary estriol excretion per 24 hours is wide, beginning with approximately 1 mg at 18 to 20 weeks, gradually increasing to between 4 and 8 mg at 28 to 30 weeks, and between 8 and 25 mg or more at 38 to 42 weeks. The curve for any given individual rises gradually to term and is roughly correlated with the fetal weight. Daily fluctuations in estriol excretion values are common, but precipitous drops below 50% of previous peak values are warning signals.

Fetal welfare is threatened when values in the range of 3 to 4 mg are found in late pregnancy, and fetal death is almost inevitable if the daily excretion is below 2 mg.

Human placental lactogen. Human placental lactogen (hPL) is a growth hormone–like substance possessing lactogenic and luteotrophic properties, which like hCG is synthesized solely by the placenta. A polypeptide, hPL shows immunologic cross-reaction, although incomplete, with human pituitary growth hormone (hGH). Greater purification of these substances has revealed features of hPL as distinguished from hGH and elucidated their different roles in normal pregnancy.

Relaxin. The nonsteroid hormone relaxin appears in the blood of women early in pregnancy and increases gradually to term. Human relaxin is secreted by the human corpus luteum and possibly by the uterine decidua. Although it has a major influence on the myometrium of the guinea pig, it does not appear to be essential to the continuation of human pregnancy. Relaxation of the pelvic ligaments and connective tissues in various parts of the body may represent a relaxin effect or a synergistic action with progesterone. The role of endogenous relaxin in causing softening and effacement of the human cervix is also uncertain. However, its use in pharmacologic doses to effect cervical ripening prior to induction of labor is intriguing and currently undergoing investigation in primates.

Adrenocorticotropic hormone. The fact that corticosteroids are normally increased as pregnancy advances indicates an increased production of adrenocorticotropic hormone (ACTH). Large quantities of ACTH have been repeatedly recovered from placental extracts, although there is some controversy as to whether the placenta acts as a repository for storage of ACTH or is the actual site of the increased gestational production.

Adrenal corticosteroid hormones. Cortisol, cortisone, 11-dehydrocorticosterone, aldosterone, and several of their degradation products have been demonstrated in placental extracts. The increased amounts of cortisone found in these placentas can be accounted for by the volume of trapped blood present and by the ability of the placenta to concentrate this hormone. Experiments in administration of radioactive cortisone to pregnant women revealed a placental concentration 2.2 times that in the peripheral blood.

The increased binding capacity of plasma globulin during pregnancy probably accounts for the fact that the high levels of 17-hydroxycorticosteroids, which equal or exceed those normally found in Cushing's syndrome, do not produce symptoms of this disease because protein-bound cortisol is biologically inactive. Aldosterone excretion begins to increase early in the second trimester and rises gradually to term.

Excretion of 17-ketosteroids shows only a slight rise during normal pregnancy. Venning found elevated values similar to those reported by several other investigators only when the method used was nonspecific and metabolites of progesterone were included in the final reading.

Placental enzymes

Given the diversity of physiologic and metabolic functions required of the placenta for maintenance and development of the fetus, it is not surprising that a large number of enzymes should be demonstrated within its substance. Attempts have been made to correlate quantitative measurements of several enzymes in maternal plasma with normal and abnormal pregnancies.

Diamine oxidase (DAO, histaminase). Diamine oxidase is an enzyme involved in the degradation of histamine and other diamines such as cadaverine and putrescine. Histamine is important in the metabolism of all growing tissues and is found in especially high concentration in fetal tissues. DAO is considered an adaptive enzyme produced by the mother in response to the increased production of the specific amine by the fetus.

Southren and co-workers studied the relative DAO activity of fetal and maternal tissues and found maximal activity in the retroplacental decidua. No significant increase in maternal DAO is induced by trophoblastic tumors. Instead, the presence of a fetus is necessary to induce enzyme production. Measurable increases in DAO can be detected within 5 to 6 weeks after the last normal menstrual period, followed by a rapid rise until approximately 20 weeks, at which time

levels tend to plateau and drop sharply within 2 to 4 days after delivery. The clinical use of DAO levels in following the course of pregnancy is limited to the first half of gestation.

Oxytocinase (cystine-amino-peptidase). Oxytocinase activity increases between 50% and 100% during normal pregnancy. The source is presumed to be the syncytiotrophoblast. Serial oxytocinase levels in the maternal serum accurately reflect the functional capacity of the placenta, but they are not useful in conditions in which fetal jeopardy is caused by fetal factors per se.

Alkaline phosphatase. Maternal serum alkaline phosphatase activity increases progressively during the last trimester of pregnancy. Both maternal and fetal sources contribute to the increase. The placental alkaline phosphatase is heat stable, whereas all other alkaline phosphatase is not. Heat-stable alkaline phosphatase (HSAP) is apparently liberated during periods of placental damage similarly to the liberation of other cellular enzymes from infarcted muscle.

Term placenta

The *placenta at term* is a discoid organ, measuring 15 to 20 cm in diameter and 2 to 3 cm in thickness. Its weight is roughly 500 g, or about one sixth the weight of the infant at term except in patients with erythroblastosis or syphilis, in whom oversized placentas are characteristic. The maternal surface is divided by decidual septa into 15 to 20 *cotyledons*. The umbilical cord is usually inserted near the central portion of the smooth fetal surface. Fetal vessels fan out from the base of the cord. These disappear into the substance of the placenta near the periphery.

The *umbilical cord* averages about 55 cm in length. Cord measurements, however, may vary considerably in thickness and in length. Connective tissue with high water content (Wharton's jelly) surrounds the single umbilical vein and two arteries and facilitates desiccation after the cord is tied. The vessels are usually longer than the cord, become folded on themselves, and give rise to false knots, which do not interfere with circulation.

Amniotic fluid. The volume of amniotic fluid

usually averages about 50 ml at 10 weeks' gestation, 200 ml at 16 weeks, and approximately 1 L at 38 weeks, with a slight decline to term and significant decreases beyond 42 weeks. Water content is about 98%, and solids comprise 2%. Reaction is alkaline. The fluid is produced by several means. Early in pregnancy, transudation across the amniotic membrane covering the placenta and cord is the major source. As pregnancy advances, fetal urination and efflux of lung fluid make an increasing contribution. Fetal swallowing is the major source of fluid removal. Thus both the volume and content of amniotic fluid represents a balance between the various mechanisms of production and removal.

It should be clear that the amniotic fluid is not a static medium but is continuously renewed. With the use of radioactive sodium and deuterium oxide tracers, a complete sodium exchange in 15 hours and water exchange in less than 3 hours has been demonstrated.

Ultrastructure of the human amnion reveals the presence of an extensive system of canals and channels within the amniotic epithelium. These channels communicate with lateral and basal vacuoles and with the extracellular space. It is a logical speculation that existence of this system is an important factor in the movement of amniotic fluid.

The rate of transfer of various substances, including drugs, is of practical importance in the management of the complications of pregnancy and in the conduct of labor and delivery of the infant. Because deglutition and respiration occur in utero from the fourth month on, amniotic fluid may afford an additional route for transmission of various substances to the fetus.

CONSTITUENTS. Sampling of amniotic fluid has become one of the most important diagnostic procedures for assessing the fetal status. Information regarding Rh isoimmunization, maturity, genetic disorders, and certain metabolic disturbances can now be obtained by cytologic and biochemical examination of the fluid at various stages of pregnancy.

Genetic information can be obtained from cells found in the amniotic fluid. Such studies are usually performed at about the sixteenth week of gestation. *Prenatal sex determination* can be made accurately and is useful in counseling regarding pregnancies in women who are heterozygous for sex-linked recessive disorders such as muscular dystrophy or hemophilia. *Chromosomal aberrations* involving the number and structure of chromosomes such as Down's syndrome have been detected, as well as chromosomal breaks in fetal cells. *Biochemical studies* of cultures derived from cells contained in amniotic fluid allow prenatal diagnosis of an increasing number of hereditary metabolic disorders, including cystic fibrosis, mucopolysaccharidosis, galactosemia, glycogen storage disease, and congenital adrenal hyperplasia.

Prediction of neural tube defects can be made with a high degree of accuracy at 14 to 16 weeks' gestation by determination of amniotic fluid alpha-fetroproteins (AFP). Levels associated with fetal anencephaly, spina bifida, and myelomeningocele are approximately ten to twenty times the values found when fetal development is normal. However, high levels of amniotic fluid AFP are not entirely specific for neural tube defects, especially in late pregnancy when markedly elevated AFP values have been found in maternal serum, as well as in amniotic fluid in association with fetal death, impending fetal death, Rh isoimmunization, omphalocele, and duodenal atresia.

DIAGNOSIS OF FETAL MATURITY. The composition of amniotic fluid reflects the metabolic activity and function of various fetal structures such as lung, kidney, liver, and skin. Measurement of the following amniotic fluid constituents, all of which show characteristic changes during and beyond the thirty-fifth week of gestation, provide the most useful indices among many methods studied for prediction of fetal maturity.

Lecithin/sphingomyelin (L/S) ratio. Pulmonary maturity is dependent on the presence of sufficient amounts of surface-active phospholipids to prevent alveolar collapse with expiration. In the immature fetal lungs, sphingomyelin concentration is greater than that of lecithin, but at 35 weeks a rapid surge in stable lecithin occurs. An L/S ratio of 2:1 or greater provides a highly reliable prediction of pulmonary maturity in normal pregnancy.

Phosphatidylglycerol (PG), a minor component of surfactant phospholipids as compared with lecithin, appears in the amniotic fluid during the thirty-fifth week of gestation. Hallman and associates demonstrated a sharp rise in this substance from 35 weeks to term, when PG comprised 10% of the total phospholipids. The presence of PG correlates well with advancing fetal lung development and, with a favorable L/S ratio, provides the best assurance available of fetal pulmonary maturity.

DISORDERS OF THE PLACENTA

Variations in shape. The outline of the placenta may appear elongated or kidney shaped, or there may be two or three incompletely separated lobes. These lobes are termed *placenta bipartita* or *placenta tripartita,* respectively. Most atypical forms occur as a result of minor alterations in the blood supply or nutritional state of the decidua early in gestation, but they have no real clinical significance.

Placenta succenturiata (Fig. 13-11). One or more accessory lobes may be found at variable distances from the main placenta. Vessels from the accessory lobe traverse the fetal membranes and continue over the surface of the placenta proper. During the third stage of labor, these vessels may be torn, and the succenturiate lobe retained within the uterus. Postpartum hemorrhage or infection may occur if the detached tissue is not recognized and removed. Diagnosis can be made if inspection of the fetal surface reveals an open vessel at the placenta edge.

Placenta circumvallata (see Fig. 13-11). Occasionally, a white fibrous ring is visible on the fetal surface at a variable distance from the margin of the placenta. The ring is formed by a folding back of the amnion and of the chorion on itself, forming a double layer of fetal membranes at this site. This is presumed to occur when the early chorionic plate is relatively small. Later the villi at the periphery grow out laterally into the decidua vera. The fetal vessels do not extend to the margin of the placenta but instead terminate at the ring. In other respects the placenta is normal.

The incidence of abortion early in pregnancy and bleeding late in pregnancy or during labor may be somewhat increased in association with this condition, but in most instances the course of pregnancy and the condition of the infant are unaffected.

Placenta membranacea. Occasionally, the villi covering the decidua capsularis persist; continue to function; and form a large, thin, membranous placenta that entirely surrounds the fetal membranes. Its attachment therefore is not confined to one portion of the uterus but, instead, covers the surface completely. Separation or expulsion of a placenta membranacea during the third stage of labor may be incomplete, and consequently the danger of immediate or delayed hemorrhage following delivery is increased.

Placental infarcts. Avascular areas of varying size and consistency can be found in almost all placentas at term. Many of these are not true infarcts. White or yellowish nodules are commonly *fibrin deposits,* indicative of the aging process in the placenta.

Small foci of degenerating trophoblasts may initiate localized thrombosis of the surrounding maternal blood. Fine laminations of fibrin are laid down usually parallel to the chorionic plate. These were formerly designated as *white infarcts,* but the term is misleading because the process is primarily degenerative rather than vascular. Fibrin deposition is rarely so extensive as to jeopardize the fetus.

True placental infarcts are localized areas of necrosis caused by obstruction of the nutritional blood supply. Because the placenta receives its nourishment through the maternal rather than the fetal circulation, infarction occurs only when the maternal side is interrupted. On cessation of the blood flow to a cotyledon, the intervillous spaces become ischemic, and the villi deprived of nutrition undergo necrosis. The lesion may appear pale, red, or grayish, depending on its age (Fig. 13-12).

Rupture of thin-walled or brittle vessels with extravasation of blood into the decidua and subsequent hematoma formation may also cause ischemic necrosis. The placenta becomes detached in the area of bleeding, and, if separation is extensive, the fetus will die in utero. Although rupture of decidual vessels may occur without obvious cause, its occurrence is most common in patients with hypertension or chronic renal disease.

Calcification. Small areas of calcification are frequently found in the normal placenta. In some in-

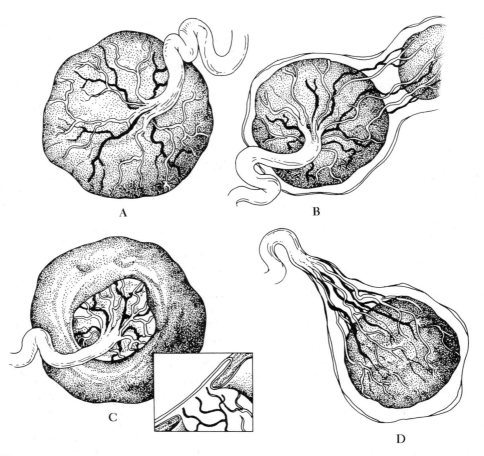

Fig. 13-11 Placental pathology. **A,** Normal; **B,** succenturiate lobe; **C,** placenta circumvallata; **D,** velamentous insertion of the cord.

stances the entire maternal surface feels sandy. Occasionally, firm white plaques are found in one or more regions. Like fibrin deposits, these are the result of degeneration of the villi, a late phase in the aging process of the placenta, and have no clinical significance.

Infection. Placental infection may occur in instances of prolonged rupture of the membranes with or without prolonged labor. An *amnionitis* develops first and may spread locally to the placenta. If the process extends through the chorionic vessels, general infection may develop in the fetus. Infection of the placenta is seldom primary, and infection resulting from a *maternal bacteremia* is relatively rare.

Syphilis frequently involves the placenta, causing thickening and clubbing of the villi. The number of villous blood vessels is reduced because of endarteritic changes. Grossly, the syphilitic placenta is large in relation to the weight of the infant and presents a greasy, yellowish surface with poorly defined cotyledons. Placental *tuberculosis* is uncommon even when the disease in the mother is advanced.

Cysts (Fig. 13-13). Cysts are frequently found on the fetal surface and arise from the chorionic membrane. They vary in size up to 5 to 6 cm and are filled with yellowish or bloody fluid. Cysts found deep in the substance of the placenta usually represent advanced de-

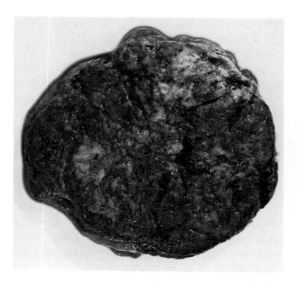

Fig. 13-12 Maternal surface of placenta showing white infarcted areas.

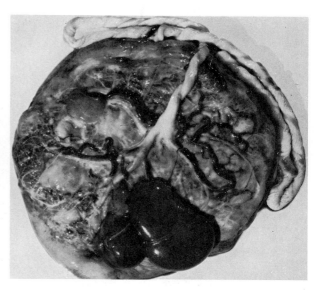

Fig. 13-13 Placental cyst.

generative changes in areas of fibrin deposition or in old infarcts.

Tumors. Neoplasms of the placenta are unusual. Of those observed, *chorioangioma* is most common. Hydramnios is often associated with these tumors.

ABNORMALITIES OF THE CORD

Variations in length of the cord between 35 and 70 cm are normal, the average length being about 55 cm. Complete absence of the cord is sometimes observed in connection with defects in the fetal abdominal wall. A *short cord* may delay descent of the fetus during labor and result in detachment of the placenta or, rarely, rupture of the cord with traction. A *long cord* predisposes to prolapse or cord entanglement. Tightening of loops about the neck or body of the infant during descent may gradually impair circulation and cause asphyxia. *True knots* are found occasionally in the cord, but unless these become tightened, fetal circulation is unimpaired.

Variations in insertion. The umbilical cord is usually inserted eccentrically but nearer the central than the peripheral portion of the placenta. A marginal insertion, designated *battledore placenta,* is relatively common

and unimportant. On the other hand, *velamentous insertion* of the cord is potentially hazardous to the fetus (see Fig. 13-11). Vessels separate from the umbilical cord and traverse the membranes for a variable distance before reaching the placenta. Tearing or rupture of the vessels during labor may exsanguinate the infant. If the vessels course over the dilating cervix in bulging membranes *(vasa previa),* pressure by the presenting part may cause fetal distress or asphyxia (Fig. 13-14).

Vascular anomalies. The cord should be checked at delivery for the presence of one vein and two arteries. A single umbilical artery is found in slightly less than 1% of cases, but this abnormality is associated with a high incidence of congenital anomalies of the newborn.

A specific type of arteriovenous shunt is seen occasionally in monozygotic twins; a fetoplacental transfusion syndrome is the result. The arterial donor twin is pale and dehydrated, whereas the venous recipient is plethoric, hypervolemic, and in greatest danger of cardiac overload.

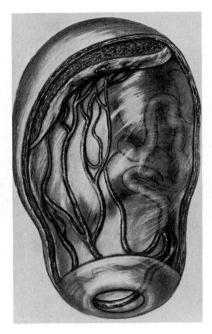

Fig. 13-14 Velamentous insertion of cord with vasa previa.

ABNORMALITIES OF THE AMNION

Hydramnios. The accumulation of amniotic fluid in excess of 2000 ml is considered abnormal. Hydramnios usually develops gradually, but in rare instances acute hydramnios occurs, and the uterus becomes remarkably distended within the course of a few days. The cause remains obscure, although various factors associated with this condition are recognized. *Fetal anomalies,* particularly those of the central nervous system and gastrointestinal tract, are more common if hydramnios is present. The occurrence of anencephaly, spina bifida, duodenal atresia, or tracheoesophageal fistula has led to the theory that an increased fetal output of fluid through the spinal fluid system or the urinary tract or failure of the fetus to ingest fluid may cause hydramnios. This theory does not explain the increased incidence of hydramnios observed with *maternal diabetes* or *erythroblastosis*. An abnormality in placental transmission of fluids from the fetal circulation or an abnormally functioning amniotic membrane may be responsible.

Symptoms are more pronounced with acute than with chronic hydramnios. The patient suffers from pain caused by overdistention of the uterus and abdominal wall, edema of the lower extremities, and severe dyspnea. The accumulation may be so rapid and so enormous that prompt evacuation is necessary to prevent maternal death.

Hydramnios should be suspected if the uterus appears larger than normal for the duration of pregnancy or if the fetal parts and fetal heart tones are indistinct. The condition must be differentiated from multifetal pregnancy. Diagnosis can be made with certainty by sonogram; at the same time certain fetal deformities involving the skull and skeletal part may be detected.

Further information can be obtained by *amniography*. This technique includes amniocentesis with removal of 25 ml of amniotic fluid under sterile conditions and insertion of 15 ml or, with severe hydramnios, 25 to 30 ml of contrast media such as Renografin-60 or Hypaque-M75. These solutions are hypertonic and may initiate labor. The fetus swallows and concentrates the material in the gastrointestinal tract. The x-ray film should be delayed and taken 1 to 2 hours after instillation of contrast material, when concentration in the gastrointestinal tract can provide information regarding gastrointestinal atresia or other soft-tissue abnormalities.

Medical treatment of hydramnios is generally ineffectual. The patient with chronic hydramnios and only mild symptoms should be kept as comfortable as possible with rest and should be permitted to go into labor spontaneously. Because contractions are sometimes of poor quality because of overdistention of the uterus, progress in labor may be slow, and the incidence of postpartum hemorrhage is increased because of atony.

Amniotomy becomes necessary if symptoms are progressive or severe. The cervix is usually effaced because of pressure. Rupture of the membrane should be carried out under aseptic conditions, and an attempt should be made to drain the fluid slowly. Free or rapid flow may encourage prolapse of the cord or a fetal part, and sudden reduction in size of the uterus may cause placental separation.

Removal of fluid by transabdominal aspiration or insertion of polyethylene tubing into the uterus has met with little success, as the fluid reaccumulates or labor ensues shortly thereafter.

Hydramnios developing in Rh-sensitized mothers or in patients with diabetes offers an unfavorable prognosis for fetal survival. If the gestation period is sufficiently advanced, delivery is often advisable, and preparations should be made for special care of the infant.

Oligohydramnios. Marked deficiency of amniotic fluid is associated with a marked increased in perinatal mortality. Oligohydramnios is defined ultrasonographically as a fluid pocket of less than 2 cm and is usually associated with obstruction of the fetal urinary system, congenital absence of or malfunctioning fetal kidneys, chronic, premature rupture of the membranes, or poor perfusion of the fetal kidney. This last circumstance may be related to hypoxia-induced redistribution of fetal blood flow and is an indication to consider prompt delivery. Oligohydramnios is seen in virtually all cases of the postmaturity syndrome and 90% of cases of intrauterine growth retardation (IUGR).

FETAL DEVELOPMENT

Organogenesis is largely completed by about the eighth week after fertilization. During this period the conceptus is designated the *embryo*, after which time it is called the *fetus*. The significant features of the various developmental stages are shown in Table 13-2.

The rate of fetal growth is proportionately more rapid in the early months of pregnancy. According to *Haase's rule,* the crown-heel length of the fetus in centimeters equals the square of the lunar month during the first 5 months, and in the last 5 months the length is equal to five times the lunar month of pregnancy.

Despite obvious difficulties in obtaining precise crown-heel measurements, the length of the fetus usually provides a more reliable index of gestation period than does the weight. The importance of an accurate estimate of fetal maturity is underscored by follow-up studies of "small-for-date" babies, "low-birth-weight infants," or intrauterine growth retardation problems. The most common cause is intrauterine malnutrition or fetal maldevelopment. Comparison of the newborn measurements with those of standard fetal growth charts

TABLE 13-2 Principal fetal characteristics at various developmental stages

Gestational age (weeks)	Crown-rump length (cm)	Weight (g)	Characteristics
12	6	14	Fingers and toes visible; appearance of ossification centers; intestines in abdomen
16	12	110	Sex revealed by external genitalia; appearance of respiratory movements and swallowing; lower limbs well developed
20	14	320	Vernix caseosa present; early toenail development
24	16	630	Fetal viability; skin wrinkled and red; fine lanugo hair over body
28	25	1000	Eyes partially open; eyelashes present
32	28	1700	Testes descending; body filled out
36	34	2500	Lanugo hair minimal; body fairly plump
40	36	3400	Prominent chest; fingernails to end of fingers; breasts protrude

such as that developed by Lubchenco and co-workers should be routine nursery practice.

Clinical evaluation of fetal growth rate is often difficult and is discussed in Chapters 20 and 29.

The *infant at term* measures 50 cm (20 inches) and weighs 3175 g (about 7 pounds). Little lanugo remains except over the shoulders. A variable amount of vernix caseosa covers the skin surfaces; this is a mixture of epithelial cells, lanugo, and the secretion of the sebaceous glands. Characteristic features of the fetal head, including suture lines, fontanels, and diameters, are of obstetric importance. The sutures and fontanels that serve as useful landmarks are the long *sagittal suture,* which separates the two parietal bones; and the *lambdoid suture,* which is between the posterior edge of the parietal bones and the occipital bone. The triangular space at the intersection of these two lines is the *posterior fontanel.* The *frontal suture* separates the frontal bones from each other, and the *coronal suture* separates the anterior edge of the parietal bones from the frontal bones. The large *anterior fontanel* is the diamond-shaped space at the junction of the sagittal, coronal, and frontal sutures (Fig. 13-15).

Respiration. Movements of the fetal chest wall have been recorded by ultrasound as early as the latter part of the first trimester of pregnancy. Rates range from 40 to 70 excursions/minute. Continuous tracings made before and during labor suggest that monitoring of human fetal breathing may be a useful adjunct to fetal heart rate monitoring. Fetal hypoxia and hypoglycemia are associated with a diminution in breathing movements and that the appearance of gasping has been noted in certain high-risk situations such as intrauterine growth-retarded babies during labor.

Circulation (Figs. 13-16 and 13-17). Initially the developing ovum derives nutrition from its own large cytoplasmic mass and then from the decidua

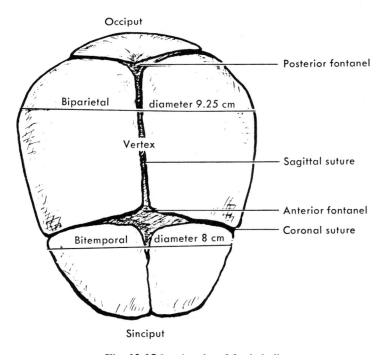

Fig. 13-15 Landmarks of fetal skull.

by activity of the trophoblastic cells. The vitelline circulation is functional in the third and fourth weeks and temporarily provides nourishment for the embryo from the yolk sac. Thereafter, connection is made between vessels developing in the chorion and those growing out from the fetus through the body stalk to establish the fetoplacental circulation.

Oxygen and nutrient substances pass from the maternal blood through the villi and are transported through small venules to the single umbilical vein. This divides at the liver edge. One branch empties into the portal vein, circulates through the liver, and enters the inferior vena cava through the hepatic vein. The larger portion passes directly to the inferior vena cava as the ductus venosus. In the right atrium, oxygen-laden blood coming through the inferior vena cava passes for the most part through the foramen ovale into the left atrium. Blood from the head region delivered by the superior vena cava is low in oxygen and tends to pass in a direct stream into the right ventricle. As the lungs are not functioning, most of this oxygen-low blood entering the

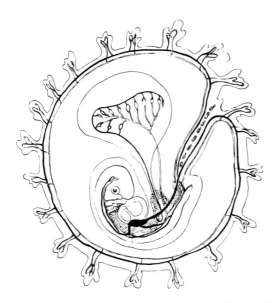

Fig. 13-16 Schema of vitelline and chorionic circulations.

pulmonary artery passes through the ductus arteriosus into the aorta and is mixed with blood of higher oxygen content pumped from the left side of the heart. In the fetus the internal iliac or hypogastric arteries send out large branches on either side, which traverse the lower abdominal wall to the umbilicus and continue through the cord as the paired umbilical arteries. Deoxygenated blood is thus transported back to the placenta.

Circulatory changes at birth (Fig. 13-17). As soon as respirations begin and the cord is clamped, circulatory changes occur:

1. The *ductus arteriosus* closes as the lungs begin to function. A large volume of blood is pumped by the right ventricle into the previously collapsed pulmonary arteries, thus reducing pressure within the lumen. The ductus arteriosus becomes occluded and forms the *ligamentum arteriosum*.
2. The *foramen ovale* closes as a result of increased tension in the left atrium and concomitant reduction in the right atrium. This is because of the increased volume of blood returned from the lungs as respirations are established and the diminished quantity of blood to the inferior vena cava when the umbilical cord is tied.
3. The functionless umbilical vein becomes the *ligamentum teres hepatis*.
4. The ductus venosus closes and forms the *ligamentum venosum*.
5. The obliterated umbilical arteries become the *obliterated hypogastric* or *lateral umbilical ligaments*.

Oxygenation. In the maternal circulation, arterial oxygen saturation is 96%, and venous oxygen saturation is 71%. Blood in the intervillous spaces is mixed, thus reducing the effective saturation.

In addition, oxygen diffuses through a wet membrane slowly. Oxygen passed to the fetus therefore provides only about 60% oxygen saturation. Fetal adaptation is effected by (1) high red cell count, (2) high hemoglobin values, and (3) differences in fetal hemoglobin as compared with the adult type. The oxygen dissociation curve of

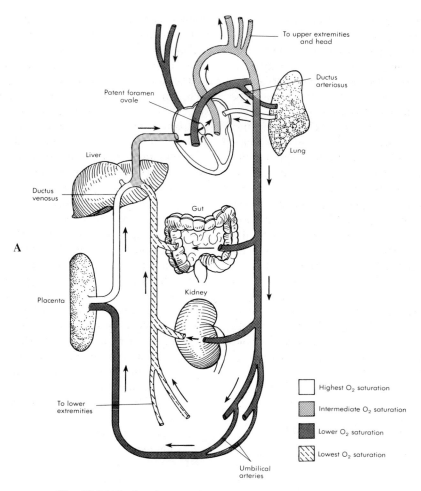

A

To upper extremities
and head

Ductus
arteriosus

Patent foramen
ovale

Lung

Liver

Ductus
venosus

Gut

Placenta

Kidney

To lower
extremities

Highest O₂ saturation

Intermediate O₂ saturation

Lower O₂ saturation

Lowest O₂ saturation

Umbilical
arteries

Fig. 13-17 Fetal and neonatal circulation. **A,** Circulation in utero.

fetal blood is shifted to the left, and, accordingly, uptake of oxygen at low gas tension is enhanced. Studies of the oxygen and carbon dioxide pressure gradients across the placenta support the hypothesis that these gases are transferred by diffusion in accordance with differences in pressure on either side of the membrane. Although the human placental membrane is wet and consists of three layers (syncytium, stroma, and capillary endothelium), it behaves like the lung.

Prystowsky, Hellegers, and Bruns obtained intervillous-space blood and umbilical vein and artery blood at cesarean section for comparison. They found an average oxygen tension of 47 mm Hg in the intervillous space, 30 mm Hg in the umbilical vein, and 18 mm Hg in the umbilical artery and oxygen pressure difference of approximately 24 mm Hg across the placenta. Carbon dioxide crosses the placenta more readily than oxygen and is found in higher concentration on the fetal than on the maternal side, with an average pressure gradient of 7 mm Hg.

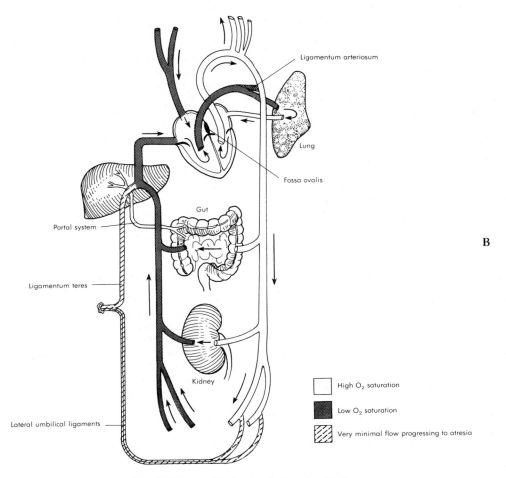

Fig. 13-17, cont'd B, circulation after birth.

It is important to recognize that the fetus possesses compensatory mechanisms that increase the margin of safety in coping with temporary periods of hypoxia, but even these have limitations. Glucose breakdown is the major source of energy, which under normal conditions includes an aerobic, as well as an anaerobic, phase. If the fetus is deprived of oxygen, it has an alternate pathway, entirely anaerobic and much less efficient, to meet requirements. In the normal pathway for glucose oxidation a total of 38 high-energy phosphate bonds are produced (eight bonds in the anaerobic and 30 bonds in the aerobic phase). In the absence of oxygen, pyruvic acid is reduced to lactic acid, using six of the eight high-energy phosphate bonds so that the net result is only two instead of 38 energy sources. An increase in hydrogen ion concentration and a corresponding decrease in base is the final result. The fetal blood pH and base deficit therefore should indicate the severity of fetal hypoxia or distress, and this is the premise on which the Saling fetal scalp blood examination is based.

Fetal blood volume averages approximately 85

ml/kg or about 300 ml at term, blood pressure averages 80/40 mm Hg, cardiac rate averages 120 to 140 beats/min, and cardiac output averages 10 to 12 ml/100 g/min, which is about three times that of a normal adult.

SUGGESTED READING

Apgar V and Patter EM: Transmission of drugs across the placenta, Anesth Analg 31:309, 1952.

Barr ML: Sex chromatin and phenotype in man, Science 130:679, 1959.

Bastide A, Manning FA, Harman C, Lange I, and Morrison I: Ultrasound evaluation of amniotic fluid volume: outcome of pregnancies with severe oligohydramnios, Am J Obstet Gynecol 154:895, 1986.

Berliner DL, Jones JE, and Salhanick HA: The isolation of adrenal-like steroids in human placenta, J Biol Chem 223:1043, 1956.

Blandau RJ and Rummary RE: Observations on the movements of the living primordial germ cells of mouse and man, Anat Rec 148:262, 1964.

Blechner JN, Stenger VG, Eitzman DV, and Prystowsky H: Effects of maternal metabolic acidosis on the human fetus and newborn infant, Am J Obstet Gynecol 100:934, 1968.

Bourne GL and Lacy D: Ultra-structure of human amnion and its possible relation to the circulation of amniotic fluid, Nature 186:952, 1960.

Cassmer O: Hormone production in the isolated human placenta, Acta Endocrinol 32(45):1, 1959.

Cheek DB, Greystone JE, and Niall M: Factors controlling fetal growth, Clin Obstet Gynecol 20:925, 1977.

Chez RA, Smith FG, and Hutchinson DL: Renal function in the intrauterine primate fetus, Am J Obstet Gynecol 90:128, 1964.

Dawes GS: Breathing before birth in animals and man, N Engl J Med 290:557, 1974.

Diczfalusy E: Endocrine functions of the human fetus and placenta, Am J Obstet Gynecol 119:419, 1974.

Doyle JB: Direct observations of ovulation by culdoscopy, Fertil Steril 5:105, 1954.

Elias S, Simpson JL, Martin AO, Sabbogha RE, Gerbie AB, and Keith LG: Chorionic villus sampling for 1st trimester prenatal diagnosis, Am J Obstet Gynecol 152:204, 1985.

Finn R: Survival of the genetically incompatible fetal allograft, Lancet 1:835, 1975.

Frandsen VA and Stakemann G: Site of production of estrogenic hormones in human pregnancy: hormone excretion in pregnancy with anencephalic fetus, Acta Endocrinol 38:383, 1961.

Fraser FC: Causes of congenital malformations in human beings, J Chronic Dis 10:97, 1959.

Grumbach MM, Kaplan SL, Sciarra JJ, and Burr IM: Chorionic growth hormone-prolactin (CGP): secretion, disposition, biologic activity in man, and postulated function as the "growth hormone" of the second half of pregnancy. In Sonenberg M, editor: Conference on growth hormone, Ann NY Acad Sci 148:501, 1968.

Hallman M, Kulovich M, Kirkpatrick E, Sugarman RG, and Gluck L: Phosphatidylinositol and phosphatidylglycerol in amniotic fluid: indices of lung maturity, Am J Obstet Gynecol 125:613, 1976.

Harris RE: Maternal and fetal immunology, Obstet Gynecol 51:733, 1978.

Head JR, Drake BL, and Zuckermann FA: Major histocompatibility antigens on trophoblast and their regulation: implications in the maternal-fetal relationship. Am J Reprod Immunol Microbiol 15:12, 1987.

Hendricks CH, Quilligan EJ, Tyler CW, and Tucker GJ: Pressure relationships between the intervillous space and the amniotic fluid in human term pregnancy, Am J Obstet Gynecol 77:1028, 1959.

Hill RM and Stern L: Drugs in pregnancy: effects on the fetus and newborn, Drugs 17:182, 1979.

Hutchinson DL, Gray MJ, Plentl AA, Alvarez H, Caldeyro-Barcia R, Kaplan B, and Lind J: The role of the fetus in the water exchange of the amniotic fluid of normal and hydroamniotic patients, J Clin Invest 38:971, 1959.

Lubchenco LO, Hansman C, Dressler M, and Boyd E: Intrauterine growth as measured by live-born birthweight: data from 24 to 42 weeks gestation, Pediatrics 32:793, 1963.

Page EW: Transfer of materials across the human placenta, Am J Obstet Gynecol 74:705, 1957.

Pierce GB Jr and Midgley AR Jr: The origin and function of human syncytiotrophoblastic giant cells, Am J Pathol 43:153, 1963.

Potter EL: Pathology of the fetus and infant, ed 2, Chicago, 1961, Year Book Medical Publishers, Inc.

Prystowsky H, Hellegers A, and Bruns P: Fetal blood studies. XV. The carbon dioxide concentration gradient between fetal and maternal blood of humans, Am J Obstet Gynecol 81:372, 1961.

Queenan JT, Thompson W, Whitefield CR, and Shah SI: Amniotic fluid volumes in normal pregnancy, Am J Obstet Gynecol 114:34, 1972.

Ramsey EM: What we have learned about placental circulation, J Reprod Med 30:312, 1985.

Ross GT: Clinical relevance of research on the structure of human chorionic gonadotropin, Am J Obstet Gynecol 129:795, 1977.

Scoggin WA, Harbert GM Jr, Anslow WP Jr, Riet BV, and McGaughey HC: Fetomaternal exchange of water at term, Am J Obstet Gynecol 90:7, 1964.

Simmons ER and MacDonald PC: Endocrine physiology of the placenta, Ann Rev Physiol 43:163, 1981.

Simpson JL: Genetic counselling and prenatal diagnosis. In

Gabbe SG, Niebyl JF, and Simpson JL, editors: Obstetrics: normal and problem pregnancies, New York, 1986, Churchill Livingston.

Simpson JL, Golbus MS, Martin AO, and Sarto GE: Genetics in obstetrics and gynecology, New York, 1982, Grune & Stratton, Inc.

Smith K, Duhring JL, Greene JW Jr, Rochlin DB, and Blakemore WS: Transfer of maternal erythrocytes across the human placenta, Obstet Gynecol 18:673, 1961.

Smith OW and Ryan KJ: Estrogens in the human ovary, Am J Obstet Gynecol 84:141, 1962.

Southren AL, Kolbayashi Y, Brenner P, and Weingold AB: Diamine oxidase activity in human maternal and fetal plasma and tissues at parturition, J Appl Physiol 20:1048, 1965.

Spellacy WN, Teoh ES, and Buhi WC: Human chorionic somatomammotropin (HCS) levels prior to fetal death in high-risk pregnancies, Obstet Gynecol 35:685, 1970.

Thompson JS and Thompson MW: Genetics in medicine, ed 3, Philadelphia, 1980, The WB Saunders Co.

Tremblay PC, Sybulski S, and Maughan CB: Role of the placenta in fetal malnutrition, Am J Obstet Gynecol 91:597, 1965.

Tyler ET: Physiological and chemical aspects of conception, JAMA 153:1351, 1954.

Venning E: Adrenal function in pregnancy, Endocrinology 39:203, 1946.

Villee CA: Regulation of blood glucose in the human fetus, J Appl Physiol 5:437, 1953.

Vosburgh GJ, Flexner LB, Cowie DB, Hellman LM, Protor NK, and Wilde WS: The rate of renewal in women of the water and sodium of the amniotic fluid as determined by tracer techniques, Am J Obstet Gynecol 56:1156, 1948.

Wislocki GB and Bennett HS: Histology and cytology of the human and monkey placenta with special reference to the trophoblast, Am J Anat 73:335, 1943.

Wynn RM and Davies J: Comparative electron microscopy of the hemochorial placenta, Am J Obstet Gynecol 91:533, 1965.

Zarrow MX, Holmstrom EG, and Salhanick HA: The concentration of relaxin in the blood serum and other tissues of women during pregnancy, J Clin Endocrinol 15:22, 1955.

14

John H. Mattox

Infertility

Objectives

RATIONALE: Infertility affects an estimated one out of every six couples; the incidence may be increasing. As many as one-fifth of the visits to the gynecologist's office may involve the management of this problem. The etiology is found more frequently when evaluating female versus male factors. Because of the importance of reproduction, it is critical to have a working knowledge of the diagnosis and therapy of infertility.

The student should be able to:

A. Define *infertility*, both primary and secondary.
B. List four possible etiologies of infertility.
C. Describe an appropriate test to evaluate each cause.

From the beginning of recorded time the problem of the barren marriage has played a major role in the lives of humans. Many ancient religious rites and social practices are specifically concerned with fertility and sterility. Magic potions and incantations are still used by primitive peoples to enhance the reproductive capacity of newlywed couples.

A frequently quoted estimate is that *one out of every six couples* in the United States is involuntarily childless, and there is concern that the problem is increasing in magnitude. The *fertility rate,* the number of live births per 1000 women of childbearing age, 15 to 45 years, has declined over recent decades and at the present time women are delaying childbearing. The number of women having their first child after 30 years of age is increasing.

Concomitantly, there have been quantum strides in the knowledge of reproductive physiology, which have served to increase the therapeutic opportunities in areas such as ovulation induction, microsurgery, and in vitro fertilization.

In order to maintain an appropriate perspective of reproductive biology, it should be recalled how inefficient the human reproductive process is. Approximately 40% of fertilized ova are lost. The generally accepted incidence of clinically recognized spontaneous abortion is 15%; approximately 7% of infants are born prematurely, and 3% to 4% have a major or minor anomaly.

DEFINITIONS

Infertility can be diagnosed if a woman has not been able to conceive during a period of 1 year of unprotected intercourse. Monthly *fecundability* (conception rate) is approximately 20%, but this is age dependent. More than 60% of normal couples who are having unprotected coitus regularly will conceive within 6 months, about 90% within 1 year, and the remainder will be pregnant by the end of the second year.

Infertility is considered to be *primary* if conception has never occurred; it is *secondary* if there has been at least one pregnancy before the present difficulty. *Sterility* implies that conception is impossible and the causative factor is irremediable.

ESSENTIAL FACTORS FOR REPRODUCTION

Normal fertility is dependent on many factors in both the man and the woman. It is appropriate to consider the couple as the "biologic unit" of reproduction. The male must produce a sufficient number of normal, motile spermatozoa that can enter the urethra through patent pathways to be ejaculated and deposited at the appropriate time for fertilization. After deposition, the male gametes must be able to penetrate and be sustained in the cervical mucus. Following *capacitation* and *acrosomal reaction,* the preparation of the spermatozoa for fertilization, they must ascend through the uterine cavity into the fallopian tube to meet the ovum.

The female must produce a healthy fertilizable ovum that enters the fallopian tube and becomes fertilized within a period of hours. The conceptus must be transported through the tubal lumen to the uterine cavity. There it must implant itself in endometrium that has been prepared to

receive it. The embryo then must grow and develop normally. This entire process requires about 5 days.

Human sperm, while capable of existing for long periods of time in the upper genital tract of the female, are thought to maintain their fertilization potential for only about 48 hours. It is believed that a healthy ovum can be fertilized for 24 hours.

If any one of these essential processes is defective or impeded, infertility may result.

CAUSES

Although the woman of an infertile couple usually consults the physician first, it is obvious that she is not necessarily totally responsible for infertility. A male factor is either the sole cause or is an important contributing cause in about 30% to 40% of infertile couples.

Cause of infertility	(%)
Male factor	40
Tubal factor	25
Ovulatory disorder	20
Cervical factor	15
Miscellaneous	5
Unknown	5

On the basis of available literature, these estimates may vary from clinic to clinic. In approximately 15% to 20% of couples, several factors are responsible, which increase patient frustration and make therapy more complex.

Faulty spermatogenesis and insemination. Like ovulation, the production of male gametes depends not only on the integration of hormone signals along the hypothalamic-pituitary-gonadal axis but also on the intragonadal hormone action. The intratesticular concentration of androgens and the relationship to specialized androgen-binding proteins is critical. The entire process from the formation of the primitive germ cell to the ejaculation of viable motile sperm takes approximately *3 months. Faulty spermatogenesis* may be the result of a number of congenital or acquired causes, some of which may be apparent after taking a history and performing a physical examination.

However, a significant number of infertile males have no clear antecedent information or genital abnormalities that would indicate a cause. About 25% of infertile males will demonstrate *oligozoospermia* (less than 20 million spermatozoa/ml); the cause is illusive, and therapy in this group of patients is disappointing. If severe oligozoospermia (less than 5 million sperm/ml), *azoospermia* (no sperm), or *aspermia* (no semen produced) is identified, more extensive assessment should be considered, including appropriate hormone studies, a vasogram, chromosomal analysis, and perhaps testicular biopsy.

A *unilateral or bilateral undescended testis,* regardless of the time of correction, can result in semen quality lower than that produced by normal males. *Significant trauma,* which could result in a break in continuity of the testicular tubule structure, can result in the formation of antisperm antibodies. Although *mumps orchitis* experienced before puberty does not appear to affect spermatogenesis, orchitis after puberty is not unusual and can seriously damage fertility. A history of *infection* such as nonspecific urethritis and chronic prostatitis or *prior genital tract surgery* such as a hydrocelectomy, repair of testicular torsion, or herniorrhaphy have all been associated with defective semen production.

Males with *gonadal dysgenesis* (Klinefelter's syndrome) may produce no sperm even though their Leydig cells are normal. *Hypogonadotropic hypogonadism with anosmia* (Kallmann's syndrome) and *severe hypothyroidism* are all associated with azoospermia. Certain medications may have a deleterious effect on sperm production. Males who were exposed to *DES* while in utero may have structural abnormalities of the ejaculatory system, as well as deficient spermatogenesis. *Nitrofurantoin* has been associated with deficient sperm production, and certain medicines to treat hypertension can result in impotence. Excessive use of *alcohol, nicotine,* or *marijuana* can all significantly alter the production of sperm. *Severe pyrexia* has resulted in transient oligozoospermia. Although great emphasis has been placed on the role of high scrotal temperature induced by constrictive underwear or long, hot baths, it is unlikely that these life habits in moderation significantly hamper fertilizing capability of an otherwise normal male. A *varicocele* has been assigned a major etiologic role in infertility. Although it is clear that reduced sperm motility may be observed and ultimately corrected following varicocelectomy, fertility is not necessarily improved. Therefore the etiologic role of the varicocele remains unclear.

Although it is essential that normal spermatozoa be present for fertilization, it is difficult to diagnose infertility accurately on the basis of sperm density alone. MacLeod and Gold found in 1951 that 5% of 1000 fertile males had counts of less than 20 million sperm/ml. There have been several additional studies to demonstrate that the normal count of fertile males is declining; the number of fertile males with counts of 20 million sperm/ml is 15% to 20%. The cause and significance of this observation are unclear.

Although sperm count, motility, and morphology are important, a major issue to be addressed is that of sperm function. Simply, can the sperm traverse the female genital tract and fertilize an ovum? *Cervical mucus penetration studies* with the use of bovine cervical mucus are presumed to complement the semen analysis. In 1976 Yanagimachi, Yanagimachi, and Rogers described a method, the *sperm penetration assay,* for evaluating human sperm penetration of specially prepared zona-free hamster ova. Cases have been described in infertile men whose sperm concentration and motility were normal but whose sperm were unable to penetrate hamster ova.

Faulty sperm transmission can be a cause of infertility. *Impotence* induced by medication or for psychogenic reasons will obviously prohibit pregnancy. The number of spermatozoa and volume of the ejaculate are definitely decreased with *frequent* (daily or greater) *coitus.* Optimum timing that allows for the replenishment of healthy sperm and adequate seminal plasma is approximately 36 to 48 hours. *Severe hypospadias or obstruction* caused by scarring of the epididymis, vas deferens, or urethra following infection may also interfere with insemination; the most frequent organism is *Neisseria gonorrhoeae*. If the penis is abnormally short, buried in fat, or malformed, emission may take place out of the vagina. Premature *ejaculation* may produce the same results. In the female, *dyspareunia, vaginismus,* or an *intact hymen* may prevent intromission and a normal deposition of the ejaculate.

Tubal factor. The fallopian tube is not merely a conduit. Although tubal patency is essential for fertility, the ascent of spermatozoa and the passage of fertilized ova require physiologic support. *Tubal obstruction,* either partial or complete, has been a cause in about 25% of women who fail to conceive. Although tubal closure is more likely caused by endosalpingitis that can be gonoccocal, chlamydial, or polymicrobial in origin, congenital anomalies are also a possibility. Tubal infertility is increased following *appendicitis,* particularly if rupture has taken place; infection associated with use of an *intrauterine device;* and pelvic surgery, particularly *ovarian wedge resection.* Peritubal scarring and immobilization of this structure can occur with *endometriosis* or *perisalpingitis* associated with a puerperal infection. Therefore mucosal damage and fimbrial compromise, as well as the kinking and mobilization that occurs from perisalpingeal involvement, can occur following infection.

After a clinically documented episode of salpingitis, a woman has an 11% to 12% chance of being infertile. After two episodes the figure increases to 23%, and after three or more episodes it is 54.3%. It has been estimated that nearly 300,000 women in the United States have been rendered sterile by salpingitis as of the year 1990.

Disorders of ovulation. An abnormality of ovulation is responsible for infertility in approximately 20% to 25% of women. The finely orchestrated events resulting in the development of a normal ovum, its periodic extrusion from the follicle, and the cyclic secretion of adequate amounts of estrogen and progesterone by the cor-

pus luteum are essential for normal fertility. In all cases of anovulation or oligoovulation, the underlying endocrine disorder has altered the hypothalamic-pituitary-ovarian interrelationship. Women who have complete absence of ovarian function as in *gonadal dysgenesis* or *premature ovarian failure* from whatever cause can be considered to be sterile, but with the possibility of donor ovum or a donor embryo these patients may have children. Although *ovarian androgen excess* (polycystic ovary syndrome) is a relatively common cause of infertility, hypothyroidism is not. *Hyperprolactinemia,* either tumor- or nontumor-related, usually produces anovulation. For a more thorough description of the disorders of ovulation, see Chapter 8. *Luteal phase deficiency,* which is found in 2% to 3% of infertile couples, is discussed in Chapter 16.

Luteinized unruptured follicle syndrome (LUF) is an uncommon cause and is characterized by the biochemical events of a normal ovulatory cycle in which the ovum is not extruded from the dominant follicle. This diagnosis is relatively difficult to make except by laparoscopy; no *stigma* can be identified on the follicle that supposedly released an egg. Lack of dominant follicle collapse assessed by ultrasonography is strong circumstantial evidence. This syndrome has been associated more commonly with endometriosis; the cause is unknown.

Cervical factor. Abnormalities in the structure or the function of the cervix are present in 10% to 15% of infertile couples. *Obstructive lesions of the cervix* such as large polyps, pedunculated leiomyomata, congenital atresia, or stenosis following cauterization or cryotherapy may interfere with ascent of spermatozoa. *Alterations in the cervical mucus* can be the result of a hormonal deficiency, a chronic infection, or medication. It is in the preovulatory cervical mucus that the sperm must undergo the process of *capacitation.* It is believed that *certain bacteria are lethal to spermatozoa.* Mycoplasma hominis infections were once thought to be an important factor in infertility. They are probably more associated with habitual abortion than with a failure to conceive.

Whether or not *chlamydial* infection plays any role at the level of the endocervix remains to be determined.

As ovulation approaches and the peak of estrogen production is reached, the cervical mucus secretion is increased and can be copious. Occasionally, certain women find this annoying. The mucus is thin and clear and can be drawn into threads 10 to 12 cm long, *spinnbarkheit*. Very few vaginal epithelial or white blood cells can be seen at this time, and if the mucus is allowed to dry on a slide, a pronounced *ferning* pattern is evident. The cervix not only is a source of cervical mucus production but also forms a *reservoir* in which sperm can live for many hours after deposition and from which they can be dispatched to the upper tract to penetrate an egg. It is this concept of the reservoir that represents the basis for the postcoital test.

Uterine factor. Malformations, malpositions, and tumors of the uterus *do not* often interfere with conception, but they may occasionally be a factor in faulty nidation and early abortion. Movable, nontender retrodisplacement of the uterus is not a factor in infertility; most of the time this should be considered a normal finding. *Submucous myomas* may obstruct the uterine ends of the tube and thus prevent fertilization or may distort the uterine cavity and interfere with nidation. Women who have been exposed to diethylstilbestrol (DES) while in utero may have characteristic cervical, uterine, and tubal deformities that can interfere with conception and lead to abortion, ectopic pregnancy, or premature labor.

Miscellaneous factors. *Chronic infections, debilitating diseases*, and *severe nutritional deficiencies* may alter the function of both male and female gonads and thus reduce fertility. *Advancing age* also may play a role; in women, fertility reaches a peak between 20 and 30 years of age and then slowly declines until the menopause. Anovulatory cycles are common in the premenopausal period.

It has long been recognized that impotence, premature ejaculation, vaginismus, and dyspareunia are likely to be associated with *psychologic dysfunction*. An example is repeated failure to have intercourse during the fertile period because of recurrent minor illness, because the woman or man is "too tired," or even because of periodic dyspareunia, vaginismus, or impotence. Other causes for impotence must be sought; medicine usage should be reviewed, and a prolactin level should be obtained.

Both men and women develop antibodies against the numerous antigens in seminal fluid and spermatozoa, but the exact mechanism whereby antisperm antibodies result in infertility is unclear. The fact that antibodies can be detected in serum does not mean that they are responsible for infertility; women and men with antisperm antibodies can achieve a pregnancy. The higher the titer of sperm antibodies, the more plausible the diagnosis of "immune infertility" becomes. It appears that a small percentage of cases of unexplained infertility may be caused by antisperm antibodies.

INVESTIGATION OF THE INFERTILE COUPLE

The investigation of infertility must be conducted systematically, according to a planned program, and within a brief time frame. Because multiple factors are common, the study of both partners should be carried out in its entirety, even though conditions that obviously would impair fertility are detected early in the investigation. Both husband and wife must be interested in the solution of their problem. The plan of study, the time, and expense involved should be explained to them during the first interview to ensure full cooperation and to prevent future misunderstandings.

The physician must not only be prepared to conduct the basic medical investigation but also be willing to expend the time and energy to deal with the couple's emotional distress. These patients, usually the women more than the men, can be frustrated, angry, and depressed. On occasion, psychotherapy should be recommended. The basic studies can usually be completed within 3 or 4 months.

INFERTILITY HISTORY

Woman

Age: Race: Religion:

Occupation:

Years of marriage: Previous marriage

Duration of involuntary infertility:

Past history   *Present history*

1. Medical   1. General
    Sexually transmitted disease   Habits
    Endometriosis   Diet
    Tumors   Work and health status
    Other medical problems   Menstrual cycle
2. Surgical   2. Sexual
    Pelvic operations   Contraception
    Appendectomy   Frequency of coitus
3. Obstetrics   Postcoital practices
    Prior pregnancies including ectopics and   Libido
    abortions   3. Personal
    Previous infertility evaluation   Motivation for childbearing
4. Menstrual history   Attitude toward partner
                                       Career aspirations

Man

Age: Race: Religion:

Occupation:

Years of marriage: Previous marriage

Past history   *Present history*

1. Medical   1. General
    Sexually transmitted infection   Diet
    Mumps orchitis   Bathing habits
    Varicocele   Work and health status
                                       Medications and drugs
2. Surgical   2. Sexual
    Herniorrhaphy   Frequency of coitus and technique used
    Hydrocele   Premature ejaculation
    Orchiopexy   Adequacy of erection
    Injury to genitals   Timing of coitus
                                  3. Personal
                                       Motivation for childbearing
                                       Attitude toward partner
                                       Career aspirations

A complete history and physical examination of both partners

History. The form on p. 177 is a useful guideline in obtaining important fertility information.

Physical examination. A complete general physical and genital examination should be performed on each partner.

Evaluation of the semen

The semen examination is one of the most important parts of the infertility study, as the man is often responsible for failure to achieve pregnancy. A complete semen analysis and study of the effects of cervical secretions on sperm motility and survival will provide the basic information necessary for evaluating the male. A single analysis may be inconclusive because the sperm count varies from day to day and is dependent on emotional, physical, and sexual activity. Three specimens at monthly intervals should usually be examined.

Semen analysis. The specimen should be collected by ejaculation into a clean, wide-mouthed, screw-top plastic container after masturbation following a 2- or 3-day period of abstinence from intercourse. Couples who cannot accept this method can collect the semen in a specialized condom. The specimen transported to the laboratory within 1 hour of its emission. No particular precaution need be taken to control the temperature, except that excessive heat and cold should be avoided.

Following are the standards for normal male semen analysis as determined by the World Health Organization:

Volume	2-6 ml
pH	7-8
Viscosity	Liquefaction within 30 minutes
Sperm concentration	20-250 million/ml
Sperm motility	>50% within 1 hour of collection
Mobility (quality of motility)	3-4+
Morphology	>60% normal oval sperm

In addition, there should be no significant sperm agglutination or pyospermia. Special staining is required to differentiate between leukocytes and immature sperm.

Determination of tubal patency

The usual test for the study of tubal patency is dependent on the injection of a radiopaque substance through the cervicouterine canal and the tubes into the peritoneal cavity. If properly performed, the tests provide accurate information concerning tubal structure and should, unless contraindicated, be included as a part of every infertility study. The assumption is made that tubal patency is equivalent to normal function. These two characteristics are not necessarily the same.

Tests for patency should never be performed in the presence of acute infections of the vagina, cervix, or tubes or during any episode of uterine bleeding, since at that time the gas or the contrast medium may enter the open blood vessels. If pregnancy is suspected, tests for tubal patency should be delayed until the diagnosis can be definitely eliminated.

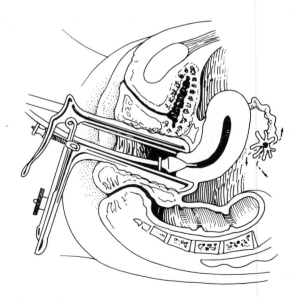

Fig. 14-1 Hysterosalpingography. Sagittal section showing technique. Contrast media flows through intrauterine cannula and out through tubes, the cervix being closed by a rubber stopper.

Hysterosalpingography. X-ray film visualization of the uterine cavity and tubal lumina after the injection of radiopaque material is the *preferred test* to evaluate the infertile female (Figs. 14-1 and 14-2). With this procedure, the site of tubal obstruction can be located accurately, and valuable information concerning the presence of tubal abnormalities such as hydrosalpinx or fixation from adhesions is provided. It also is possible to demonstrate small submucous fibroids or other congenital or acquired defects that may be present in the uterine cavity.

If the hysterosalpingogram is normal, the patient has about a 75% chance of having normal pelvic structures and no peritubal involvement. To replace this valuable test by laparoscopy and dye instillation as a routine initial approach negates the diagnostic effect and the therapeutic value, increases the risk to the patient, and is not cost-effective.

Water-soluble media are preferable to oil-soluble types because they are absorbed from the peritoneal cavity rapidly. A small amount of medium is injected, under fluoroscopic control, to fill the normal uterine cavity without distending it. This may outline small irregularities that would be obscured by a larger amount. Additional contrast medium, which should distend the uterus and flow through the tubes, is then injected.

Laparoscopy. Direct observation of the passage of methylene blue dye from the uterus through the fimbriated ends of the tubes is possible with the laparoscope and may be used for the determination of tubal patency by those experienced in the use of the instruments. An added advantage of this method is it provides an opportunity for direct visualization of the pelvic structures, supplementing the other methods for evaluating normalcy.

Disorders of ovulation

The production of normal ova and their release from the ovary, as well as their pickup by the fallopian tube, are primary requirements for female fertility. Documentation of when ovulation occurs is an important part of an infertility investigation. The majority of clinical tests used to assess ovulation are indirect and determine more specifically

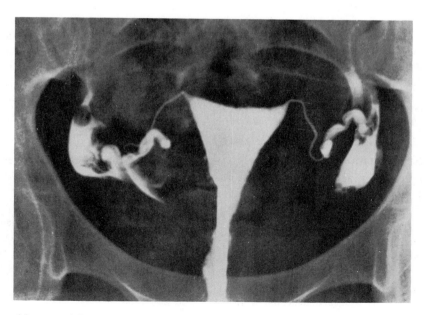

Fig. 14-2 Normal hysterosalpingogram showing passage of radiopaque material through fimbriated ends of tubes.

whether or not *progesterone* is secreted in significant concentrations.

Ovulation probably is occurring if the *basal body temperature curve is typically biphasic* with a sustained rise of at least 0.6° F during the last 2 weeks of the cycle (Chapter 2). *Luteal phase deficiency* can be suspected if the thermal rise is maintained for less than 11 days.

The adequacy of progesterone secretion can be estimated by *a serum progesterone assay*. At least one and preferably three assays are made between the second day after ovulation is presumed to have occurred and the onset of menses. A midluteal progesterone concentration of at least 12 ng/ml of serum suggests normal luteal function. A concentration of at least 3 ng/ml implies that ovulation has occurred.

An *endometrial biopsy* performed late in the luteal phase, cycle day 24 to 26, can determine whether changes in the glands, stroma, and vasculature correspond to the cycle day the sample was obtained. Agreement between the histologic dating and the menstrual cycle timing with ±2 days occurs normally. If progesterone secretion is inadequate, lag in endometrial development will be greater than 2 days.

Ovulation predictor kits can be purchased over the counter by the patient. Utilizing an immunocolorimetric assay for LH in the urine, the LH surge can be identified. Ovulation will occur in approximately 24 hours in 88% of women using the most accurate kits. These kits assist in timing of coitus, diagnostic testing, and certain therapies.

Cervical factor evaluation

After fertility potential in the husband has been established by semen analysis, it becomes necessary to determine the effect of the vaginal and cervical secretions on the activity of the sperm. Spermatozoa can penetrate the cervical mucus during a period of only 24 to 72 hours in the entire menstrual cycle. This occurs in the ovulatory phase of the cycle when the mucus is copious, thin, and watery and exhibits maximal spinnbarkheit and arborization.

The *postcoital examination of cervical mucus (Sims-Huhner test)* provides information concerning the number of spermatozoa that have entered the cervical canal and the percentage that retain their motility in the cervical mucus, but it gives minimal information regarding the adequacy of the semen specimen. It is therefore not a substitute for semen analysis. It is essential that the postcoital test be performed when the secretions should be optimal for sperm penetration and survival; the day before ovulation is most appropriate. The test can be correctly interpreted only at the end of the cycle to ascertain that the timing of the examination was appropriate. The urinary LH predicator kits have greatly facilitated the timing of this test.

The patient is instructed to report for examination about 6 to 8 hours after coitus without having used a precoital lubricant or a postcoital douche. At least 2 days' abstinence before the test is desirable. Endocervical mucus is aspirated through a small plastic suction catheter or a tuberculin syringe. The material is examined for clarity, viscosity, and spinnbarkheit, and the pH is determined. The specimen is then spread on a clean glass slide and examined for the presence of sperm and, after it has dried, for arborization of the mucus. The cervical environment is clearly normal if there are 10 or more highly motile spermatozoa. The most common explanation for a poor postcoital examination is that the specimen was obtained at the wrong time.

TREATMENT

The treatment of infertility often begins with the first consultation, although no specific therapeutic program can be outlined until all data obtained from the complete investigation of the couple have been analyzed and correlated. A significant percentage of women conceive after the initial visit or after assessment of tubal patency; Grant reported "spontaneous" cures of primary infertility in 35% of 1415 patients. Similar results were obtained in 1166 women with secondary infertility.

In general the treatment of infertility must be directed to the factors that the investigative procedures have indicated to be responsible for the failure to conceive.

Failure of insemination. Obvious abnormalities such as an intact hymen, developmental defects, or obesity should be corrected if possible. If failure of insemination occurs because of penile abnormalities, therapeutic insemination with the husband's semen should be considered. Impotence, vaginismus, and dyspareunia are seldom of organic origin; and psychotherapy usually is necessary for their correction. Faulty sexual techniques can be corrected by discussing the coital technique with both partners and suggesting necessary modifications.

Coitus every 48 hours during the period starting 3 days before and ending 2 days after the anticipated time of ovulation should cover minor deviations from the expected ovulatory pattern. If temperatures are being recorded, the couple should have intercourse on the day the temperature falls and the day after.

Failure of spermatogenesis because of *destructive testicular disease* cannot be improved, and the inability to transport the sperm because of *occlusion in the ductal system* is difficult to correct surgically. *Oligozoospermia* can sometimes be improved by thyroid therapy if decreased thyroid function is the responsible factor, but other endocrine preparations, with the possible exception of clomiphene, are usually ineffectual in stimulating spermatogenesis. Any *documented infection* of the male reproductive system should receive appropriate antibiotic therapy.

Cervical infections should be eradicated, and the cervix returned to as normal a state as possible. The treatment of benign disease of the cervix is discussed in Chapter 5.

Viscous cervical mucus, which can interfere with the ascent of the sperm through the cervical canal, may be the result of a diminished effect or production of estrogen. The administration of oral estrogen daily from the fifth to the twelfth day of the cycle may decrease the viscosity of the cervical secretions; if the primary defect lies in ovulation, pregnancy cannot be expected to occur. Supraovulation with menotropins (Pergonal) has been used successfully to treat deficient cervical mucus production.

THERAPEUTIC INSEMINATION. Therapeutic or artificial insemination refers to the artificial injection of semen into the cervical canal. It is termed *homologous* insemination (AIH) if the husband's semen is used and therapeutic donor insemination (TDI) if the semen is from a donor other than the husband.

Homologous insemination is indicated if the husband is normally fertile but is unable to ejaculate the semen over the cervix because of obesity or a penile defect. If a cervical abnormality appears to prevent the invasion of a sufficient number of sperm, intrauterine insemination (IUI) with processed ejaculate has proven successful. Neither type of insemination should be considered unless a reasonable study of the female partner proves her to be free from defects that might be partially responsible for the failure to conceive and without the expressed written consent of both partners.

Insemination with the husband's semen presents no legal problem, but heterologous insemination involves a great many emotional, ethical, legal, and religious considerations. If the male partner is solely responsible for the failure to conceive, the couple can be offered adoption, insemination, or in vitro fertilization in selected cases.

Healthy donors with physical characteristics and a blood type compatible with that of the infertile husband should be selected. Donors should be screened thoroughly for infection, including AIDS, chlamydia, hepatitis, and other sexually transmitted diseases. A complete genetic history and physical examination are necessary. Routine karyotyping is not productive and is unnecessary. As of February 1988, the standard for TDI was changed from fresh to quarantined frozen and thawed ejaculate because of the HIV transmission potential. Frozen ejaculate can be purchased commercially. The specimens are more costly.

Tubal abnormalities. Although restoration of tubal patency is equated with restoring tubal function, that is not necessarily the case. Attempts to force open diseased and damaged tubes with the use of contrast media, antibiotic preparations, or adrenal cortical substances have been uniformly unsuccessful and place the patient at risk for developing a serious tubal infection. Surgical procedures are preferred, but the results are not spectacular. The outcome of *tuboplasty* is determined by the cause of the occlusion, the extent of the damage, and the experience of the surgeon. It is easier to restore patency in tubes that have been occluded by a sterilizing operation, *tubal reversal*, than in those that have been damaged by infection. With the use of microsurgical techniques, reversal of sterilization can result in pregnancy rates as high as 65%. If pregnancy occurs following tubal surgery, the patient should be monitored closely because her chances of having a tubal pregnancy are increased.

Selective tubal cannulization under fluoroscopic guidance is a new technique that may avert the need for a major tubal operation with cornual occlusion.

Disorders of ovulation. Women who have ovarian failure, as evidenced by at least two serum FSH levels in the menopausal range, are sterile. Such patients would include those with *gonadal dysgenesis* (Turner's syndrome) and *premature ovarian failure*. There is no known way to restore ovarian function. However, it is possible to use donor ova and the partner's ejaculate and, after in vitro fertilization, effect zygote transfer into the patient's uterus, which has been appropriately stimulated by estrogen and progesterone. Donor embryos are also an option. Women who are oligomenorrheic or amenorrheic should be thoroughly evaluated before the institution of any therapy. The assessment is discussed in detail in the chapters relating to menstruation and its abnormalities (Chapters 7 and 9).

More often the cause of the ovulatory disturbance is related to hypothalamic-pituitary dysfunction, and *clomiphene citrate* is the initial drug of choice. This latter medication sends a "message" of estrogen deficiency at the level of the hypothalamus by preventing the replenishment of estrogen receptors and activates the negative feedback relationship between estrogen and gonadotropins. Because of the perceived reduction in estradiol, GnRH is secreted, stimulating the release of FSH and LH.

Clomiphene is available as a 50-mg tablet (Clomid or Serophene) and is administered initially 5 days each cycle following uterine bleeding occurring spontaneously or induced by progesterone. Most of the pregnancies occur after three consecutive ovulatory cycles, and the incidence of side effects is low. This medicine should not be used in women who have hepatic disease and should be discontinued in those who experience scotomata and severe ovarian hyperstimulation while taking the preparation. Clomiphene is of minimal value in women who are estrogen deficient.

If a pregnancy does not occur within three to six ovulatory cycles, other fertility factors should be assessed or reassessed. Individuals with *polycystic ovarian syndrome* (PCO) are often hyperresponsive to clomiphene, and a smaller dose of the medication may be required initially to induce ovulation.

Luteal phase defects can be treated by supplementing the deficiency of progesterone. Some clinicians use clomiphene because enhancing follicular development will result in normal corpus luteum function and progesterone output. Others prefer *progesterone vaginal suppositories,* 25 mg twice a day, or *progesterone in oil,* 12.5 mg intramuscularly once a day. Treatment is started 1 to 2 days after ovulation and is continued until menstruation.

As a general rule, individuals who do not respond to clomiphene therapy are candidates for *menotropin therapy* (Pergonal), which contains equivalent amounts of FSH and LH, 75 IU per ampule, and is administered parenterally. This medication is expensive and needs to be monitored closely by individuals familiar with its usage. Human chorionic gonadotropin is administered to simulate the LH surge after the ovarian follicles are stimulated and a dominant follicle is developed. Ovarian hyperstimulation, multiple pregnancies, and an increased number of spontaneous abortions are a few of the complications. Before instituting this therapy, other causes of infertility should have been eliminated.

Miscellaneous. *Uterine myomas* are rarely responsible for the failure to conceive, and *myomectomy* is seldom indicated to improve fertility. If the myomas obstruct the cornual ends of the tubes or distort the endometrial cavity, removal should be considered if no other cause of infertility can be found. *Congenital fusion defects* of the müllerian system, that is, bicornuate and septate uterus, rarely cause infertility; spontaneous abortion and premature labor are more characteristic problems of these developmental anomalies. However, it is reasonable to consider *metroplasty,* a uterine reconstruction, if no other cause of infertility can be identified. It must be remembered, though, that approximately 10% of women with a uterine anomaly will have a luteal phase defect and that this should be excluded before any surgery is performed.

Infertility caused by development of *antisperm antibodies* does not occur often. Condom therapy for several months has been shown to reduce antibody concentrations but has not necessarily resulted in a greater number of pregnancies than in those individuals who are left untreated. Cyclic *corticosteroid therapy* for the male or female who is producing antisperm antibodies has resulted in higher pregnancy rates, but the use of this medicine can produce some serious complications.

Although *in vitro fertilization* and *embryo transfer* (IVF-ET) is a form of therapy that was initially developed to treat women with obstructive tubal disease, it is clear that the indications are expanding. In some IVF centers severe oligozoospermia, disorders of ovulation, immune infertility, and unexplained fertility are considered reasonable indications after all other therapies have failed. Gamete intrafallopian transfer (GIFT) is a procedure wherein eggs and sperm are replaced into healthy-appearing tubes at laparoscopy. Pregnancy rates tend to be higher than in IVF-ET.

Emotional care. Couples with an infertility problem usually are depressed and anxious and have decreased libido. Referral to a counselor, an appropriate support group, or RESOLVE (a national lay group that provides information and support to couples with infertility problems) and, occasionally, psychotherapy will be helpful. Although it is obvious to the practitioner that the couple is under significant stress during the fertility evaluation, the distress does not seem to have any bearing on the couple's ability to function as parents when pregnancy is achieved.

Although adoption remains a theoretic option, the number of available infants is small; thus other therapeutic modalities should be pursued as long as it is emotionally and financially feasible for the couple to do so.

SUGGESTED READING

Beer AE and Neaves WB: Antigenic status of semen from the viewpoints of the female and male, Fertil Steril 29:3, 1978.

Grant A: Spontaneous cure rate of various infertility factors or post hoc and propter hoc, J Obstet Gynecol 9:224, 1969.

Katayama KP, Ju KS, Manuel M, Jones GS, and Jones HW Jr: Computer analysis of etiology and pregnancy rate in 636 cases of primary infertility, Am J Obstet Gynecol 135:207, 1979.

MacLeod J and Gold RZ: The male factor in fertility and infertility. II. Spermatazoon counts in 1000 men of known fertility and in 1000 cases of infertile marriages, J Urol 66:436, 1951.

Moghissi K: Cyclic changes in cervical mucus in normal and progestin-treated women, Fertil Steril 17:663, 1966.

Westrom L: Incidence, prevalence, and trends of acute pelvic inflammatory disease and its consequences in industrialized countries, Am J Obstet Gynecol 138:880, 1980.

15

J. Robert Willson

Family planning

Objectives

RATIONALE: Primary care physicians are frequently called upon to provide counseling regarding methods of contraception. An understanding of the medical as well as the personal issues involved in a couple's decisions regarding contraceptive methods is necessary to adequately advise these patients.

The student should be able to:

A. For each method of contraception, demonstrate a knowledge of the physiologic or pharmacologic basis of action, effectiveness, advantages, disadvantages, contraindications, and complications.
B. Describe methods of male and female surgical sterilization and the advantages, disadvantages, contraindications, and complications of each method.
C. Demonstrate knowledge of the role of elective abortion in family planning and its advantages, disadvantages, contraindications, and complications.

There is little to indicate that uncomplicated pregnancy and delivery are harmful to normal women, but one cannot logically conclude that uncontrolled reproduction is desirable. Increasing social and economic demands make it essential that each couple reach a decision as to when pregnancy is appropriate and the number of children for which they can assume responsibility. Physicians, family-planning clinics, and governmental social agencies share the responsibility for making effective and appropriate contraceptive methods available to those who want them.

Physicians should bring up the subject of contraception during premarital examinations, when they are consulted by young married couples, during gynecologic examination of teenagers as well as more mature women, after each delivery, and with patients near the menopause. Some women hesitate to ask about contraception even though fear of pregnancy is a constant concern and a source of marital discord. Unless the subject is introduced by the physician, these problems may remain unresolved.

Physicians who choose not to provide contraception for their patients should refer them to another physician or to an agency for this essential service.

CONTRACEPTION IN TEENAGERS

Pregnancy in teenagers is a major problem and one that has not decreased, in spite of the availability of effective contraceptive techniques. About half of unmarried women between the ages of 15 and 19 have had intercourse and many, even among those who are regularly sexually active, do not use any contraceptive method. Each year 1 of 10 women between the ages of 15 and 19 (a total of about 837,000) conceive. An additional 23,000 pregnancies occur in girls younger than age 15. Elective abortion is chosen as a solution by 14,000 of those under age 15 and by 162,000 (about 50%) of those between 15 and 17. The emotional trauma and the cost of many of these pregnancies could be avoided if accurate information and contraception were made available to young women approaching menarche and to teenagers. The usual courses in sex education given in schools are often inadequate; as many as a third of those who have had such courses are not aware of when they are most likely to conceive during the menstrual cycle. Courses in reproductive physiology, pregnancy, and contraception should be complemented by individual contraceptive counseling.

It is difficult to ignore one's personal biases when dealing with teenage sexuality. Regardless of one's beliefs, however, such requests cannot logically be handled by a curt refusal even to consider the problem. One should learn as much as possible about the circumstances that led to the request for contraception. Some young girls may be confused by the pressures being put on them by their peers who are already sexually active. They may be asking for help in understanding and resisting the pressures rather than for contraceptive counseling. Others who already are having intercourse need a reliable contraceptive method. It takes a great deal of courage for a young girl to ask a physician for contraception. Many feel guilty but are wise enough to want to avoid the problems inherent in pregnancy. A cold refusal, particularly when accompanied by a moralistic lecture, will be so embarrasing that many will not risk exposing themselves to similar experiences by consulting another physician. The inevitable result is preventable pregnancies.

Although a 1983 Supreme Court ruling stated that minors do not need parental consent to obtain contraceptive counseling through federally funded services, there are times when it is appropriate to include parents in the decision. It is unnecessary for young women in their late teens. However, the parents of young teenagers who seek contraceptive advice should be involved. Before approaching the parents, however, one must learn all one can about the girl and her need for contraception and be ready to support her in her decision.

There is no ready answer to teenage contraception. The solution is determined by the individual problem, which will never be clarified if the physician either complies with the request or denies it without exploring the situation.

Contraceptive methods

The many contraceptive methods range from relatively simple forms to operative procedures that interrupt the continuity of the fallopian tubes or of the ductus deferens. No single method is uniformly satisfactory, and the physician must be familiar with several types so that individual couples can select the one best suited to their needs after analyzing all the factors involved. Zatuchni has illustrated the factors involved in selecting a contraceptive method (Fig. 15-1).

The effectiveness of any contraceptive method is determined by its usage. *Theoretic effectiveness* refers to the protection offered by a technique when it is used perfectly by a human couple. *Use effectiveness* refers to the protection offered to large groups of couples, many of whom may use the method carelessly or irregularly.

High use effectiveness is determined by the theoretical effectiveness of the method, how ap-

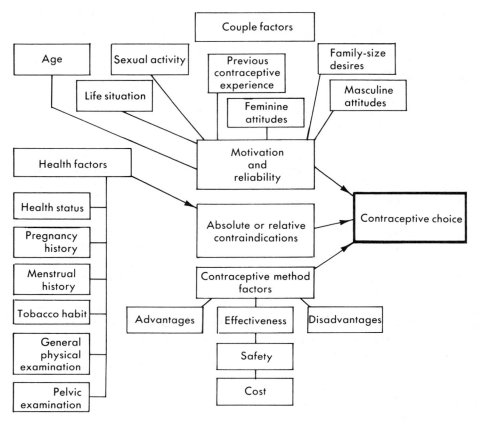

Fig. 15-1 Factors involved in selection of contraceptive method. (Modified from Zatuchni GI: The Female Patient 3[5]:48, 1978.)

propriate it is for an individual couple, how important it is that they prevent pregnancy, and how consistently the method is used. A method that is too difficult for a couple to use or one that is unacceptable for one reason or another will have low use effectiveness. In contrast, use effectiveness is high in couples who are strongly motivated to prevent pregnancy and who are using an effective method that is acceptable to both partners.

The use effectiveness for any contraceptive method can be calculated by determining the number of pregnancies per 100 years by use of *Pearl's formula,* which permits comparison of methods:

$$\text{Pregnancy rate/100 yrs} = \frac{\text{Total number of conceptions} \times 1200}{\text{Total months of exposure}}$$

For example, if 100 couples use a method for a total of 3600 months and 12 pregnancies occur, the pregnancy rate is 4:

$$\frac{12 \times 1200}{3600} = \frac{14,400}{3600} = 4/100 \text{ yrs}$$

In general, contraceptive methods can be divided into (1) physiologic, (2) chemical, (3) barrier, (4) intrauterine, (5) hormonal, and (6) surgical. All attempt to prevent the union of the sperm and ovum or to interfere with nidation.

PHYSIOLOGIC CONTRACEPTION

In physiologic contraception, no chemical or mechanical device is used. The two methods are coitus interruptus and avoiding coitus during the period of greatest fertility.

Coitus interruptus (withdrawal)

The penis is withdrawn from the vagina just before ejaculation occurs. This method does not afford maximum protection because fertilization can occur if live sperm are present in the seminal fluid that leaks from the urethra during coitus and if the withdrawal is delayed so that part of the semen is discharged within the vagina.

Coitus interruptus is the oldest and probably the most frequently used contraceptive method throughout the world. If properly used, the pregnancy rate can be kept low, but the average is probably about 16 pregnancies/100 years of use.

Natural family planning (rhythm or safe period)

Couples who use natural family planning prevent conception by confining coitus to the phases of the menstrual cycle during which conception is unlikely to occur.

The human ovum can be fertilized no later than 24 to 48 hours after it is extruded from the ovary. Although motile spermatozoa have been recovered from the uterus and the oviducts as long as 60 hours after coitus, their ability to fertilize the ovum probably lasts no longer than 24 to 48 hours. Pregnancy is unlikely to occur if a couple refrains from intercourse for 4 days before and for 3 or 4 days after ovulation *(fertile period)*. Unprotected intercourse on the other days of the cycle *(safe period)* should not result in pregnancy. The principal problems with natural family planning are that the exact time of ovulation cannot be predicted accurately and that couples may find it difficult to exercise restraint for several days before and after ovulation.

Ovulation usually occurs about 14 days (12 to 16) before the onset of menstruation. The fertile period can be anticipated by calculating the time at which ovulation is likely to occur by the length of the menstrual cycles *(calendar method)*, by recording the rise in basal body temperature caused by the thermogenic effect of progesterone *(temperature method)*, by recognizing the changes in cervical mucus at different phases of the cycle *(cervical mucus method)*, or by combinations of all three.

With the *calendar method* the fertile period is determined after accurately recording the number of days of a menstrual cycle for a year. The fertile period for a woman with 27- to 30-day cycles extends from the ninth to the nineteenth day; for one with 25- to 35-day cycles, from the seventh to the twenty-fourth day of each cycle (Fig. 15-2). Pregnancy rates as high as 40/100 years of use have been reported when the calendar method is used alone.

With the *cervical mucus method* couples are taught to recognize the characteristic changes in cervical mucus at the different stages of the menstrual cycle. Observations are made on secretions that are collected by wiping the vaginal introitus daily with white toilet tissue. During the first few days after menstruation there is little discharge and the introitus is dry. As estrogen stimulation increases, the secretions become sticky and cloudy. Ovulation occurs soon after the peak estrogen production, when the mucus at the introitus is abundant, clear, thin, and watery. The last day of the "wet" phase is known as the *peak symptom day*. Progesterone reduces mucus secretion, and that which is present is scant and sticky. Infertile days include those during and shortly after menstruation when the introitus is dry and those starting 3 or 4 days after the peak symptom day, when the vulva again becomes dry.

Couples should not engage in coitus after tacky mucus is first recognized and until the watery discharge characteristic of ovulation disappears. Although this method provides greater protection than does the calendar method, the average pregnancy rate may be as high as 20 to 25/100 years of use.

The *symptothermal method* is a combination of basal

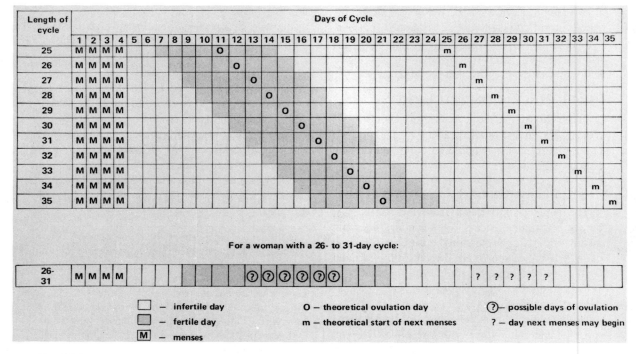

Days of Cycle

Length of cycle	1	2	3	4	5	6	7	8	9	10	11	12	13	14	15	16	17	18	19	20	21	22	23	24	25	26	27	28	29	30	31	32	33	34	35
25	M	M	M	M							O														m										
26	M	M	M	M								O														m									
27	M	M	M	M									O														m								
28	M	M	M	M										O														m							
29	M	M	M	M											O														m						
30	M	M	M	M												O														m					
31	M	M	M	M													O														m				
32	M	M	M	M														O														m			
33	M	M	M	M															O														m		
34	M	M	M	M																O														m	
35	M	M	M	M																	O														m

For a woman with a 26- to 31-day cycle:

| 26-31 | M | M | M | M | | | | | | | | | | (?) | (?) | (?) | (?) | (?) | (?) | | | | | | | | ? | ? | ? | ? | ? | | | | |

☐ — infertile day   O — theoretical ovulation day   (?)— possible days of ovulation
☐ — fertile day   m — theoretical start of next menses   ? — day next menses may begin
M — menses

Fig. 15-2 Day of ovulation and fertile period during cycles of varying length. (From Population Reports: Periodic abstinence, series 1, no 1, Baltimore, June 1974, Population Information Program, The Johns Hopkins University.)

body temperature and evaluation of cervical mucus. The period of abstinence begins with the appearance of the estrogen effect on the mucus and continues until the fourth day after the temperature rise. The pregnancy rate can be kept as low as those with conventional methods but is usually between 11 and 20/100 years of use.

Natural family planning is satisfactory for those who cannot use other methods and for those who are planning more pregnancies sometime in the future. It is not certain enough for those in whom pregnancy must be prevented.

CHEMICAL CONTRACEPTION

The chemical methods of contraception consist of the deposition of a spermicidal substance in the vagina before coitus. This material coats the vaginal wall and the cervix and collects in the for-

nices, thus exposing the spermatozoa to its destructive action.

This method in general affords better protection than does the rhythm method but less than condoms and the diaphragm with contraceptive jelly. Pregnancy rates as low as 2 and as high as 39/100 years have been reported. The average is probably about 15 to 20.

Aerosol foams, which contain spermicidal chemicals, provide protection as good as condoms provide if they are used properly and consistently. The protection can be increased almost to that provided by oral contraceptives by using both a condom and aerosol foam during the few days before and after ovulation and foam alone the rest of the month.

Other chemical methods include the use of *foaming tablets* and *suppositories*. Neither is as effective as aerosol foams or spermicidal jellies and creams.

An advantage of spermicidal contraception is that it appears to reduce the risk of gonococcal and other sexually transmitted infections.

In spite of the fear that spermicides increase the risk of spontaneous abortion and congenital malformations, no proof of such an association exists.

Postcoital douches offer no protection against conception. Large numbers of spermatozoa enter the cervix within a few seconds after ejaculation, and there is no way they can be removed by a vaginal douche.

BARRIER CONTRACEPTION

Before oral contraceptives were developed, the most frequently prescribed method was a combination of an *occlusive vaginal diaphragm* and a *spermicidal jelly*. A diaphragm is a dome-shaped rubber cup with a flexible rim. It fits in the vagina with its anterior edge behind the pubic bone, its lateral edges against the vaginal walls, and its posterior edge against the posterior vaginal fornix. The cervix is covered by the diaphragm, and the external os rests in a pool of spermicidal jelly, which immobilizes any spermatozoa that get past the barrier (Fig. 15-3).

It is necessary that the physician fit the diaphragm, instruct the patient in its use, and make certain, by having her return with the diaphragm in place after practicing using it at home, that she can insert it properly. For many women the insertion of a diaphragm is distasteful and too much trouble, but for those who use one regularly and properly, a diaphragm offers good protection. The diaphragm must be inserted before intercourse and left in place at least 6 hours after ejaculation.

The theoretic effectiveness of this method should be comparable to that of the intrauterine device (1.5 to 3 pregnancies/100 years), and for motivated couples it is. The general use effectiveness, however, is much less; that is, between 10 and 20 pregnancies/100 years. The principal reasons for failure are inconsistent use, improper in-

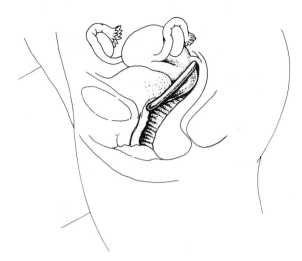

Fig. 15-3 Occlusive contraceptive diaphragm in place.

sertion, improper size, and displacement during coitus caused by expansion of the upper vagina.

Possible *side effects* in diaphragm users are irritation from the spermicidal cream or jelly and an increased incidence of urinary tract infections.

The *condom* is a common form of barrier contraceptive that offers good protection but has disadvantages. It may break or slip off the penis. It provides better protection when used in conjunction with a vaginal spermicidal jelly. The pregnancy rate with condoms can be as low as 1 to 3 pregnancies/100 years of use, but the general rate is about 15. The reasons for failure are inconsistent use, leakage of semen if the condom is put on late in coitus or as the deflated penis is withdrawn, and breakage.

The regular use of condoms should reduce the chance of contracting gonorrhea, chlamydia, or HIV infections. To accomplish this it is essential that the condom be used throughout the entire act and that there be no unprotected contact with the female genitals.

Contraceptive sponges made of polyurethane saturated with a spermicidal substance, nonoxynol-9, were introduced in the United States in 1983. The sponge has three effects: (1) it releases the spermicide slowly, (2) it covers the external cervical os, and (3) it absorbs semen. It may be inserted several hours before coitus and need not be changed during repeated episodes of coitus within a 24-hour period. It should be removed 6 hours after intercourse.

The thimble-shaped latex rubber *cervical cap* fits snugly over the normal cervix and is held in place by suction. Additional protection is provided by a spermicide placed within the cap before it is inserted. The cap must be fitted, but because there are only four sizes all women cannot use it. It may not be appropriate if the cervix is short or distorted, and it may be difficult to insert and remove. It can be left in place for 2 days, but, because of the risk of toxic shock syndrome, it should be removed during menses.

INTRAUTERINE DEVICES

The prototype intrauterine device (IUD) was the German silver Graefenberg ring, which was first used during the 1920s. The method was abandoned by most physicians because the rings caused ulceration of the uterine wall and infection.

In 1959 Oppenheimer reported on his use of a silkworm gut coil that effectively prevented conception with few ill effects. Subsequently several different plastic devices were developed and used successfully. The IUDs are inserted into the uterine cavity by a physician and are allowed to remain in place, offering constant protection against pregnancy without need for preparing for each individual coital act. Most IUDs have a fine plastic thread that protrudes through the cervix into the vagina. Only two types of IUDs are now available: the Progestasert, a **T**-shaped device containing a synthetic progesterone that is released slowly, and the Paragard T 380A, a **T**-shaped device, the stem and arms of which are partially covered with copper wire.

Copper-coated IUDs provide better protection against pregnancy than do the pure plastic types. The copper, which is absorbed slowly by the endometrium, adds to the protective effect of the device itself by altering local enzymes, DNA con-

tent, glycogen metabolism, and estrogen uptake. They must be replaced every 6 years.

Progesterone-containing devices decrease menstrual flow, but they may produce annoying intermenstrual spotting. They also appear to be associated with a higher rate of ectopic pregnancies. An additional disadvantage is that they must be replaced yearly.

The *pregnancy rate* is 1.5 to 3 pregnancies/100 years of use. Some pregnancies occur because the patient is not aware that the device has been expelled from the uterus. These accidents can be prevented if the patient feels for the thread, which is attached to the device and comes through the cervical canal into the vagina, at the end of each menstrual period, when expulsion most often occurs, and again just before ovulation is expected. If she cannot feel the thread, she should use another form of contraception until she can see her gynecologist. The uterus expels the device in about 10% of women, and in another 10% to 15% it is removed because of a complication or because of a vague concern over the presence of a foreign body in the uterus. The continuation rate is between 50% and 80% at the end of 1 year.

Selection of patients

Although intrauterine devices can be used by either nulliparous or parous women, they are more suitable for the latter. Women who have never been pregnant are more likely to experience unacceptable cramping and bleeding than are those whose uteri have been enlarged by pregnancy. Women who are not motivated enough to use ordinary contraceptive methods consistently and those in whom oral contraceptives are contraindicated are suitable candidates for IUDs.

Contraindications to the use of IUDs include active pelvic infection, acute cervicitis, undiagnosed bleeding, abnormal uterine size or shape, and suspected pregnancy. *Relative contraindications* include recurrent attacks of pelvic infection, multiple sexual partners, severe dysmenorrhea, and hypermenorrhea. IUDs should be used with caution in women with diabetes who are prone to develop infections and in women with valvular heart disease.

Complications

The most common complications are intermenstrual spotting, increased menstrual bleeding, increased cramping during menstruation, perforation of the uterus, and infection. Because of increased bleeding, most women using IUDs should take iron regularly, and the hemoglobin should be checked periodically. *Cramping* can usually be controlled with prostaglandin inhibitors. Women who have had severe dysmenorrhea that was relieved by oral contraceptives will usually not continue using an IUD unless the pain can be controlled.

Perforation of the uterus probably occurs during the insertion of the device. The perforation may be *incomplete,* with the tip of the device protruding through the serosa and its proximal end in the uterine cavity. Uterine contractions may eventually expel the device into the peritoneal cavity. With *complete perforation* the tip of the inserter is pushed through the uterine wall, and the device is inserted directly into the peritoneal cavity.

If the tail of an intrauterine device that once was visible can no longer be seen, the device has been expelled through the cervix, it has entered the peritoneal cavity, or the tail has been drawn upward into the uterine cavity. If the device is still in the uterus, it can be located by probing the uterus or by sonography. Intraperitoneal IUDs should be removed.

Perforation can almost always be prevented by careful selection of patients, care during insertion, and experience. Perforation is more likely to occur with insertion during the first 6 to 8 weeks after delivery than after the tenth.

Bacteria are inevitably introduced into the uterus during insertion; hence, *infection* may develop. The patient with a mild, localized infection usually experiences low abdominal discomfort, dyspareunia, thin vaginal discharge, and perhaps low-grade fever for as long as 2 to 3 weeks. The uterus and parametria may be tender, suggesting a low-grade endometritis and cellulitis. They can be treated effectively with a broad-spectrum antibiotic. Tubal infections, which usually do not appear for several months, are more often due to sexually transmitted diseases than solely to the presence of the IUD. Rarely, an overwhelming bacteremia may appear soon after insertion, and this can be lethal.

The incidence of infection varies with the socioeconomic class of the user and with the number of sexual partners. Willson, Ledger, and Lovell found that 1.3% of 706 private patients who were using Lippes Loops developed infections. Of the nine, two were caused by gonorrhea and cannot be related to the device. In contrast, 8% of 623 women of the lowest socioeconomic classes developed infections; many of these were of gonococcal origin. One can assume that most private patients are more likely to be monogamous and less exposed to sexually transmitted diseases than are those with many partners.

About 50% of *intrauterine pregnancies* that occur with an IUD in place are *aborted*. Removal of the device reduces the abortion rate to 25% or less. When pregnancy is diagnosed, the device should be removed. If the tail is not visible, it may have been drawn upward into the enlarging uterus or extruded before conception. An IUD can be located by sonography if there is a question as to whether it has been expelled. If the device cannot be removed, the patient should be informed of the possibility that serious infection may develop and be given the option of abortion.

Because IUDs lie outside the amniotic sac, they do not disturb embryonic differentiation and development.

IUDs prevent 97% to 98% of intrauterine pregnancies, but *tubal* and *ovarian pregnancies* still occur. About one in 20 pregnancies in IUD users is extrauterine. Women who are at risk of developing ectopic pregnancies should use another form of contraception if possible.

In terms of mortality, the death rates of healthy young women using oral contraceptives is twice that for those who use IUDs. For those predisposed to developing cardiovascular disorders, the risk from oral contraceptives is three to five times that for IUDs. The risk of death from complications of pregnancy, particularly in women over the age of 30, is far greater than from IUDs.

Action

The *method by which IUDs prevent pregnancy* is not completely clear. Ovulation continues, and spermatozoa can be recovered from the fallopian tubes, but there is no evidence to suggest that IUDs cause repeated abortions of normally implanted blastocysts. The most likely explanation is that the device creates an intrauterine environment unfavorable for implantation. The local endometrial changes, stromal edema, increased vascularity, and a sterile inflammatory reaction may alter the tissue enough so that it cannot support the blastocyst. In addition, products from the breakdown of inflammatory cells may be toxic to both spermatozoa and blastocysts.

HORMONAL CONTRACEPTION

The most popular form of steroidal contraception is provided by *oral contraceptive agents.* Oral contraceptive preparations contain varying amounts of an *estrogen,* either mestranol or ethinyl estradiol, and a *progestin,* which usually is a 19-nor derivative of testosterone. The progestational, estrogen, antiestrogen, and androgenic effects of the various progestins vary considerably; hence one needs to consider these, as well as the estrogen content, when prescribing oral contraceptives.

Combined oral contraceptives contain both an estrogen and a progestin. The hormones interfere with orderly GN RH release from the hypothalamus, thereby suppressing anterior pituitary function and inhibiting ovulation. The hormones also have a direct stimulatory effect on the endometrium, so that from 1 to 4 days after the last tablet is taken the endometrium sloughs and bleeds as a result of hormone withdrawal. The bleeding usually is less profuse than that during a normal period and may last only 2 to 3 days. Some women have no bleeding at all.

The contraceptive action is a combined effect of ovulation inhibition, endometrial changes, an alteration in cervical mucus, and perhaps altered tubal function.

The constant daily dosage of the estrogen-progestogen compound produces *changes in the endometrium* that are different from those that occur during the normal cycle. Under the stimulus of an estrogen-progestogen–containing oral contraceptive, the endometrial glands are fairly widely scattered and remain straight throughout the cycle. Secretory activity can be detected in the gland cells after a few days of treatment, but by about the twentieth day the cells appear inactive. The stroma remains dense throughout. The

reduction in menstrual bleeding is probably a direct result of the unphysiologic endometrial stimulus; the stroma remains thin, compact, and relatively avascular compared with the normal changes.

The *cervical mucus* remains thick as a result of the effect of the progestogen and does not provide as suitable an environment for sperm penetration and survival as does the thin, viscid mucus at ovulation.

Progestin-only pills, *the minipill,* also reduce the risk of pregnancy and may be appropriate when estrogen is contraindicated. The progestin in the pills now available is either norethindrone (0.35 g) or norgestrel (0.075 g). The major contraceptive effects are on cervical mucus and the endometrium; inhibition of ovulation is less predictable.

Complications

Side effects. Undesirable side effects are common but fortunately are transient, usually lasting for no more than three or four cycles. They include nausea, vomiting, breast engorgement, headache, vertigo, and fluid retention, which may result in a weight gain of 3 or more pounds. If these disagreeable side effects do not disappear spontaneously after a few cycles, one should consider trying another pill with a different hormone distribution. Those in which estrogen is dominant are more likely to cause nausea, fluid retention, and breast tenderness than are those with a relatively high progestin content. These side effects are less common and less annoying in women taking pills with an estrogen content of 35 mg or less.

Depression, which may be severe and incapacitating, occurs in some women who are taking oral contraceptives. Occasionally, it is necessary to discontinue oral contraceptives completely to relieve depression.

The total incidence of *breakthrough bleeding* is about 8% to 10%, but it occurs more often during the first few cycles than later. It also occurs more often when progestin-dominant products or those with low estrogen content are used. If the bleeding is slight and occurs only occasionally and particularly if it consists only of slight spotting during the last few days of pill ingestion, the physician should reassure the patient that it means nothing and attempt to convince her to ignore it. More persistent breakthrough bleeding can usually be controlled by prescribing a preparation with a higher estrogenic effect or by adding conjugated estrogens 1.25 to 2.5 mg daily for 7 days while the bleeding is present.

The lower the amount of hormone, the less the endometrial stimulation and growth and the greater the possibility of *amenorrhea*. This concerns both the patient and the physician because of the possibility of pregnancy. Although it is unlikely that one who has taken her pills regularly and fails to menstruate has conceived, some women will not tolerate the uncertainty and will discontinue the method. A pregnancy test should be ordered with the first episode or two of amenorrhea; if the failure to bleed persists, repeated tests are probably not necessary.

Most of the complications are inconsequential when compared to the ease with which pregnancy can be prevented, but others may be more significant.

Cardiovascular diseases. Concern that oral contraceptives increase the risk of cardiovascular diseases appears no longer to be tenable. Increased instances of myocardial infarction and cerebrovascular accidents reported during the 1960s and 1970s were based on studies of women who were using formulations containing 50 μg or more of estrogen. Preparations containing 35 μg or less were introduced in 1974, and their use has increased steadily until now relatively few of the higher-dose pills are prescribed.

Estrogen increases high-density lipoprotein cholesterol and decreases low-density lipoprotein cholesterol and thereby offers some protection against myocardial infarction. However, the synthetic estrogens in oral contraceptives stimulate an increased liver production of serum globulins. One of these, angiotensinogen, may increase angiotensin II in some women and thereby increase blood pressure. Increased blood pressure associated with the use of oral contraceptives is not permanent; the blood pressure returns to its regular level when oral contraceptives are discontinued.

The progestogens in oral contraceptives have androgenic potential and may counteract some of the beneficial effects of estrogen. Some progestogens decrease high-density lipoprotein cholesterol concentrations and increase low-density lipoprotein levels. These undesirable effects are counterbalanced by estrogen, so the net result is no change.

No evidence supports the concept that oral contraceptives are responsible for atherosclerotic changes. There is no increase in myocardial infarction in women who have used oral contraceptives in the past, and there is no relationship between duration of use and heart attacks. Any increase in cardiovascular deaths seems to be related to thrombosis rather than to atherosclerosis.

Recent studies of oral contraceptive users aged 20 to 44 revealed no increase in myocardial infarctions or cerebrovascular accidents after 36,248 women-years of use. The risk for venous thrombosis was 0.9. In a later study of women between 15 and 44, there were no myocardial infarctions, one stroke, and three episodes of venous thrombosis during 36,807 woman-years of use. There was a steadily increasing use of low-dose oral contraceptives during the study periods.

Moreover, even in the early studies, increases in heart attacks occurred primarily in older women who smoked more than 15 cigarettes daily and who had preexisting risk factors for coronary artery disease.

We can conclude from these studies that healthy women, even those up to age 45, who do not smoke and who are using low-dose oral contraceptives are not at increased risk of developing strokes or heart attacks. There is a slight increase in venous thromboembolism, but this can be kept at a minimum if only low-dose preparations are used.

Other complications. Oral contraceptives containing less than 50 µg of estrogen do not alter *carbohydrate metabolism*. There is no indication that oral contraceptives cause diabetes, and most women with well-controlled diabetes can take oral contraceptives without deleterious effects on the disease. However, there may be an increased risk of cardiovascular diseases.

Women who have had *cholestasis and jaundice* during pregnancy may respond in the same manner to oral contraceptives. The incidence of *cholecystitis and cholelithiasis* is almost doubled during the first years of oral contraceptive use. After 4 years, the rate may actually decrease. The most serious complication affecting the liver is the development of *liver tumors*, principally focal nodular hyperplasia and hepatic adenomas. The main danger is from rupture of the tumor with intrahepatic or intraperitoneal hemorrhage and death unless the blood loss is controlled promptly. Malignant liver neoplasms have not been related to the use of oral contraceptives.

There is no evidence to suggest that combined oral contraceptives increase the risk of cancer of the cervix, endometrium, breast, or any other organ.

Oral contraceptives actually protect against *endometrial* and *ovarian cancer*. Although they do decrease the risk of *benign breast disease*, there is still controversy as to the relationship between the use of hormonal contraceptives and *breast cancer*. An increase in *cervical cancer* has been observed in only one study.

Most women *ovulate* soon after discontinuing oral contraceptives, but in some there may be a delay of several weeks before ovulation and menstruation are resumed. One to three percent are amenorrheic for as long as 6 months. Eventually almost all of those who want to conceive will do so. There is no difference in fertility between those using oral contraceptives and those who use other contraceptive methods. Because of the uncertainty as to when ovulation may resume, women who discontinue oral contraceptives to become pregnant should be advised to use another form of contraception until menstrual cycles resume their normal pattern. There is no increase in spontaneous abortion, chromosomal abnormalities, or congenital defects in women who have used oral contraceptives as compared to those who have not.

Advantages

Much has been written about the complications related to the use of oral contraceptives, but the advantages, other than protection against pregnancy, have had little publicity. Mishell lists the *noncontraceptive health benefits of oral contraceptives* as decreased menstrual blood loss and resultant iron-deficiency anemia, regulation of irregular cycles, decreased menstrual discomfort, protection against endometrial adenocarcinoma, reduced incidence of benign breast disease, protection against the development of functional ovarian cysts, protection against acute salpingitis, and possible protection against ovarian cancer.

Limitations and cautions

Nevertheless, because there is still so much question concerning the physiologic effects of estrogen-progestogen combinations, it seems wise to limit their use to perfectly normal healthy young women who choose them over other methods after the risks have been described to them.

As a general rule, there is no reason why healthy women below the age of 35 cannot take oral contraceptives, even though they smoke. Healthy women between the ages of 35 and 45 can continue to use low-dose oral contraceptives as long as they do not smoke and have no factors that increase the risk of cardiovascular diseases, such as diabetes and hypertension. For women over age 35, it is wise to obtain a lipid panel before prescribing pills.

Each woman taking oral contraceptives should be examined before the medication is prescribed and yearly thereafter. The examination should include medical and family history, weight, blood pressure, general physical and pelvic examination, screening cervical cytologic analysis, and hemoglobin determination.

All women who take oral contraceptives should be encouraged to stop smoking. Those who continue must be made aware of the risks involved.

If contraceptive tablets are taken accordingly to the recommended schedule, the incidence of unplanned pregnancy should be close to zero. If they are taken irregularly during the cycle, ovulation and fertilization may occur.

Selection of an oral contraceptive

The estrogen and progestin contents of the oral contraceptives vary considerably. Although preparations with relatively large amounts of estrogen are available, those containing no more than 35 μg are appropriate for most women.

Standard combined oral contraceptives do not actually mimic the normal cycle. The daily estrogen-progestogen content does not vary during the 21 days during which the pills are taken.

Biphasic preparations contain varying amounts of progestin, making their effects more like those that occur during normal cycles. The estrogen content remains constant throughout; but the progestin content, which is low during the first 10 days, is increased during the last 11 days. These preparations are designed to provide relatively low estrogen.

Triphasic preparations attempt to mimic the normal menstrual cycle by providing small amounts of progestogen during the first 11 days with an increase during the last 10 days. In contrast to biphasic preparations, the estrogen content varies, being low during the first 6 days, higher during the next 5 days, and reduced during the last 10 days. These preparations provide excellent protection against conception with a low incidence of breakthrough bleeding despite relatively small amounts of both estrogen and progestogen.

Injectable steroids

Depomedroxyprogesterone acetate (DMPA), when injected intramuscularly in doses of 150 mg every 3 months, inhibits ovulation. Pregnancy rates comparable to those achieved with oral contraceptives have been reported in large numbers of women. The only metabolic effect associated with this preparation is a possible decrease in insulin tolerance and an increase in plasma insulin. Bleeding may occur irregularly during the first few months, but it gradually decreases, and many women become amenorrheic.

In spite of its proven effectiveness and safety, DMPA has not been approved for contraceptive use by the FDA, but it can be prescribed for women who cannot use other methods. It is particularly advantageous for women in the perimenopausal period.

Contraindications to oral contraceptives

There are women for whom oral contraceptives should not be prescribed. The *absolute contraindications* include:

1. Coronary artery disease, stroke, or thromboembolism either present or in the past
2. Severe hypertension
3. Lupus erythematosus
4. Hemoglobin SS disease
5. Insulin-dependent diabetes with vascular disease
6. Impaired liver function
7. Estrogen-dependent neoplasms and breast cancer
8. Suspected pregnancy
9. Smokers over age 35, particularly obese women

Relative contraindications include:

1. History of cholestasis during pregnancy
2. Migraine headaches or headaches associated with oral contraceptive use
3. Depression
4. Seizure disease

Pregnancy interception

Another method of pregnancy prevention is the use of *large doses of estrogen after coitus*. This should be considered as an emergency measure to be used after unprotected coitus during the fertile period rather than as a regular method of contraception. The exact mechanism by which postcoital estrogen prevents pregnancy is not yet known, but it does produce a premature fall in corpus luteum progesterone production and changes in the endometrium, which may provide an unacceptable implantation site for the fertilized ovum.

Ovral, two tablets repeated once in 12 hours, is most often prescribed. Because estrogen ingested by the mother is related to the subsequent development of vaginal adenosis and clear cell carcinoma in their daughters, it is essential that each patient be examined to make certain that she is not already pregnant before the drug is prescribed. Repeat examinations to make certain that the patient did not conceive despite the drug also are essential. Abortion should be available if pregnancy occurs.

SURGICAL CONTRACEPTION

Termination of fertility by an operative procedure is the most common form of contraception in the United States. As many as 15 million couples may rely on this method. Elective sterilization is appropriate for normal women who have completed their childbearing careers and who still have several years of fertility ahead. It may be particularly important for those who cannot use an effective contraceptive method, and it usually is preferable to many years of using oral hormonal contraceptives.

The fallopian tubes can be occluded or severed in conjunction with any indicated abdominal operation or as a primary procedure. This may be accomplished by *laparoscopic tubal cautery,* by the application of *rings* or *clips,* or by removing a segment of each tube through a *vaginal* or *small abdominal incision (minilaparotomy).* All of these procedures can be performed in an ambulatory setting. *Puerperal sterilization,* usually during the first day or two after delivery, is easy and safe and often is an appropriate choice.

The patient should understand that it is unlikely that she will conceive after the operation but that she is being sterilized (termination of fertility), not castrated (removal of gonads).

Vasectomy can be performed in an outpatient facility with a local anesthetic. There are few complications and a minimal period of disability. Spermatozoa may remain in the reproductive tract for several weeks; consequently, an additional method of contraception should be used until aspermia has been proved. Recanalization occurs in a small percentage of cases, probably less than 5%.

One must always consider the possible emotional effects of permanent elimination of procreative ability. It is not easy, even for a woman who wants no more children, to relinquish her ability to conceive. Men who are somewhat uncertain in their masculine roles may be impotent after vasectomy. These potential effects of sterilization must be explored before the operation is performed because, even though each member of the couple may verbally agree, they may be unconsciously resisting.

FUTURE METHODS

The currently available methods for controlling conception leave much to be desired. With the exception of IUDs and surgical procedures, each requires a considerable amount of motivation—particularly the taking of oral medication daily or the use of a physiologic or mechanical method consistently year after year. The current research in immunologic methods, by which it will be possible to provide temporary immunity against spermatozoa, is promising, as are hormonal methods that require single injections at long intervals. The ideal is a method that is completely effective and without danger but reversible and that requires no preparation for individual acts of coitus.

LEGAL ABORTION

The term *legal abortion* refers to the termination of early pregnancy by a qualified physician in an approved medical facility.

Until about 1965 termination of pregnancy was considered only when it was likely that the mother would die if she remained pregnant (therapeutic abortion). Such abortions were legal in most states. Abortion was seldom considered because of fetal conditions, even if one could anticipate a fetus being born with a lethal or incapacitating condition, or for social reasons. These abortions were illegal.

Restrictive laws did not prevent women for whom pregnancy was a personal disaster from obtaining abortion. They usually had to seek assistance from illegal operators, and many developed serious complications or even died as a result of the procedures. Before 1970, when abortion became legal in New York, more than 50% of maternal deaths in New York City followed illegally induced abortion. During the 5-year period 1955 to 1959, 21% of maternal deaths in Michigan were attributed to illegally induced abortions. During the next 5-year period, 37% of maternal deaths followed abortion.

In January 1973 the United States Supreme Court declared all restrictive abortion laws unconstitutional. As a consequence, abortion became legal in all states. The number of illegal abortions and the accompanying deaths fell precipitously after abortion became legal. During the 5-year period from 1975 to 1979, only 17 women died after illegal abortion in the United States.

The decision included directives concerning the performance of abortions, as well as decision making. During the *first trimester* the decision for abortion can be made by a patient and a physician, but the operation can be performed only by a licensed physician. States may develop regulations concerning who performs *second trimester* pregnancy terminations and where they can be done, but the decision for the procedure still rests with the patient and a physician. States may develop regulations for *third trimester* termination of pregnancy and may even proscribe termination, except to preserve the life and health of the mother.

Repeated attempts have been made to reverse the Supreme Court decision and to limit the availability of elective abortion or even to prohibit it. If these are successful, we can anticipate a resurgence of illegal abortions and their accompanying deaths.

Indications

Legal abortions include those performed because of a disorder that makes pregnancy hazardous *(medical indications)* and those performed for social or economic reasons *(nonmedical indications)*.

Medical reasons (therapeutic abortion). Therapeutic abortions are performed in women with se-

rious medical diseases that make pregnancy hazardous, fetal conditions that interfere with normal growth and development, and serious psychiatric disorders.

The *maternal medical conditions* for which abortion is most often performed are *chronic hypertension* or *renal disease,* especially when there is considerable vascular degeneration and reduced renal function; *diabetes,* especially when there are associated degenerative vascular changes; and advanced *heart disease.*

Termination of pregnancy can be considered whenever the *fetus* has little chance of developing normally because of maternal disease such as rubella, when it has been exposed to teratogenic stimuli, or when it is destined to die at an early age from a lethal hereditary condition. Certain chromosomal and metabolic abnormalities that, if present, may influence a decision for abortion can be detected by appropriate amniotic fluid studies early in pregnancy.

Therapeutic abortion for *psychiatric conditions* is justified when the pregnancy interferes with necessary psychotherapy or when the psychopathologic condition of the patient and her family is severe enough to suggest that a baby reared in the atmosphere of the home would have a small chance for normal emotional development.

Nonmedical reasons (elective abortions). The *nonmedical* reasons for abortion are primarily social or economic, and the decision as to the advisability of terminating pregnancy will be one made individually by the woman and her physician.

Physician responsibility

Physicians who choose to perform *nonmedical abortions* make the decisions concerning the advisability of the procedure with individual patients. The request for the operation always originates with the patient. One important responsibility is to recognize the occasional woman for whom termination of pregnancy may not be appropriate.

It is obvious that a woman with an undesired pregnancy may think first of termination without considering other options. Therefore, it is essential that a physician not agree to perform an abortion without a thorough review of the situation with the patient. The doctor or a specially trained nurse, social worker, or counselor should discuss with the patient the advantages and disadvantages of keeping the pregnancy. An important aspect to be considered is what effect a baby will have on her life or on members of her family. Abortion is difficult for many women to accept with equanimity; hence counseling, even for those who are adamant concerning interruption, is an important part of the treatment.

The responsibility of physicians in dealing with *medical abortions* is somewhat different. They must be able, with the help of appropriate consultants, to evaluate the severity of the systemic disease and to establish the potential risk of permitting the pregnancy to continue. In contrast to elective abortion, physicians must recommend termination for medical reasons. In many instances this is difficult for the patient to accept because she wants the pregnancy.

The need for medical abortions can be kept at a minimum by *prepregnancy examinations*. If a condition that contraindicates pregnancy is found, a suitable contraceptive method can be prescribed for temporary use if the condition can be corrected, or permanently if there is no possibility of improving it.

Complications

Complications associated with abortion occur inevitably, but they can be kept at a minimum if the procedures are performed on carefully selected patients by skillful operators in properly equipped facilities. Complications most likely to occur during early abortion are perforation of the uterus, hemorrhage, and infection. As these cannot be anticipated in advance, it is essential that provision be made to treat them promptly when they occur.

The risk of serious complications as a result of abortion during the first 12 gestational weeks for women of all ages is about one to two per 100,000 procedures. The more advanced the pregnancy when the operation is performed, the greater the risk of serious complications. Uncomplicated induced abortion appears to have little effect on the outcome of subsequent pregnancies.

At best, abortion is an unsatisfactory way of controlling reproduction. When effective contraceptive methods are used regularly, abortion is not necessary.

Technique

Blood-typing and a check for Rh antibodies are important preabortion laboratory procedures. Women who are Rh negative but who have no evidence of isoimmunization should be treated with *human anti-D gamma globulin (RhoGAM)* to prevent immunization by the fetal red blood cells that enter the maternal bloodstream during abortion.

During the first trimester of pregnancy the uterus can usually be evacuated by dilating the cervix and removing the products of conception by suction curettage. Preoperative dilation of the cervix several hours before the uterus is evacuated will soften the cervix and reduce the need for forcible dilation. Laminaria sticks made of seaweed that absorbs water, swells, and gently opens the cervix are inserted through the internal os the day before the operation is performed. They are removed just before the uterus is evacuated.

After the twelfth week the safest way to terminate pregnancy is by dilating the cervix and extracting the fetus and placenta with ring forceps and a large curet. This is far more difficult than is suction curettage during the early weeks and should be done only by individuals who are experienced in the technique.

Prostaglandins, given by intraamniotic or intravenous infusion or by intravaginal suppositories will stimulate uterine contractions at any stage of pregnancy. The placenta is often retained after the fetus is expelled and must be removed surgically.

Progesterone antagonists, which block progesterone receptor sites in the decidua, will induce bleeding in pregnant women within a few days. An additional effect of these substances is to sensitize the uterus to prostaglandins. The available progesterone antagonist, RU 486, plus a prostaglandin preparation, will induce abortion in 95% of women who have been amenorrheic for up to 49 days. It is not available in the United States, and it is not likely to be soon.

The *death rate* associated with legal abortion is determined by the stage of pregnancy, the method of induction, and the experience of the operator. Between 1972 and 1978 more than 6 million legal abortions were reported to the Centers for Disease Control. The lowest death rate, 0.5/100,000, was for abortions performed on pregnancies of 8 weeks' duration or less. The death rate increased progressively to 2.3 at 11 to 12 weeks, 6.7 at 13 to 15 weeks, and 13.9 at 16 to 20 weeks. During 1983 there were nine maternal deaths following 811,063 legal abortions at all stages of pregnancy.

When pregnancy is terminated because of a chronic condition such as heart disease, diabetes, or essential hypertension, *sterilization* should be considered, because there is little hope that the condition will improve enough to permit pregnancy in the future. This is not true of abortions performed for other reasons.

Care of patients after abortion

The patient who has had an uncomplicated elective abortion and little blood loss may be discharged a few hours after the uterus has been evacuated. Those with serious medical disorders and those in whom intraoperative complications develop should remain in the hospital until they are stabilized. Normal activity may be resumed whenever the patient feels able to carry out her usual duties. Involution usually is complete in 1 month, and menstruation begins 4 to 6 weeks after the abortion has occurred.

The most important aspect of postabortion care is to help women deal with the *grief reaction,* which may occur even in those who have been counseled extensively preoperatively. Although most women have few symptoms, some experience deep depression. Physicians who perform abortions should encourage patients to express their feelings about the procedure and help them resolve any problem resulting from it.

SUGGESTED READING

Abortion surveillance: 1982-83, Centers for Disease Control Morbidity and Mortality Weekly Report 36:1155, 1984.

Austin H, Louv WC, and Alexander J: A case-control study of spermicides and gonorrhea, JAMA 251:2822, 1984.

Boston Collaborative Drug Surveillance Program: Surgically confirmed gallbladder disease, venous thromboembolism, and breast tumors in relation to postmenopausal estrogen therapy, N Engl J Med 290:15, 1974.

Bracken MB: Spermicidal contraceptives and poor reproductive outcomes: the epidemiological evidence against an association, Am J Obstet Gynecol 151:552, 1985.

Cates W Jr, Schulz KF, and Grimes DA: The risk associated with teenage abortion, N Engl J Med 309:6211, 1983.

Connell E: Barrier contraceptives, Clin Obst Gynec 32:377, 1989.

Daling JR and others: Primary tubal infertility in relation to the use of an intrauterine device, N Engl J Med 312:938, 1985.

Faich G, Pearson K, Fleming D, and others: Toxic shock syndrome and the vaginal contraceptive sponge, JAMA 255:216, 1986.

Grimes DA and Schulz KF: Morbidity and mortality from second-trimester abortions, J Reprod Med 30:505, 1985.

Hogue CJR, Cates W Jr, and Tietze C: Impact of vacuum aspiration abortion on future childbearing: a review Fam Plan Perspect 15:119, 1983.

Inman WNW and Vessey MP: Investigation of deaths from pulmonary coronary and cerebral thrombosis and embolism in women of childbearing age, Br Med J 2:193, 1968.

Kelaghan J and others: Barrier-method contraceptives and pelvic inflammatory disease, JAMA 248:184, 1982.

Labbok MH and Queenan JT: The use of periodic abstinence for family planning, Clin Obst Gynec 32:387, 1989.

Malhotra N and Chadbury RR: Current status of intrauterine devices. II. Intrauterine devices and pelvic inflammatory disease and ectopic pregnancy, Obstet Gynecol Surv 37:1, 1982.

Mishell DR Jr: Contraception, NEJM 320:777, 1989.

Mishell DR Jr: Correcting misconceptions about oral contraceptives, Am J Obst Gynec 161:1385, 1989.

Oppenheimer W: Prevention of pregnancy by the Graefenberg ring method, Am J Obstet Gynecol 78:446, 1959.

Ory HW, Forrest JD, and Lincoln R: Making choices: evaluating the health risks of birth control methods, New York, 1983, Alan Guttmacher Institute.

Petitti DB and Wingerd J: Use of oral contraceptives, cigarette smoking and risk of subarachnoid hemorrhage, Lancet 2:234, 1978.

Population Reports: Intrauterine devices, series B, no. 3, July 1982, Baltimore, Population Information Program, The Johns Hopkins University.

Potts M: Birth control methods in the United States, Fam Plan Perspectives 20:288, 1988.

Ramcharan S, Pellegrin FA, Ray RM, and Hsu JP: The Walnut Creek contraceptive drug study of the side effects of oral contraceptives, J Reprod Med 25:349, 1980.

Rosenberg L, Hennekens CH, Rosner B, Belanger C, Rothman KJ, and Speizer FE: Oral contraceptive use in relation to nonfatal myocardial infarction, Am J Epidemiol 111:59, 1980.

Schwartz DB, Wingo PA, Antarsh L, and Smith JC: Female sterilizations in the United States, 1987, Fam Plan Perspectives 21:209, 1989.

Segal SJ and others: Absence of chorionic gonadotropin in sera of women who use intrauterine devices, Fertil Steril 44:214, 1989.

Sandmire HF and Cavanaugh MD: Long-term use of intrauterine contraceptive devices in a private practice, Am J Obstet Gynecol 152:169, 1985.

Tatum HJ and Connell-Tatum EB: Barrier contraception: a comprehensive overview, Fertil Steril 36:1, 1981.

Trussell J: Teenage pregnancy in the United States, Fam Plan Perspectives 20:262, 1988.

Willson JR, Ledger WJ, and Lovell J: Intrauterine contraceptive devices: a comparison between their use in indigent and private patients, Obstet Gynecol 29:59, 1967.

Zakin D, Stern WZ, and Rosenblatt R: Complete and partial uterine perforation and embedding following insertion of intrauterine devices. I. Classification, complications, mechanism, incidence, and missing string, Obstet Gynecol Surv 36:335, 1981.

Zakin D, Stern WZ, and Rosenblatt R: Complete and partial uterine perforation and embedding following insertion of intrauterine devices. II. Diagnostic methods, prevention and management. Obstet Gynecol Surv 36:401, 1981.

Zatuchni GI: Current methods of contraception, The Female Patient 3(5):48, 1978.

16

John H. Mattox

Spontaneous abortion

Objectives

RATIONALE: Approximately 15% to 20% of clinically recognized pregnancies are aborted spontaneously. While this event can be considered a part of the quality control process in human reproduction, it is important to understand the other possible etiologies and when therapy might prevent pregnancy loss.

The student should be able to:

A. Define *spontaneous abortion, threatened abortion, incomplete abortion,* and *habitual abortion.*

B. List the three most common etiologies for spontaneous abortion.

C. Describe symptoms, physical findings, and the clinical course of a patient with a threatened abortion versus an incomplete abortion, including potential complications.

D. List four causes of habitual abortion.

Abortion is the expulsion of the products of conception before the end of the twentieth week, when the fetus weighs less than 500 g. Abortions that occur during the first 12 weeks are *early abortions;* those that occur from the end of the twelfth through the twentieth week are *late abortions.* Abortions that occur because of some maternal, genetic, or embryonic defect are termed *spontaneous,* whereas those that are produced intentionally are said to be *induced.* An induced abortion is *legal* if performed by a physi-cian in an approved facility or *illegal* if performed by an individual not approved by the law. Abortions that are accompanied by infection are termed *septic.* There are significant religious, ethical, and societal issues involved with the elective termination of a pregnancy that will not be addressed in this chapter.

Early abortions are estimated to occur in 15% of clinically recognized pregnancies, but the actual rate is higher. Some occur after a slight delay in the onset of menstruation and cause so few symptoms that medical aid is not sought. About 40% of implanted fertilized eggs terminate spontaneously and most are not recognized clinically.

ETIOLOGY

The causes of spontaneous abortion are multiple and include fetal, maternal, and probably paternal factors. A definite reason for a specific spontaneous abortion cannot always be established because a complete analysis of all causative factors is impossible.

Genetic factors

Many early abortions of so-called *blighted ova* are actually a result of chromosomal aberrations. Boué, Boué, and Lazar, studying tissue from 1500 spontaneous abortions, identified chromosomal anomalies in 61%. On the basis of their material, they estimate that 150 of every 1000 pregnancies will terminate in recognizable spontaneous abortion. Utilizing banding techniques shows that about 52% are autosomal trisomies; the next most common is the monosomy 45 X, at about 20%. The remainder will demonstrate a mixture of karyotypic abnormalities.

Late abortions are more often associated with defective placental implantations than with defects in the embryo. However, Haxton and Bell in detailed study, including karyotyping of abortuses, at 12 to 26 weeks, found major somatic anomalies in 20% and minor abnormalities in 14%.

Maternal factors. The maternal factors that may be responsible for abortion include both local and systemic conditions.

INFECTIONS. Acute febrile illnesses may be responsible for death of the embryo and abortion, whereas tuberculosis and other chronic diseases generally do not disturb pregnancy. Syphilis may cause fetal death, but it rarely causes abortion. Generalized peritonitis, appendiceal and pelvic abscesses, and other serious local infections often, but not invariably, cause abortion.

Ordinary cervical infections, with the possible exception of *Mycoplasma hominis* and *Ure-*

aplasma urealyticum, do not usually cause abortion, but *genital herpesvirus* infection may.

NUTRITIONAL DEFICIENCIES. A nutritional deficiency sufficient to cause pronounced loss of weight may interfere with both fertility and the maintenance of pregnancy, but the role of subclinical deficiencies is less clear.

GENITAL TRACT ABNORMALITIES. *Cervical lacerations* that extend through the internal os may be responsible for repeated second-trimester abortion and immature labor. As pregnancy advances, the support provided by the intact cervix is lacking; the internal os dilates and retracts, the membranes rupture, and labor begins.

Developmental abnormalities of the uterus, especially the more advanced duplication defects, increase the premature delivery rate. The septate uterus can be responsible for spontaneous abortions.

The incidence of abortion associated with *uterine leiomyomata* also is increased if submucous tumors distort the uterine cavity and reduce the area in which normal placental implantation and growth can take place. Subserous and intramural tumors are less likely to interfere with the progression of the pregnancy. An increased incidence of spontaneous abortion has also been documented in women with *endometriosis*.

ENDOCRINE FACTORS. Disturbances in the secretions of reproductive hormones undoubtedly are responsible for some abortions, but probably are less important than they have been considered to be. Reduced hormone secretion may be a result of abnormal trophoblastic secretion rather than a primary factor in abortion.

If the ovum is fertilized, hCG from the trophoblast stimulates the corpus luteum to continue to produce estrogen and progesterone rather than to regress as it does during the normal menstrual cycle.

If the secretion of progesterone by the corpus luteum is inadequate, the endometrium may be so poorly prepared for nidation and for support of the fertilized egg that early abortion may result. It has been postulated that corpus luteum regression may be a result of defects in the trophoblast. If the trophoblast fails to develop normally, for example, when the embryo is defective, the secretion of hCG may be too low to support the corpus luteum, and production of estrogen and progesterone is inadequate to maintain normal decidua. After the *tenth gestational week,* the trophoblast usually provides enough estrogen and progesterone to maintain pregnancy.

Normal function of other endocrine glands (for example, adrenal, thyroid, pancreas) is important for maintenance of a healthy gestation. However, it appears that only when there is a clinically serious dysfunction could one ascribe the pregnancy loss to an endocrine abnormality.

PHYSICAL TRAUMA. Surgical removal of the corpus luteum or direct uterine trauma before 6 weeks' gestation increases the chances of spontaneous abortion significantly. If pelvic surgery is required, it should be postponed until early in the second trimester if it is medically feasible. Abdominal trauma rarely interrupts a normally implanted pregnancy. In many instances, pregnancy has continued despite fractures or crushing injuries to the pelvic girdle. Although a minor bump or fall can almost always be remembered by the patient to have preceded an abortion, it seems highly unlikely that injury often is a responsible factor.

MISCELLANEOUS CAUSES. Many of the miscellaneous causes for abortion are even less well understood than those already listed. Advanced maternal age, poor socioeconomic status and/or malnutrition, infertility, and ABO blood type incompatibility probably result in a hostile environment for an early pregnancy. The male contribution to abortion has been inadequately explored, but it may account for some instances of pregnancy failure. Daughters of women exposed to DES run an increased risk of abortion.

Exposure to *anesthetic agents* may be a factor in abortion. Cohen, Belville, and Brown reported abortion rates of 38% among anesthetists and 30% among operating room nurses as contrasted to a rate of 10% among general duty nurses.

Many studies suggest that *cigarette smoking* is responsible for a variety of reproductive failures, one of which may be abortion. Kline and colleagues reported that 41% of 574 women who aborted spontaneously were smokers as compared with 28% of 320 whose pregnancies continued for at least 28 weeks. *Excessive alcohol consumption* and *cocaine abuse* have also been implicated in an increased incidence of spontaneous abortion.

MECHANISM

The precipitating cause of the majority of abortions is death of the embryo or its failure to develop normally. The demise usually occurs an average of 6 weeks before expulsion. The loss of the stimulus of the growing embryo results in a gradual diminution in trophoblastic production of hCG, and subsequently ovarian estrogen, and progesterone. This is followed by spasm of the spiral arterioles, ischemic necrosis of the decidua, and bleeding into the decidua vera and the choriodecidual space. The accumulation of blood separates the placental tissue, at least partially, from its attachment to the decidua basalis. Uterine contractions, which are induced by increasing prostaglandin synthesis in the disintegrating decidua, complete the placental separation and expel the ovum completely or in part.

CLINICAL STAGES AND TYPES

As an abortion progresses, it advances through a series of fairly characteristic stages that can usually be recognized clinically. These are classified as *threatened, inevitable, incomplete,* and *complete* (Figs. 16-1 and 16-2). Abortion may also be *missed* or *habitual.*

Threatened abortion. At some time during early pregnancy, usually after having missed one or two periods, the patient becomes aware of bleeding, which is slight and usually consists of the spotting of bright blood or of dark brown discharge. She may also experience some slight cramping pain. The symptoms may subside within a day or two, but in about half the cases both the cramps and the amount of bleeding increase. The eventual outcome is uncertain and pregnancy may continue uneventfully. *No change is observed in the cervix during this stage.*

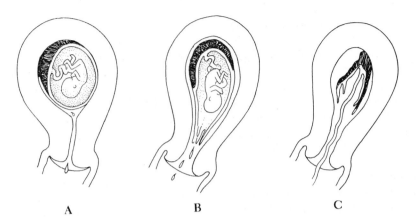

A   B   C

Fig. 16-1 **A,** Threatened abortion. Edge of placenta has separated, but cervix is closed. **B,** Inevitable abortion. Placenta has separated, cervix is effaced and partially dilated, and membranes may be ruptured. **C,** Incomplete abortion. Fetus and part of placenta have been expelled.

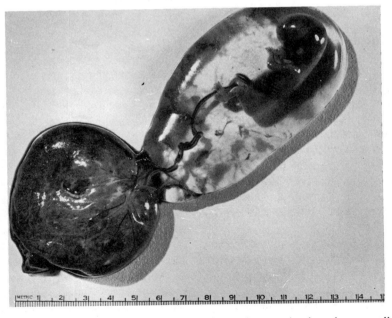

Fig. 16-2 Complete abortion. The entire products of conception have been expelled.

Inevitable abortion. If the pregnancy loss progresses, the cramps become more severe, the cervix first becomes effaced and then begins to dilate; more of the placenta is separated from the uterine wall. The bleeding increases and often is accompanied by the passage of clots. The term *inevitable abortion* implies that the changes are irreversible and that any attempt to maintain pregnancy is useless.

Incomplete abortion. In the majority of spontaneous abortions, except those that occur before 8 weeks, varying amounts of placental tissue may remain within the uterus either attached to the wall or lying free in the cavity. The patient usually reports the passage of some type of tissue, but she rarely observes the fetus because it either has never developed or has died and degenerated some time before the contractions began. Pain associated with the cramps is severe, and the amount of bleeding in some instances may be sufficient to produce profound anemia, shock, and even death. The bleeding will continue until the remaining tissue has been removed or expelled because only then can the uterine muscle contract to compress the bleeding vessels and control the hemorrhage.

Complete abortion. A complete abortion is one in which the uterus empties itself completely of the fetus and its membranes, the placenta, and the decidual lining. This usually occurs only during the first 6 weeks.

Missed abortion. Occasionally, the products of conception are retained within the uterus long after the fetus has died. As fetal death occurs sometime before the products are expelled in the usual abortion, it has been suggested that the term *missed abortion* should not be applied unless the products are retained for at least 8 weeks. The cause for the delay is unknown, but eventually spontaneous evacuation almost always occurs.

Missed abortion usually occurs during the early weeks of the second trimester, which is usually after 14 weeks of gestation. The clinical picture is that of a threatened abortion that seems to have subsided spontaneously. The amenorrhea persists, but in most patients brown vaginal discharge occurs intermittently. The symptoms of normal pregnancy disappear, the breasts become smaller, uterine growth ceases, and eventually the size of the uterus diminishes. Currently, with the use of serial ultrasound determinations and serum beta hCG levels to monitor early suspected abnormal pregnancies, missed abortion is diagnosed more often and earlier than by clinical observation alone.

Habitual abortion. Although isolated instances of spontaneous abortion are fairly common and do not necessarily recur in subsequent pregnancies, repeated abortions may be the result of a permanent maternal or paternal defect and are of greater significance. The term *habitual abortion* should be reserved for patients who have lost *three* or more pregnancies *consecutively*.

The term *recurrent pregnancy wastage* has been applied when women have lost at least two pregnancies perhaps at different stages of gestation. Because of the emotional burden produced with pregnancy loss, some patients require investigation before they will be assured that the chances of losing the next pregnancy are not extreme.

MANAGEMENT

Because the treatment of each of the various uterine stages and types of abortion is different, an accurate evaluation must be made before treatment can be planned. A properly performed pelvic examination does not adversely influence the course of the abortion and is necessary to establish the presence of a pregnancy, to eliminate tubal pregnancy as a cause of the symptoms, and to determine how far the abortive process may have advanced. The examination should include gentle digital and visual examination of the cervix and bimanual palpation of the uterus and of the adnexa. The degree of cervical effacement and dilation can be determined by palpation. Because pathogenic organisms may be carried directly to the placental site, gloves, instruments, and materials used in the examination must be sterile.

Threatened abortion. In patients with a small amount of bright red bleeding after a period is missed, when the fertilized ovum is actively invading the uterine epithelium, bleeding can occur. This spotting can occur in 30% of women, only half of whom experience pregnancy loss. Later in pregnancy, bleeding may follow mechanical separation of the edge of the normally developing placenta. This type of bleeding usually is of short duration and does not recur, but occasionally it becomes progressively more severe, particularly if it is caused by separation of a placenta implanted low in the uterine cavity. Benign lesions of the cervix such as polyps and cervicitis, as well as invasive cancer, may be a source of bright red bleeding. Such lesions can be detected by visual examination of the cervix.

Many women want to go to bed because they have heard that bed rest is important whenever bleeding occurs during pregnancy. Although this need not be discouraged, one should not make patients think it is essential because bedrest will not prevent the progression of abortion. Physicians also should not permit themselves to be pressured into administering progesterone at this stage of the process; the only effect exogenous progestogens have on the course of abortion is to delay evacuation of the uterus.

The bleeding associated with threatened abortion may be associated with uterine cramping; bleeding usually ceases in 1 to 2 days or rapidly increases in amount as other symptoms appear, whereas that from cervical or vaginal lesions is more likely to continue unchanged from day to day. Vaginal examination, including inspection of the cervix to eliminate local lesions as a cause, should be performed if the bleeding continues for more than a week.

Ultrasonic scanning may be helpful in determining the probable outcome of bleeding during early pregnancy. With an intact, normal-appearing sac containing a normal embryo or fetus, the prognosis is favorable. If the sac is broken or empty, there is no chance of a normal pregnancy, and the uterus should be emptied promptly. If the sac is smaller than is anticipated for the stage of pregnancy and does not grow, missed abortion can be diagnosed. Use of an endovaginal probe provides earlier documentation of pregnancy than a transabdominal scan.

A combination of serial ultrasonic screens and hCG assays provides the best prognostic information in women who bleed during early pregnancy. A favorable outcome can be anticipated if the embryo continues to grow at the anticipated rate and has normal heart action and if hCG secretion increases steadily. Conversely, low or falling concentrations of hCG coupled with inadequate embryonic growth are associated with a high probability of abortion.

Inevitable abortion. Because the diagnosis of inevitable abortion implies that irreversible progress toward uterine evacuation has already taken place, treatment should be directed toward reducing blood loss and pain. *The administration of oxytocics is unnecessary* because these substances do not hasten the process and serve only to increase the discomfort. When the abortion occurs between the tenth and the fourteenth weeks, uterine evacuation will usually be incomplete whether uterine stimulants are given or not. In the event of profuse bleeding it is preferable to empty the uterus surgically as soon as a moderate amount of cervical dilation has occurred or earlier. Intramuscular analgesia will not retard the progress of the abortion and may be given as needed to relieve the pain.

Incomplete abortion. Placental tissue remaining in the uterus after an incomplete abortion should be removed because it often becomes infected and, in addition, may be responsible for continued and excessive bleeding. The majority of clinically recognized abortions occur between the eighth and the twelfth weeks of pregnancy, and, as the passage of the products at this period is likely to be incomplete, a planned program for their management will keep complications at a minimum.

Patients with incomplete abortions require uterine evacuation with suction technique. The procedure can often be performed in an office or outpatient setting with paracervical anesthesia and some sedation.

Surgical evacuation of the uterus should be considered for most patients with early abortions even though the material that has been passed appears to represent the entire conceptus. Many who have had "complete" abortions between the eighth and the fourteenth weeks of pregnancy continue to bleed until the remaining placental tissue has been removed surgically.

The uterus should be evacuated promptly unless there is evidence of endomyometritis or parametritis. When infection is present, the operation should be delayed, unless excessive blood loss cannot be controlled, while antibiotics are being administered. In these cases hospitalization of the patient is necessary.

Complete abortion. During the first 7 weeks after the onset of the last period, nearly all abortions are complete and require no operative therapy. After the sixteenth week, delivery of the placenta may be delayed after expulsion of the fetus, but in most instances the placenta is passed intact, and no further treatment is required.

Missed abortion. In the past, missed abortions were generally treated expectantly until the products were expelled spontaneously, after which the uterus was curetted. It is possible to speed the process in carefully selected patients.

Before one evacuates the uterus, the diagnosis must be confirmed. Missed abortion can be suspected when the uterus is smaller than it should be for the presumed duration of pregnancy, if the uterus becomes smaller from week to week, when fetal heart sounds that have been clearly audible can no longer be heard, when fetal heart activity cannot be demonstrated by sonography, and when placental hormone concentrations are subnormal or decreasing.

Coagulopathy, initiated by the release of tissue thromboplastin into the maternal bloodstream from the necrotic decidua and placenta, may occur after prolonged retention of a dead fetus *(dead fetus syndrome).* Clotting defects rarely occur in association with missed abortion during the first half of pregnancy, but become progressively more likely if the pregnancy is advanced. The defect develops slowly and is not often seen unless the dead fetus is retained for at least 6 weeks. Fibrinogen, fibrin degradation products, and platelet levels should be checked periodically after fetal death has been diagnosed because the coagulopathy usually develops without any evidence of abnormal bleeding.

Habitual abortion. The outlook for women who have aborted more than once is considerably less bleak than the 80% rate after three consecutive abortions that was initially suggested. Warburton and Fraser calculated the risk of a repeated abortion to be about 25%. There was no appreciable increase in the risk after subsequent abortions, except for couples who had had no living children.

ETIOLOGY. The etiologic factors responsible for repeated abortion include congenital and acquired structural defects in the uterus and cervix, chromosomal abnormalities, chronic infections, perhaps psychogenic factors, hormonal deficiencies, and causes such as immunologic deficiencies that are even less clearly delineated.

A significant etiologic factor or combination of factors responsible for habitual aborters can be identified in only 60% of couples. Although the specific mechanism of action can be speculated for the "known" entities, the exact pathogenesis is often unclear. Finally, it must be remembered that a disease associated with a single spontaneous abortion is not necessarily the explanation for habitual abortion.

DIAGNOSIS. Stray-Pedersen and Stray-Pedersen categorized the causes in 195 couples who had a history of three or more consecutive spontaneous abortions. A summary of their observations can be seen in Table 16-1. *Structural abnormalities* can include uterine anomalies or the presence of a leiomyoma, usually submucosal. Either condition can reduce the available endometrial surface or provide the endometrial surface with abnormal vascularization and presumably inhibit normal implantation and placentation. Some *uterine fusion defects* limit the capacity of the uterus to enlarge

TABLE 16-1 Causes of habitual abortion — a
retrospective study of 195 couples

Cause	Rate (%)
Uterine abnormalities	28.2
Corpus (15.4%)	
Cervix (12.8%)	
Infection	14.9
Endocrine dysfunction	5.1
Chromosomal disorders	2.6
Miscellaneous	5.6
Sperm disorders (4.1%)	
Systemic illness (1.0%)	
Smoking (0.5%)	
Total "known" causes	56.4
Total "unknown" causes	43.6

Modified from Stray-Pedersen B and Stray-Pedersen S: Am J
Obstet Gynecol 148:140, 1984.

as the pregnancy grows. A cervix that has been injured during a prior pregnancy or surgical procedure or one that is congenitally defective may be unable to remain closed as the pregnancy advances, *incompetency of the internal os.* Characteristically, the patients have had pregnancies that have terminated in the second trimester in a characteristic manner; the cervix effaces and dilates painlessly with the membranes rupturing and labor being initiated. On the basis of the work of Danforth, it has been postulated that there are some patients who have an excessive amount of uterine muscle in the cervix and a decrease in the normal concentration of fibrous tissue. This muscle relaxes, as does other smooth muscle in the body during pregnancy, and the cervix dilates prematurely. If the characteristic history is present, the diagnosis becomes more probable if a no. 8 Hegar cervical dilator can be passed through the cervical canal in the nonpregnant state without meeting resistance.

Although *chromosomal abnormalities* were identified in only 2.6% of the couples in the Stray-Pedersens' series, most authors report between a 5% to 10% incidence of chromosomal problems, predominantly of *balanced translocation.* It should be remembered that if the couple has a history of recurrent pregnancy wastage and a fetus with a malformation, the probability of a chromosomal abnormality increases fivefold. Simpson has postulated that the mutant genes produce metabolic errors that interfere with some process essential to embryonic development and that polygenic factors may disturb the normal differentiation of embryonic structures.

Although *hormonal abnormalities* have long been considered to be a major cause of early pregnancy wastage, they probably are responsible for only about 5%. Diabetes mellitus and hypothyroidism receive the greatest attention. If either of these endocrinopathies is present, it would not necessarily be the only cause. A *luteal phase deficiency* has been suggested as a probable cause. Premenstrual endometrial biopsy that lags histologically more than two days behind the menstrual dates is considered the most reliable method of making this diagnosis. Serial progesterone levels have also been used. It is important that more than one cycle be studied before a diagnosis is made and therapy instituted. Once pregnancy has occurred, it is difficult to make the diagnosis of a progesterone deficiency.

Endometrial and cervical infection or, more correctly, colonization of the latter areas should probably receive greater attention. Identification of *Ureaplasma urealyticum* has been identified in up to 44% of the women with recurrent pregnancy wastage; *M. hominis* is cultured less frequently. Although significant systemic bacterial infections and viral infections have been associated with single pregnancy losses, it appears unlikely that they play a significant role in consecutive abortions.

There has been a group of *miscellaneous disorders* that have been postulated as an explanation, such as systemic illness; that is, ulcerative colitis, nutritional deficiency, semen abnormalities, and excessive smoking. Although one should attempt to identify these problems and correct them if possible, again the pathogenesis remains unclear.

Women who are habitual aborters may have several problems under this classification of immune disorders. They may share more HLA antigens with their partners, have reduced cell-mediated immune response, lack maternal blocking antibody, and have lower lymphocytotoxic antibody titers. Frequently ANA titers are elevated, requiring further evaluation to exclude systemic lupus erythematosus.

Lupus anticoagulant, an abnormal immunoglobulin, probably IgM, has been identified in women having recurrent abortions or unexplained fetal deaths. How this IgM results in the demise of an embryo or fetus is unclear, but it is thought to facilitate thrombus formation through its effect on prostaglandins. Anticardiolipin antibodies should also be measured.

A summary of the assessment of the couples who have experienced repeated abortions can be seen in the box at right.

THERAPY. The effective treatment of habitual abortion must be instituted before conception. It is not unusual for these couples to achieve pregnancy during the course of the workup; therefore the physician may wish to advise the couple to use some contraceptive measure for a brief period during the course of the evaluation. The physician can approach this assessment in a positive manner. If the cause can be identified, most of the problems can be treated. If no cause can be found, the couple can be reassured that they have approximately a 75% chance of carrying the next pregnancy to completion. It seems prudent to attempt to correct any nutritional deficiencies and eliminate excessive smoking or alcohol or drug consumption.

SURGERY. Surgical procedures are seldom required to treat habitual abortion and should not be considered until the entire assessment has been completed and other potential possible causes have been corrected. More evidence is being accumulated that the *correction of a septate uterus* via hysteroscopy is feasible and offers patients satisfactory repair without transabdominal metroplasty; concomitant laparoscopy is required to ensure safety of the hysteroscopic approach. In carefully

---

EVALUATION OF THE HABITUAL ABORTER

History
Include documentation of pregnancy loss, symptoms of systemic illness

Physical exam
Emphasis on pelvic examination to detect leiomyomata or uterine anomaly

Hysterosalpingogram
Hysteroscopy may be used

Karyotype
Special banding technique required to identify translocations

Hormonal
TSH
Hgb/AIC

Premenstrual endometrial biopsy
At least two cycles assessed; collated with BBT recordings

Immune assessment
Lupus anticoagulant
HLA typing*
ANA
Anticardiolipin antibody

Cervical cultures

---

*Applicable to the male and female.

selected patients, *removal of a submucous leiomyoma* may return the cavity to a normal configuration.

The *correction of cervical incompetence* is usually performed in the second trimester as the cervix shows evidence of effacement and dilation. The risk of ruptured membranes and infection are increased during the second half of pregnancy. Although *cervical cerclage* has been recommended by several authors with a variety of suture material, the McDonald type of repair, with a large monofilament nonabsorbable suture, is commonly preferred (Fig. 16-3).

HORMONE THERAPY. The most common entity to be treated in this category is *luteal phase deficiency*. This problem is characterized by a deficiency in progesterone, but there are several causes ranging from poor follicular development to a progesterone receptor deficiency in the endometrium. During pregnancy, estro-

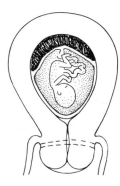

Fig. 16-3 Incompetent internal cervical os. Suture is in place to assist in the retention of the fetus.

gen and progesterone are secreted by the corpus luteum and later by the trophoblastic cells. It is more likely that progesterone is the most important for the maintenance of an early human pregnancy. Clomiphene citrate, 50 mg daily, for 5 days in the early follicular phase will enhance follicular recruitment and development. Progesterone therapy should be used only in patients who have a documented progesterone deficit on the basis of study of at least two cycles. Progesterone vaginal suppositories, 25 mg twice a day, or progesterone in oil, 12.5 mg IM daily, have been used. Although there is no scientific evidence to support that these substances are teratogenic, they are not currently approved for use during pregnancy by the Federal Drug Administration. Other progestogens such as medroxyprogesterone acetate and the 19-norsteroids, norethindrone, and ethisterone should not be used. Their androgenic activity has been associated with masculinization of the external genitalia of female fetuses.

PSYCHOTHERAPY. Women who undergo pregnancy loss have extremely intense grief reactions. The most significant response is characterized by self-guilt. It is logical to assume that some compounding of this emotional distress takes place with frequent and consecutive pregnancy wastage. Every woman who has aborted will certainly become anxious and fearful as soon as she realizes that she is pregnant again. A sympathetic approach with a special sensitivity to the problem accompanied by patience on the part of the physician are potent factors in the ultimate successful outcome of every case of repeated abortion, regardless of the cause.

There are two noteworthy studies of the treatment of women who were habitual aborters with psychother-apy. Mann studied 160 women who had aborted repeatedly. Of the 145 women who did not have a demonstrable organic cause and were treated with psychotherapy, 81% completed the pregnancy successfully. Tupper and Weil treated a group of habitual aborters, regardless of the cause, with psychotherapy and also had a similar pregnancy rate.

OTHER THERAPY. In *culture-proven infections* involving ureaplasma, an appropriate course of tetracycline therapy may result in improved pregnancy outcome. If a *male has been identified as carrying a balanced translocation*, donor insemination may be discussed as an option. In those *individuals who share major histocompatibility antigens*, transfusion of paternal leukocytes have been associated with a successful outcome. This therapeutic approach should be considered experimental, as there may be some significant risks.

High daily doses of corticosteroids combined with low doses of aspirin have resulted in increased embryo and fetal salvage in women who have lupus anticoagulant present.

SUGGESTED READING

Boué J, Boué A, and Lazar P: Retrospective and prospective epidemiological studies of 1500 karyotyped spontaneous human abortions, Teratology 12:11, 1975.

Gleicher N and Friberg J: IgM gammopathy and the lupus anticoagulant syndrome in habitual aborters, JAMA 253:3278, 1985.

Haxton MJ and Bell J: Fetal anatomical abnormalities and other associated factors in middle-trimester abortion and their relevance to patient counselling, Br J Obstet Gynaecol 90:501, 1983.

Simpson JL: Genes, chromosomes, and reproductive failure, Fertil Steril 33:107, 1980.

South J and Naldrett J: The effect of vaginal bleeding in early pregnancy on the infant born after the 28th week of pregnancy, J Obstet Gyanecol Br Comm 80:236, 1973.

Stray-Pedersen B and Stray-Pedersen S: Etiologic factors and subsequent reproductive performance in 195 couples with a prior history of habitual abortion, Am J Obstet Gynecol 148:140, 1983.

Tupper C and Weil RJ: The problem of spontaneous abortion: IX, the treatment of habitual aborters by psychotherapy, Am J Obstet Gynecol 83:421, 1962.

Warburton D and Fraser FC: Spontaneous abortion risks in man: data from reproductive histories collected in a medical genetics unit, Am J Hum Genet 16:1, 1964.

17

John H. Mattox

Ectopic pregnancy

Objectives

RATIONALE: Over the past three decades the incidence of ectopic pregnancy has increased dramatically. It was responsible for 14% of the maternal deaths in 1980 and is the most common cause of death in the first trimester. After a ruptured tubal pregnancy only about one-third of women will eventually have a live birth. A complete understanding of this condition will result in an earlier diagnosis, fewer deaths, and improved fertility.

The student should be able to:
A. List five factors predisposing patients to ectopic pregnancy.
B. Enumerate the symptoms and physical findings suggestive of ectopic pregnancy.
C. Describe the use of serial hCG determinations and ultrasound to diagnose this condition.
D. List the therapeutic alternatives.

An ectopic pregnancy, *eccyesis,* is one in which an impregnated ovum implants and develops outside the uterine cavity (Fig. 17-1). It is sometimes referred to as an extrauterine pregnancy, but this term would not apply to the occasional cornual and cervical pregnancies that are not in actual fact outside of the uterus. Although ovum fertilization occurs in the distal ampulla, implantation may occur at any point in its journey from the ovary to the uterine cavity.

SITES OF IMPLANTATION

Implantation sites of ectopic pregnancies in order of their frequency are:
1. Tubal (97% of all ectopic pregnancies)
   a. Ampullar
   b. Isthmic
   c. Fimbrial
2. Ovarian
3. Abdominal
4. Uterine
   a. Cornual
   b. Cervical

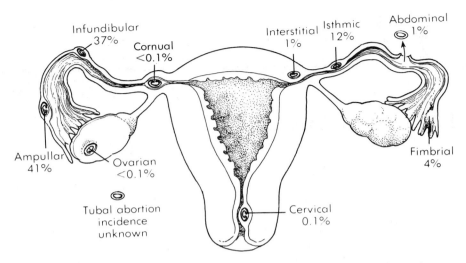

Fig. 17-1 More than 97% of ectopic pregnancies are located in the fallopian tube.

Twins and even triplets have been found in one tube, and bilateral tubal pregnancies have been reported. Combined tubal and intrauterine gestation, *heterotopic pregnancy,* used to be rare, occurring in one of 30,000 pregnancies; the use of supraovulation and in vitro fertilization, and increased frequency of tubal infection has made the event more likely.

Based upon the occurrence of ectopic pregnancy per live birth in hospital, the incidence of eccyesis has increased dramatically over the past decade. Of the several contributing factors, the increase in sexually transmitted diseases resulting in tubal destruction is the most significant factor. Depending upon the geographical location and the patient mix, the incidence can be as high as one in 60 deliveries (range is one in 60 to 200 pregnancies). The rates at all ages are higher for black women than for white women.

In the 1970s ectopic pregnancy tended to occur in women in their late twenties who had a prior pregnancy. Unfortunately, the problem is now being encountered in younger women for whom the ectopic pregnancy is their first. An ectopic pregnancy, particularly if tubal rupture and significant intraperitoneal hemorrhage occurs, bodes poorly for future fertility. Also, eccyesis is the leading cause of maternal mortality in the first half of pregnancy in the United States.

ETIOLOGIC FACTORS

Under normal conditions the ovum is fertilized in the outer third of the fallopian tube, after which it descends through the tube and enters the uterus at the blastocyst stage. If the progress of the fertilized ovum toward the uterus is delayed, it is still in the tubal lumen when it becomes capable of implanting. The trophoblast then invades the tubal epithelium, and implantation occurs there rather than in the uterus.

The following conditions within or around the oviduct retard or prevent the passage of the fertilized ovum and may be responsible for ectopic gestation:

1. *Endosalpingitis,* the single most significant factor, may be a result of sexually transmitted infections, puerperal infections causing agglutination of the fimbria and the folds of the mucosa or diverticula, or constriction of the tubal lumen.

Vasquez, Winston, and Brosens, studying tubal epithelium by scanning electron microscopy, found the proportion of normally ciliated epithelial cells to be reduced in 25 women with tubal pregnancies as compared to tubal biopsies at the time of sterilization procedures. Ciliated cells were also reduced in eight women who had previously had tubal pregnancies and in four who developed tubal pregnancies after salpingoplasty. They proposed that the reduction in ciliated epithelial cells delayed transportation of the ovum through the tube.

2. Scarring from *tubal surgery* performed to restore patency in tubes already damaged by infection.
3. *Peritubal adhesions* that may kink or immobilize the tube, which may occur after infections following abortion or puerperal infections, appendicitis, a result of endometriosis, or pelvic surgery.
4. *Congenital tubal abnormalities* such as diverticula or atresia. Similar changes can occur as a result of intrauterine exposure to DES. Salpingitis isthmica nodosa may also be a factor.
5. The fact that as many as 50% of pregnancies that occur after *surgical sterilizations* are tubal.

According to Tatum and Schmidt, the tubal pregnancy rate after laparoscopic coagulation alone is 42.9%, after coagulation and transection it is 14.5%, and after occlusion by loops and rings it is only 4.4%.

6. *Transmigration of the fertilized ovum,* a condition in which an ovum produced in one ovary enters the opposite fallopian tube. The corpus luteum is in the ovary opposite the involved tube. With *external migration* the ovum presumably is fertilized in the cul-de-sac, where it begins to develop before it is picked up by the fallopian tube. With *internal migration* the fertilized ovum enters the uterine cavity but by some means crosses and enters the opposite fallopian tube. In either case the delay in entering the tube permits the ovum to develop to a point at which it can implant.

7. Although the *presence of an IUD* does not appear to increase the risk of tubal pregnancy, those pregnancies that do occur are more likely to be either in the tube or in the ovary than in the uterus. According to Tatum and Schmidt, tubal pregnancy occurs five and one-half times more often in women who are using progesterone-releasing devices than with copper-bearing types. In addition, oral contraceptives containing only progesterone increase the risk of tubal implantation.
8. *Ovulation induction* with menotropins (Pergonal) produces an increased incidence of ectopic pregnancy. The mechanism is unclear.
9. *Assisted reproductive technologies,* such as in vitro fertilization (IVF) or gamete intrafallopian transfer (GIFT), result in a higher incidence of ectopic pregnancies, including heterotopic pregnancy.

PATHOLOGIC ANATOMY

For a better understanding of the pathogenesis of ectopic pregnancy, a review of normal fertilization and implantation (Chapter 13) is recommended.

Implantation

Conflicting evidence exists concerning implantation. Undoubtedly the location of the tubal pregnancy and the predisposing factors (such as a diverticulum or endosalpingitis) can explain some of the controversy. *Does the fertilized ovum attach itself to the tubal epithelial surface and develop within the tubal lumen, or does the developing trophoblast burrow beneath the epithelial surface and develop submucosally, breaking the tubal epithelial continuity at the time of rupture?*

Both situations exist. Intraluminal growth is unlikely in the very narrow isthmus and is more likely in the distal infundibular portion of the tube.

Pauerstein and colleagues examined 25 complete tubes that contained pregnancies and that were fixed by a technique that made them transparent so the internal anatomy could be seen in three dimensions. This permitted accurate sectioning of the tube to include the implantation site and the adjacent tubal wall. They found the trophoblastic spread to be predominantly intraluminal in 67%; in the rest the trophoblast had eroded through the mucosal surface and had extended into the muscularis between the serosa and the tubal epithelium. In all but two of the 15 unruptured tubes, the growth was intraluminal. In seven of the ten that were ruptured, the growth was predominantly extraluminal.

Uterine changes. The uterine endometrium is converted to decidua similar to that of normal pregnancy even though the ovum is implanted in the tube. The decidua develops in response to the stimulus of placental estrogen and progesterone without regard for the implantation site. Decidual growth continues as long as the trophoblast is actively producing the gestational hormones, but when the placenta separates from the tubal wall or degenerates and can no longer function, the hormonal stimulation of the uterine endometrium is withdrawn, and it degenerates and sloughs. *The external bleeding that accompanies tubal pregnancy is almost entirely the result of decidual slough and indicates failing placental tissue.*

The size and consistency of the uterus may change even though the pregnancy is in the tube. Both the cervix and the body of the uterus soften, and the corpus may enlarge to a size comparable to that of an intrauterine pregnancy of 6 to 8 weeks, but often it changes little. Uterine growth is caused by estrogen and progesterone.

Arias-Stella reaction is an exaggerated endometrial response with gland hypertrophy, crowding, and polymorphism. It needs to be distinguished from neoplastic epithelium and at one time was considered pathognomonic of ectopic pregnancy. It is now understood that these unique changes are seen in a variety of clinical settings including normal pregnancy.

Other sites

Abdominal pregnancy. Abdominal pregnancy is unusual, occurring in one in 3000 to 8000 deliveries. The fertilized ovum may implant directly on a peritoneal surface without entering the tube *(primary abdominal pregnancy)*. If the primary implantation site is just within the distal tubal opening, the developing placenta may grow through the ostium, attaching itself to the peritoneal covering of the pelvic viscera as it advances *(secondary abdominal pregnancy)*. If the embryo is properly nourished, the pregnancy continues to develop, gradually extending from the tube until the entire structure is in the abdominal cavity. An abdominal pregnancy may continue to term, but the infant usually dies before the fortieth week.

Cornual pregnancy. Cornual pregnancy occurs when the implantation site is in that portion of the tube that transverses the uterine wall, *the intramural portion* of the tube, near the tubouterine junction. Characteristically, these pregnancies produce few symptoms, because the thick uterine wall in the cornual area can enlarge more before it ruptures than can the narrow tube. Eventually the uterus will rupture, but in contrast to tubal pregnancies, rupture is usually delayed until 14 to 16 gestational weeks. Because the cornual area of the uterus contains many large blood vessels, extensive intraperitoneal hemorrhage is inevitable.

Cervical pregnancy. Cervical implantations occur only once in 15,000 to 16,000 pregnancies. They often are confused with cervical malignancy because the cervix is enlarged and friable. Profuse bleeding occurs if the cervix is biopsied.

Ovarian pregnancy. With ovarian pregnancy the ovum is fertilized before it is extruded into the peritoneal cavity, and the trophoblast develops within the ovary itself.

COURSE AND TERMINATION

The duration of tubal pregnancy and the eventual outcome are determined primarily by the area of the tube in which the pregnancy is situated.

If the ovum implants in the relatively large and distensible ampullary portion of the tube, the pregnancy will usually continue longer than it does in the narrow isthmus; however, it almost always terminates within 8 to 10 weeks after the onset of the last normal period.

Local bleeding caused by the destructive action of the trophoblastic invasion continues and increases, and eventually the hemorrhage separates the ovular sac from the tubal wall. With complete early separation, the entire sac and surrounding trophoblast may be extruded from the end of the tube, *tubal abortion,* and, unless a major vessel is injured, the bleeding ceases. This event occurs over a more protracted time.

When trophoblastic cells proliferate and invade the tubal wall, the growing conceptus and the hemorrhage cause destruction of the tubal tissue and gradually distend the peritoneum covering the oviduct. The placenta may grow directly through the peritoneum, or the wall may become so thin and distended that *tubal rupture* may occur during examination or coitus or as the patient strains to defecate.

Pregnancy in the tubal isthmus usually terminates 6 to 8 weeks after the onset of the last period. The tube usually ruptures into the peritoneal cavity, and its perforation is accompanied by sudden and profuse bleeding.

Many tubal pregnancies, probably more than become clinically obvious, undergo *spontaneous regression.* Either the ovum dies at an early stage, or it implants so close to the tubal ostium that it is soon extruded. The woman may have a slight delay in menses and mild discomfort, but one does not usually suspect tubal pregnancy, much less make an accurate diagnosis.

SYMPTOMS

The entire focus of the diagnosis of eccyesis has changed over the last decade. In the past, the traditional historical information and physical findings were based upon a more advanced clinical picture with impending or already evolved tubal rupture. The current emphasis should be upon making the diagnosis earlier, before tubal architecture has been markedly distorted and tubal rhexis has taken place. This approach minimizes the risk of morbidity and mortality and improves the chances of tubal salvage, thereby increasing future fertility potential.

The basic symptoms that should alert one to the possibility of ectopic pregnancy are a delay of menses, abnormal uterine bleeding, and pelvic pain.

Paramount to an early diagnosis is keeping predisposing factors in mind. Any woman in the reproductive age range who experiences a *delay in menses* must be evaluated not only for pregnancy but also for the possibility of tubal pregnancy. Two to 4 weeks after the missed period, a small amount of *reddish or brownish vaginal discharge* may appear, along with *lower abdominal or pelvic pain.* The pain may be slight, episodic, or quite sharp. The pain is thought to be caused by the stretching of the peritoneum covering the tube related to the growing conceptus. Intraperitoneal leakage of blood is also believed to be associated with dull discomfort. If the patient experiences extremely sharp sudden pain, particularly with a *syncopal episode,* tubal rupture should be feared. The patient may lapse into shock. Although tubal abortion may present with similar symptomatology, the acute pain and bleeding tend to be less. *Suprascapular pain,* "aching in the shoulder," signifies phrenic nerve irritation by the resultant hemoperitoneum.

Some women with tubal pregnancies are unaware of having missed a period because they interpret bleeding or spotting from the decidua as a menstrual period.

PHYSICAL SIGNS

Pelvic examination ordinarily discloses the usual *signs of early pregnancy* such as cyanosis and softening of the cervix and perhaps slight uterine enlargement.

Although a *tender adnexal mass* may be present, it could be a corpus luteum, an infected tube-ovarian complex created by the fibrin attachment of the involved tube and adjacent ovary, or the sausage-shaped tubal mass detectable in some patients with ectopic pregnancy. In very early cases of tubal pregnancy, no mass is palpable.

Unilateral adnexal tenderness is a common finding. Pain in the affected tube may be induced by putting it under tension either by elevating the cervix or moving the uterus from side to side.

Bulging of the cul-de-sac can usually be detected by vaginal or rectal examination if a pelvic hematoma has formed or if the cul-de-sac is distended with fluid blood. *Signs of peritoneal irritation* and *of free fluid in the abdomen* may be present if there has been profuse or prolonged bleeding within the peritoneal cavity.

Fever is slight or absent except in the rare patient with a secondary infected pelvic hematocele. Orthostatic changes in *pulse rate* and *blood pressure* are dependent on the amount of bleeding and are a very important part of the exam.

LABORATORY FINDINGS

The leukocyte count may be normal or slightly elevated to about 15,000 mm^3. The hemoglobin concentration or hematocrit falls slowly with chronic bleeding from the tube or rapidly with tubal rupture.

Chorionic gonadotropin (hCG) is secreted by the syncytiotrophoblast 7 to 8 days after fertilization and can be detected in small amounts in the maternal serum shortly thereafter. The use of serial *quantitative* hCG determinations that detect as little as 5 mIU/ml aids significantly in the early diagnosis of ectopic pregnancy. (For a more detailed description of hCG testing, review Chapter 2.) With the current sensitivity, the quantitative test will be negative in fewer than 1% of the cases. In addition, during the first 6 to 7 weeks of pregnancy, the circulating hCG concentration should double approximately every 48 hours. A leveling off or a decline in chorionic gonadotropin levels alerts the clinician to an abnormal pregnancy.

The *discriminatory zone*, a concept developed by Kadar and co-workers, refers to the level of hCG that must be associated with the identification of an intrauterine gestational sac by abdominal ultrasound; they pointed out that a serum level of 6500 mIU/ml detected in the absence of a sac presents a very high probability that the patient has an ectopic pregnancy. Utilizing the more sensitive endovaginal ultrasound probe has lowered the discriminatory zone to 1800 mIU/ml, which will probably continue to decline.

DIAGNOSIS

The diagnosis of an unruptured tubal pregnancy is not too difficult to make when classic symptoms and signs are present. Unfortunately, symptoms are often atypical, and pelvic findings may be misleading. In general, the diagnosis can be made with a considerable degree of accuracy if one has a high index of suspicion for this condition and is alerted by the history (Fig. 17-2).

Special studies

Ultrasound. *Sonography*, particularly with the endovaginal probe, is very helpful in making the diagnosis of tubal pregnancy. A direct diagnosis can be made if a typical gestational sac is identified outside the uterus. Unfortunately, this is not always possible, so the diagnosis is often made by exclusion. A characteristic and normally situated gestational sac within the uterine cavity virtually excludes ectopic pregnancy, except in rare instances of combined tubal-intrauterine pregnancies.

If the scan is performed too early, the gestational sac may be too small to detect in the uterus. Occasionally, an image that looks like an intrauterine pregnancy or a blighted ovum can be seen in women who have a tubal pregnancy or who have aborted an intrauterine gestation. This structure, a *pseudogestational sac*, is produced by blood clots in the uterine cavity.

The *double ring sign* outlining a portion of the gestational sac and the decidua basalis can be detected early and is reassuring that the gestation is intrauterine.

The combination of a positive pregnancy test without ultrasonic evidence of an intrauterine pregnancy 6 weeks or more after the onset of the last menstrual period is very suggestive of tubal pregnancy.

Culdocentesis (Fig. 17-3). Hemoperitoneum or a cul-de-sac hematoma can be detected by *needle culdocentesis*, which can be performed in the out-

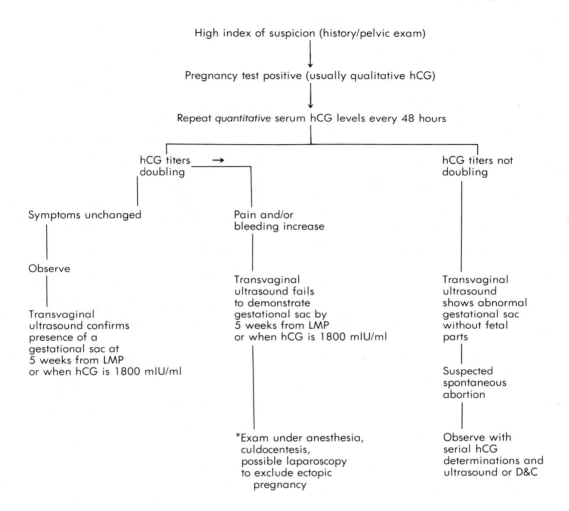

Fig. 17-2 Diagnostic approach to ectopic pregnancy.

patient or hospital examining room using local infiltration anesthesia. If dark or bright red nonclotting blood flows freely through the needle, the presence of intraperitoneal bleeding is confirmed. The hematocrit of the aspirate is usually above 15%. If only a small amount of bright red blood can be aspirated, the needle may have perforated a blood vessel and should be withdrawn and reinserted. Failure to obtain blood does not rule out ectopic gestation. If serosanguineous fluid is obtained, eccyesis is less likely. Culdocentesis is a painful procedure and therefore is not applicable to

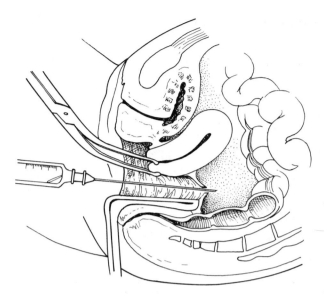

Fig. 17-3 Culdocentesis. An 18-gauge needle, with attached syringe, is being inserted into the cul-de-sac.

every patient. Medical judgment must be exercised when selecting patients. Performing it in the operating suite with the patient anesthetized is sometimes preferable.

If nonclotting blood is aspirated from the cul-de-sac, one may proceed directly to laparotomy. If blood cannot be aspirated from the cul-de-sac in a patient with a positive pregnancy test and without sonographic evidence of an intrauterine pregnancy, it is essential that the diagnosis be confirmed or excluded by looking at the pelvic organs. This can be accomplished by *laparoscopy*.

Dilation and curettage. A D&C should be performed if vaginal bleeding has been profuse and prolonged. This affords an opportunity for careful pelvic examination under anesthesia and may rule out an ectopic pregnancy if placental tissue is obtained from the endometrial cavity. If the material grossly resembles normal endometrium, further investigation, usually by laparoscopy, is indicated. Sometimes a frozen-section preparation for microscopic review can be helpful in distinguishing decidua from trophoblastic tissue.

DIFFERENTIAL DIAGNOSIS

Although it is usually possible to diagnose tubal pregnancy with reasonable accuracy, uterine abortion, adnexitis, appendicitis, and ruptured corpus luteum or follicular cysts may produce symptoms so similar that differentiation is difficult.

Threatened or incomplete abortion. The period of amenorrhea preceding the onset of symptoms usually is longer, the amount of vaginal bleeding is greater, the pain usually is more severe than in early ectopic pregnancy and is in the midline and crampy in nature, and no adnexal mass and tenderness are present. Serial hCG determinations and ultrasound will usually establish the diagnosis.

Adenexitis. The symptoms accompanying acute tubal infection, which usually involves the adjacent ovary and parametrium, usually appear at the time of menstruation rather than after a period of amenorrhea. However, with either salpingitis or ectopic pregnancy, the bleeding may be irregular, prolonged, and more painful than usual. The pain, tenderness, and palpable tubal enlargement usually are bilateral with salpingitis. The temperature ordinarily is elevated, and leukocytosis is much greater than with ectopic pregnancy. The pregnancy test is negative.

Appendicitis. There is usually a history of digestive disturbances such as nausea and vomiting, there is no amenorrhea or abnormal bleeding, and there is no adnexal mass unless an appendiceal abscess has developed. The pregnancy test is negative.

Corpus luteum cysts. The mass in corpus luteum cysts usually is larger and more globular than in ectopic pregnancy. Unless the cyst has ruptured, there is no evidence of intraperitoneal bleeding. The pregnancy test is negative unless there is an intrauterine pregnancy and the cyst can be visualized with ultrasound.

Ruptured graafian follicle with excessive bleeding. Usually amenorrhea is not associated with ruptured graafian follicle, and the rupture occurs most often at midcycle, at the time of ovulation. The pregnancy test is negative. With the utilization of ultrasound, particularly the endovaginal probe, the diagnosis can be made easily.

TREATMENT

The usual treatment of tubal pregnancy is surgical, but the exact procedure is determined by the duration of pregnancy, the site, the condition of the tube, and the condition of the patient. If the pregnancy has been diagnosed early, it often is possible to preserve the tube *(salpingostomy or segmental resection).* Conversely, if there has been delay in making the diagnosis, the tube may be so damaged that it cannot be salvaged and must be removed *(salpingectomy).* If the patient's condition is stable, and the operator is an accomplished laparoscopic surgeon, ectopic pregnancy may be treated by *operative laparoscopy.*

Because Rh-negative women can be sensitized by Rh-positive blood from extrauterine embryos, they should be treated with Rh immunoglobulin as part of the treatment of tubal pregnancy. This is particularly important when the pregnancy is advanced.

The patient with ruptured tubal pregnancy and massive intraperitoneal hemorrhage must be operated on as soon as she can be transported to the hospital and the operating room can be prepared. If she is in deep shock, a surgical procedure without preliminary blood transfusion will increase the mortality. Consequently, type-specific blood must be administered while the patient is being prepared and anesthetized.

In *linear salpingostomy,* an incision is made through the tubal wall over the gestational sac, which is then removed. The defect can be closed or left open. With *segmental resection,* the area of the tube containing the conceptus is removed, and the cut ends are either anastomosed immediately or at a later operation. These operations are justified when tubal distortion is slight and are particularly useful if the other tube has already been removed or is extensively damaged.

It may be possible to express the gestational sac from the ampulla without removing the tube if the diagnosis is made early.

Treatment of ectopic pregnancy with medical therapy (methotrexate) has been successful in other countries and in research protocols in the United States. It may be possible to treat women with systemic chemotherapy or with ultrasound-guided injection of the gestational sac, eliminating the need for a major surgical procedure.

PROGNOSIS

Mortality. Although almost 10% of maternal deaths each year in the United States are caused by ectopic pregnancy, the death rate has decreased steadily. According to statistics from the Centers for Disease Control, the death rate (deaths from ectopic pregnancy/1000 ectopics) was 3.5 in 1970, 1.6 in 1975, and 0.9 in 1980. Fortunately these rates continue to decline. Death rates were consistently higher for black than for white women.

Subsequent pregnancies. Many women who have had a ruptured tubal pregnancy either do not conceive again or have another pregnancy in the remaining tube. The reason is that the tubal lesions responsible for the first abnormal pregnancy may also be present in the opposite tube. Schenker, Eyal, and Polishuk studied the reproductive performance of 277 women who had been operated on for tubal pregnancy. Of these women, 114 (41.4%) had 219 pregnancies subsequent to the tubal gestation, which terminated in 114 live births, 37 spontaneous abortions, 29 induced abortions, and 39 recurrent ectopic pregnancies (16.2%).

The outlook after conservative surgery is much better than after salpingectomy. Sherman and co-workers reported an intrauterine pregnancy rate of 85% in women with normal fertility and normal pelvic organs. In patients who had had difficulty conceiving or whose pelvic organs were abnormal, the subsequent intrauterine pregnancy rates were 67% after salpingotomy and 44% after salpingectomy. He also observed more successful pregnancies in women who had been operated on when the tube was intact as compared to those in whom the tube already had ruptured.

SUGGESTED READING

Breen JL: A 21-year survey of 654 ectopic pregnancies, Am J Obstet Gynecol 106:1004, 1970.

Budowick M, Johnson TRB Jr, Genadey R, Parmley TH, and Woodruff JB: The histopathology of the developing tubal ectopic pregnancy, Fertil Steril 34:169, 1980.

Pauerstein CJ, Croxatto HB, Eddy CA, Ramzy I, and Walters MD: Anatomy and pathology of tubal pregnancy, Obstet Gynecol 67:301, 1986.

Romero R, Kadar N, Janty P, and others: Diagnosis of ectopic pregnancy: value of discriminatory human chorionic gonadotropin zone, Obstet Gynecol 66:357, 1985.

Schenker JG, Eyal F, and Polishuk WZ: Fertility after tubal pregnancy, Surg Gynecol Obstet 135:74, 1972.

Sherman D, and others: Improved fertility following ectopic pregnancy, Fertil Steril 37:497, 1982.

Weckstein LN: Current perspective on ectopic pregnancy, Obstet Gynecol Surv 40:259, 1985.

18

Michael P. Hopkins

Gestational trophoblastic neoplasms

Objectives

RATIONALE: Although gestational trophoblastic neoplasms are relatively uncommon, they are important because of their malignant potential and because of the risk of death from hemorrhage and infection.

The student should be able to:

A. List symptoms and physical findings suggesting the disease.
B. Demonstrate knowledge of methods of confirming the diagnosis.
C. State the principles of management and followup of women with gestational trophoblastic neoplasms.

Gestational trophoblastic neoplasms encompass a wide range of malignant degeneration of trophoblastic tissue. These diseases are best viewed as a continuum with hydatidiform mole as benign and progressing through invasive mole to choriocarcinoma. This is a pathologic description that attempts to predict the potential for metastases. From a historical standpoint, it was once extremely important to determine which patients required hysterectomy in the hopes of complete surgical removal before metastasis occurs. The present management of this disease, however, has been completely changed by the advent of an accurate tumor marker (hCG) and chemotherapy. In fact, this disease, which previously was one of the most lethal, is now one of the most curable. Currently, the metastatic potential is monitored by serial hCG levels, and almost all patients with persistent titers or progressive disease are managed by chemotherapy. Hysterectomy now plays a limited role in the management of this disease. Thus, whereas gestational trophoblastic neoplasia was once managed by light microscopy clinicopathologic correlations with early aggressive surgery, this has been replaced by biochemical tumor markers and medical management. The distinctions between hydatidiform mole, invasive mole, and choriocarcinoma are presented as a framework for understanding this disease. The most benign-appearing mole, however, can metastasize and is then considered a choriocarcinoma; on the other hand the most aggressive-looking choriocarcinoma can regress after D&C without metastasizing.

HYDATIDIFORM MOLE

Hydatidiform mole is a neoplastic proliferation of the trophoblast in which the terminal villi are transformed into vesicles filled with clear viscid material (Fig. 18-1). Hydatidiform mole usually is benign, but at times it has malignant potential and can precede the development of choriocarcinoma.

The exact frequency with which hydatiform moles develop is not known. They are presumed to occur once in 1500 to 2000 pregnancies in the United States and more often in Asian countries. That these figures may be inaccurate is suggested by a report of 10,929,354 pregnancies in 3,089,399 women from 26 provinces in China, in which the overall incidence of hydatidiform mole was 1 in 1238 pregnancies. The question concern-

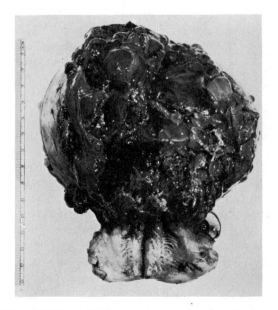

Fig. 18-1 Hydatidiform mole at approximately hundredth day of pregnancy. Note uneffaced, undilated cervix with deep molar penetration into myometrium. Patient is a 43-year-old primigravida.

ing the exact frequency exists because of the way rates are determined and because of differences in the frequency with which pregnancy and its termination are reported. Even in more advanced nations, all the events of pregnancy are underreported. There are even greater inaccuracies in developing countries, where most births occur at home and may be unreported and where the number of early pregnancy terminations certainly is unknown. The presumed rates are based upon known pregnancies and on women who are treated for hydatidiform moles in hospitals.

Etiologic factors

Approximately half the specimens of tissue from spontaneous abortions may have pathologic ova. Early hydatidiform placental degeneration can be present in two thirds of the specimens with abnormal ova. These vesicles may develop because of the absence of fetal circulation. The physiologic activity of the trophoblast continues, but the fluid accumulates and distends the villi because it cannot be removed by a normal embryo.

Moles in which normal placental tissue or fetal structures can be identified are called *partial*. Those that have no fetal or normal placental tissues are *complete*. The latter are the more likely to become malignant.

The effect of nationality or race on the incidence of hydatidiform mole is not completely clear. There is a high incidence in Asian women that some believe may be related to a dietary protein deficiency, although this is not completely established.

Age seems to be a significant factor in the genesis of the lesion. Hydatidiform mole develops 10 times more often in women over the age of 45 than in those who are younger.

The chromosome pattern of most hydatidiform moles is 46 XX, and the entire genome of hydatidiform moles is of paternal origin. The most likely explanation is that an "empty egg"—one without genetic material—is fertilized by a haploid sperm (23 X), which restores the diploid number (46 XX) by duplicating itself, and grows.

Moles with 46 XY configuration may occur because of fertilization with two spermatozoa, one an X and the other a Y. A triploid chromosomal pattern (usually XXX) is found in partial moles.

Trophoblastic disease may also have a familial component. Instances in monozygotic twins and a propensity for the neoplasm to develop in certain families have been reported. Additionally, there is a tendency for recurrence. A woman with one molar pregnancy has an approximately 2% to 3% chance of developing a subsequent molar pregnancy. In one report, 52 episodes of trophoblastic disease in 22 (1.33%) of 1648 women were reported.

Pathologic findings

The trophoblast is converted into a mass of vesicles, which vary in size from a few millimeters to a maximum diameter of about 3 cm. The entire mass may be small, or it may enlarge the uterus to the size of a normal 24- to 26-week gestation. If a fetus can be identified (partial or incomplete mole), it is small and malformed, although occasionally a normal baby may be born at or near term with a considerable amount of the placenta having undergone hydatidiform degeneration. They may be twin pregnancies with hydatidiform degeneration of one placenta and normal development of the other.

The histologic pattern of a benign complete mole is characterized by trophoblastic proliferation, hydropic degeneration of the stroma, and absence of blood vessels. When the mole is benign, the villous pattern is maintained, and there is neither anaplastic change nor epithelial penetration into the stroma or the myometrium.

Potentially malignant moles are characterized by more pronounced trophoblastic activity and anaplastic change. Attempts have been made to establish histologic criteria for estimating the degree of malignancy, but the most accurate method is still the clinical course.

The ovaries can respond to the stimulation of the elevated levels of chorionic gonadotropic hormones (hCG) by the development of theca-lutein cysts. The cysts, which develop in 30% to 50% of hydatidiform moles and are usually bilateral, vary in size from those that barely enlarge the ovary to those 20 cm or more in diameter. Definite ovarian enlargement is recognized clinically only in a minority of hydatidiform moles. The change probably reflects the stage of molar development and the amount of gonadotropin being produced. After the uterus is evacuated, the ovaries gradually return to normal size as hormone levels decrease. The same change may occur during normal pregnancy.

Symptoms

After a period of amenorrhea during which the patient considers herself to be pregnant, bright red spotting or dark brown vaginal discharge appears. It may be followed rather rapidly by cramps and expulsion of the mole, or discharge and bleeding may continue intermittently for several weeks. Patients who have bled for long periods of time may become anemic. Partial spontaneous evacuation, during which bleeding may be profuse, eventually occurs. These patients are often diagnosed as having a threatened or missed abortion until the characteristic vesicles are passed.

All symptoms of early pregnancy may be exaggerated in women with hydatidiform mole. Nausea and vomiting may begin earlier, be more severe, and last longer than during normal pregnancy. Severe pregnancy-induced hypertension may develop during the early part of the second trimester of a molar pregnancy; this is the only situation in which this condition is diagnosed before the twenty-fourth week. Hypertension is most likely to occur when the uterus enlarges rapidly and is considerably larger than might be expected for that stage of gestation. Plasma thyroxine concentrations often are elevated, but obvious signs of hyperthyroidism occur in only about 2% of women with hydatidiform moles.

Diagnosis

Most patients with moles are first diagnosed with a threatened or inevitable abortion unless typical vesicles are passed. The diagnosis is usually made preoperatively when ultrasound is performed; otherwise, the correct diagnosis may be made when the physician begins to evacuate the uterus.

Hydatidiform mole can be suspected if the uterus is inappropriately enlarged for the calculated duration of pregnancy. In about half of the cases, the uterus is larger than expected. Usually, the discrepancy is not great, but in some the uterus may be as large as that of a 24- to 26 week pregnancy during the early second trimester. In the remainder of the cases, the uterus is either appropriately enlarged or smaller than that anticipated for the gestational age. One must, of course, consider other conditions that may cause what seems to be inappropriate uterine enlargement. The most common are an uncertain date for the last menstrual period, multifetal pregnancy, and myomas.

Between the sixteenth and twentieth weeks of normal pregnancy, it is almost always possible to identify a fetus by hearing fetal heart sounds. However, the absence of these signs does not eliminate normal pregnancy.

A positive diagnosis of hydatidiform mole is almost always made by sonography. The characteristic pattern, when it is present, cannot be confused with normal pregnancy (Fig. 18-2). The pattern during early molar pregnancy may be less distinctive because the cysts are smaller. A repeat examination in 2 to 3 weeks usually clarifies the diagnosis.

Assays for hCG may be helpful in suspected hydatidiform mole because the serum concentration of hCG is usually much higher than during comparable stages of normal pregnancy. This alone is not a reliable diagnostic measure, however, because the levels at the time of peak secretion in normally pregnant women, at about the

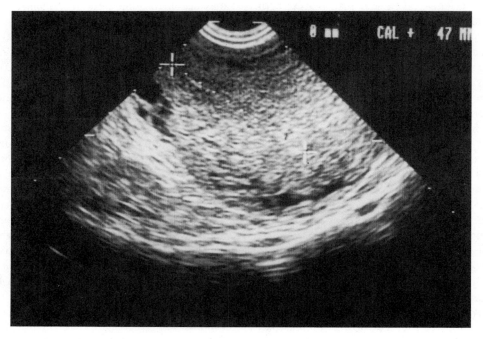

Fig. 18-2 Sonogram of hydatidiform mole. The mottled, snowstormlike appearance caused by cystic villi is typical and distinct from an intrauterine pregnancy.

sixtieth to seventieth day, may be in a range consistent with a mole.

The serum values of hCG rise during early normal pregnancy and reach about 50,000 mIU/ml at 45 days and a maximum of as much as 600,00 mIU/ml at about 60 days. The titer then decreases rapidly and is rarely above 20,000 mIU/ml after 100 days. The levels with multiple pregnancy are higher than those with a single fetus. The values for hydatidiform mole often reach 1.5 to 2 million mIU/ml, but they can also be low if the mole is regressing rather than growing.

It is evident that it would be hazardous to diagnose hydatidiform mole at the sixtieth day of pregnancy in a patient with a history suggesting threatened abortion and a uterus larger than anticipated gestational age simply on the basis of a serum gonadotropin concentration of 500,000 or even 1 million mIU/ml.

Some authors have suggested using both ultrasound and hCG assay to assist in diagnosing early hydatidiform moles. Usually fetal cardiac motion is seen on ultrasound by the sixth to eighth week of pregnancy when the hCG concentration is in the range of 80,000 mIU/ml.

Treatment

The uterus should be evacuated as soon as possible after the diagnosis is made. The molar tissue can be removed in almost every instance by suction curettage. This method is appropriate even though the uterus is as large as that of a late-second-trimester normal pregnancy. Suction is preferable to a standard D&C because the uterus can be emptied more rapidly and its wall is less likely to be injured. An oxytocin infusion during surgery stimulates the uterus to contract and reduce blood loss. The operation is completed by carefully curetting the uterine wall with a large, sharp curet. Tissue from the implantation site may provide more information concerning myometrial invasion and malignancy than do the vesicles.

As many as 10% of women develop acute pulmonary complications after curettage. They are characterized by tachycardia, tachypnea, and hypoxia. The condition is thought to result from pulmonary embolization with trophoblastic tissue combined with fluid overload, which is caused by physiologic dilutional hypervolemia, pregnancy-induced hypertension, and hyperthyroidism. The patient's condition can be monitored by measuring pulmonary wedge pressure, and the pulmonary symptoms are treated with administration of diuretics and oxygen and limitation of fluid administration. Primary treatment by hysterectomy can be considered for women who have completed childbearing.

Follow-up

Between 15% and 25% of women develop persistent trophoblastic disease after complete moles are evacuated. The risk of malignancy is somewhat less with partial moles, approximately 10%.

Every patient treated for hydatidiform mole must be kept under observation until the physician can be certain that she does not have malignant trophoblastic disease. If the mole has been evacuated completely, uterine bleeding should cease within a week and the uterus should return to its normal size within 4 to 6 weeks. If bleeding persists and involution is delayed, another curettage should be performed in an attempt to determine whether the cause is residual benign molar tissue or a chorionic malignancy.

A more precise method for detecting continuing trophoblastic activity is by the weekly measurement of gonadotropin concentration in the serum. If the mole has been removed completely, the chorionic gonadotropin production will cease, and the material will gradually be excreted. It usually has all disappeared from the serum within 100 days after removal of the mole (Fig. 18-3). If active molar tissue remains or if a malignant trophoblastic lesion has developed, gonadotropin secretion will persist or increase, and the concentration will plateau or rise.

A test for the beta subunit of hCG is performed at weekly intervals until the hormone cannot be detected in two consecutive specimens. If the level has fallen steadily at the expected rate to

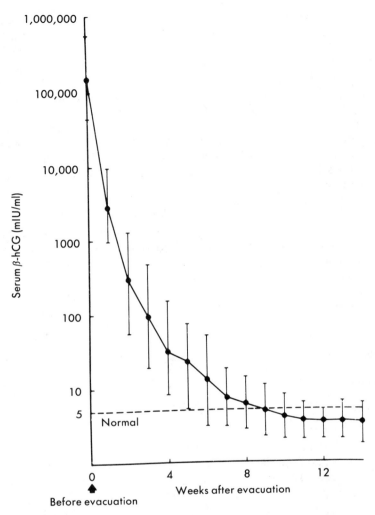

Fig. 18-3 Regression curve for hCG after evacuation of hydatidiform mole. (From Morrow CP, Kletzky OA, Disaia PJ, Townsend DE, Mishell DR, and Nakamura RM: Am J Obstet Gynecol 128:424, 1977.)

nondetectable levels, it should then be checked monthly for 1 year.

An effective contraceptive method is essential during the follow-up period because hCG from a new pregnancy will mask any activity from the neoplasm. Low-dose oral contraceptives do not interfere with the interpretation of hCG assay, nor do they increase the risk of trophoblastic disease. A chest x-ray film should be obtained after the

mole is evacuated in search of pulmonary metastases that already may have occurred. It should be repeated during the follow-up period.

The regression of hCG to nondetectable levels occurs at varying intervals. Approximately 60% to 80% of women have nondetectable levels by 8 weeks after evacuation. Regression to nondetectable levels can, however, take as long as 6 months. These women need careful evaluation when the regression time is extended to the limit and should be given individual recommendations. In general, short plateaus of 2 to 3 weeks can be a normal variation, whereas longer plateaus usually signify the necessity for therapy.

Standard pregnancy tests are inadequate for following patients who have been treated for hydatidiform mole or choriocarcinoma because only positive tests are significant. Even the most sensitive will not detect low levels of hCG, which may be present with residual active mole.

The quantitative beta-subunit radioimmunoassay is the most accurate of the assay techniques and should be used during follow-up. It is the only one that differentiates between LH and hCG; hence it measures only trophoblastic activity. It is so sensitive that it detects concentrations of hCG to which no other test responds. This test is now routinely available in all clinical laboratories.

No active treatment is necessary as long as there is a progressive decline in the level of hCG. If the level plateaus or rises, one can assume that there still is active trophoblastic disease and that treatment is indicated.

INVASIVE MOLE

Invasive mole is similar to hydatidiform mole, from which it arises, but its malignant potentials are much greater. It invades the myometrium, in some instances penetrating the uterine wall completely and extending into the broad ligament or the peritoneal cavity. In half or more of all cases, invasive mole metastasizes through the peripheral circulation to distant sites, most characteristically the lung.

Pathologic findings

The histologic pattern is similar to that of hydatidiform mole in that the villous architecture is maintained, even in metastatic implants. The most important differences are the excessive trophoblastic proliferation and invasiveness. The degree of anaplasia is variable; in some patients the metastatic tissue looks completely benign, and in others the cells are anaplastic. The preservation of the villous pattern serves to differentiate invasive

mole from choriocarcinoma, which is so anaplastic that villi cannot form.

Clinical course and diagnosis

Bleeding may continue after the evacuation of a mole if the lesion is relatively superficial; there may be no blood loss if the trophoblast lies deep in the myometrium. The first evidence of the disorder may be coughing or hemoptysis from metastatic lung lesions.

Invasive mole or choriocarcinoma can be suspected if the gonadotropin titers fail to regress or continue to rise after evacuation of a hydatidiform mole. When this occurs, repeat curettage is indicated, but it may not be conclusive. If the lesion is superficial, a diagnosis may be possible; if it lies deep in the muscle, the curet will not reach it. A chest x-ray film will reveal metastatic lesions if they are present.

The potential for persistent disease or metastatic spread from invasive mole is greater than that from benign mole but less than that from choriocarcinoma.

Treatment

Treatment is identical to that for choriocarcinoma.

CHORIOCARCINOMA

Choriocarcinoma is a malignant trophoblastic tumor that may follow hydatidiform mole, abortion, or normal pregnancy. Approximately 50% of choriocarcinomas are preceded by hydatidiform mole, but only about 15% to 25% of the latter have malignant propensities. About 25% follow abortion, and about 25% develop after delivery at term or an ectopic pregnancy. Small foci of choriocarcinoma have been identified in otherwise normal term placentas.

Pathologic findings

The tumor appears as an irregular or circumscribed hemorrhagic growth in the uterine wall. The ulcerating surface usually opens into the endometrial cavity, but on occasion the entire tumor is embedded in myometrium. It sometimes grows

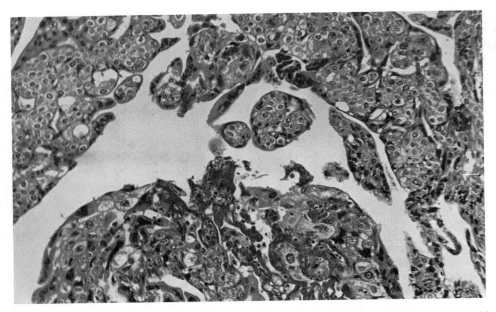

Fig. 18-4 Section through viable choriocarcinoma. Neoplastic trophoblastic cells are of both syncytial and Langhans type. There is no necrosis or hemorrhage in this field.

entirely through the uterus into the broad ligament or the peritoneal cavity. There may be dark red, blood-filled metastases in the vagina or the vulva.

Masses of anaplastic trophoblastic cells invade the uterine wall and destroy blood vessels and muscle tissue as they grow. Necrosis and hemorrhage are prominent in the histologic appearance. The cells proliferate in masses and sheets, and villi cannot be recognized. The same pattern is retained in metastases (Fig. 18-4).

Clinical course and diagnosis

Irregular bleeding continues after the passage of a hydatidiform mole, abortion, or delivery unless the growth is situated deep in the uterine wall. Bleeding usually increases as more tissue is destroyed. Malignant tumor cells enter the circulation through open blood vessels and are transported to the lungs, brain, or other organs and soft tissues. The first evidence of an abnormality may be the appearance of symptoms caused by pulmonary lesions or the discovery of a metastatic nodule in the vagina or vulva.

Choriocarcinoma must be suspected as a possible reason for continued bleeding after any pregnancy. A less serious lesion is more often the cause, but if each patient who bleeds is studied by curettage and tests for chorionic gonadotropin, malignant trophoblastic disease will be diagnosed as early as possible.

Curettage may be deceptive; if the tumor is situated deep in the myometrium, it cannot be reached with the curet. It may not even be possible to make an accurate histologic diagnosis from tissue curetted directly from a large ulcerating lesion because the material may represent only necrotic tissue from the surface.

The measurement of chorionic gonadotropin is the most important single diagnostic aid. Choriocarcinoma must be suspected whenever the concentration of this hormone remains high or is increasing and retained molar or placental tissue has been eliminated as its source. One can expect the serum hCG to fall to less than 10 mIU/ml in about 30 days after induced abortion of early pregnancy, in about 19 days after spontaneous abortion, and in about 8 to 9 days after an ectopic pregnancy is removed. If the level remains elevated or continues to rise, the diagnosis is almost certain, and it is reinforced by the presence of characteristic lung lesions. In any woman of reproductive age with unexplained lung or brain metastases, choriocarcinoma should be considered in the differential diagnosis. Compared to other malignancies, choriocarcinoma is very responsive to chemotherapy.

Treatment

Until chemotherapeutic drugs that specifically destroyed trophoblast became available, 80% to 85% of women with choriocarcinoma died within a year. Total hysterectomy with bilateral salpingo-oophorectomy, irradiation, and resection of local metastases were the only treatment before chemotherapy became available. They were generally ineffective because by the time therapy was instituted, the tumor had already metastasized widely.

The prognosis for choriocarcinoma has improved considerably as a result of chemotherapeutic drugs. The response rate is determined by the extent of the lesion and the quality of treatment. When the diagnosis of metastatic disease is established, a metastatic evaluation consisting of chest x-ray and head and abdominal CT scan is instituted. Classification into low- or high-risk categories determines the chemotherapy protocol. Those with low-risk disease can be treated with single-agent chemotherapy (methotrexate or actinomycin D), whereas those with high-risk disease require aggressive multiagent chemotherapy (see box at right). The tumor can be completely eradicated in almost every patient with localized or with low-risk metastatic disease. Although the results are less satisfactory when the tumor is more extensive and is widely disseminated, 80% to 90% of those with high-risk disease respond well to treatment.

CRITERIA FOR DELINEATING LOW-RISK FROM HIGH-RISK METASTATIC GESTATIONAL TROPHOBLASTIC DISEASE

Low risk requires single-agent chemotherapy, whereas high risk requires multiagent therapy.

Good prognosis (low risk)
hCG <40,000 mIU/ml pretreatment
No brain or liver involvement
No prior chemotherapy
Less than 4 months duration
Poor prognosis (high risk)
hCG >40,000 mIU/ml
Brain or liver metastases
Failed chemotherapy
Following term pregnancy

The outcome greatly depends on the initial management and initial therapy. The best results, especially in high-risk patients, are obtained when women with gestational trophoblastic neoplasms are treated in centers that provide the necessary diagnostic facilities and expert personnel who are experienced in managing this disease.

The drugs most often used in treating gestational trophoblastic neoplasms are amethopterin (methotrexate) and actinomycin D (dactinomycin). Methotrexate, a folic acid analog that interferes with normal metabolism, was the first drug to eradicate abnormal trophoblast effectively. Its principal action appears to be the prevention of synthesis of thymidylate, an essential component of DNA. Actinomycin D is an antibiotic with an action similar to that of alkylating agents. Treatment of patients with nonmetastatic or low-risk metastatic disease can be started with one of these drugs.

Women whose hCG titers plateau or rise during postevacuation follow-up or those with metastatic disease should receive chemotherapy. The regimen is selected on the basis of a pretreatment survey to determine the extent of the disease. The survey includes a complete blood study with differential and platelet counts, serum biochemical determinations, liver function studies, thyroid studies, chest x-ray film examinations, an intravenous pyelogram, liver and brain CT scans, and hCG assay.

Nonmetastatic gestational trophoblastic neoplasms are usually treated with a single agent, which is continued until the tumor has been eradicated. Usually, the first drug is methotrexate. Side effects from the medication include stomatitis, dermatitis, leukopenia from bone marrow depression, gastrointestinal ulceration, and alopecia. They can be kept minimal by a regimen that includes larger doses of methotrexate and folinic acid. Methotrexate, 1 mg/kg body weight, is given on days 1, 3, 5, and 7; and 0.1 mg/kg of body weight of folinic acid is given on days 2, 4, 6, and 8. This treatment regimen is very effective and, with the folinic acid, the side effects are reduced to a minimum. Because of its effectiveness and decreased side effects, many now consider this the treatment of choice for low-risk disease. Patients with liver or kidney dysfunction and those who cannot tolerate repeated courses of methotrexate can be treated with actinomycin D. This drug is given intravenously 0.5 mg for 5 days. Daily monitoring for toxic effects is essential. Courses are repeated at 14-day intervals for as long as necessary. There is a high rate of stomatitis with this regimen.

The regimen that is selected for the treatment of metastatic disease is determined by the extent of the tumor and the location of the metastases. Treatment of patients classified as *good prognosis/low risk* is begun with methotrexate or actinomycin D in the same doses as for nonmetastatic disease. Serum beta-subunit hCG concentrations are determined at weekly intervals. If the tumor fails to respond, as indicated by plateauing or rising hCG titers, a change to the high-risk treatment protocol is indicated.

Patients classified as *poor prognosis/high risk* are usually treated with a combination of methotrexate, actinomycin D, and chlorambucil or cyclophosphamide. A variety of combinations of other chemotherapeutic drugs have also been employed. Recently, combinations with etoposide (VP16) and cisplatinum have proven to be highly effective.

Additional surgery or irradiation may be necessary for patients who fail to respond to the drugs. Such intensive therapy is highly toxic and must be carried out in treatment centers.

Chemotherapeutic agents have almost completely replaced surgical treatment of malignant trophoblastic disease. Not only was hysterectomy ineffective in the management of metastatic choriocarcinoma but also it eliminated all hope of future childbearing in young women. If the primary tumor and the metastases can be eradicated by drug therapy, there is no reason to remove the uterus. Menstruation will be normal, and pregnancy can occur. Chemotherapeutic agents used to treat malignant trophoblastic disease will not affect the growth and development of the embryo during subsequent pregnancies.

In a few patients, chemotherapeutic regimens are unsuccessful, either because the cells are unresponsive or because the drug fails to reach the primary tumor in the uterine wall. Hysterectomy to remove the local lesions may be performed. The ovaries need not be removed. Chemotherapy should be continued after surgery according to the criteria noted previously.

Hysterectomy can be part of the treatment of women with localized or metastatic disease if they do not want to retain their reproductive capacities. The operation can be performed soon after chemotherapy is started, and those who undergo hysterectomy require fewer courses of treatment and recover faster.

Chemotherapy is less effective in eradicating brain metastases than those in other parts of the body. Radiation therapy sometimes destroys lesions in the brain that have not responded to drugs. Radiation therapy may also be used to treat liver metastases.

Follow-up examinations

Women who have been treated for invasive mole or choriocarcinoma should be checked frequently for 1 year after the gonadotropin concentration has returned to normal. The essential studies are pelvic examination every 3 months, chest x-ray film examination as indicated, and tests for serum chorionic gonadotropin on a monthly basis. The pulmonary lesions usually regress slowly and, with successful treatment, disappear completely.

After the first year, the examinations are repeated at 4-month intervals. If there is no evidence of recurrence by the end of the second year, one can assume that the lesion has been eradicated. An effective contraceptive method should be used during the follow-up period.

PLACENTAL SITE TROPHOBLASTIC TUMOR (PSTT)

This variant of gestational trophoblastic disease, described as a pseudotrophoblastic tumor, was initially thought to be a benign process arising from the placental site. The trophoblastic cell type is described as an intermediate cell that on light microscopy is between a cytotrophoblastic and syncytiotrophoblastic cell. Not unexpectedly, then, this intermediate cell produces less hCG. Approximately 50 patients have now been reported in the world's literature, and most have followed a benign course. Approximately 10 patients have been reported to have developed metastases and died from this disease leading to a change in the nomenclature to PSTT. Unlike choriocarcinoma, which is very sensitive to chemotherapy, this disease is resistant to chemotherapy. Therefore, hysterectomy after diagnosis is the usual treatment.

SUGGESTED READING

Berkowitz RS, Goldstein DP, and Bernstein MR: Natural history of partial molar pregnancy, Obstet Gynecol 6:677, 1985.

Bracken MB: Incidence and aetiology of hydatidiform mole: an epidemiologic review, Brit J Obstet Gynaecol 94:1123, 1987.

Eddy GI and others: Postmolar trophoblastic disease in women using hormonal contraception with estrogen, Obstet Gynecol 62:736, 1983.

Franks HR and others: Plasma human chorionic gonadotropin disappearance in hydatidiform mole: a central registry from the Netherlands, Obstet Gynecol 62:467, 1983.

Grimes DA: Epidemiology of gestational trophoblastic disease, Am J Obstet Gynecol 150:309, 1984.

Hammond CB, Weed JC Jr, and Currie JL: The role of operation in the current therapy of gestational trophoblastic disease, Am J Obstet Gynecol 136:844, 1980.

Hertig AT and Mansell H: Hydatidiform mole and choriocarcinoma, Washington DC, 1956, Armed Forces Institute of Pathology.

Jacobs PA, Wilson CM, Sprenkle JA, Rosenshein NB, and Migeon BR: Mechanism of origin of complete hydatidiform moles, Nature 286:714, 1980.

Kajii T and Ohama J: Androgenic origin of hydatidiform mole, Nature 268:633, 1977.

Lurain JR and Brewer JI: Treatment of high-risk gestational trophoblastic disease with methotrexate, actinomycin D and cyclophosphamide chemotherapy, Obstet Gynecol 63:830, 1985.

Lurain JR, Brewer JI, Torok EE, and Halpern B: Natural history of hydatidiform mole after primary evacuation, Am J Obstet Gynecol 145:591, 1983.

McCorrison CC: Racial incidence of hydatidiform mole, Am J Obstet Gynecol 101:377, 1968.

McDonald TW and Ruffolo EH: Modern management of gestational trophoblastic disease, Obstet Gynecol Surv 38:67, 1983.

Patillo RA, Sasaki S, Katayama KP, Roesler M, and Mattingly RF: Genesis of 46,XY hydatidiform mole, Am J Obstet Gynecol 141:104, 1981.

Song HZ and Wu PC: Hydatidiform mole in China: a preliminary survey of incidence on more than three million women, Bull World Health Organ 65(4):507, 1987.

Trophoblastic disease, Clinical Obstet Gynecol, vol 27, 1984.

19

Russell K. Laros, Jr.

Physiology of normal pregnancy

Objectives

RATIONALE: An understanding of the physiologic changes accompanying normal pregnancy is essential to the diagnosis and treatment of abnormalities that may occur.

The student should be able to:
A. Describe the maternal physiologic changes that occur during pregnancy.

Profound local and systemic changes in maternal physiology are initiated by conception and continue throughout pregnancy. After expulsion of the placenta, many of these changes are rapidly reversed, although certain alterations, particularly those affecting the generative tract, are more gradual in their return to the nongravid state. For purposes of evaluating any system, whether genital, renal, cardiovascular, endocrine, or other, it is important to realize that the effects of pregnancy are not fully reversed until at least 6 weeks after the baby is born.

GENERATIVE ORGANS

Uterus. The *size of the uterus* increases five to six times (from 7 by 5 by 3 cm to 35 by 25 by 22 cm) (Fig. 19-1), the *weight* undergoes a twentyfold increase (from 50 to 1000 g at term), and the capacity increases spectacularly one thousandfold (from 4 to 4000 ml).

Uterine growth is caused almost entirely by hypertrophy of the muscle cells. In addition, an increase in the amount of elastic connective tissue adds considerably to the strength of the uterine wall, and a remarkable increase in the size and number of blood vessels provides the rapidly growing tissues with an adequate supply of oxygen and nutritive substances (Fig. 19-2).

The initial stimulus to uterine hypertrophy is hormonal. Thus in the first 6 weeks the size of the uterus is similar in either intrauterine or extrauterine pregnancy. Enlargement thereafter depends on the size of the conceptus and the actual growth of the muscle fibers.

Related uterine and fetal weights throughout gestation show that the greater part of the uterine

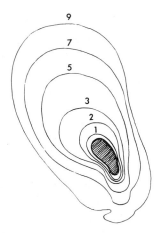

Fig. 19-1 Growth of uterus during successive months of pregnancy.

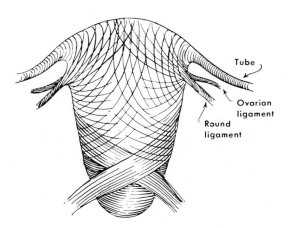

Fig. 19-2 Diagram showing interwoven pattern of uterine muscle fibers.

weight is gained before the twentieth week, during which time the myometrial walls become progressively thicker. In the last half of pregnancy, when the fetal growth is accelerated, the myometrium is thinned out to accommodate the fetus. Late in pregnancy and particularly during labor, myometrial contractions with shortening of the muscle fibers cause progressive thickening of the upper uterine segment as the lower segment develops.

The *position* of the gravid uterus changes as gestation advances. Early, an exaggerated anteflexion is usual; and then as the uterus rises from the pelvis, varying degrees of dextrorotation develop because the rectosigmoid occupies a relatively fixed position in the left posterior aspect of the pelvis.

Uterine blood flow in normal term pregnancy measured during cesarean section averages 500 ml/min, as opposed to 50 ml/min in the nonpregnant state. Oxygen consumption of the gravid uterus is 25 ml/min (5 ml/kg/min), and the carbon dioxide production, 22 ml/min. On the basis of these determinations the average respiratory quotient of the uterus at term is 0.91.

LOWER UTERINE SEGMENT. The uterus is differentiated into an upper and a lower segment. The wall of the upper contractile portion of the uterus becomes thicker during labor as the lower uterine segment, which must undergo circumferential dilation to permit passage of the presenting part, becomes thinned out and about 10 cm in length.

From the beginning of the second trimester until the last few weeks of pregnancy, the isthmic portion hypertrophies and becomes incorporated or indistinguishable from the rest of the uterine muscle. Late in pregnancy and most particularly during labor the lower uterine segment becomes thinned out, and its upper pole is more clearly demarcated from the thick upper segment.

UTERINE CONTRACTILITY. The uterus contracts irregularly throughout pregnancy. Uterine activity, the increase in intrauterine pressure generated by a contraction, is measured in Montevideo units, the sum of the intensity of all the contractions in mm Hg during a 10-minute period. From early pregnancy until 30 weeks, uterine activity is less than 20 Montevideo units. Irregular, painless contractions (Braxton Hicks contractions) increase gradually thereafter from about 30 to 80 Montevideo units as the cervix ripens. At the onset of labor, intrauterine activity averages between 80 and 120 Montevideo units. At peak activity near the end of labor, when the intrauterine pressure during each contraction is increased to about 50 mm Hg and the frequency to 5 contractions/10 minutes, an average of 250 Montevideo units is reached.

Cervix. Changes in the cervix are apparent by the sixth week. Softening and congestion are a result of increased vascularity. The glands hypertrophy, mucus secretion is greatly increased, and the consistency is altered by steroid hormone activity. Inspissation of the water content of cervical mucus results in the formation of the thick mucous plug that acts as a barrier, protecting the conceptus against mechanical or bacterial invasion throughout pregnancy. Progesterone overshadows the effects of increased estrogen production on cervical mucus; hence ferning, or arborization, does not occur when corpus luteum activity is sufficient to support a normal intrauterine pregnancy.

The cervical epithelium is far less responsive to estrogen and progesterone than is the endometrium. The cervical stromal cells show a decidual reaction in about half of pregnant women; but, aside from this change, the increased vascularity, and the edema, no alterations can be considered characteristic of specific pregnancy effects. The squamous epithelium is often thicker, and the basal layer may be increased from one- to four-cell strata. Growth of the endocervical epithelium is more pronounced, and squamous metaplasia is common. Frequently, the columnar proliferation advances beyond the external os for a variable distance on the surface of the cervix. This so-called erosion is actually a *cervical ectropion* or *eversion* of the cervical canal. Its gross appearance may be indistinguishable from pathologic conditions of the cervix. Cytologic or histologic examination is necessary.

One concern is the interpretation of basal cell hyperactivity when this change is found in the gravid cervix. Coloscopic examination can be just as informative in pregnant as in nonpregnant women, and the diagnosis of any type of epithelial abnormality must be made on the basis of changes in the cellular characteristics, particularly those of the nuclei, whether or not the patient is pregnant.

Fallopian tubes and round ligaments. The *round ligaments* are hypertrophied and elongated. Because their relationship to the uterine fundus is retained, their position in late pregnancy is almost vertical. The round ligaments help stabilize the uterus and tend to keep the heavy organ closer to the abdominal wall.

The *fallopian tubes* are also elongated and ultimately lie almost parallel to the long axis of the uterus, but unlike the round ligaments their muscular coats are not hypertrophied.

Ovaries. Because of the increased vascularity, both ovaries become somewhat enlarged and elongated. The enlargement is more pronounced in the ovary containing the corpus luteum, which reaches its maximum development during the third month. Ovulation is suspended during pregnancy because of pituitary inhibition.

At cesarean section, one often sees patchy, reddened areas and elevated ridges on the surface of the ovary that represent a decidualike reaction of the stroma and hyperplasia of the surface epithelium, respectively. These reactions are probably related to some hormone of chorionic origin, either chorionic gonadotropin or progesterone from the same source.

The infundibulopelvic ligament is enlarged during pregnancy, mainly because of the great distension of the ovarian veins. The capacity of these veins increases more than 60 times. Such a vast change in diameter is possible because the ovarian veins are not confined within fascial sheaths as are the veins in the extremities. Compensatory hypertrophy of the smooth muscle of the vein media provides protection against spontaneous rupture.

Vagina. The vagina becomes deeply congested and cyanotic (Chadwick's sign) because of the greatly increased vascularity. In preparation for the great distension that the vagina must undergo during delivery, the mucosa thickens, the connective tissue becomes less dense, and the muscular coat hypertrophies to such an extent that the vault is considerably lengthened and the lower portion may protrude through the introitus, giving the appearance of a cystocele even in the primigravida.

Secretions present in the vaginal vault during pregnancy have a highly acid pH (3.5 to 5.5) because of the increased glycogen content of the vaginal epithelium.

GENERAL CHANGES

Abdominal walls. Tension and stretching of the anterior abdominal wall and the tissues over the outer aspect of the thighs frequently cause changes in the collagen and elastic fibers of the deep layer of the skin, producing reddish, irregular lines, the *striae gravidarum*. Microscopic studies of striae show that collagen and elastic fibers lose their crisscross appearance and become thinned and straightened out longitudinally but do not become disrupted. Thus striae appear to be caused by the loss of the adhesive property of ground substance because of the effect of adrenocortical hyperactivity. After delivery, the discoloration gradually fades, but the scarred lines do not disappear.

In the latter part of pregnancy, the rectus abdominis muscles are under considerable strain, and their tone is reduced. Wide separation of the muscles *(diastasis recti)* develops when the linea alba gives way to the stress and permits abdominal contents to protrude in the midline.

Breasts. The breasts become enlarged and sensitive by the eighth week of pregnancy. The primary areola deepens in color, and a more lightly pigmented secondary areola develops at the periphery. Sebaceous glands located in the primary areola undergo hypertrophy, forming *Montgomery's tubercles.*

Colostrum can be expressed from the nipples after about the tenth week, but lactation is inhibited by the high estrogen-progesterone levels. Growth of the mammary apparatus is a direct response to hormone stimulation. Estrogen stimulates proliferation of the ducts; progesterone causes proliferation of lobule-alveolar tissue. Development is functionally complete by midpregnancy. As the breasts enlarge, the vascular supply is increased, engorged veins are frequently visible beneath the surface of the skin, and striae may appear over the outer aspects.

After delivery, anterior pituitary *prolactin* stimulates synthesis and secretion of milk (see Chapter 41).

Skin. Pigmentation of the skin in areas other than the breasts is a common finding. The *linea nigra,* a brownish black streak down the midline of the abdomen, is especially prominent in brunettes. Occasionally, pigmentation occurs in a characteristic distribution over the face, forming the "mask of pregnancy," or *chloasma,* which may persist for many months after delivery. The external genitals are similarly affected.

Palmar erythema and *spider nevi* or *telangiectases* sometimes appear over the face and upper trunk and are related to the increased concentration of estrogen.

CIRCULATORY SYSTEM

Vast alterations in hemodynamics occur as a result of (1) the increased metabolic demands of new tissue growth; (2) the expansion of vascular channels, particularly those of the generative tract; and (3) the increase in steroid hormones, which exert a positive effect on sodium and water balance.

Blood. The *total blood volume* increases approximately 30% to 40% (Fig. 19-3). The range is wide, and increases up to 50% are reported. Although the *red cell volume* and the *total hemoglobin* increase during pregnancy, the expansion of plasma volume is approximately three times greater than that of the red cell mass. Studies using red cells labeled with radioactive iron (^{59}Fe) indicate an average increase in red cell mass of 495 ml at term and calculated the concomitant whole blood rise at 1800 ml. If dietary iron supplements are withheld, the expected red cell increase is lessened by as much as 30% to 40%.

Erythropoiesis during pregnancy is to a large extent regulated by the kidneys. Renal erythropoietic factor (REF) is produced in response to the demand by the tissues for oxygen, and this in turn

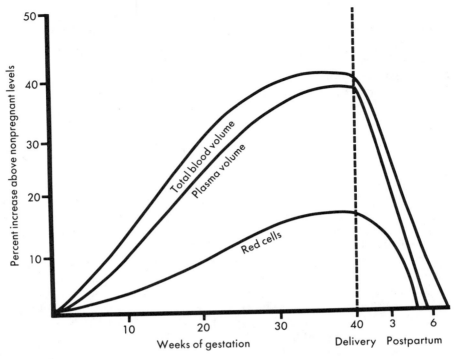

Fig. 19-3 Changes in total blood volume, plasma volume, and red cell mass during pregnancy and puerperium, based on compilation of reported data.

activates production of erythropoietic hormone in the plasma. Human placental lactogen (hPL) and prolactin have also been shown to enhance the stimulatory effect of endogenous erythropoietin.

The disparity between the increase in fluid and cellular elements is reflected in the peripheral blood count as an apparent or dilution anemia, as both hemoglobin and hematocrit determinations are usually decreased in the third trimester as compared with the first. The average reduction in hematocrit is 15%, whereas the decrease in viscosity is 12% as a result of this dilution. True anemia is present if the hemoglobin is less than 12 g/dl and the hematocrit less than 32%.

The *plasma volume* begins to increase during the first trimester, reaches a peak approximately 40% above normal at 32 to 34 weeks, and remains elevated to term. During and immediately after the third stage of labor there is a sharp temporary rise in plasma volume, followed by a rapid drop toward the normal nonpregnant range, although the original level is not actually reached until 3 or 4 weeks after delivery. On the contrary, the red cell mass continues to rise until the end of pregnancy and does not decline to its original level until the eighth postpartum week.

Most of the increase in plasma volume occurs between the sixth and the twenty-fourth week of gestation. These findings parallel the curve of increases in cardiac output. Thus maximal risk for the patient with heart disease is reached earlier in pregnancy than previously thought and persists throughout gestation. Plasma volume correlates well with reproductive performance.

Interstitial fluid volume expansion is less pronounced than the plasma volume rise during the first and second trimesters. The rate is accelerated in the latter part of pregnancy and continues until term, when the maximum increase of 40% is reached. Return to original levels occurs gradually by 6 to 8 weeks after delivery.

The *bone marrow* is hyperplastic throughout pregnancy and remains so for about 2 months after delivery. The white cells and the erythrocytes are increased. A *leukocytosis* in the range of 10,000 to 12,000 is normal in gravid women.

Serum protein concentrations are approximately 1 to 1.5 g/dl lower in pregnant than in nonpregnant women. It is not unusual to obtain values of 5.5 to 6 g/dl. The colloid osmotic pressure of the plasma is thereby reduced by about 20%. This is in part but not entirely a result of dilution. There is a significant drop in the albumin fraction that is incompletely compensated for by the rise in alpha and beta globulin. The albumin-globulin ratio is reduced from 1.5 to 0.8. In normal mothers, total plasma protein concentration decreases by about 13% by the third trimester. The albumin and gamma globulin concentration decrease progressively, but at the same time the alpha-1, alpha-2, beta fraction, and fibrinogen increase. The lipoproteins also increase.

Serum lipids. Total serum lipid increases by 46% during the latter part of pregnancy. There is a marked increase in triglycerides resulting primarily from a rise in the very-low-density lipoproteins. Total cholesterol and free fatty acids are also increased; however, there is no increase in esterified cholesterol.

Fibrinogen concentration increases progressively to term. Chemical values show an increase from 300 mg/dl to 400 to 600 mg/dl. Electrophoresis values are approximately 100 mg/dl higher. *Urea* and *creatinine* are found in lower concentrations in the plasma during pregnancy because of the normal increase in renal filtration fraction.

Alpha-fetoprotein is produced primarily in the fetal liver with lesser amounts coming from the yolk sac and the gastrointestinal tract. The fetal serum level reaches a maximum at 13 weeks' gestational age, declines thereafter, and becomes virtually absent after the age of 2 years. Amniotic fluid levels parallel the fetal serum levels in a ratio of about 1:150, with the maximum occurring at 12 to 14 weeks. The maternal serum levels are lower than the fetal by a factor of 10,000. However, the maternal levels increase progressively until week 32 of pregnancy and then decline modestly to term. Normal values are usually defined at a given gestational age based on multiples of the median (MOM). Values greater than 2.5 MOM are considered abnormally high, and those less than 0.4 MOM as low.

Screening programs aimed at detecting fetal neural tube defects are now a standard part of prenatal care. This approach takes advantage of the fact that amniotic fluid and maternal serum levels are substantially elevated if the fetus has an open neural tube defect. Women not at increased risk of carrying a fetus with a neural tube defect are offered serum screening at 16 to 18 weeks. Although the primary purpose of maternal serum screening is the detection of neural tube defects, other fetal conditions are associated with either an abnormally high or low level (see box on p. 238).

SERUM ENZYMES. During the prenatal period a profound change in the maternal serum enzymes is found in the increase in serum alkaline phosphatase. Individual variation is considerable, but in normal pregnancy values rise steadily to term. Serum aspartate transaminase (AST) and serum alanine transaminase (ALT) concentrations show significantly increased activity only during labor.

Serum cystine aminopeptidase (oxytocinase) is the primary oxytocin-inactivating enzyme of pregnancy plasma. A relatively steady rise in the enzyme is noticed beginning at about 6 weeks' gestation to term in normal pregnancies. The enzyme appears to be mainly of placental origin, but it is of limited clinical value in assessing placental function and, more particularly, fetal welfare.

Heart. Serial studies at various stages of pregnancy reveal an actual alteration in position and apparent increase in size of the cardiac silhouette.

CONDITIONS ASSOCIATED WITH
ABNORMAL MATERNAL ALPHA-
FETOPROTEIN LEVELS

Elevated
Neural tube defects
Multiple gestations
Fetal death
Abdominal wall defects—omphalocele and
　gastroschisis
Esophageal and duodenal atresia
Congenital nephrosis
Cystic hygroma
Subsequent intrauterine growth retardation and
　poor fetal outcome
Renal anomalies
Sacrococcygeal teratoma
Underestimation of fetal age
Low
Chromosomal abnormalities, especially trisomies
Fetal death
Subsequent poor fetal outcome
Overestimation of gestational age

The heart is rotated slightly anteriorly and displaced upward and to the left. The factors responsible for these alterations are controversial, although recognized changes in the chest wall doubtless play an important role. The rib cage is flared out so that its circumference is increased at the base. The diaphragm is pushed up as the uterus enlarges, but it may or may not appear disproportionately elevated.

The fact that the heart appears enlarged on x-ray film examination long before the uterus is large enough to push the abdominal contents upward raises the question as to whether the cardiac muscle undergoes some hypertrophy during pregnancy. If it does so, it is likely that the hypertrophy is in proportion to the increase in total body weight. Because the cardiac output is increased by about 75 ml, it is likely that the increased blood volume is accompanied by slight cardiac dilation.

In addition to the altered x-ray film appearance of the heart, functional changes simulating organic heart disease in nonpregnant patients must be recognized and carefully evaluated. A soft systolic *murmur* at the base or over the precordium is demonstrable in more than 50% of patients. *Extrasystoles* are common, and the *pulse rate* is slightly increased. There is a distinct change in heart rate immediately after delivery, when bradycardia is the rule, unless blood loss has been excessive. These findings and the frequent occurrence of dyspnea make the diagnosis of cardiac disease during pregnancy more difficult.

Blood pressure. *Arterial blood pressure* does not increase in normal pregnancy. The level remains unchanged or may decrease during the second trimester and return to the normal range during the third trimester. The maximal *pulse pressure* occurs during the twenty-eighth to thirty-second week, at about the time of the maximal pulse rate. *Venous pressure* measured in the antecubital region remains constant and normal. Elevated venous pressure in the upper extremity is indicative of cardiac overload. Femoral venous pressure rises 10 to 15 cm H_2O above normal in the upright or supine position as a result of increasing pressure by the enlarging uterus on the pelvic veins, a factor that contributes to the development of ankle edema and varicose veins. Femoral pressure is normal in the lateral recumbent position.

Late in pregnancy, patients often complain of feeling faint in the supine position, when venous pressure may rise to at least 20 cm H_2O. The syncope is attributed to the *vena cava syndrome.* When the heavy uterus falls back on the inferior vena cava, venous return to the heart is sufficiently impeded to cause a precipitous drop in blood pressure. The patient appears pale and apprehensive, but if she can turn on her side, which she usually does promptly, symptoms disappear almost immediately. This phenomenon is accentuated when the patient is unable to move about after an anesthetic is administered. We have seen a few patients exhibit a profound drop in blood pressure after low-dose spinal anesthesia given for cesarean section, although the level of anesthesia was no higher than the eighth or ninth thoracic segment. When pressure was exerted against the lateral abdominal wall, thus displacing the uterus to one side of the inferior vena cava, the blood pressure rose without any other aids. In such cases, delivery should be carried out without delay. If initial hypotension is caused by this condition, there is no difficulty in maintaining blood pressure once the uterus is emptied.

Capillary permeability remains unchanged except with the increased hydrostatic pressure in the lower extremities.

Cardiac output. Increased tissue demands for oxygen may be met physiologically by (1) an increase in cardiac output of oxygenated blood or (2) an increased extraction of oxygen from blood at the capillary level. Measurements of cardiac output during normal pregnancy indicate a rise, primarily in stroke volume, with the maximal increase of about 30 to 35% being observed at about the twenty-eighth week. The heart rate follows the same general course but with a much lower increment of rise. Cardiac output is increased slightly during the first stage of labor and appreciably increased during the second stage with the bearing down efforts. Immediately after delivery there is a sudden increase amounting to about 29% as the uterus contracts and forces a large volume of blood into the circulation. During these periods the patient with a diseased heart experiences further increased cardiac strain.

Measurements of cardiac output taken in the supine position show diminution amounting to 10 to 25% of the peak output in the last stages of pregnancy. Serial studies of cardiac output performed in the lateral recumbent position show no significant reduction of output, and therefore of ventricular work, in late pregnancy.

As the overall increase in *oxygen consumption* is between 10 and 20% during pregnancy, it is evident that the heightened cardiac output exceeds this demand until the last trimester. The arteriovenous oxygen difference is reduced to 3.4/dl during the fourteenth to thirtieth weeks. This adjustment would appear to favor the margin of safety for fetal oxygenation. However, in the last trimester, when the cardiac output decreases, a larger percentage of oxygen must be removed at the uterine level, and the arteriovenous oxygen difference increases to values similar to or exceeding values found in nonpregnant women (4.4/dl).

RESPIRATORY SYSTEM

Functional changes in the respiratory tract are demonstrable early in pregnancy, whereas anatomic alterations become evident later when intraabdominal pressure is increased. The lower half of the thoracic cage is pushed upward and widened, and the diaphragm is accordingly elevated, especially at the periphery. The central portion may appear flattened, and its excursion reduced; hence breathing is more costal than abdominal.

The *vital capacity* remains unchanged or undergoes a slight increase. A decrease in vital capacity should always be considered significant. In gravidas with pulmonary or cardiac disease, particularly with mitral stenosis, reduced vital capacity is one of the earliest signs of impending failure. Serial testing should be initiated early in pregnancy to permit valid interpretation of changes with advancing gestation.

Hyperventilation. The respiratory rate is slightly increased, and tidal volume rises. These changes may increase the margin of safety for the fetus. Hyperventilation lowers the carbon dioxide content of alveolar air, and, in turn, reduced carbon dioxide tension favors diffusion of carbon dioxide from fetal to maternal circulation. Thus all changes in the respiratory system during pregnancy are well compensated, and pulmonary function is not impaired in normal patients. Nevertheless, pulmonary diseases are often more serious during pregnancy when oxygen requirements of gestation are increased.

URINARY SYSTEM

Pregnancy exerts a profound influence on the entire urinary tract. The outstanding anatomic effect is a dilation of the *ureter* and *renal pelvis* and *hydronephrosis,* all more pronounced on the right. The capacity of a dilated kidney pelvis and ureter increases from an original 10 or 15 ml to 60 ml.

Changes appear early and are progressive until the last month or two of pregnancy. The ureter is elongated and widened, and, although it becomes curved and tortuous, actual kinking is rare. The flow of urine is reduced because ureteral peristalsis and tone are diminished. All these alterations, especially those affecting ureteral function, are basically hormonal influences, mainly of progesterone. As pregnancy advances, pressure from the enlarged uterus may be a contributory factor. Dilation is frequently considerably more pronounced in the right ureter than in the left, probably because of the cushioning effect of the rectosigmoid and the dextrorotation of the uterus. The muscular wall of the lower third of the ureter undergoes hyperplasia similar to that involving most structures within the broad ligament. Reduction of the lumen at this level may also contribute to dilation of the ureter above.

Renal function. Changes in renal function during normal pregnancy follow a recognized pattern, although the extent of the alteration may vary from one individual to another. Serial studies of para-aminohippurate (PAH) and inulin clearances demonstrate the following: (1) *effective renal plasma flow* increases approximately 25% during the first and second trimester and then falls to normal nonpregnant levels in the last trimester (600 ml/min); (2) *glomerular filtration* increases by about 50% and remains in this range until the last 2 to 3 weeks of pregnancy, when the rate declines somewhat but does not fall to normal (125 ml/min) until early in the puerperium; and (3) the *filtration fraction* is elevated throughout pregnancy, particularly in the third trimester, when renal plasma flow decreases while glomerular filtration remains elevated. The filtration fraction at this time is approximately 40% above control levels.

The late pregnancy regression of renal blood flow and glomerular filtration may be related to position. The PAH and inulin clearances and so-dium and chloride excretion are all depressed in the supine position as compared with the lateral position. Potassium excretion does not change. The fact that the lateral position is conducive to optimal function provides good reason for recommendation of programmed rest periods in this position in patients with borderline or diminishing renal function.

The alterations in renal function are most probably a result of increased maternal and chorionic hormonal secretions. Hormones capable of increasing renal function include ACTH, antidiuretic hormone (ADH), aldosterone, cortisone, growth hormone, and thyroid hormone. The part played by each of these and by the increased plasma volume of pregnancy needs further study before the final answer can be given.

The known anatomic and physiologic changes in the kidney have important clinical implications. *Glycosuria* is common because of the increase in glomerular filtration, but, before its occurrence can be assigned to a physiologic change, a glucose tolerance test is indicated. *Amino acids* are excreted in larger amounts during pregnancy. This is particularly true of histidine, the glomerular filtration of which is raised by more than 50%, whereas tubular reabsorption appears to be partially inhibited. Blood concentrations of *urea, uric acid,* and *creatinine* are lowered as a result of increased clearance rates, but the clearance of *sodium* is not significantly altered in normal pregnancy. Renal *iodide clearance* is increased, and the plasma inorganic iodine level is reduced, which increases the physiologic demands on the thyroid.

Allowances must be made for changes in the genitourinary system in the interpretation of renal function tests. The results of the *phenosulfonphthalein (PSP) test* can be misleading because the dye may be excreted normally, but dilation of the renal pelvis and ureter and the relative stasis of this system may delay its arrival in the bladder. The test is better avoided during pregnancy. *Concentration tests,* when positive, are significant. If the urine does not show concentration, it may be related to the positive nitrogen balance, sodium retention, and low-sodium intake, particularly if the salt has been restricted for a time before the test is performed. It should be performed in the late puerperium before a final diagnosis of failure of concentrating power is made.

Serial determinations of 24-hour renal clearance of endogenous creatinine are useful and practical in evaluating renal function during pregnancy. Collection and timing of the sample are important. Values are lower in 24-hour tests than in those performed during short test periods with fluids administered. In normal ambulatory gravid women, clearance rates range between 130 and 160 ml/min until the last 2 to 4 weeks of pregnancy, when values usually range between 100 and 110 ml/min.

The *bladder* is pulled up into the abdomen as the uterus enlarges. In the early weeks of gestation, pressure of the uterus on the bladder, traction at the vesicle neck, and hyperemia of the trigone cause frequency of urination. The vascularity of the bladder is greatly increased, and on cystoscopy engorged vessels or small varicosities are sometimes visible. Trauma that occurs late in pregnancy or during delivery may cause hemorrhage from these areas.

The hormonal influences responsible for dilation of the structures of the urinary tract above the bladder exert a similar influence on the smooth muscle of the bladder. There is a decrease in bladder tone and a progressive increase in capacity of up to 1300 to 1500 ml during pregnancy and in the postpartum period. Overdistension of the bladder in the postpartum period is a troublesome, often protracted complication of labor and delivery in which this physiologic reduction in tone plays an important role.

Renin-angiotensin-aldosterone system. The activity of the proteolytic enzyme *renin,* produced largely but not entirely by the kidney, is increased during normal pregnancy. The enzyme acts on *renin substrate, angiotensinogen,* to form *angiotensin* in two steps. Vascular reactivity to angiotensin II is reduced during pregnancy so that elevation of blood pressure does not normally occur with the increased levels of this substance, but in pregnancies complicated by preeclampsia, this relative resistance to angiotensin is lost. Angiotensin II is a major stimulus for adrenocortical secretion of *aldosterone,* which together with antidiuretic hormone favors salt and water retention during pregnancy.

GASTROINTESTINAL TRACT

An alteration in the normal *alkaline pH of the saliva* toward the acid side is common in pregnancy. It is this change rather than withdrawal of calcium that predisposes to tooth decay. The quantity of saliva is frequently increased, sometimes excessively so (hyperptyalism), but the cause of the increased secretion is not yet known. Occasionally, the gums become hypertrophied and spongy and tend to bleed easily. This is attributed to a hormonal effect, although vitamin C deficiency may contribute to the disturbance. Gingivitis tends to disappear spontaneously after delivery.

Gastric acidity is usually reduced, particularly in the first trimester, although the degree of hypochlorhydria is variable. Certain cases of otherwise unexplained severe anemia are occasionally related to an exaggerated gastric hypochlorhydria.

Gastric motility is somewhat diminished throughout pregnancy, and during labor the emptying time of the stomach is so slow that oral feedings are contraindicated. Nausea and vomiting of early pregnancy may well be influenced by these functional alterations.

Reduced peristaltic activity and *diminished tone* are evident in bowel function, as well as in the stomach. These effects are a result of the same hormonal influences, mainly progesterone, that induce atony in the smooth muscle of ureters, arteries, veins, and various other structures during pregnancy. Constipation, so common in pregnant women, usually results from these functional changes, although the condition is undoubtedly aggravated by pressure of the uterus on the rectosigmoid.

During the last half of pregnancy, the stomach is gradually pushed upward into the left dome of the diaphragm. Hormonal effects may cause relaxation or dilation of the hiatus and predispose to the development of *hiatal hernia*. The condition is usually reversed after delivery. The cecum also undergoes a progressive upward displacement, beginning during the third month and continuing until term, when the *appendix* is located out toward the right flank above the level of the iliac crest.

Gallbladder. Gallbladder emptying time is increased during pregnancy. Serum cholinesterase activity is reduced by about 25%. Relative biliary stasis and increased cholesterol levels may contribute to the formation of biliary calculi in gravid women. The ratio of women to men with calculous disease is approximately 4:1.

Liver. Measurements of liver function in human pregnancy remain in the normal range. Liver biopsies show no characteristic morphologic changes in normal mothers. However, in patients with existing liver disease, high levels of estrogens and overall added work of the liver during gestation may adversely affect hepatic function.

BONES AND JOINTS

The sacroiliac synchondroses and symphysis pubis are widened and rendered movable beginning about the tenth to twelfth week of gestation. This alteration is believed to be almost entirely caused by the action of the hormone relaxin. The blood concentrations of relaxin in pregnant women average 0.2 guinea pig U/ml of serum at 7 to 10 weeks' gestation, with a maximum concentration of 2 guinea pig U/ml at 38 to 42 weeks.

Posture changes become evident as pregnancy advances. The upper spine is thrown backward to compensate for the increased size of the abdomen. Disturbances arising from altered weight bearing and from relaxation of the pelvic articulations are discussed in Chapter 25.

ENDOCRINE SYSTEM

Thyroid. The thyroid gland is palpably enlarged in more than 50% of persons during pregnancy. This is caused by a diffuse hyperplasia of glandular elements, new follicle formation, and increased vascularity.

An increase in *basal metabolic rate* is evident by the sixteenth week and rises 10 to 30% above the prepregnant rate during the third trimester. Because the basal metabolic rate measures total oxygen consumption rate, the growing fetal and maternal tissues logically increase the oxygen demand. The increase in thyroid activity and in the size of the thyroid gland is more likely to represent compensatory changes because of the increased renal iodine clearance and resulting reduced plasma inorganic iodine level and the protein binding of thyroxine (T_4).

Thyroid function is affected in a major way by the elevated estrogen levels of pregnancy. Estrogens increase the response of pituitary thyroid-stimulating hormone (TSH) to hypothalamic thyrotropin-releasing hormone (TRH) and also cause significant increases in thyroxine-binding globulin (TBG), the alpha globulin moiety of serum proteins. The thyroid gland secretes T_4 and small amounts of triiodothyronine (T_3). In the free form, both are biologically active hormones. Most of the circulating T_3 is derived from monodeiodinization of T_4, and a major portion of T_4 is protein bound. Hence circulating levels of free T_4 are not appreciably different from or only slightly higher than nonpregnancy levels.

The most useful means of evaluating thyroid function during pregnancy is by direct assay for T_4. This method eliminates contamination errors caused by ingested iodides or radiographic dyes. Values during pregnancy range from 5.0 to 10.5 μg/dl as compared with normal nonpregnant values of 3.0 to 7.5 μg/dl. Additional thyroid function tests are usually necessary when thyroid dysfunction is suspected. These include determination of the free T_4 index in a suspected hyperthyroid or TSH in a hypothyroid state, which are discussed in Chapter 21.

Evaluation of thyroid activity by radioactive iodine (^{131}I) uptake is contraindicated during pregnancy, since fetal thyroid follicles are differenti-

ated by the fourth lunar month and may be damaged by ^{131}I.

Parathyroid glands. The parathyroids undergo hypertrophy as the fetal demands for calcium increase. Although more parathormone is secreted at this time, many pregnant women show a relative deficiency or a predisposition to parathyroid tetany in late pregnancy. Chvostek's sign is frequently positive in the latter part of gestation. Increasing calcium intake readily corrects relative deficiencies. One quart of milk daily is protective.

Pituitary gland. The *anterior lobe of the pituitary gland* increases 20 to 40% in size during pregnancy. The increase is largely in a single cell type, the "pregnancy cell," which is a prolactin-containing cell.

Serum levels of *human prolactin* (hPr) rise steadily from 10 ng/ml at the onset of pregnancy to about 200 ng/ml at term. Despite high, late pregnancy levels of prolactin and hPL, which also has some lactogenic activity, lactation does not occur before delivery. Friesen, Fournier, and Desjardins present good evidence that high levels of placental steroids inhibit the secretory activity of the breast by blocking the peripheral action of hPr and hPL on the breast.

The *posterior lobe* does not hypertrophy during pregnancy. The secretion of oxytocin and vasopressin—antidiuretic hormone is presumably increased. However, the measurements are made indirectly on the basis of increasing quantities of oxytocinase, which can be determined by electrophoresis.

Adrenal glands. Enlargement of the adrenal glands occurs progressively throughout the prenatal period because of *hyperplasia of the cortex.* A significant increase in corticosteroid secretion can be detected in the first trimester; and, a second higher peak reaching values similar to those found in patients with Cushing's disease normally occurs at about 200 days. The peak in corticosteroid secretion corresponds with the period during which water retention is maximal.

Not all functions of the adrenal cortex are equally stimulated during pregnancy. Corticosteroids that influence carbohydrate metabolism show the predominant and most universal rise, but, at the same time, binding protein (transcortin) is also increased as a result of the stimulus provided by increasing amounts of estrogen. As a consequence, significant amounts of otherwise excessive levels of corticosteroids are rendered biologically less active. However, there is a small actual increase in free cortisol in late pregnancy.

An increase in aldosterone levels is noted by the fifteenth week of pregnancy. Increased and fluctuant levels are attributable to the control of aldosterone secretion effected by the renin-angiotensin system.

The 17-ketosteroids associated with androgenic activity are relatively unchanged or increase only slightly in the last trimester.

Adrenal medullary activity is slightly increased in normal pregnancy. The mean values for urinary-free catecholamines expressed as norepinephrine equivalents in micrograms per hour are as follows: 12.5 in normal nongravid women of reproductive age, 13.2 in normal gravid women during the first and second trimesters, and 18.5 in normal gravid women during the third trimester. Further increases in epinephrine secretion during the stress of labor might be expected. However, studies of plasma epinephrine and norepinephrine during the third trimester, in labor, and after delivery show no significant change in either catecholamine. The mean plasma value of epinephrine is 0.1 µg/L and of norepinephrine, 1.5 µg/L.

METABOLISM

Proteins. A positive nitrogen balance demonstrable early in gestation increases progressively through the third trimester when fetal requirements are greatest. Nitrogen accumulates during pregnancy far beyond the needs of the conceptus. Nitrogen accumulation during the last half of pregnancy totaled 446 g. Net gain after delivery was 310 g. A negative balance continues in the puerperium with blood loss, lactation, and involutional changes in the uterus and other maternal tissues. Maternal protein intake should be at least 65 g/day throughout pregnancy.

Good maternal protein nutrition plays a key role in providing for normal fetal growth and development and may well be related to the actual condition of the newborn. Urinary urea nitrogen/total nitrogen (UN/TN) can be used as an index of maternal protein nutrition. When prenatal dietary protein intake is adequate, the UN/TN ratio is in the range of 60 to 80. On low-protein diets, the ratio usually ranges between 20 and 40. Birth weights of babies born to mothers with high UN/TN ratios average more than 1 pound higher than the weight of babies born to mothers with low UN/TN ratios. The differences in well-matched subjects are highly significant. The test is relatively simple and provides a tool for identifying the protein-deficient mother and assessing her response to dietary therapy.

Carbohydrates. Reducing substances can be found in the urine at some time or other during pregnancy in about 30% of persons. In most instances the reducing substance is glucose. The presence of lactose in the urine is unusual except for the 2- to 3-week period preceding the onset of labor, although during the puerperium lactosuria is common.

The renal threshold for glucose may be reduced from normal nonpregnant levels, which range between 150 and 200 mg/dl, to a range of 100 to 150 mg/dl because of the increased glomerular filtration that normally occurs during pregnancy. This phenomenon accounts for many cases of glycosuria and may contribute to the relatively low fasting level of blood sugar found in gravid women. However, in some instances glycosuria during pregnancy provides the first evidence of a diabetic state. Fasting blood sugar determination alone is not sufficient for diagnosis. Instead, a glucose tolerance test is essential for differentiation of physiologic and abnormal glycosuria of pregnancy. These problems are discussed in detail in Chapter 21.

A maternal glucose sparing effect noted in pregnancy is related to the demands of the fetus. Although secretion of insulin during pregnancy is increased, resistance to insulin by elevated free fatty acids and destruction of insulin by the placenta is also increased. The level of growth hormone per se is not appreciably increased, but its counterpart, chorionic hPL, is greatly elevated and is probably responsible for the elevated free fatty acids (FFA) and increased insulin resistance. Increases in corticosteroid and T_4 levels in normal gravid women may have some effect on carbohydrate metabolism, but protein binding of these substances is sufficiently increased so that actual biologic activity related to the free form of each is only slightly elevated during pregnancy. Plasma insulin antagonists are found in latent and overt diabetic women during pregnancy, but no such antagonists are detectable in the plasma of normal pregnant women.

Fats. Fat metabolism is altered during pregnancy in concert with the changes in carbohydrate metabolism just described. Metabolic alterations include an increase in maternal use of fat stores and a related increase in insulin resistance. The hPL plays an important role in mobilization of FFA. The elevated level of FFA exerts an antiinsulin effect by interfering with peripheral use of glucose. Oxidation of fats provides an alternate maternal source of energy, and glucose sparing ensures that the critical needs of the fetus for this energy source are met.

Estrogen is known to increase the production of the alpha globulins, including lipoproteins, and the glucocorticoids are known to increase serum cholesterol. The lipoproteins are significantly increased during pregnancy, particularly the beta lipoproteins. Neutral fats are approximately doubled. The level of free cholesterol progressively increases until the thirtieth week of pregnancy. Ketonuria occurs more readily in pregnant than in nonpregnant women when carbohydrate production is reduced or when dietary fat is increased.

The normal values for maternal and cord plasma glucose and nonesterified fatty acids (NEFA) have been established in a group of rigidly controlled normal pregnancies. Maternal values average 92.9 mg/dl for glucose and 881.8 mEq/L for NEFA; umbilical cord values average 61.9 mg/dl and 536.0 mEq/L, respectively. The differences in maternal-to-newborn ratios of glucose (1.3:1) and NEFA (1.7:1) suggest independent homeostasis in this biologic system. Because various metabolic diseases are known to influence blood glucose and NEFA levels, alterations in the ratio of these substances may provide a useful tool in the investigation of these disorders.

Minerals. Demands for inorganic substances necessary for growth rise sharply at about the fourth lunar month, when the fetus begins to increase rapidly in weight. Materials used for blood and skeletal formation continue to increase progressively to term.

CALCIUM AND PHOSPHORUS. Requirements for calcium and phosphorus are approximately doubled during pregnancy. These demands are satisfied by the daily intake of 1.5 g of calcium and 2 g of phosphorus. Total storage during the course of pregnancy is approximately 50 g and 35 to 40 g, respectively. Only about half of these amounts are used by the fetus; the remainder is stored in maternal tissues. Total serum calcium levels fall in the last half of pregnancy as a result of the decrease in serum albumin to which calcium is bound. However, free ionized calcium level remains within the normal range unless there is a relative or actual deficiency in parathyroid function. Because most of the fetal calcium deposition takes place in the latter part of pregnancy, relative deprivation or a deficiency in parathyroid function will cause a decrease in concentration of ionized calcium.

During pregnancy, calcium is more rapidly exchanged between the maternal circulation and bone. The bone therefore can be considered part of the metabolic calcium pool and can be drawn on when calcium supplies are low. The skeletal system is protected by a delicate balance in the rise of parathyroid hormone, which causes withdrawal of calcium from bone in response to hypocalcemia, and the rise in thyroid secretion of calcitonin during pregnancy, which inhibits this response when circulating calcium levels are elevated.

Osteomalacia, a condition in which softening and distortion of the long bones occurs as a result of excessive mobilization of calcium, is almost never found in the United States. Dentin does not contribute to the metabolic pool, and thus dental caries associated with pregnancy are not caused by the removal of calcium from the teeth but by local changes in pH and oral bacteria flora.

IRON. The demand for iron is increased, especially in the last trimester of pregnancy, because fetal absorption is far greater at that time. In addition, the hemoglobin mass continues to increase until term, and a small amount is necessary for other maternal tissues such as the uterus. Many women in an apparently good nutritional state have less than the normal 1 g of available iron in storage, and therefore iron supplements are necessary in most to prevent a nonanemic iron deficiency state or an obvious iron deficiency anemia. An appropriate dose is 30 to 60 mg/day of elemental iron.

Folic acid. Folates play an essential role in the metabolism of several amino acids and in the synthesis of nucleic acids. During pregnancy, rapid tissue growth of trophoblastic, maternal, and fetal origins creates an increased demand for folic acid. The undisputed example of maternal folic acid deficiency is seen in the development of megaloblastic anemia resulting specifically from inadequacy of folate and not from vitamin B_{12} deficiency. Association of less severe depletion of folic acid with other obstetric complications has been suggested but not confirmed.

The daily requirement of folic acid during pregnancy is about 300 to 500 μg. Green vegetables, some fruits, liver, and kidney are the principal sources.

Acid-base balance. Maternal plasma bicarbonate and total base are normally reduced during pregnancy. The values for total base average 146 mEq/L in normal gravid women as compared with 154 mEq/L in nonpregnant control subjects. At term the average carbon dioxide combining power value is about 45 ml/dl as compared with the nonpregnant average of approximately 60 ml/dl or plasma bicarbonate values of 22 to 25 mmol/L, respectively. Because the blood pH is unchanged, the alkali deficit is well compensated. The specific cause for this alteration remains unknown. It is probable that the normally increased ventilation effects the change, but whether the hyperventilation of pregnancy is of sufficient magnitude to reduce the carbon dioxide and induce the compensatory increase in renal excretion of sodium is as yet uncertain.

SUGGESTED READING

Assali NS, Douglass RA, Baird WW, Nicholson DB, and Suyemoto R: Measurement of uterine blood flow and uterine metabolism, Am J Obstet Gynecol 66:248, 1953.

Bartter FC, Casper AGT, Delea CS, and others: On the role of the kidney in control of adrenal steroid production, Metabolism 10:1006, 1961.

Beydoun SN, Cuenco VG, Evans LP, and Aubry RH: Maternal nutrition. I. The urinary urea nitrogen/total nitrogen ratio as an index of protein nutrition, Am J Obstet Gynecol 114:198, 1972.

Caton WL, Roby CC, Reid DE, and others: The circulating red cell volume and body hematocrit in normal pregnancy and the puerperium, Am J Obstet Gynecol 61:1207, 1951.

Chesley LC, Sloan DM, and Wynn RM: Effects of posture and angiotensin 2 upon renal function in pregnant women, Am J Obstet Gynecol 90:281, 1964.

Davidson JM: The physiology of the urinary tract in pregnancy, Clin Obstet Gynecol 28:257, 1985.

Friesen HG, Fournier P, and Desjardins P: Pituitary prolactin in pregnancy and normal and abnormal lactation, Clin Obstet Gynecol 3:25, 1973.

Hibbard BM and Hibbard ED: Folate metabolism and reproduction, Br Med Bull 24:10, 1968.

Hodgkinson CP: Physiology of the ovarian veins during pregnancy, Obstet Gynecol 1:26, 1953.

Hytten FE and Leitch I: The physiology of human pregnancy, ed 2, London, 1971, Blackwell Scientific Publications, Ltd.

Jepson JH: Endocrine control of maternal and fetal erythropoiesis, Can Med Assoc J 98:844, 1968.

Komins JI, Snyder PJ, and Schwarz R: Hyperthyroidism in pregnancy: a review, Obstet Gynecol Surv 30:527, 1975.

Laros RK Jr: Blood disorders in pregnancy, Philadelphia, 1986, Lea & Febiger.

Lewis BV: Uterine blood flow: a review, Obstet Gynecol Surv 24:1211, 1969.

Lowenstein L and Bramlage CA: The bone marrow in pregnancy and the puerperium, Blood 12:261, 1957.

Lund CJ and Donovan JC: Blood volume during pregnancy: significance of plasma and red cell volumes, Am J Obstet Gynecol 98:393, 1967.

Metcalfe J, Romney SL, Eamsey LH, Reid DE, and Burwell CS: Estimation of blood flow in normal human pregnancy at term, J Clin Invest 34:1632, 1955.

Milunsky A and Flyate E: Prenatal diagnosis of neural tube defects: problems and pitfalls. Analysis of 2495 cases using the alpha-fetoprotein assay, Obstet Gynecol 48:1, 1976.

Pitkin RM: Calcium metabolism in pregnancy: a review, Am J Obstet Gynecol 121:724, 1975.

Poidevin LOS: Histopathology of striae gravidarum, J Obstet Gynaecol Br Commonw 66:654, 1959.

Reynolds WA, Williams GA, and Pitkin RM: Calcitropic hormone responsiveness during pregnancy, Am J Obstet Gynecol 139:855, 1981.

Whaley WH, Zuspan FP, and Nelson GP: Glucose and nonesterified fatty acid levels in maternal and cord plasma, Am J Obstet Gynecol 92:264, 1965.

Yeomans ER and Hankins GD: Cardiovascular physiology and invasive cardiac monitoring, Clin Obstet Gynecol 32:2, 1989.

20

J. Robert Willson

Diagnosis and duration of pregnancy and prenatal care

Objectives

RATIONALE: Appropriate prenatal care promotes maternal and fetal well-being. It includes the initial and ongoing evaluation of the patient with a history, physical examination, laboratory studies, and other methods of assessment as needed. Such care promotes patient education and provides ongoing risk assessment and development of an individualized patient management plan.

The student should be able to:

A. Diagnose pregnancy.
B. Assess gestational age.
C. Distinguish the normal from the at-risk pregnancy.

D. Assess fetal growth, well-being, and maturity.
E. Demonstrate a knowledge of appropriate diagnostic studies.
F. Discuss patient education programs.
G. Perform physical examinations of obstetrical patients.
H. Answer commonly asked questions concerning pregnancy, labor, and delivery.
I. Develop a problem list and management plan based upon the initial assessment and ongoing evaluation.

Prenatal care can be defined as a program of examination, evaluation, observation, treatment, and education of pregnant women directed toward making pregnancy, labor, and delivery as normal and as safe as possible for mothers and their infants. Physical abnormalities and emotional disturbances that might alter the course of pregnancy can be detected and often corrected so that the mothers approach the time for delivery in as perfect health as possible.

The current program of prenatal care, which was developed early in the twentieth century, was designed to help reduce maternal, fetal, and neonatal deaths by giving the physician an opportunity to diagnose conditions such as preeclampsia-eclampsia soon after their onset rather than in their terminal stages. The effectiveness of systematic prenatal care is evidenced by the reduced mortality from such disorders.

The general improvement in health, particularly of middle-class women, has permitted a change in the emphasis of prenatal care. One important objective of prenatal care is to identify women who have unusual emotional responses to reproduction and to support them in their areas of need.

Educational programs relating to general health care can be made available to prenatal patients. Most women return for prenatal visits periodically for 5 to 6 months, which provides time for a fairly extensive program. Appropriate subjects for discussion include nutrition, infant and child care, general health care, and contraception.

Conditions that may constitute temporary or permanent contraindications to pregnancy can be detected by *prepregnancy examination.* Ideally, every woman who is contemplating pregnancy should be examined before she attempts to conceive. At this time the physician should obtain a detailed personal and family medical history, perform a complete physical examination, and order appropriate laboratory tests. The physician should also attempt to evaluate her emotional reactions toward pregnancy and to initiate an educational program that may help her learn more about reproduction and her own responses to it. The *premarital examination* can serve as the initial prepregnancy examination if it is properly structured.

One of the most important aspects of prenatal care is *risk assessment.* Several systems have been designed to quantitate the risks that individual women assume when they become pregnant. A variety of medical and obstetric conditions are scored numerically according to their potential for placing either the mother or the fetus in jeopardy; the higher the score, the greater the risk. Actually, one does not need a numerical score to recognize a patient with a *high-risk pregnancy.* Any condition that is known to interfere with normal growth, development, and delivery of the fetus or any maternal disease that may be present at conception or develop during pregnancy increases the risk. Many of these conditions can be recognized during a prepregnancy examination or at the first prenatal visit, and others that develop during pregnancy at subsequent visits. A special program of care should be developed for each patient with a high-risk pregnancy. Following are the most important risks:

I. Sociodemographic risks
   A. Age and parity
      1. Under age 15
      2. Age 35 to 45, birth order 1 and 5+
   B. Lowest social classes
   C. Illegitimacy
II. Medical-obstetric risks
   A. Conditions present at conception
      1. Previous abortion, ectopic pregnancy, fetal death, neonatal death, or congenital anomaly
      2. Previous low-birth-weight infant
      3. Less than a year since last pregnancy terminated
      4. Difficulty in conceiving
      5. Chronic cardiovascular-renal or collagen diseases
      6. Diabetes mellitus
      7. Malnutrition and anemia
      8. Chronic urinary tract infection
      9. Seizure disorders
      10. Congenital malformation of reproductive organs
      11. Syphilis
      12. Herpes virus, papilloma virus, and chlamydia infections
      13. Tuberculosis
      14. Tobacco, drug, or alcohol addiction
      15. Abnormal pelvis
      16. Uterine or ovarian neoplasms
   B. Conditions developing during pregnancy
      1. Pyelonephritis
      2. Preeclampsia-eclampsia
      3. Bleeding
      4. Acute infectious diseases

5. Malnutrition
6. Sexually transmitted diseases
7. Multifetal pregnancy
C. Conditions during labor and delivery
   1. Premature labor
   2. Premature rupture of membranes
   3. Abnormal labor
   4. Abnormal fetal position
   5. Cesarean section
   6. Hemorrhage following delivery

Neither prepregnancy nor prenatal care can be expected to compensate for inferior care during labor and delivery. To achieve the lowest maternal and perinatal morbidity and mortality, the responsible physicians and their associates must maintain careful supervision of the entire pregnancy and delivery.

Too often prenatal "care" consists of a series of visits during which a patient is weighed, the blood pressure is recorded, and an abdominal examination is performed. She is told that her weight gain is just right (which she knows) and that the baby is alive and growing (which she also knows) and is directed to return in 2 weeks. She hesitates to ask questions because she knows there are many other women to be seen. As a consequence she may make 10 to 15 prenatal visits and learn little about pregnancy, labor, delivery, and infant care and nothing about general health measures.

Because the healthy woman with a normal pregnancy needs little medical care, it seems appropriate that health professionals other than obstetrician-gynecologists play a major role in providing pregnancy care. An appropriate method for accomplishing this is through an *obstetric team,* consisting of a physician and one or more nurse midwives or obstetric nurse practitioners. Each patient is evaluated at the first prenatal visit to determine the level of care she needs. Thereafter, responsibility is divided; the physician concentrates on women with problems, and the nurses provide most of the care for those who are normal and the educational program for all patients.

With such a distribution of responsibilities, it is possible to provide appropriate care for every woman. Nurses will have sufficient time to spend with healthy women, and physicians can concentrate their efforts on women who need special medical care.

INITIAL EXAMINATION

Ideally, each patient should be examined as soon as it is reasonably clear that she is pregnant, usually about 2 weeks after she has missed a menstrual period. Unfortunately, the initial examination often is delayed either because the patient does not call or because the first open appointment is several weeks in the future. This presents no great problem for the healthy woman, but it may have serious consequences for those with complicated medical conditions or those who may need or want an abortion.

The problem can be solved by scheduling each initial prenatal visit with an obstetric nurse, usually within a few days of her first call. The nurse evaluates risk by obtaining a complete history, records the weight and blood pressure, determines the approximate duration of pregnancy, and orders the necessary laboratory studies. If the patient is normal, the nurse schedules the next visit with a physician who will have all the necessary information available. If any problem is suspected or if the patient wants an abortion, consultation is obtained before the patient leaves.

The *obstetric history* includes a general medical and social review with particular reference to diseases or conditions in the patient or her family that might affect the course of pregnancy and a detailed analysis of gynecologic function. The details of alcohol, tobacco, and drug use should be noted.

One should record the *date of onset and the duration of at least the last two periods.* It is particularly important to determine specifically whether the last period of bleeding was normal and came at the expected time. Many women report any bleeding, even spotting, as a "menstrual period" unless questioned in detail. One should also record the *contraceptive method* the patient was using before she conceived. Ovulation is often delayed for some time after oral contraceptive pills are discontinued. The "last period," the episode of withdrawal bleeding, may have preceded conception by several weeks.

Information concerning *previous pregnancies* should include their duration at delivery; the length of labor; the type of delivery; the size, condition, and subsequent development of the infant; the occurrence of complications; and the patient's emotional reaction to the event. For those who have delivered by cesarean section, it is important to obtain a copy of the operative note to identify the type of uterine incision. Previous pregnancy failures such as abortion, ectopic pregnancy, and fetal and neonatal deaths should be recorded also.

A *general medical examination* is performed after the patient has been interviewed. The *pelvic examination* includes bimanual palpation of the reproductive organs and inspection of the external genitals, the vagina, and the cervix. It is particularly important to determine uterine size as accurately as possible and relate it to the menstrual history. Manual measurements of the bony pelvis are usually obtained during the initial pelvic examination, but it often is appropriate to postpone this part of the examination until later in pregnancy, when the pelvic structures are more relaxed.

Basic laboratory studies in the normal patient include determinations of the hemoglobin level or hematocrit, blood type, and Rh; a serologic test for syphilis; urine tests for protein and sugar; and a screening cytologic examination for cervical abnormalities.

A *screening antibody test,* which is nonspecific in that it indicates the presence of any abnormal antibody rather than the precise type, should be run. If it is positive, further tests are necessary to identify the specific factor involved. A *rubella antibody titer* should also be obtained if it has not already been done.

Skin tests for reaction to tuberculin are appropriate for women who are at ordinary risk for tu-

berculosis infection. *Chest x-ray film examination,* with proper protective shielding, should be ordered for those from populations in which the incidence of tuberculosis is high, those whose skin tests are known to have been negative in the past and are now reactive, and for individuals with a history or physical findings suggesting active disease.

Because about 7% of all pregnant women have asymptomatic bacteriuria, and because most urinary tract infections before and after delivery occur in women with bacteriuria, it is wise to screen all pregnant women by testing for nitrates and leukocyte esterase. Urine culture is indicated for those with positive reactions. This is particularly important in women who have had urinary tract infections.

Fasting and *2-hour postprandial blood sugar concentrations* should be determined on women whose history suggests the possibility of diabetes. Patients at risk for hepatitis should be screened for *hepatitis B antigen.*

Serum alpha fetoprotein screening at about the sixteenth week of pregnancy may help to identify neural tube defects. Positive results should be repeated. If the second specimen also is positive, an ultrasound examination is appropriate to exclude multifetal pregnancy, intrauterine fetal death, or incorrect estimation of fetal age.

Genetic amniocentesis is recommended for women whose fetuses are likely to have chromosomal or biochemical abnormalities (Chapter 2).

After the examination has been completed and the diagnosis of pregnancy has been established, the findings are discussed with the patient. This portion of the interview should be unhurried and presented in words that she can understand easily. The physician first confirms the fact that she is pregnant, if this is possible, and indicates the date at which delivery can be expected. Unless there is some abnormality, she should be assured that her physical condition is satisfactory, that her pelvis is adequate, and that no complications are anticipated.

It is impossible for most women to understand

the full implication of pregnancy and to realize that they are going to have a baby, in contrast to being pregnant, until they actually can feel fetal activity. As a consequence, it is preferable to discuss specific problems at appropriate times during the pregnancy when the patient has some interest in them and when they are applicable. It usually is helpful to have printed instructions to which the patient can refer.

DIAGNOSIS OF PREGNANCY

The clinical diagnosis of pregnancy is made on the history of the *subjective symptoms,* which are the sensations experienced by the patient, and the detection of the *objective signs,* which are evident to the examiner. It may be difficult to establish an accurate diagnosis early, but the physician who uses all available aids will make few mistakes.

Subjective symptoms

It is not possible to make a diagnosis of pregnancy on the basis of symptoms alone. Each of the characteristic symptoms can be associated with conditions other than pregnancy, and some gravid women have none of them except amenorrhea.

Amenorrhea. Cessation of menstruation should always suggest the possibility of pregnancy, but it should not be concluded that the patient is pregnant only because amenorrhea is present. A few women bleed at irregular intervals throughout pregnancy because of some abnormality, and others may cease menstruating for reasons other than pregnancy. *Regular cyclic menstruation cannot occur during pregnancy because ovarian function is suspended.*

Morning nausea and vomiting. Morning nausea and vomiting usually appear a week or two after the period is missed and continue until about the tenth or twelfth week. The severity varies from mild nausea, which is easily relieved by ingesting food, to persistent vomiting, which depletes fluid and electrolytes (Chapter 23).

Although some degree of nausea and vomiting is experienced by more than half of all pregnant women, it is not diagnostic of pregnancy. Women who are not pregnant, as well as husbands of women who are, may have morning nausea and vomiting.

Bladder disturbance. Frequency of urination is caused by pressure or tension on the bladder by the enlarging uterus.

Breasts. Enlargement, tingling, or actual discomfort in the breasts is the result of hormonal stimulation of alveolar and ductal structures. This may also occur premenstrually.

Quickening. *Quickening* is a term that indicates the perception of fetal motion by the mother. Multiparas first feel movement at about the seventeenth week, and primigravidas about 2 weeks later. Women with pseudocyesis also experience "quickening."

The first sensation is usually described as a slight fluttering or a feeling similar to gas passing through the bowel. As the fetus grows and becomes more active, the sensation becomes stronger and may even be painful.

Objective signs

Breasts (Fig. 20-1). The breasts are firm and distended, and Montgomery's glands are prominent. The nipple and areola become darker as pregnancy advances and are surrounded by an area of increased pigmentation in the normal skin, the *secondary areola.* Colostrum can be expressed from the nipples, but it is not a reliable sign, because it may also be produced in pseudocyesis, with anterior lobe pituitary tumors, and in multiparas between pregnancies.

Genitals. The most remarkable changes take place in the genital organs.

VAGINA. The vaginal wall becomes cyanotic and congested (Chadwick's sign). This may also be detected before menstruation or with increased local congestion from any cause.

CERVIX. Softening in the tip of the cervix (Goodell's sign) can be detected soon after the onset of pregnancy. The entire cervix eventually is softened.

UTERINE ISTHMUS (Fig. 20-2). The isthmus of

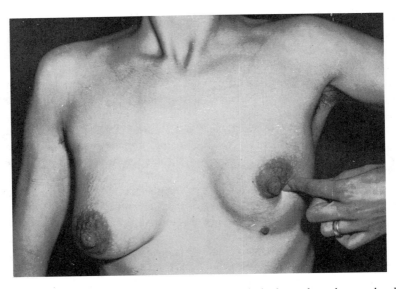

Fig. 20-1 Breast changes. Montgomery's glands are prominent, and nipples and areolae are deeply pigmented. Accessory nipple beneath left breast is also pigmented.

the uterus is soft at 6 to 8 weeks and can be compressed between the fingers on bimanual examination (Hegar's sign). Within a few weeks the entire cervix and the corpus become much softer, and the difference can no longer be detected.

UTERUS (Fig. 20-2). The consistency and shape of the firm, pear-shaped nonpregnant uterus change as pregnancy advances. Soon after the fertilized ovum implants, a soft bulge can be detected in half of the uterus, usually fairly high in the fundus, whereas the other side remains firm. The softened area probably indicates the implantation site.

The consistency of the uterus becomes soft and doughy rather than firm as pregnancy advances, and a progressive increase in size can be detected by repeated examinations.

Demonstration of the fetus (Fig. 20-3). The fetal parts can usually be *palpated* by the twentieth week of pregnancy unless the patient is too obese, the abdomen is tender, or there is an excessive amount of amniotic fluid (hydramnios). It may be possible to feel the fetus slightly earlier by *ballot-*

tement through the vagina. The examining fingers in the vagina push the anterior vaginal wall and lower uterine segment sharply upward, and the fetus first rises and then falls back, bumping against the fingertips.

Fetal motion can usually be seen, felt, or heard by the physician after the eighteenth week. Quickening is subjective and therefore unreliable.

The *fetal heart tones* can be heard first with an ordinary stethoscope at about the eighteenth to twentieth week low in the midline. The normal rate varies from 120 to 160 beats/minute, and usually it is not difficult to differentiate the double beat of the fetal heart from the maternal pulse. The sounds may be obscured by obesity, hydramnios, or an unusual fetal position. With the Doppler apparatus, one can detect the fetal heart consistently by the twelfth week and sometimes a week or two earlier.

Pregnancy can be confirmed much earlier by sonography than by physical examination. A *gestational sac* can usually be identified 5 to 6 weeks after the beginning of the last period, a *fetal pole*

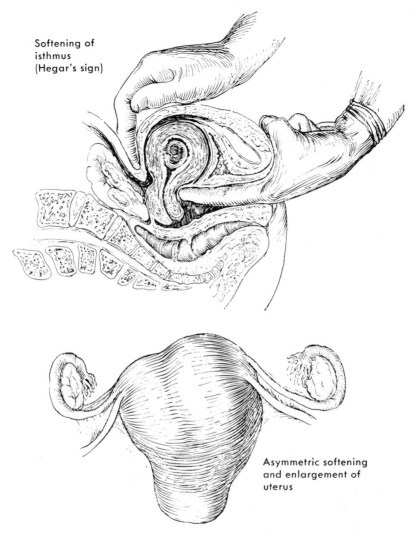

Softening of
isthmus
(Hegar's sign)

Asymmetric softening
and enlargement of
uterus

Fig. 20-2 Uterine changes in early pregnancy.

1 to 2 weeks later, and the *skull and thorax* can be identified by about the fourteenth week. With real-time ultrasound techniques *fetal heart motion* can be detected by 6½ to 7 weeks.

The embryonic structures can be detected earlier with an *endovaginal ultrasound probe* than with an abdominal transducer. The yolk sac can be seen within the gestational sac about 5½ to 6 weeks after the onset of the last period. A fetal pole can often be seen a few days later.

Pregnancy tests. The laboratory tests for pregnancy are based on the identification of chorionic gonadotropic hormones (Chapter 2). Because similar hormones are produced by certain teratomas

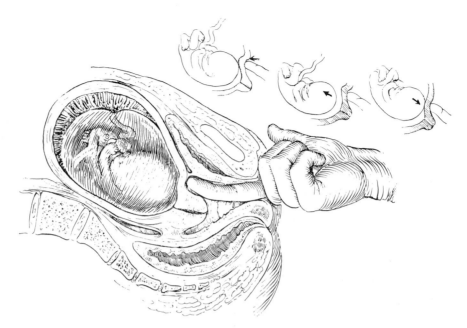

Fig. 20-3 Ballottement of fetus.

of the ovary and testes, choriocarcinoma, and hydatidiform mole, as well as by normal placenta, a positive test does not necessarily indicate the presence of normal pregnancy.

Positive diagnosis

A positive diagnosis of pregnancy can be made only if the fetus is identified by palpating its parts, by hearing its heart, by palpating motion, or by sonography. This can be accomplished during the first trimester of pregnancy only by sonographic techniques.

Differential diagnosis

Typical uterine changes must make the physician suspect pregnancy even though the patient denies the possibility.

Cystic ovarian neoplasms situated either in the posterior cul-de-sac or in the anterior pelvis may simulate a pregnant uterus. Ovarian neoplasms alone do not often cause amenorrhea. They usually can be separated from the uterine fundus, and they do not increase in size as rapidly as the pregnant uterus.

Sonography may be helpful. If the patient is not pregnant, one can expect to see an adnexal mass separate from a normal uterus without any evidence of pregnancy.

Uterine fibromyomas, particularly a large single tumor situated in the fundus of the uterus, may be almost impossible to differentiate from a normal pregnancy. Uterine tumors do not cause amenorrhea; and, as they grow slowly, one can detect little or no change in the uterus by repeated examinations at intervals of 2 to 3 weeks.

Pregnancy and fibromyomas or ovarian tumors often occur simultaneously. In situations of this kind, it may be necessary to use every possible diagnostic aid. Pregnancy must be considered in women who have missed one or more periods and in those whose periods have been normal but who are now bleeding irregularly, even though an ovarian cyst, a fibroid tumor, or another obvious lesion is present. In such women, pregnancy tests and sonography may be particularly helpful in diagnosing early pregnancy.

PSEUDOCYESIS

Pseudocyesis (spurious or pseudopregnancy) is an outstanding example of emotional control of physiologic function. Women with pseudocyesis may be amenorrheic or have significantly reduced menstrual flow, and the breasts may become firm, enlarge, and secrete colostrum. The abdomen enlarges, but, in contrast to pregnancy during which the umbilicus becomes flattened or even everted, the navel retains its normal depression. The abdominal enlargement is in part caused by weight gain, which often is greater than that during normal pregnancy. Patients with pseudocyesis experience all the symptoms of normal pregnancy; in fact they may be exaggerated. They also report "quickening" but frequently earlier than one would anticipate if the pregnancy were normal.

Pseudocyesis may appear at any age but is more common in older women. It usually represents an emotional need for an infant in an attempt to maintain a failing marriage, proof for herself that she can conceive, or a similar psychologic reason.

The diagnosis can be suspected if the physician cannot detect characteristic pregnancy changes in the pelvic organs and can be confirmed if the pregnancy test is negative or by sonography.

Because of the emotional factors involved, it does no good and in fact may be harmful simply to tell the patient that she is not pregnant. An attempt must be made to uncover the underlying emotional problem that makes pregnancy necessary to her. In some instances she should be interviewed several times before she is even told that she is not pregnant. Intensive psychotherapy may be necessary.

SIGNS OF LIFE OR DEATH OF THE FETUS

During the first 16 to 18 weeks of pregnancy the physician must rely on progressive uterine growth, detection of fetal heart activity by an ultrasonic instrument, or sonography to determine whether the fetus is alive and growing.

If *fetal motion suddenly ceases* and cannot be detected by the mother or the physician and if the *fetal heart can no longer be heard,* the fetus may have died. Occasionally, the fetal heart cannot be heard with an ordinary stethoscope because the fetus has assumed an unusual position and its chest wall is not in contact with the anterior uterine wall. A positive answer can be obtained by real-time ultrasonography; if fetal heart motion can be detected, the fetus is alive.

If the fetus has died, *uterine growth ceases,* or the size of the uterus may even regress. When placental function is disturbed, the breasts become softer and smaller.

The trophoblast may continue to secrete hCG for some time after fetal death, but repeated assays will demonstrate falling levels of the hormone.

DURATION OF PREGNANCY

The duration of pregnancy extends over an approximate period of 280 days from the first day of the last normal menstrual period or 268 days from fertilization. The duration of pregnancy therefore is about 40 weeks when calculated from the onset of the last period and 38 weeks when calculated from conception.

The exact time of fertilization can only be determined accurately by women who are recording basal body temperatures or by those who conceive by artificial insemination; consequently, *the first day of the last normal menstrual period is used as a starting point.* The thirteenth week of pregnancy therefore is the thirteenth week after the onset of the last normal period, not the thirteenth week after conception. Because most women do not keep calendar records of menstruation, this calculation is far from precise, but it is acceptable for clinical use.

There is no accurate method for determining exactly when labor will begin; however, the patient will want some day toward which to point—*the expected date of delivery, or EDD*—and this may be provided by the following methods:

1. The date of the first day of the last normal menstrual period minus 3 months plus 7 days gives the day of expected delivery. Since the date of the last menstrual period

often is unreliable, and since the last period of bleeding recognized by the patient may or may not have been true menstruation, this date does not necessarily indicate the day delivery will occur, but it usually is within 2 weeks on either side.

This calculation often is inaccurate in women with irregular cycles and when conception occurs after discontinuing oral contraceptives. Ovulation and conception may not occur for several weeks after the last withdrawal bleeding.

2. The EDD may also be calculated by adding 268 days to the day of ovulation as determined by basal temperature recordings or to the date of presumed fruitful coitus. The latter may well be inaccurate.

The physician can eliminate much confusion concerning the accuracy of the EDD of women who are first seen early in pregnancy by means of the following:

1. Comparing uterine size with the presumed duration of pregnancy on the basis of menstrual history at the first examination
2. Comparing uterine size with dates at specific weeks of pregnancy when the size of the uterus can be determined reasonably ac-

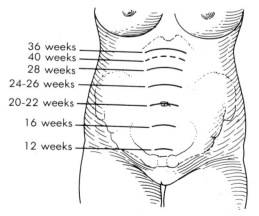

Fig. 20-4 Height of uterus above pubis at various weeks of pregnancy.

curately (Fig. 20-4). At the end of the twelfth week, the uterine fundus can usually be felt above the upper border of the pubis; by the sixteenth week, it is about halfway between the pubis and the umbilicus; and by the twentieth week, it has reached the level of the umbilicus. Between 20 and 30 weeks, the height of the fundus in centimeters, measured from the top of the uterus around the curve of the abdomen to the upper border of the symphysis pubis, approximates the week of gestation. This measurement becomes less accurate during the last weeks of pregnancy. *Measurements must be made with an empty bladder.*

3. Recording the exact date of quickening and the uterine size when fetal motion was felt
4. Recording the date when the fetal heart was first heard with an ordinary stethoscope

When this information is not available (for example, when conception occurs before the menses have returned after abortion or delivery, before a patient has had a normal period after discontinuing oral contraceptives, or when her periods are grossly irregular), it still is possible to arrive at a reasonable approximation of fetal age and maturity by using *sonography.*

During the first trimester, fetal age can be estimated with reasonable accuracy between the sixth and eighth weeks by *measuring the crown-rump length of the embryo.* After the sixteenth week one can measure the *biparietal diameter of the fetal skull.* At 16 weeks the average variation between gestational age on the basis of an accurate menstrual history and that calculated from the biparietal diameter is ±7 days. This increases to about ±10 days between weeks 17 and 26, to ±14 days during weeks 27 and 28, and to as much as ±21 days after week 29.

Amniotic fluid analysis. An amniotic fluid examination may be helpful in determining fetal maturity, but not actual fetal age.

LECITHIN/SPHINGOMYELIN (L/S) RATIO. The concentrations of lecithin and of sphingomyelin in amniotic fluid are about equal before the thirty-fifth week of pregnancy. After that time the lecithin concentration rises rapidly until term, whereas the sphingomyelin concentration decreases. High lecithin concentration indicates fetal lung maturity. Consequently, if the L/S ratio is at least 2:1, the lung is probably mature, despite fetal size, and there is little likelihood that serious respiratory distress will develop.

PHOSPHOTIDYLGLYCEROL. The presence of the surfactant activity of this substance gives evidence of lung maturity and provides reasonable reassurance that the infant, if delivered, will not develop respiratory distress syndrome. Its absence, however, is a less positive indication that respiratory distress syndrome will occur. The test for phosphotidylglycerol is not influenced by the presence of blood, meconium, or amniotic fluid.

These tests are more sensitive indicators of pulmonary maturity and the risk of the newborn infant developing respiratory distress syndrome than are other evaluations of amniotic fluid.

DIET AND WEIGHT GAIN

Weight gain. An increase of about 9 kg (20 pounds) over the prepregnancy weight can be accounted for by the products of conception and physiologic changes in the maternal organs. The weight of these components averages as follows:

	Kilograms	Pounds
Fetus	3600	7.5
Placenta	720	1.5
Amniotic fluid	960	2
Uterus	960	2
Breasts	480	1
Plasma volume	1440	3
Extracellular fluid	1440	3

Most women gain more than this, the *average weight gain during normal pregnancy* being about 11.5 kg (24 pounds). Those who gain an average amount usually return to their prepregnancy weights after involution is complete. According to Naeye, the lowest perinatal mortality occurs when the weight gain is about 20 pounds in normally proportioned women and about 30 pounds in those who are underweight.

Gains greater than 11.5 kg (24 pounds) can usually be accounted for by the ingestion of a diet too high in calories, the result of which is a residual increase in fat stores, or by the accumulation of fluid in the extravascular spaces. The former is responsible for many of the overweight women who find it difficult to lose the excess fat later and who repeat the same process during each of several pregnancies.

Excessive storage of fluid is not likely to be a cause of obesity but has a more serious immediate significance because it is one of the warning signs that preeclampsia may be developing. Excessive weight gain per se is not a cause of toxemia, but most women with preeclampsia do gain abnormally because of fluid retention. Conversely, the majority of women who store an excessive amount of fluid during pregnancy do not develop preeclampsia.

There is a definite relationship between maternal weight gain and the weight of the baby. Eastman and Jackson studied the records of 6675 white women and 5236 black women who were delivered of normal, living, single infants between the thirty-ninth and forty-second weeks of uncomplicated pregnancies. The mean weight gain for white women was 10.6 kg (22.1 pounds) and for black women, 9.8 kg (20.5 pounds). The mean birth weight of white infants was 3395 g, and progressive increases in maternal weight gains were accompanied by progressive increments in infant birth weights. The mean infant birth weights and maternal weight gains were as follows:

Maternal weight gain (kilograms)	(pounds)	Birth weight (grams)
0-4.8	0-10	3278
5.3-9.6	11-20	3301
10.1-14.4	21-30	3426
14.9-19.2	31-40	3562
+19.7	+41	3636

An interesting finding is that the mean birth weights of 61 infants whose mothers had lost weight during pregnancy was 3360 g.

The infants of black women followed a similar

pattern but weighed less in each group than did the white babies.

It is illogical to recommend that the mother gain excessively solely in an attempt to increase the size of the baby. It is equally as illogical to try to restrict the infant's weight by drastically curtailing the mother's caloric intake. This can only lead to impaired fetal development.

The *rate of gain* may have prognostic significance. The weight gain during the first trimester of normal pregnancy may be no more than 0.7 to 1.4 kg (1.5 to 3 pounds), even though there is no nausea. During the last two trimesters the gain usually is fairly steady at a rate of less than 0.48 kg (1 pound) per week. Excessive weight gain that begins during the first trimester and continues throughout pregnancy is almost always a result of excessive caloric intake. During the last 16 weeks of pregnancy, sudden increases in weight or gains of more than 1 kg (2 pounds) weekly are almost always an indication of excessive fluid accumulation.

Women who are *underweight* may be malnourished. Whenever possible, the nutritional deficit should be corrected before pregnancy, but generally, these patients are not seen until the first prenatal visit. At this time each underweight patient should be impressed with the importance of altering her diet to one that is suitable for pregnancy. Underweight patients can gain more than 11.5 kg (24 pounds), but the diet must provide the ingredients necessary for fetal growth.

Overweight women are also likely to be malnourished; their diets may be deficient in everything except calories. The pregnancies of obese women are more often complicated by hypertension and abnormal glucose metabolism than are those of more normal-weight mothers. Overweight women have a higher incidence of excessively large babies; conversely, they deliver fewer low-birth-weight infants.

It would appear that the weeks of pregnancy when a woman is under regular medical observation might be an appropriate time for controlled weight reduction, but this is not true. The primary nutritional objective should be to prevent excessive weight gain rather than to reduce or even to maintain weight. Excessive caloric reduction may require elimination of some essential nutrients, interfere with use of protein, produce ketonuria caused by catabolism of stored fat, and restrict fetal growth. Naeye calculated that the lowest perinatal mortality in infants who are born to overweight women occurs when the weight gain is about 16 pounds.

Some pregnant women gain at an excessive rate because they become progressively less active as pregnancy advances and continue to ingest the same amount of food. Pregnant women should be encouraged to remain active and to exercise.

NUTRITIONAL REQUIREMENTS

One can predict with reasonable certainty that the diets of most *teenagers* are deficient and that many of them are malnourished. Nutrition may be one of the most important factors determining the outcome of pregnancy in teenagers.

The adolescent who conceives before she has reached maximum longitudinal growth is at even greater risk of malnutrition than are those who become pregnant several years later. The dietary intake of the pregnant teenager must include the nutritional requirements for her own continuing growth as well as for the pregnancy.

The caloric content of the diet influences fetal growth. Delgado and associates supplemented the inadequate basic diets of two groups of mothers: one with an increase in both calories and protein and one with an increase in calories alone. The weights of the newborn infants were similarly increased in both groups. One can conclude from this study that calories are essential for fetal growth, but that the birth of a large baby does not indicate conclusively that the mother's diet was optimal.

It is desirable that the pregnancy diet contain an *adequate amount of good-quality protein* because protein is required for fetal development and for many of the basic maternal changes during pregnancy. There is no information, however, to suggest that a high-protein diet is essential for either maternal or fetal well-being. Zlatnik and Burmeister could find no differences in birth weight and anthropometric indices of infants born to mothers with mean protein intakes of 0.7 g/kg/day as compared to those of mothers whose mean intake of protein was 1.5 g/kg/day.

Many women survive on *vegetarian diets* that may be either vegan, which exclude fish, meat, poultry, eggs, and milk; or ovolacto, which exclude only fish, meat, and poultry. The former may be quite inadequate for pregnancy, whereas the latter may provide the necessary food elements.

Normal pregnancy diet. If the necessary ingredients for fetal growth and development are not supplied in the mother's diet, the fetus will obtain them at the expense of maternal tissues. During the winter of 1944-1945, the caloric intake of the population of the Netherlands was reduced to as little as 450 kcal/day. The median birth weight of infants born to mothers who were pregnant during this time was reduced by about 240 g, but perinatal mortality was not increased. A diet that provides the materials required for fetal growth prevents depletion of maternal tissue.

The daily dietary requirements for mature women and the additions necessary during pregnancy and lactation are listed in Table 20-1.

It is helpful to provide pregnant women not only with a list of optimal dietary requirements but also with menus and strategies they can use to help ensure an appropriate diet. Nutritional counseling is often helpful. Periodic reviews of food

TABLE 20-1 Recommended daily dietary allowances for mature women with added allowances for pregnancy and lactation

	Recommended daily allowances for nonpregnant women	Recommended daily allowances added for pregnancy	Recommended daily allowances added for lactation
Calories (kcal)	2100	300	500
Protein (g)	44	30	20
Vitamin A (RE)	800	200	400
Vitamin D (μg)	7.5	5	5
Vitamin E (mg equiv)	10	2	3
Ascorbic acid (mg)	60	20	40
Folacin (mg)	0.4	0.3	0.1
Niacin (mg equiv)	14	2	5
Riboflavin (mg)	1.3	0.3	0.5
Thiamine (mg)	1.1	0.4	0.5
Vitamin B (mg)	2	0.6	0.5
Vitamin B_{12} (μg)	3	1	1
Calcium (g)	800	400	400
Phosphorus (g)	800	400	400
Iodine (μg)	150	25	50
Iron (mg)	18	Supplement	0
Magnesium (mg)	300	150	150
Zinc (mg)	15	5	10

Based on data from Recommended dietary allowances, ed 9, Washington, DC, 1979, National Academy of Sciences.

intake identify those whose diets are inadequate. *Multivitamin supplements* are certainly essential for those whose diets are deficient. They usually are recommended for all pregnant women because few actually follow diets consistently.

Pica. The term *pica* indicates the ingestion of materials not ordinarily considered as foods. The most common are laundry starch, clay, and coal. Pica is more prevalent in black than in white women and is usually increased during pregnancy. The ingestion of large amounts of these materials often leads to malnutrition, iron deficiency anemia, and even bowel obstruction. Pregnant women from population groups in which pica is common should be questioned in detail about their eating habits.

Low-sodium diets. Low-sodium diets have been used extensively in an attempt to prevent or to control edema during pregnancy and in the treatment of preeclampsia-eclampsia. The accumulated evidence suggests that sodium restriction during pregnancy, even in women with edema and preeclampsia-eclampsia, may be harmful. As a consequence, low-sodium diets are usually not appropriate for pregnant women.

PRENATAL INSTRUCTIONS

In addition to needing advice concerning diet, the patient must know what she is permitted to do and what she should avoid doing during her pregnancy. The normal individual does not need to alter her activities much because she is pregnant.

Exercise. The amount of physical activity permitted is determined by the tolerance of the individual patient, what she is used to doing, and whether she has a complication that would ordinarily require rest rather than activity. Any usual activity, including walking, jogging, golf, tennis, and cycling can be continued by normal pregnant women. They become less agile as pregnancy advances and must consider the possibility of injury with more strenuous activities. Women who gain weight excessively should be encouraged to increase physical activity.

Swimming is an excellent form of exercise that can be continued throughout pregnancy. Snorkeling in reasonably calm water is permissible, but *scuba diving* should be avoided. The effects of diving on fetal development have not yet been determined.

Most of the studies on the effects of exercise on the fetus have been performed on animals. Although uterine blood flow is decreased and maternal temperature is increased during strenuous activity, there is no evidence to suggest that maternal exercise, within the tolerance of the individual, has a deleterious effect on the fetus. Certainly, pregnant women should not exercise to a point of fatigue.

Work. Pregnant women can continue working until term if the pregnancy is normal and if the environment in which they work and the physical activity involved pose no threat to the fetus or to the pregnancy. Women who develop complications and those with multiple fetuses usually should stop working.

Naeye and Peters reported that women who continue to work throughout pregnancy, particularly those who must stand for long periods of time, have more placental infarcts and babies whose weights are reduced by 150 to 400 g than do women who do not work. The overall maternal weight gain did not correspond to newborn weights. This suggests that women whose jobs require prolonged periods of standing, repeated stooping and bending, climbing ladders or stairs, and heavy lifting might be advised to stop working several weeks before term. It is not certain, however, whether the outcome is primarily a result of working or whether socioeconomic factors that require women to work are responsible.

Travel. The only danger in travel for the normal patient is that she may develop an acute complication, abort, or go into labor while away from home. Those who have aborted previously or who have abnormal pregnancies should not travel. Train, airplane, or automobile trips are permissible, but pregnant women should not sit for long periods of time. On long automobile trips, for example, they should stop and walk about for 10 minutes every 2 hours.

Wearing *seat belts* should be a routine. The

belt should encircle the bony pelvis, not the abdomen, to reduce the possibility of injury to the uterus in case of an accident.

Intercourse. Although there is conflicting information concerning the effects of coitus during pregnancy, it seems likely that normal women can continue intercourse without fear of injury or infection. Women who have aborted previously and those who are threatening to abort should be advised against coitus at least until it is clear that the pregnancy is proceeding normally. The desire for intercourse may be reduced during pregnancy, but it usually returns after delivery.

Some women are aware of uterine contractions that occur after orgasm, and fetal bradycardia has been reported. Chaven and associates recorded fetal heart patterns during intercourse in two normal pregnant women between the twenty-eighth and fortieth gestational weeks. Both mothers were aware of uterine contractions and increased fetal movements after orgasm. Fetal heart patterns included late decelerations, loss of short-term variability, periods of bradycardia lasting from 5 to 7 minutes, and periods of tachycardia lasting as long as 10 minutes. Since contractions occur with orgasm, produced either by coitus or masturbation, it seems likely that orgasm rather than prostaglandins from the ejaculate stimulates the uterine activity.

Bathing. Tub or shower baths are permitted throughout pregnancy. As pregnancy advances, the patient must take care not to lose her balance as she climbs into and out of the tub.

Bladder. Pubococcygeus exercises, if performed daily and if continued after delivery, will aid in preventing urinary incontinence after delivery.

Bowel. Constipation, which is probably caused by the physiologic decrease in peristalsis during pregnancy, can usually be corrected by adding bulky foods to the diet, an adequate fluid intake, and the judicious use of prune juice, milk of magnesia, and stool softeners.

Breast care. The nipples may be massaged and stretched with fingers lubricated with cocoa butter if the patient wishes, but this probably will not influence their response to nursing. She must be careful not to injure the nipples, particularly if they are inverted or abnormal. During the last weeks of pregnancy, nipple stimulation may induce uterine contractions.

Clothing. No special clothing is necessary, but all clothes should be loose and hang from the shoulders. *Circular garters* may promote the development of varicose veins. *Low-heeled shoes* increase stability and decrease backache. High heels rotate the body forward, thereby increasing the normal pregnancy lordosis and strain on the back muscles to balance the protuberant abdomen. A *maternity brassiere* that may be used after delivery should be worn if breast support is required. A *maternity girdle* is necessary only to control unusual discomfort caused by backache, pelvic pressure, or a pendulous abdomen.

Dental care. The teeth should be examined and any necessary repairs performed at least twice during pregnancy. Necessary extractions are permissible. Only local anesthesia should be used.

Alcohol. Fetal alcohol syndrome has been described in the offspring of human alcoholics. The affected infants have a variety of craniofacial, limb, and neurologic anomalies. They are below normal in intelligence, and they may develop behavioral problems. The effects of high blood alcohol levels may be enhanced by excessive smoking, drug use, and malnutrition, all of which may accompany alcoholism.

There is as yet no exact correlation between the amount of alcohol ingested and fetal growth and development, but the offspring of heavy drinkers are in greater jeopardy than are those whose mothers drink moderately. Although there is no precise information concerning the effects of "social" drinking, it seems prudent to suggest that pregnant women refrain from drinking, particularly during the early weeks when fetal anomalies can be produced. If possible, women who abuse alcohol should be identified before they conceive and be encouraged to stop drinking, at least during pregnancy.

Tobacco. The babies of women who smoke heavily are smaller than those of nonsmokers. Perinatal death rates among infants born to smoking mothers also are increased.

According to Underwood and co-workers, the mean birth weight of babies of 4856 nonsmokers was 3395 g; that of women who smoked one to 10 cigarettes daily, 3286 g; that of women who smoked 11 to 30 cigarettes daily, 3196 g; and that of even heavier smokers, 3182 g. Other studies confirm the decreased birth weights associated with maternal smoking.

Butler, Goldstein, and Ross reported a 30% increase in late fetal mortality and a 26% increase in neonatal death rate in infants born to mothers who smoked after the fourth month of pregnancy. Rush and Kass concluded that perinatal mortality is increased by 34.4% in infants of smoking mothers and that smoking rather than socioeconomic status is the cause.

The effect on the fetus may result from hypoxia caused either by reduced placental perfusion from the vasoconstrictive effects of nicotine or because carbon monoxide reduces oxygen capacity of both maternal and fetal hemoglobin. Another possible factor is that smoking reduces appetite and may be responsible for decreased maternal caloric intake.

One can only conclude that smoking is harmful to the fetus and that it may represent the difference between life and death when other factors that may influence survival also are present.

Drugs. It has long been known that fetal anomalies can be produced experimentally by the administration of certain drugs at appropriate times during embryonic development. Drugs such as thalidomide, methotrexate, and testosterone, together with many other presumably innocuous preparations, are known to produce anomalous development of the human fetus.

As a general rule, no drugs should be prescribed during the first trimester of normal pregnancy. Only medications that are essential to the health of the patient should be permitted. The use of drugs during pregnancy is discussed in detail in Chapter 32.

SUBSEQUENT VISITS

Although the adequacy of care cannot be gauged by the number of visits to the physician, frequent observation is necessary. For many years it has been customary to space prenatal visits at 3- to 4-week intervals during the first 28 weeks, at 2-week intervals between the twenty-eighth and thirty-sixth weeks, and then weekly until delivery. This schedule may be appropriate for the primigravida who has little responsibility at home, who will have many questions concerning the pregnancy, and who may need a considerable amount of support and reassurance. It generally is completely inappropriate for healthy multiparas whose previous pregnancies have been uncomplicated. These women have little to learn about the course of pregnancy, and their prenatal visits often are social calls rather than significant medical consultations.

If one can be assured after the first two or three visits that there are no abnormalities and that the fetus is growing at a normal rate, the subsequent examinations can be scheduled at 6-week intervals until the twenty-eighth or thirtieth week, at 3- to 4-week intervals until the thirty-sixth week, and at 2-week intervals until delivery. One should schedule a visit for about the twelfth week and another for about the twentieth week because these are good times to compare uterine size and duration of pregnancy. In addition, one should be able to hear the fetal heart at the twentieth week and can also record the quickening date. Such a schedule is appropriate only if the patient is comfortable with it and understands that she can see the obstetrician whenever she thinks it necessary and that she must call at once if there is any question of an abnormality.

At each visit the following are done:

1. The patient is weighed, and not only the total gain but the gain since the last visit are calculated. The diet is reviewed and any necessary adjustments made.
2. The blood pressure is recorded and compared with the previous readings.
3. A urine specimen is examined for protein and sugar.
4. The patient is questioned regarding symptoms.
5. Any change in treatment indicated by the findings is suggested.

The *pelvic examination* may be repeated if the first was inconclusive, if any abnormality was encountered, or if pelvic symptoms appear. *Vaginal examinations* may be performed in the office at any time during normal pregnancy. During the last weeks or whenever there is a question of early labor, one should use sterile gloves and instruments to decrease the possibility of introducing pathogenic bacteria.

The *abdomen is usually examined* at each visit. During the first 30 weeks the principal information one can gain from abdominal examination is the rate at which the uterus is enlarging. The fetal heart can be heard with an ordinary stethoscope after 20 weeks, and the position and presentation can be determined with reasonable accuracy in normal women after 30 weeks. During the final weeks before labor starts, one can chart the descent of the presenting part into the pelvic inlet.

The *breasts* should be examined at least once during the last trimester of pregnancy. This provides a good opportunity to discuss breast-feeding.

Certain *laboratory examinations* should be repeated even though they were normal during early pregnancy. The hemoglobin, hematocrit, and antibody screen should be ordered between 26 and 30 weeks. A 2-hour postprandial blood sugar test should be obtained at the same time. Serologic tests for syphilis and cervical cultures for gonorrhea and chlamydia should be repeated in late pregnancy when exposure to venereal disease is likely.

The administration of 300 µg of Rh immunoglobulin to unsensitized Rh-negative women at 28 to 32 weeks of pregnancy will aid in preventing Rh sensitization during late pregnancy.

Symptoms that appear during the prenatal period must be thoroughly investigated, making use of any physical or laboratory test that may be indicated. The problems most often encountered during pregnancy (nausea, vomiting, heartburn, backache, separation of the symphysis, and varicosities of the legs and vulva) are discussed elsewhere.

High-risk pregnancy. Women with proven or suspected abnormalities that may interfere with the course of pregnancy must be seen more often than normal women. The spacing of visits is determined by the complication. It usually is advisable to see *high-risk patients* on a special day when the efforts of all the office staff can be directed toward them and their specific problems.

Patient education. Too many obstetricians consider only the medical aspects of prenatal care and think little of *patient education.* Healthy women need a minimum of medical attention during pregnancy, and the outcome for most healthy middle- and upper-class women would probably be changed little if prenatal care were unavailable to them. This is not true for those with medical conditions that may complicate pregnancy or for women of lower socioeconomic classes; for these individuals a well-designed prenatal program may be essential in determining the outcome of pregnancy. Unfortunately, those who need the least medical care (that is, healthy middle- and upper-class women) usually make the greatest number of prenatal visits and gain the least from them.

Too little effort is made to use the prenatal period as an educational experience. Prenatal "education" too often consists of the physician outlining at the first visit what the patient can expect during pregnancy or recommending a book to read. Later in the pregnancy the physician may advise the patient and her husband to attend a prenatal class, which often is nothing more than a large group lecture given by a house officer who is assigned the task. Such lectures are often contracted courses in obstetrics and are inappropriate for an individual patient with personal problems. These problems are usually not covered in the lectures, and the patient may be given no opportunity to discuss them with her busy obstetrician.

The most effective educational programs are those conducted in an office or a clinic that are designed to meet individual as well as group needs. Because obstetricians are generally too busy to devote adequate time to teaching sessions, they are best conducted by nurse midwives or trained obstetric nurses. The essential information concerning reproduction, motherhood, nutrition, and general health care can be considered in small group discussions led by the nurse. Individual problems are often brought up by patients and discussed by the group. Much can be learned of the reactions of a patient to pregnancy by her interaction with other members of the group. Individual counseling sessions for patients who need them can be arranged.

The nurse can perform prenatal examinations on women in the educational groups on the days they meet, thus relieving the obstetrician of this responsibility.

Each obstetrician should conduct two prenatal programs, one for healthy women and one for those at risk. The major responsibility for the examination and education of healthy women can be delegated to nurse midwives or trained obstetric nurses. The obstetrician should assume immediate responsibility for all women with complications and serve as consultant to the nurses for well women, whom the physician can also see occasionally. Such a program can meet individual needs of all patients while making appropriate use of the skills of the professionals who are conducting it.

SUGGESTED READING

Andersen FH, Johnson TRB Jr, Barclay ML, and Flora JD Jr: Gestational age assessment. I. Analysis of individual clinical observations, Am J Obstet Gynecol 139:173, 1981.

Andersen FH, Johnson TRB Jr, Flora JD Jr, and Barclay ML: Gestational age assessment. II. Prediction from combined clinical observations, Am J Obstet Gynecol 140:770, 1981.

Butler NR, Goldstein H, and Ross EM: Cigarette smoking in pregnancy; its effect on birth weight and perinatal mortality, Br Med J 2:127, 1972.

Chaven B and others: Fetal heart rate changes during coitus (Abstr. 22). Las Vegas, 1985, Society of Perinatal Obstetricians.

Delgado H and others: Maternal nutrition: its effects on infant growth and development and birth spacing. In Moghissi KS and Evans TN, editors: Nutritional impacts on women, New York, 1977, Harper & Row, Publishers.

Eastman NJ and Jackson E: Weight relationships in pregnancy. I. The bearing of maternal weight and pre-pregnancy weight on birth weight in full-term pregnancies, Obstet Gynecol Surv 23:1003, 1968.

Gross T, Sokol RJ, and King KC: Obesity in pregnancy: risks and outcome, Obstet Gynecol 56:446, 1980.

Hadi HA, Hill JA, and Castillo RA: Alcohol and reproductive function, Obst Gynec Survey 42:69, 1987.

Henderson GI and others: Fetal alcohol syndrome: overview of pathogenesis, Neurobehav Toxicol Teratol 3:73, 1981.

Kleinman JC and others: The effects of maternal smoking on fetal and infant mortality, Am J Epidemiol 127:274, 1988.

Lotgering FK, Gilbert RD, and Longo LD: Maternal and fetal responses to exercise during pregnancy, Physiol Rev 65:1, 1985.

Mahan CS and McKay S: Let's reform our antenatal care methods, Contemp Obstet Gynecol vol. 147, 1984.

Mills JL and others: Maternal alcohol consumption and birth weight. How much drinking during pregnancy is safe. JAMA 252:1875, 1984.

Naeye RL: Weight gain and outcome of pregnancy, Am J Obstet Gynecol 135:3, 1979.

Naeye RL and Peters EC: Work during pregnancy: effects on the fetus. Pediatrics 69:724, 1982.

Nyirjesy I, Lonergan WM, and Kane JJ: Clinical significance of total weight gain in pregnancy. Obstet Gynecol 32:391, 1968.

Reamy K and White SE: Sexuality in pregnancy and the puerperium: a review. Obstet Gynecol Surv 40:1, 1985.

Rosett HL and others: Patterns of alcohol consumption and fetal development, Obstet Gynecol 61:539, 1983.

Rush D and Kass EH: Maternal smoking: a reassessment of the association with perinatal mortality, Am J Epidemiol 96:183, 1972.

Ryan GM Jr, Sweeney PJ, and Solola AS: Prenatal care and pregnancy outcome, Am J Obstet Gynecol 137:876, 1980.

Sabbagha RE: Diagnostic ultrasound applied to obstetrics and gynecology, New York, 1980, Harper and Row, Publishers.

Seager KG: The onset of labor in relation to the length of the menstrual cycle, J Obstet Gynecol Br Commonw 60:92, 1953.

Shiono PH, Klebanoff MA, and Rhoads GG: Smoking and drinking during pregnancy: their effects on preterm birth, JAMA 255:82, 1986.

van der Velde WJ, Copius Peereboom-Stegeman JHJ, Treffers PE, and James J: Basil lamina thickening in the placentae of smoking mothers, Placenta 6:329, 1985.

Zlatnik FJ, and Burmeister LF: Dietary protein in pregnancy: effect on anthropometric indices of the newborn infant, Am J Obstet Gynecol 146:199, 1983.

21

Russell K. Laros, Jr.

Endocrine disorders during pregnancy

Objectives

RATIONALE: Abnormal function of the thyroid, parathyroid, adrenal, pancreatic, and pituitary glands can coexist with pregnancy. A knowledge of diagnosis and treatment of these disorders and their effect on the fetus is important to good prenatal care.

The student should be able to:
A. Diagnose and treat diabetes mellitus.
B. Diagnose and treat gestational diabetes.
C. Diagnose and treat hypothyroidism and hyperthyroidism.

Physiologic alterations in secretions of the endocrine glands are so essential to the reproductive process that even minor abnormalities in pituitary, ovarian, thyroid, placental, or other hormone production may seriously affect fertility, nidation, or the maintenance of pregnancy.

DIABETES MELLITUS

The steady increase in the number of patients with diabetes complicating pregnancy is the result of (1) insulin therapy, (2) improved management of the obstetric problems peculiar to diabetic mothers, and (3) the hereditary tendency of the disease. In the preinsulin era the reproductive potential of women with diabetes was incredibly poor. Menstrual disturbances were common, and sterility was the rule. The maternal mortality in the few patients who did conceive was 25% to 30%, and the fetal loss was as high as 60% to 70%. At present the perinatal mortality is at least 10% throughout the United States, but it is much lower in perinatal centers where women with diabetes can be given special attention. The danger to the mother is no different from that for nondiabetic mothers.

Incidence. Frank diabetes occurs in about one in 300 deliveries. In one large study 20,070 pregnancies were screened and abnormalities in carbohydrate tolerance that met the criteria for diagnosis of gestational diabetes were found in one in 116 prenatal registrants. Progression to frank diabetes occurred in 28.5% of these patients within 5½ years.

Diagnosis. Pregnancy may precipitate rapid onset of diabetic symptoms, leading to acidosis in women with undiagnosed diabetes. The renal threshold for glucose is reduced during pregnancy, in part at least, from the physiologic increase in glomerular filtration rate. This accounts for many instances of glycosuria, but the exact cause can be determined only by glucose tolerance tests.

Most patients with frank diabetes have already been identified before they become pregnant. In fact, a key element of preconception counseling for these patients is to stress the importance of good glucose control during the first trimester.

Influence of pregnancy on diabetes. Metabolic control of diabetes is more difficult during pregnancy. *Vomiting* disturbs chemical balance, and acidosis may develop with little warning. *Lowering of the renal threshold for glucose* is variable; a large amount of sugar may be excreted, even though the blood glucose concentration is only slightly elevated; hence urine tests for sugar may fail to provide an accurate index on which to base insulin dosage. *Carbohydrate tolerance is altered,* but the direction and the degree of change is unpredictable. As a rule, glucose tolerance is reduced in the latter half of pregnancy. In relatively few patients the status is unchanged or improved.

Insulin requirements are increased in approximately 70% of patients, beginning about the twenty-fourth gestational week. Studies of fetoplacental function indicate that the fetus and placenta are specifically implicated in this change. Anabolic and diabetogenic properties of a lactogenic growth hormone–like substance (human placental lactogen, hPL) are now well recognized. Contrainsulin effects of hPL and, in addition, active degradation of insulin by placental proteolysis may well account for the increased insulin demands of pregnancy.

Evidence for placental degradation of insulin is clear-cut. A proteolytic enzyme (insulinase), which is present in the soluble cytoplasm of placental elements, has the ability to cleave insulin into constituent peptide and amino acid residues. Inactivation or increased destruction of insulin is only part of the picture. The hPL plays a key role in the metabolic adjustments of pregnancy. Large amounts of hPL secreted by the syncytiotrophoblast pass unidirectionally into the maternal circulation. The rise in plasma free fatty acids (FFAs) is at least in part induced by hPL. Elevated FFAs act as a specific peripheral antagonist to insulin in normal gravid women, but in diabetic mothers insulin resistance is exaggerated. Glucagon levels rise slightly during pregnancy, but this small increase plays little if any role in maternal gestational insulin resistance, and no significant amount reaches the fetus.

In normal pregnant women, fasting glucose levels are approximately 20 mg/dl lower than in nonpregnant subjects, a reflection of the increased glucose space and the mandate of the fetus, in addition to the maternal brain, for glucose.

A decrease in peripheral use of glucose is indicated by a diminution of the normal degree of hypophosphatemia after an intravenous glucose load. Plasma FFA levels are considerably higher in the maternal circulation during late pregnancy, whereas fetal plasma FFA levels are low. Concurrently, an increase in maternal insulin resistance is clearly evident in lower reactivity to both insulin and tolbutamide tests.

Reduction in insulin requirements after delivery can be anticipated because the contrainsulin effects of hormones and placental destruction are halted abruptly. *Hypoglycemic shock* occurs more often in the immediate period following delivery than at any other time in pregnancy. This can be prevented by appropriate reduction in insulin dosage and frequent chemical and clinical observations.

Influence of diabetes on pregnancy. The adverse effects of diabetes on pregnancy can be greatly reduced but not entirely prevented by good chemical control. Maternal *acidosis* is frequently disastrous to the fetus. Although chemical derangement may occur at any stage, particularly if vomiting or infection develops, it is most common during the last half of pregnancy, when insulin demands are increased. Although severe acidosis is still a major cause of fetal loss, it is a preventable complication.

Water balance is readily disturbed. Both fetal and maternal edema are common complications.

Hydramnios occurs in 10% of diabetic mothers—an incidence 20 times that observed in nondiabetic mothers.

The incidence of *hypertensive disorders of pregnancy* may be as high as 50%. The risk from preeclampsia to the mother with severe diabetes is greatly increased if vascular sclerosis or renal damage already exists. Fetal loss associated with preeclampsia-eclampsia per se is increased in diabetic pregnancies.

The harmful effects of diabetes may be demonstrable in the fetus of the patient exhibiting the earliest manifestations of the disease. *Excessive size of the infant is so common a finding that unrecognized maternal diabetes should be suspected in patients who deliver babies weighing more than 4320 g (9 pounds). There is an actual increase in both splanchnic and somatic growth.*

The cause for macrosomia in the infant of a diabetic mother is not yet fully understood. Insulin is capable of promoting growth in experimental animals, and *hyperplasia of the islets of Langerhans* is a consistent finding in postmortem examinations of affected infants. The combination of increased human growth hormone (hGH) common to all newborns and the fetal islet cell hyperplasia with a significant hyperinsulin response to glucose in the newborn infant of a diabetic mother bears certain similarities to the situation found in studies of growth hormone and serum insulin levels in obese subjects.

In the human, insulin does not pass the placental barrier freely; therefore it is unlikely that the increased fetal insulinogenesis is of much significance to the diabetes of the mother. On the contrary, glucose is readily transferred, and thus hyperglycemia in the mother probably serves as an important stimulus for pancreatic islet cell hyperplasia in the fetus.

Stillbirth and *neonatal death rates* are increased, even with mild maternal diabetes. The risk of intrauterine fetal death rises sharply after the thirty-sixth week.

It is difficult to predict impending fetal death on the basis of clinical evidence alone. A mother may notice a *reduction in activity of the fetus* as its metabolic disturbance increases. In addition, a *rapid increase in the amount of amniotic fluid* and *decreasing insulin requirements* suggest that the condition of the fetus and placenta, respectively, are deteriorating. Any of the maternal complications arising in late pregnancy may jeopardize the fetus.

The newborn infant of a diabetic mother exhibits certain characteristic signs. *Excessive size* and *a puffy, plethoric, "Cushinglike" appearance* is most common. However, the more advanced the diabetes, the smaller the baby is likely to be. *Newborn infants of mothers with diabetic vasculopathy may actually exhibit intrauterine growth retardation.*

Until recently, *respiratory distress syndrome* posed the greatest threat to infants of diabetic mothers. This threat has been greatly reduced by the many advances in prenatal management that permit individualization of the time for delivery and by advances in neonatal intensive care for the sick infant who must be delivered before maturity is complete. Perinatal mortality caused by birth asphyxia and trauma, particularly in vaginal delivery of the oversized infant, has also decreased and should be largely preventable.

Liveborn infants who subsequently become ill show *evidence of acidosis at birth* as demonstrated by high Pco_2 and low pH of arterial cord blood and a *hypoglycemia at 2 to 4 hours of birth* that is more profound and more persistent than the hypoglycemia common to infants of normal mothers. There is an increased incidence and intensity of *hyperbilirubinemia* and hypocalcemia.

Major congenital anomalies occur in 4% to 12% of infants of overtly diabetic women. Anomalies observed include the caudal regression syndrome, anencephaly, spina bifida and hydrocephalus, cardiac anomalies (transposition of the great vessels, atrial and ventricular septal defects), anal and rectal atresia, situs inversus, and renal anomalies (agenesis, cystic kidneys, and ureteral duplication). All of these anomalies occur primarily as a result of the influence of hyperglycemia on the developing embryo during the fifth to eighth week after conception. Measurement of glycosylated hemoglobin serves as an indicator of the degree of hyperglycemia over the preceding 4 to 6 weeks. There is a strong correlation between first trimester glycohemoglobin levels and the incidence of congenital anomalies in infants of diabetic women.

To decrease the frequency of congenital anomalies, one must assure excellent glucose control from the onset of pregnancy. To achieve this requires the attention and effort of the diabetic woman's primary care provider, who should inquire about the woman's pregnancy plans and method of contraception. The diabetic woman should be informed about the risk of congenital anomalies and their prevention. If not already doing so, the patient should be taught diabetic self-management skills, including management of capillary blood glucose levels with visual strips or meters in anticipation of starting a pregnancy. The goal for capillary blood glucose is a post-prandial value of 115 to 140 mg/dl. A variety of dietary and insulin regimens can be used to achieve this goal.

Other alterations include a more frequent occurrence of *renal vein thrombosis, enlargement of the liver and spleen* with extramedullary erythropoiesis, *cardiomegaly,* and a *higher than average incidence of hyaline membrane disease for gestational age. Beta cell hyperplasia of the pancreatic islets* is the most common pathologic finding in infants who fail to survive. The islet cell hyperplasia with infiltration of eosinophils is the most consistent evidence of diabetic embryopathy. Its appearance is identical in stillborn infants of mothers with diabetes irrespective of the mildness or severity of the disease.

Management. Principles of management of diabetic pregnancies, which are responsible for the remarkable improvement in outcome for both mother and baby, are (1) experienced team care; (2) accurate diagnosis, preconceptual counseling, and risk assessment; (3) rigid metabolic control

TABLE 21-1   White's classification of diabetes in pregnancy

Class	Characteristics	Management considerations
Gestational diabetes	Abnormal glucose tolerance during pregnancy	Diagnosis and treatment during second trimester to prevent macrosomia
A	Chemical diabetes diagnosed before pregnancy and managed by diet alone	Management as above
B	Onset at age 20 or later; duration <10 years; control with insulin or oral agents	Some endogenous insulin secretion may persist; fetal and neonatal risks as with type C or D; can be type I or II
C	Onset age 10-20 or duration 10-20 years	Type I diabetes
D	Onset before age 10; duration >20 years; or presence of chronic hypertension or retinopathy	Fetal macrosomia or intrauterine growth retardation (IUGR) possible; retinopathy may progress during pregnancy
F	Diabetic nephropathy with proteinuria	Anemia and hypertension common; IUGR common; perinatal survival 85%-90% with optimal care
H	Coronary artery disease	Increased maternal mortality
R	Proliferative retinopathy	Neovascularization with risk of retinal hemorrhage or detachment

with home glucose monitoring; (4) screening for congenital anomalies including maternal serum alpha-fetoprotein determination at 16 weeks' gestation and level three ultrasonic evaluation of the fetus at 18 to 20 weeks; (5) fetal surveillance; (6) allowing the pregnancy to continue until fetal lung maturity is demonstrated, unless contraindicated by deterioration of mother or fetus; and (7) neonatal intensive care.

Table 21-1 outlines White's classification of diabetes during pregnancy. Maternal risk and neonatal morbidity increase as the class progresses.

Study of each patient early in pregnancy should include the laboratory tests essential to metabolic regulation and those necessary for detection of cardiovascular or renal disease and retinopathy. The blood pressure record, 24-hour urine protein determination, creatinine clearance, and funduscopic examination are requisite baseline studies of the vascular system. Electrocardiographic study is indicated when evidence of vascular disease is found or in any case of long-standing diabetes. Renal function tests are mandatory in women with kidney disease because the prognosis is determined in large measure by the ability of the kidney to respond to the demands of pregnancy. The outlook for the diabetic patient with severe renal damage is so unfavorable that termination of pregnancy may be advisable. Retinopathy may be revealed and intensified, and vision may be threatened during pregnancy.

All prenatal patients with diabetes should be examined by the obstetrician and the internist at least every 2 weeks during the first half of pregnancy and weekly thereafter.

DIET. Total caloric allowance must be adjusted in accordance with the patient's nutritional status. A diet containing 25 to 30 kcal/kg of ideal body weight with a lower limit of 1700 kcal and an upper limit of 2000 kcal is prescribed. Approximately 125 g (500 kcal) of protein are included, with the remainder of the calories equally divided between fat and carbohydrate. Four feedings per day are advised. Supplementary vitamin and mineral preparations should be prescribed.

INSULIN. In the past few years many studies have demonstrated that stricter metabolic control than was previously considered acceptable is a major factor in improving perinatal morbidity and mortality. Rigid control aims at maintaining euglycemia between 60 and 120 mg/dl whole body glucose levels.

Better techniques have been developed to achieve good metabolic control even on an ambulatory basis. A steadier state is obtained by combining intermediary NPH and regular insulin for both the prebreakfast and the predinner doses, using two thirds of the total in the morning in the ratio of 2:1 and the other third in the evening in the ratio of 1:1. Some patients will require a third dose consisting of preprandial regular insulin at lunchtime.

Regulation of insulin dosage is greatly enhanced by the use of glucose oxidase reagent strips and a small reflectance meter either in the clinic or by the patient at home. The postprandial blood sample is more informative than the preprandial, which is generally well below the peak. The goal for the postprandial capillary blood glucose is <140 mg/dl at 1 hour or <115 mg/dl at 2 hours.

FETAL SURVEILLANCE. Techniques for monitoring maternal metabolic control and fetal welfare and maturity have made possible individualization of prenatal care and timing of delivery and in many cases reduced the need for long hospitalizations. However, monitoring of the fetus does not minimize the importance of clinical observations and judgment. The threat to the fetus is greatly increased at any stage of pregnancy by neglect or by development of any of the complications commonly associated with maternal diabetes: ketoacidosis, hypertensive disorders of pregnancy, progressive hypertension, pyelonephritis, or polyhydramnios.

Ultrasound scanning is useful in detecting abnormalities in fetal growth, gross anomalies, placental site, and polyhydramnios. The first scan should be done at about 20 weeks as a baseline to permit a meaningful interpretation of growth later in pregnancy.

Maternal *estriol determinations,* using either the 24 hours estriol/creatinine ratio or the unconjugated plasma estriol provides the best of the various biochemical tests of both fetal and placental metabolic activities. Early baseline values should be obtained beginning at about 28 weeks and repeated at weekly intervals until the thirty-fourth week if estriol production is steadily increasing. The test may need to be repeated much more frequently thereafter depending on clinical conditions, the preceding estriol level, and the results of electronic fetal monitoring.

Electronic fetal monitoring should begin at 30

TABLE 21-2 Tests of fetal well-being useful in managing the pregnant diabetic

Test	Abnormal result
Kick counts	Decreasing count day to day or absence of movement for three 20-min periods in one day
Urinary estriol	Decline of 35% over the previous three highest values
Plasma estriol	Decline of 40% over previous three highest values
Nonstress test	Fewer than four fetal movements with accelerations of the fetal heart of at least 10 beats per minute in a 20-min period
Contraction stress test	Persistent late decelerations in the fetal heart rate
Biophysical profile	Nonstress test Interpreted as above Fetal breathing Absence of a 1-min episode of fetal breathing in a 30-min time span Fetal body movement Less than three movements in a 30-min time span Fetal tone Less than one episode of extension in a 30-min time span Amniotic fluid volume Less than a 1-cm pocket of fluid
Doppler flow studies	Abnormal systolic/diastolic ratio

weeks. Fetal heart rate testing using the *nonstress test (NST)* provides a good and relatively simple screening method for predicting fetal distress or morbidity. The *contraction stress test (CST)* is positive if decelerations occur with contractions. Alternatively, the biophysical profile can be used. Abnormal results for the various tests of fetal surveillance are summarized in Table 21-2.

LABOR AND DELIVERY. The loss of the infant of an insulin-dependent mother when delivery has been carried out needlessly early is a disaster that should rarely occur today. If one can be certain of the gestational age and can demonstrate adequate fetal pulmonary maturity, problems related to prematurity are not an issue after 38 weeks. An amniocentesis performed during weeks 37 to 38 should reveal an *L/S ratio* of 2 or greater and the presence of *phosphatidylglycerol*. The latter substance represents the final step in maturation and is a particularly useful addition to the L/S ratio in diabetic pregnancies.

More well-controlled, uncomplicated diabetic pregnancies can now continue to term if all monitoring techniques indicate fetal well-being. On the other hand, it is not uncommon for signs of fetal distress to appear in some apparently uncomplicated diabetic pregnancies; intervention then is essential. Maternal complications that cannot be readily reversed, fetal distress, or both frequently mandate delivery well before term. Fetal pulmonary maturation often appears to be accelerated in connection with certain maternal complications, particularly hypertension, but meticulous neonatal intensive care is the critical factor for intact survival in these cases.

Vaginal delivery may be both difficult and dangerous because of the size and fragility of the infant and the need for early intervention. Delivery by the normal route is feasible if the diabetes is uncomplicated, if the pelvis is normal, if the size of the infant is not excessive, and if the cervix is favorable for induction. A normal oxytocin challenge test provides a measure of assurance that vaginal delivery is appropriate and safe. Electronic monitoring should be continued throughout the labor.

Cesarean section is indicated if the disease is severe, if pregnancy complications exist, if induction is unsuccessful, or if the progress in labor is poor. *Regional anesthesia* is preferable, and narcotics should be withheld until the baby is delivered.

Readjustment of insulin dosage is required during labor, delivery, and the period following delivery. It is best to withhold long-acting insulin on the day of delivery and administer all insulin as a drip. The patient is given an intravenous infusion of 5% glucose in normal saline, and the insulin dosage is regulated on the basis of regular blood sugar determinations. The usual requirement will be from 0.5 to 2 U/hour. Because the insulin requirement will frequently drop dramatically during the first few days after delivery, long-acting insulin should be reinstituted with care and a significantly decreased dosage.

Subsequent course. Despite the difficulties encountered during the course of pregnancy and the immediate puerperium, frank maternal diabetes is generally not made worse by pregnancy. Furthermore, a previous intrauterine or neonatal loss should not discourage the mother from attempting another pregnancy unless her diabetes is complicated by cardiovascular renal disease. Although perinatal losses may be repeated, meticulous management of the prenatal course, optimal timing of delivery, and skillful care of the newborn infant can provide the diabetic mother with a reasonably good prognosis.

Management of the newborn patient. Infants of diabetic mothers are often of necessity subjected to the cumulative effects of prematurity, delivery by cesarean section, and acidosis and hypoglycemia. Since the incidence of hyaline membrane disease is increased, every effort should be made to prevent or reduce respiratory distress. Treatment begins at delivery and consists of aspiration of mucus and other material from the respiratory passages, administration of oxygen, removal of the gastric contents by suction through a small tube, and treatment in an intensive care nursery.

Intensive care and laboratory and clinical support measures are essential. Correction of acid-base abnor- malities and maintenance of optimal hydration, glucose levels, and oxygenation are often critical matters. Observations for development of hyperbilirubinemia and hypocalcemia must be made, and appropriate treatment initiated if dangerous levels are reached.

SUBCLINICAL DIABETES

Glucose intolerance of pregnancy or gestational diabetes is the presence of glucose intolerance during pregnancy that reverts to normal in the nonpregnant state. Women who subsequently develop type II diabetes tend to produce oversized infants and to suffer a high fetal loss rate for many years before their diabetes becomes apparent. Macrosomia can be reduced substantially if this metabolic disorder is recognized and treated before the thirtieth week of gestation.

Diagnosis. Because diabetic symptoms in the mother are virtually absent in the early stages of the disease, a glucose screening test should be performed in patients whose records include one or more of the following: (1) a family history of diabetes, (2) previous stillbirth or unexplained neonatal loss, (3) oversized infants, (4) glycosuria during pregnancy, (5) hydramnios, and (6) repeated abortions. The presence of obesity in a patient with any of these disorders is often significant.

We recommend glucose screening in all pregnant women. Women who have not been found to have glucose intolerance before the twenty-fourth week should be screened between the twenty-fourth and twenty-eighth weeks. The screen consists of a 50-g oral glucose load given without regard to the time of the last meal or the time of day. Venous plasma glucose is measured 1 hour later; a value of greater than 140 mg/dl is abnormal and dictates the performance of a standard glucose tolerance test.

The glucose tolerance test should follow the recommendations of O'Sullivan and Mahan. The test is performed in the morning after an overnight fast of 8 to 14 hours and after at least 3 days of an unrestricted diet containing at least 150 g of carbohydrate. A 100-g oral glucose load is given, and the venous plasma glucose measured fasting and at 1, 2, and 3 hours. An abnormal test requires that two or more of the following glucose values be exceeded: fasting, 105 mg/dl; 1 hour, 190 mg/dl; 2 hours, 165 mg/dl; and 3 hours, 145 mg/dl.

The abnormality improves rapidly after the uterus is emptied in the same way that insulin requirements are decreased after delivery in the patient with clinical diabetes. Hence glucose tolerance tests obtained during the puerperium are usually uninformative of conditions existing during pregnancy. However, postpartum measurement of glycohemoglobin, which reflects the mean blood glucose level during the 2 months or so before testing, may be more informative. Hemoglobin A_{1c}, the most abundant of the minor hemoglobins, is formed by slow glycosylation of hemoglobin A. The process is relatively irreversible and persists throughout the life span of the cell. Normal values range from 3 to 6%. A clearly elevated value is significant in detection of previously unrecognized maternal diabetes, but a normal value would not rule out the diagnosis.

In general, an abnormality in carbohydrate metabolism found during one pregnancy tends to become increasingly abnormal in a subsequent pregnancy.

Management. The condition of many patients can be controlled by dietary restrictions alone during the early stages of diabetes. Insulin should be added if the 2-hour blood glucose level cannot be kept within normal range on the prescribed diabetic diet.

Oral hypoglycemic agents, which in contrast to insulin pass the placental barrier with ease, should be avoided. Severe and protracted hypoglycemia of the newborn has been encountered, particularly with use of the long-acting agents, a situation that carries considerable risk of death or cerebral damage in surviving infants.

Many patients with subclinical diabetes can be carried to term uneventfully and delivered normally. Early delivery is justifiable in patients with a previous poor obstetric history, those in whom obstetric complications arise that cannot be readily reversed, and those in whom a significant fall in estriol levels or abnormalities in fetal monitoring tests or both give evidence of failing fetoplacental function.

DIABETES INSIPIDUS

Diabetes insipidus is seldom associated with pregnancy because the disease is relatively rare. However, the reproductive capacity of patients with this condition is not necessarily reduced. Symptoms may be aggravated, improved, or unchanged during pregnancy. But for the most part these alterations can be met by adjusting the dosage of antidiuretic hormone. The disease may appear transiently during the course of pregnancy and must be differentiated from psychogenic polydipsia. Labor and delivery do not differ significantly from normal pregnancies, and there is no increase in fetal loss.

Treatment throughout pregnancy is with lysine vasopressin used 2 to 4 times daily as a nasal spray. In some acute situations an injection of 5 to 10 units of aqueous vasopressin may be helpful and does not cause an increase in uterine activity. The course of diabetes insipidus during pregnancy is variable, with some women requiring significant increase in their dose of vasopressin. No problems have been reported in the infants of women with diabetes insipidus.

DISEASES OF THE THYROID GLAND

Thyroid disease occurs four times more often in women than in men. The female reproductive functions can be adversely affected by any of the various types of thyroid disorders. Fortunately, effective treatment is available for hypothyroid and hyperthyroid states, including those complicating pregnancy. However, special problems in diagnosis and management are encountered during pregnancy that must be taken into account in the interest of both the mother and her offspring.

Accurate evaluation of thyroid activity may be difficult during pregnancy. Levels of thyroxine (T_4) and triiodothyronine (T_3) are elevated during pregnancy as a result of increases in specific binding proteins induced by high levels of estrogen. The T_3 resin uptake (T_3RU), which measures the unoccupied sites on the circulating thyroid-binding proteins, is decreased. The free thyroxine index (FTI) should therefore remain in the normal range. The FTI can be estimated by the following formula:

$$FTI = \frac{T_3RU}{T_4 \times 100}$$

In hyperthyroid patients the index is elevated, and in hypothyroid patients it is decreased in relation to the normal range of 1.0 to 3.5. Measurement of thyroid-stimulating hormone (TSH) is highly significant if the values are well above the top normal of 10 μU/ml. Borderline values are not definitive, since TSH cross-reacts with chorionic gonadotropin in pregnancy testing.

Thyroxine-binding globulin (TBG) can now be measured directly, and values obtained throughout pregnancy confirm the fact that the fraction of bound hormone is significantly larger as the binding globulin concentration increases.

Simple colloid goiter

The basic disturbance in simple goiter is an iodine deficiency resulting in reduced transport of thyroxine to the tissues. In response, thyrotropic stimulation is increased, and the thyroid undergoes hypertrophy followed by involution and increased storage of colloid. As a rule, thyroid function remains within normal limits, and neither the pregnancy nor the condition of the infant at birth is affected, although the gland frequently undergoes further enlargement during pregnancy when iodine intake is borderline. If thyroid function tests reveal thyroid deficiency, patients with colloid goiter should receive thyroid substance and iodine supplement throughout pregnancy to prevent congenital goiter or frank cretinism in the infant.

Hypothyroidism

Menstrual disturbances, sterility, and repeated abortions are common in women with thyroid deficiency. In some cases, conception and maintenance of the pregnancy proceed uneventfully, but untreated hypothyroidism in the mother is a potential cause for cretinism or congenital goiter in the infant. Preconceptional diagnosis and replacement therapy continued throughout the prenatal period are highly effective in preventing pregnancy complications because of thyroid deficiency.

The need for an increased production of thyroid hormones is evident by 6 weeks' gestation. Abortion is likely in patients with antecedent borderline hypothyroidism who fail to compensate for this demand. Substitution therapy with T_4 is indicated and highly effective if given before the rise in TBG occurs.

Myxedema

The infertility rate is so high that only a few cases of pregnancy in women with proven myxedema have been reported. The outstanding features of six offspring of a myxedematous mother were multiple congenital anomalies and mental retardation.

Hyperthyroidism

The incidence of hyperthyroidism complicating pregnancy is about 0.2%. Views concerning the influence of pregnancy on the development of this disorder differ. One series reported the initiation of hyperthyroidism during the gestation period was rare. Another, however, reported the onset of symptoms concurrent with pregnancy in 12 of their 21 patients. In either event the course of hyperthyroidism is essentially the same in gravid and in nongravid patients, but the pregnancy may be affected. Fetal loss is higher, particularly in early pregnancy, if the disease is untreated.

Diagnosis. The recognition of mild degrees of hyperthyroidism may be difficult. Nervousness, some increase in pulse rate, and thyroid enlargement are frequently found in normal pregnant women. A serum T_4 value above 12 μg/dl with a normal T_3RU will best establish the diagnosis.

Since amenorrhea is a relatively common symptom of hyperthyroidism, radioactive iodine should not be used for diagnosis of this condition until pregnancy has been ruled out. Fetal tissues have higher avidity for ^{131}I than do maternal tissues. Ill effects in fetal life have resulted not only in hypothyroidism and mental retardation but also in increased incidence of congenital anomalies and in the occurrence of thyroid carcinoma during childhood.

Treatment. Thyrotoxicosis can be adequately controlled during pregnancy and therefore does not provide an indication for therapeutic abortion. Certain safeguards must be observed in the interest of the fetus. Generally, these are concerned with avoidance of overtreatment, causing myxedema in the mother and thus increasing the risk of abortion or of inducing goiter in the infant. On the contrary, hyperthyroidism in the mother does not produce permanent effects on the fetus, although the newborn infant may exhibit symptoms of hyperthyroidism at birth and may require antithyroid treatment temporarily.

Thyroidectomy after medical preparation with iodine or antithyroid drugs seldom affects the pregnancy, particularly if surgery is performed during the second trimester. Postoperative deficiency should be anticipated and corrected by the administration of desiccated thyroid.

Antithyroid drugs such as propylthiouracil may be used during pregnancy without resorting to surgery, but they must always be used with caution. These drugs cross the placental barrier with ease. This treatment consists of administering antithyroid drugs until normal pregnancy levels of T_4 are reached.

Thyroid hormone does not cross the placental barrier to any significant degree. Hence if a maternal level of T_4 appropriate for pregnancy is maintained during treatment, the addition of thyroid substance to the maternal antithyroid therapy provides no added benefit to the fetus.

Poorly controlled hyperthyroidism of a pregnant woman risks development of a thyroid crisis with tachycardia, cardiac arrhythmia, fever, sweating, widened pulse pressure, and tremulousness. An excessively high T_4 level is the usual finding, but in a small percentage T_3 is remarkably elevated with not much change in T_4. Occasionally, both are elevated. In addition to intravenous fluids, antithyroid therapy, cooling, and intravenous propranolol may be necessary for control. Although the condition and the treatments put the fetus in some jeopardy, stabilization must be fully achieved before any thought of delivery is considered.

Breast-feeding is inadvisable in patients taking antithyroid compounds or iodine, since these drugs are secreted in maternal milk.

The clinical diagnosis of mild or moderate degrees of hypothyroidism and mental retardation is admittedly difficult in the newborn infant. Cord blood or blood levels of thyroid hormones should be obtained in any newborn infant in whom potential depression exists. These levels should be only slightly lower than those obtained in the mother (Table 21-3). Several states have instituted required screening programs for detection of neonatal hypothyroidism.

TABLE 21-3 Normal values for thyroid function tests in nonpregnant and pregnant women and in cord blood*

	Nonpregnant women	Pregnant women	Cord blood
T_4 (µg/dl)			
By displacement	5-12	9-15	6-13
By column	3-7.5	5-10.5	
T_3 (ng/dl)	50-175	140-200	40-60
TBG (mg/dl)	3-5	7-9	
T_3RU (percent)	25-35	>20	10-15
Free T_4 (ng/dl)		1.6-2.4	1.5-3
PBI (µg/dl)	4-8	6-11	4.5-5

*Values in various laboratories may differ, but the relationship should remain the same.

DISEASES OF THE PARATHYROID GLANDS
Hypoparathyroidism

During normal pregnancy, circulating levels of calcium are lowered mainly in the protein-bound fraction because of the decrease in serum albumin concentration. The ionized calcium that controls parathyroid hormone secretion is essentially unchanged.

Changes in calcium metabolism during pregnancy and lactation may predispose to *parathyroid tetany*. Calcium requirements are doubled after the fourth month of gestation, and consequently the need for parathyroid hormone is increased. Relative deficiency of parathyroid hormone may interfere with phosphorus excretion and permit the serum level of ionized calcium to drop below 6 mg/dl. Latent tetany is aggravated by inadequate intake or low absorption of calcium and by hyperventilation, which causes a diminution in ionizable calcium through alkalosis.

Treatment consists of regulation of the intake with a high-calcium, low-phosphorus diet supplemented by calcium lactate, 2 to 4 g daily. Aluminum hydroxide can be used to reduce the absorption of phosphorus from the gastrointestinal tract. During an acute attack, 10 to 20 ml of 10% calcium gluconate given intravenously will effect prompt temporary control.

An increase in fetal morbidity and mortality is associated with this disease. The major problems of the newborn are tetany and convulsions and occasionally heart block with electrocardiographic changes characteristic of hypocalcemia. All of these symptoms are reversed with prompt calcium replacement.

Hyperparathyroidism

This condition has been considered relatively rare, although it does occur in women of child-bearing age, usually because of a single parathyroid adenoma. In recent years hypercalcemia has been observed after renal transplantation. Renal stones are common, and pregnancy losses are frequent in patients with hyperparathyroidism. Neonatal tetany occurs in at least 50% of the infants and may be the first evidence of unrecognized maternal hyperparathyroidism. The tetany is thought to result from suppression of the fetal parathyroid glands by the high levels of calcium that readily cross the placenta. Mild cases can be treated medically with oral phosphates to create a calcium-phosphorus balance, but most require parathyroid surgery.

DISEASES OF THE ADRENAL GLANDS
Adrenal insufficiency (Addison's disease)

Properly treated Addison's disease poses no threats to the pregnant woman and her fetus. Difficulties in control are encountered early in pregnancy if nausea and vomiting ensue and again during labor and delivery. However, adrenal crisis occurs most frequently in the period immediately following delivery. Acute vascular collapse at this time is caused by a combination of several factors, including poor tolerance to the stress of labor or cesarean section, depletion of carbohydrate reserves, blood loss superimposed on low blood volume, and removal of placental hormones.

Treatment is by substitution therapy with special provision made for salt and carbohydrate replacement during labor and delivery. Because of the specific salt- and water-retaining properties of deoxycorticosterone acetate, cortisone plus additional salt in the diet is preferable for control during the prenatal period. A daily maintenance dose of 30 mg of cortisone is usually sufficient. At the onset of labor, 100 mg of hydrocortisone should be given and repeated every 6 hours.

Patients with hypoadrenalism have an exceedingly low tolerance to analgesics and anesthetics. Oversedation occurs if more than half the usual dosage of narcotics is administered. An intravenous drip of 5% or 10% glucose in physiologic saline solution offers protection against the hypoglycemia and dehydration common to these patients under stress. Cortisone should be reduced gradually after delivery until the maintenance dose is reached on the sixth or seventh day. The infant is unaffected by the maternal disorder.

Acute adrenocortical failure

Sudden collapse, persistent shock, and finally death can occur as a result of acute adrenal failure during pregnancy or in the puerperium. This rare condition should be considered when severe obstetric shock occurs, as death can be prevented by recognition and prompt treatment of adrenal failure. The pathologic lesions found in women who die of adrenal insufficiency are hemorrhage, necrosis, or infarction of the adrenal glands. Preeclampsia, late vomiting, hemorrhage, and infection frequently are precipitating causes, but at autopsy such deaths are proved to be primarily of adrenal origin. In addition to treatment with hydrocortisone and with other measures, as outlined in the discussion of Addison's disease, it may be necessary to administer dopamine intravenously by slow drip as a temporary measure to maintain blood pressure.

Adrenal atrophy

The administration of adrenocortical hormones may suppress adrenal function and induce adrenal atrophy, presumably through inhibition of pituitary production of ACTH. Impairment of adrenal function persists for varying periods of time after hormone therapy is discontinued. The increasing use of cortisone and similar drugs for many varied disorders is cause for concern. Suppression of the patient's own adrenal function may be sufficient to prevent a normal response to sudden stress. Death has followed relatively simple operations in patients with induced adrenal atrophy. Patients who have taken cortisonelike drugs for a protracted period, even if discontinued within 3 months, should be treated prophylactically with 100 mg of cortisone at the onset of labor, and treatment should be continued in gradually decreasing dosage after delivery.

Adrenal hyperfunction

Adrenocortical hyperplasia (Cushing's syndrome). Although patients with adrenocortical hyperplasia are relatively infertile, there is one report of seven pregnancies in four patients with this disturbance. The primary threat to pregnancy was chronic hypertension, and the resultant fetal loss was high (43%).

Medullary hyperfunction (pheochromocytoma). Maternal and fetal mortalities associated with pheochromocytoma are appalling. The largest series reports 30 pregnancies in 20 patients with this condition. Of the 20 women, 10 died; one died undelivered, and the other nine died within 72 hours after delivery. There were eight stillborn and three nonviable fetuses. Hypertension is extreme, may be paroxysmal or persistent, and is likely to progress during pregnancy. The usual symptoms are headache, anxiety, substernal pain, and nausea and vomiting, followed by exhaustion and profuse sweating. Profound and irreversible vascular collapse is the great threat and occurs most commonly soon after delivery.

When symptoms are found in late gestation they are usually confused with those of a severe hypertensive disorder of pregnancy; and, since pheochromocytoma is generally a benign tumor, it is important to make the diagnosis before its effects are disastrous. Pharmacologic tests are helpful but not definitive. Histamine vasopressor and phentolamine tests are associated with severe side reactions, particularly in pregnancy. However, side reactions are not severe with the tyramine test, and false-positive reactions are rare, although false-negative reactions sometimes occur. Final diagnosis is dependent on increased production of catecholamines or their major metabolites, and metanephrines (MN) or vanillylmandelic acid (VMA). Accuracy of diagnosis is so important that specific tests for these substances must be used; no reliance should be placed on some of the crude screening tests currently available. Values must be elevated distinctly above the normal pregnancy levels for these substances.

SUGGESTED READING

Burrow G: The management of thyrotoxicosis in pregnancy, N Engl J Med 313:562, 1985.

Cousins L: Pregnancy complications among diabetic women: review 1965-1985, Obstet Gynecol Surv 42:140, 1987.

Fisher DA: Maternal-fetal thyroid function in pregnancy, Clin Perinatol 10:615, 1983.

Gabbe SG: Definition, detection, and management of gestational diabetes, Obstet Gynecol 67:121, 1986.

Hunt AB and McConahey W: Pregnancy associated with diseases of the adrenal glands, Am J Obstet Gynecol 66:970, 1953.

Kitzmiller JL, Gavin LA, Gin GD, and Newman RB: Managing diabetes and pregnancy, Curr Prob Obstet Gynecol Fertil 11:107, 1988.

Komins JI, Snyder PJ, and Schwarz RH: Hyperthyroidism in pregnancy: a review, Obstet Gynecol Surv 30:527, 1975.

Lemons JA, Vargas P, and Delaney JJ: Infant of the diabetic mother: review of 225 cases, Obstet Gynecol 57:187, 1981.

Mennuti MT: Teratology and genetic counseling in the diabetic pregnancy, Clin Obstet Gynecol 28:486, 1985.

Momotani N, Nok J, Oyanagi H, Ishikawa N, and Ito K: Antithyroid drug therapy for Grave's disease during pregnancy, N Engl J Med 315:24, 1986.

Montoro MN, Collea JV, and Mestman JH: Management of hyperparathyroidism in pregnancy with oral phosphate therapy, Obstet Gynecol 55:431, 1980.

Mussey RD, Harris SF, and Ward E: Hyperthyroidism and pregnancy, Am J Obstet Gynecol 55:609, 1948.

O'Sullivan JB and Mahan CM: Criteria for the oral GTT in pregnancy, Diabetes 13:278, 1964.

Parer JT: Handbook of fetal heart rate monitoring, Philadelphia, 1983, WB Saunders Co.

Peacock I, Hunter JC, Walford S, Allison SP, Davison J, Clarke P, Symonds EM, and Tattersall RB: Self-monitoring of blood glucose in diabetic pregnancy, Br Med J 2:1333, 1979.

Pederson LM: Pregnancy and diabetes, a survey, Acta Endocrinol 94(suppl 238):13, 1980.

Peelen JW and De Groat A: Pheochromocytoma complicated by pregnancy, Am J Obstet Gynecol 69:1054, 1955.

Ramsay I, Kaur S, and Krassas G: Thyrotoxicosis in pregnancy: results of treatment by antithyroid drugs combined with T_4, Clin Endocrinol 18:73, 1983.

Selenkow HA, Birnbaum MD, and Hollander CS: Thyroid function and dysfunction during pregnancy, Clin Obstet Gynecol 16:66, 1973.

Thomas R and Reid R: Thyroid disease and reproductive dysfunction: a review, Obstet Gynecol 70:789, 1987.

White P: Diabetes mellitus in pregnancy, Clin Perinatol 1:331, 1974.

Zucker P and Simon G: Prolonged symptomatic neonatal hypoglycemia associated with maternal chlorpropamide therapy, Pediatrics 42:824, 1968.

Russell K. Laros, Jr.

22

Diseases of the respiratory system, the circulatory system, and the blood during pregnancy

Objectives

RATIONALE: Diseases of the respiratory, circulatory system, and blood occur commonly during pregnancy. An understanding of their pathophysiology, diagnosis, and treatment is important for optimal prenatal care.

The student should be able to:
A. Describe the relevant signs, symptoms, and diagnostic methods.
B. Discuss the approach to the patient with asthma, with symptomatic heart disease, or with anemia.

Diseases affecting the lungs, the heart, the blood vessels, and the hematopoietic system are encountered in only a small percentage of pregnant women, but they are potentially more serious than are many other complications. Most disorders affecting the cardiovascular system are not difficult to recognize and can be detected by the usual prenatal studies.

DISEASES OF THE RESPIRATORY SYSTEM

Pulmonary function is not impaired during pregnancy in women of normal health, even though functional and anatomic changes occur that produce significant alterations in respiration (Chapter 19). However, both the mother and the fetus can be compromised if pulmonary function is decreased significantly.

Pulmonary tuberculosis (TB). Tuberculosis is now relatively rare during pregnancy. In the United States, most cases of active TB occur as reactivation of old disease in immigrants from countries with endemic disease or in women with chronic diseases leading to immunosuppression, such as AIDS. At-risk populations of women should be screened with a tuberculin skin test in early pregnancy. A chest x-ray should be performed on tuberculin reactors with known prior negative reactions, tuberculin reactors with a indeterminate history of prior reactivity, and those who have a history or physical findings of active disease. A definite diagnosis depends on demon-

278

stration of *Mycobacterium tuberculosis* by culture (or smear in certain situations) in sputum, tissue, or other body fluids.

Whereas the primary goal of therapy is to eliminate the TB bacillus, choosing agents that will not be harmful to the fetus is equally important. The efficacy of short-course chemotherapy (9 to 12 months of isoniazid [INH] and rifampin [RFM] with ethambutol [EMB] or streptomycin [SM] added for the first month or two) has been well documented. However, SM causes ototoxicity, and RFM appears to cause an increase in the frequency of limb reduction defects. Thus, a combination of INH and EMB is both safe and effective during pregnancy. If a triple regimen is required by drug resistance or extrapulmonary TB, rifampin can be added after the first trimester. When INH is used during pregnancy, supplemental vitamin B_6 is recommended to prevent the potential neurotoxicity in the fetus.

Typically, patients with documented or suspected conversion of their tuberculin test are treated with INH for 6 months to 1 year. However, both the Centers for Disease Control and the American Thoracic Society recommend that prophylactic therapy be withheld during pregnancy and then started postpartum. A possible exception is documented recent conversion, in which case treatment should be started after the first trimester.

Although congenital infection can occur as a result of either hematogenous spread or aspiration of the bacillus during the birth process, most infection comes from postpartum maternal contact; BCG vaccination of newborns of women with active tuberculosis is recommended. An alternative regimen is INH prophylaxis; however, compliance can be difficult.

Asthma. Bronchial asthma is encountered in 3% to 5% of adults. During pregnancy approximately 50% of patients experience no change in the severity of their disease, while 25% improve and 25% worsen. When asthma worsens, triggers that include respiratory tract infection, medications, allergens, GI reflux, and exercise should be sought.

The degree of expiratory wheezing and the use of accessory muscles of respiration are good physical signs that mirror the severity of decompensation. However, they may be misleading, and simple bedside or office testing of the forced vital capacity and the forced expiratory volume in 1 second are extremely useful.

The goal of long-term therapy is to reduce the number and severity of attacks, and the goal of acute therapy is to alleviate hypoxia and to improve ventilation. The agents commonly used for chronic maintenance include B_2-agonists delivered by aerosol or orally, theophylline, and cromolyn. The last inhibits mast cell degranulation and is most useful as a single-agent treatment for young adults with exercise-induced asthma. During episodes of acute decompensation, treatment with an inhaled beta-agonist, subcutaneous epinephrine, subcutaneous terbutaline, or epinephrine suspension should be used. Failure to terminate an attack within an hour will require the addition of intravenous theophylline and corticosteroids. During pregnancy, special effort should be directed at maintaining the Po_2. Short courses of steroids may give the quickest relief of exacerbations with the fewest real or potential side effects on the fetus.

Acute respiratory infections

Upper respiratory disease. Pregnant women are somewhat more susceptible to the development of the common cold, and upper respiratory infections tend to last longer than in nonpregnant women. The usual symptomatic treatment can be administered.

Although there is no evidence to suggest that the usual viruses that presumably cause the common cold have a teratogenic effect, some viral diseases that are characterized by respiratory symptoms may. There is a significant increase in congenital heart lesions in the infants of mothers who had coxsackievirus B, types 3 and 4, infections during pregnancy.

Pneumonia. Pneumonia is far less serious since the development of the antibiotic drugs than it was in the past, but when it occurs during pregnancy it may prove fatal to the mother or her fetus. The choice of an antibiotic is determined by the responsible organisms.

Reduced pulmonary function

Pregnancy is not necessarily contraindicated in women who have had pulmonary resections if there is enough normal lung tissue to meet the requirements for pregnancy. Even women who have had pneumonectomies may be able to tolerate pregnancy with little difficulty. The principal risk for those with limited capacity is the possibility of losing much of the remaining function from an acute attack of pneumonitis; hence respiratory infections should be treated vigorously.

Adult respiratory distress syndrome. The adult respiratory distress syndrome (ARDS) presents as acute respiratory failure resulting from noncardiogenic pulmonary edema. The general pathophysiology appears to be an increased alveolar capillary permeability leading to hypoxemia secondary to decreased O_2 transport across the alveolus. Additionally, there is often a significant degree of right-to-left intrapulmonary shunting. Attenuated alveolar type I cells are replaced by proliferating type II cells, and the interstitium becomes infiltrated with inflammatory cells. Pulmonary fibrosis follows rapidly, leading to obliteration of pulmonary capillaries and alveoli. During pregnancy, ARDS is seen in association with various infection, severe preeclampsia/eclampsia, disseminated intravascular coagulation (DIC), and malignancy.

Even in young, healthy women the mortality of ARDS exceeds 50%. Hypoxemia is treated with O_2 in concentrations of 75% to 100%. If the Pao_2 does not increase to above 60 mm Hg, a mechanical ventilator should be used. The addition of positive end expiratory pressure (PEEP) both decreases shunting and capillary leak but at the expense of an increased risk of pneumothorax and a decreased cardiac output. Infection, if present, should be treated, as should any treatable cause of DIC. Although commonly used, high-dose corticosteroids do not appear to be of benefit in reducing the mortality from ARDS.

DISEASES OF THE CIRCULATORY SYSTEM
Heart disease

About 1% of all pregnant women have organic heart disease. In the past almost all were of rheumatic origin, but improvements in the treatment of rheumatic fever have decreased the incidence of significant valvular lesions. As a consequence, there has been a reduction in the total number of pregnancies complicated by heart disease, but the proportion caused by congenital malformation has increased.

Diagnosis. The diagnosis of heart disease is made on the basis of clinical history and examination, electrocardiographic recordings, echocardiography, and cardiac x-ray film examination. A more precise diagnosis can be made with cardiac catheterization. It may be difficult to make an accurate diagnosis of heart lesions during pregnancy by clinical examination alone. At least half of all women develop systolic murmurs during pregnancy, and the heart sounds, particularly those of the apex, are altered. The changes, which are caused by the increase in plasma volume and cardiac output, altered viscosity of the blood, and changes in the shape of the heart, begin during the early second trimester and reverse rapidly after delivery.

Patients suspected of having a cardiac lesion should be treated as are those who actually have one, even though a precise diagnosis cannot be made until after delivery. The lesions are classified according to the functional classifications of the New York Heart Association as follows:

Class I: Patients with cardiac disease that does not limit activity. Ordinary physical activity does not cause discomfort. The patients have neither symptoms of cardiac insufficiency nor anginal pain.
Class II: Patients with cardiac disease that produces slight limitation of activity. They are free from symptoms while at rest, but ordinary activity is accompanied by undue fatigue, palpitation, dyspnea, or anginal pain.
Class III: Patients with cardiac disease that produces

marked limitation of activity. Less than ordinary activity is accompanied by undue fatigue, palpitation, dyspnea, or anginal pain.

Class IV: Patients with cardiac disease that prevents them from carrying out any activity without discomfort. Symptoms of cardiac insufficiency or anginal pain are present at rest, and any activity increases them.

Prognosis. The prognosis for a patient with cardiac disease is determined by the functional capacity of the heart and its ability to meet the increased demands placed on it by the normal physiologic changes of pregnancy, the most important of which are the expanded pregnancy, plasma volume and the great increase in the total vascular bed in the enlarging uterus. Another physiologic change that adds to the cardiac load is a gradual rise in heart rate, with a maximum increase of 10 to 15 beats per minute near term. Additional factors that influence the outcome are the ability of the patient to adhere to the physical restrictions necessary during pregnancy, the quality of the medical care available to her, and the possibility that added complications such as serious infections may develop.

To maintain an adequate circulation, the cardiac output begins to rise at about the tenth week and reaches a maximum, at least 30% above that of nongravid women, between the twenty-eighth and thirty-second weeks. It remains elevated until term. The changes in output occur mostly in response to alterations in stroke volume. The curve for cardiac output roughly parallels that for plasma volume. Plasma volume, however, continues to increase until at least the middle of the third trimester and often until term. If an adequate output can be maintained, the patient will progress through pregnancy and delivery without difficulty, but if cardiac reserve is limited, the heart will be unable to respond to the increasing demands.

Maternal mortality is approximately 0.4% in class I or II and 6.8% in class III or IV of the New York Heart Association's classification. Pa-

tients with pulmonary hypertension appear to be at greatest risk. *Most deaths are caused by heart failure.* Although this can occur at any time, it is most common when the maternal blood volume is at a maximum. The normal heart has no difficulty in increasing its output as the plasma volume expands, but, if there has been significant valvular damage, the heart may be unable to respond to this and other demands.

Plasma volume and cardiac output decrease slightly, if at all, during the last weeks of pregnancy, and general physical demands increase. Failure can occur at this time if cardiac reserve is limited.

Heart failure occurs during labor when demands are greater than they have been during pregnancy. Cardiac output increases 25% to 30% during each first-stage uterine contraction if the patient is supine. However, if she is on her left side, the increase is only 7.6%. The difference is accounted for by caval compression with consequent alterations in venous return and arterial pressure.

Cardiac output reaches a maximum during labor and delivery and then declines slightly during the first few hours after delivery. During each contraction 250 to 300 ml of blood is forced from the uterine into the systemic circulation. After delivery, there is a permanent redistribution of blood from the uterine into the general circulation.

Maternal heart disease alone does not increase *perinatal mortality,* but intrapartum death from hypoxia may occur from circulatory changes accompanying decompensation, paroxysmal tachycardia, and similar complications. Infants born of mothers with heart disease are likely to weigh less than those whose mothers are normal. This suggests that the heart lesion and the reduced ability to increase cardiac output in response to exercise may reduce uterine perfusion and interfere with fetal growth.

Treatment during pregnancy. The patient with heart disease should be examined before she becomes pregnant so that the lesion can be accurately diagnosed and cardiac function evaluated. A patient with a serious lesion (class III or IV) should usually be advised against pregnancy. If a patient with heart disease is first seen during pregnancy, it often is wise to admit her to a hospital for study; this is particularly important with severe lesions. In most instances consultation with a cardiologist is indicated, but the fact that the cardiologist offers a good prognosis should not alter the physician's care of the patient. She may decompensate during pregnancy even though the lesion seems relatively innocuous.

With proper treatment, the mortality should be minimal, even in those with advanced lesions; if the cardiac abnormality is ignored or if she cannot or will not follow instructions, however, the death rate will be high.

Acute infections, particularly those of respiratory origin, often precipitate failure; consequently, most women with active infections other than uncomplicated upper respiratory infections should be treated in the hospital until they have recovered.

It is usually recommended that patients with class IV heart disease be admitted 10 to 14 days before delivery is anticipated for controlled rest in preparation for labor.

Rest is of utmost importance, and a specific plan should be developed for each individual. Rest periods each morning and afternoon and at least 10 hours in bed each night are advisable. Although light tasks around the home are permissible if they do not produce symptoms, unusual activity such as stair climbing, shopping, and heavy cleaning should be avoided; this is particularly true after the middle of pregnancy. Patients who have decompensated or those in whom slight exertion causes symptoms should remain in bed or in a chair at the bedside almost all the time. If the cardiac reserve is limited, coitus should be avoided after the twentieth week.

There is no need to reduce salt intake or to prescribe diuretics unless they are essential to the management of the heart lesion. A reduced salt intake may limit the normal expansion of plasma volume that is essential for adequate circulation.

An *iron supplement* is important because anemia increases the demands on the heart. *Digitalis* is used when indicated. Women with class III lesions must be considered to be partially decompensated; consequently, they, as well as those with class IV lesions, usually should take digitalis throughout the pregnancy.

THERAPEUTIC ABORTION. Termination of pregnancy is unnecessary in women with milder lesions and even in those of classes III and IV if they can be provided proper care during the entire pregnancy. Unfortunately, this is not always possible, and if a patient cannot or will not follow advice, the risk from continuing pregnancy may offer a serious threat to her life. If proper treatment cannot be administered, termination of pregnancy and tubal sterilization are justifiable for the following patients.

1. Those who have decompensated previously, particularly those who have been in failure between pregnancies (about two thirds of these will decompensate during pregnancy)
2. Those with atrial fibrillation
3. Those in functional classes III and IV (the incidence of failure is high, particularly with the more advanced lesions)
4. Those over age 35 years with serious lesions
5. Those with pulmonary hypertension

Interruption should be performed as early as possible because a major operative procedure may prove too much for the heart already burdened with gestational demands. In fact, the operation may actually contribute to the patient's death. Interruption should never be performed in a patient who is already in failure; the decompensation should be corrected first.

VALVULOTOMY AND HEART VALVE PROSTHESES. Operations to correct heart lesions are seldom necessary during pregnancy, as is indicated by the excellent results that can be obtained by medical treatment alone. Occasionally, however, mitral commissurotomy is warranted in a woman with stenosis if the constricted opening prevents the necessary increase in blood flow through or from the heart. The mortality is less than 3%, and there should be no effect on the fetus if all phases of the operative procedure are managed properly. Whenever possible, the operation should be performed during the first trimester; but, when necessary, it can be done later.

Although the experience in treating women with heart valve prostheses is limited, it appears that they are reasonable candidates for pregnancy but require even more care than do other women with heart disease. Most of them must be treated with antibiotics and maintained on heparin throughout pregnancy. Warfarin (Coumadin) sodium crosses the placenta, is teratogenic, and should not be used during pregnancy.

Care during labor. Induction of labor for heart disease alone is contraindicated. If the patient is allowed to start labor spontaneously, the physician can be assured that labor will more likely be short and normal than if induction is attempted early. Heart disease does not alter the length of labor.

Although failure usually does not occur during labor, it may set in soon after delivery; in most instances there is adequate warning that cardiac function is deteriorating. The best index of the condition of the heart during labor is offered by the pulse and respiratory rates, which, with the blood pressure, should be checked and recorded every 15 minutes. Failure is likely to occur if the pulse rate increases above 110 and the respiratory rate above 24 during the first stage. If there are any signs of beginning decompensation, oxygen should be administered, and the patient should be given digitalis rapidly unless she already is receiving an adequate dosage of digitalis. A pulmonary artery catheter (Swan-Ganz) and a radial artery catheter should be placed at the onset of labor in patients with hemodynamically significant heart disease and in all cases of pulmonary hypertension. A number of clinically significant cardiovascular parameters can then be monitored continuously, and pharmacologic agents used to alter preload, afterload, and contractility as needed.

Pain, anxiety, and muscular activity add to the burden on the heart, and the physician should try to eliminate them. This is best achieved with an epidural anesthetic if it can be administered safely. These techniques usually have little effect on blood pressure; therefore oxygenation is maintained. The anesthetic is started when the patient becomes uncomfortable, if she is making satisfactory progress in labor, and can be continued for delivery.

If caudal or epidural anesthesia is not available, the discomfort can be relieved with morphine sulfate or meperidine (Demerol). Scopolamine may increase both heart rate and muscular activity and is contraindicated. Phenothiazine derivatives should be used with caution because they may cause hypotension, particularly when a general anesthetic agent also is administered.

The American Heart Association no longer recommends prophylactic antibiotics to prevent subacute bacterial endocarditis in uncomplicated vaginal deliveries. Broad-spectrum coverage with penicillin and an aminoglycoside (vancomycin for women with penicillin allergy) are indicated for operative vaginal deliveries and cesarean sections. However, in view of the simplicity of prophylaxis and the serious consequences of subacute bacterial endocarditis, many cardiologists and perinatologists continue to recommend prophylaxis in all cases of congenital or acquired heart disease.

Delivery. Vaginal delivery is usually preferred to cesarean section unless there is an obstetric reason for the latter. A test of labor is ordinarily contraindicated for patients with moderate or severe cardiac disease because it increases the risk of infection or decompensation if labor is prolonged or if cesarean section becomes necessary after several hours of ineffectual labor.

The choice of anesthesia is one of the most important considerations when cesarean section must be performed on women with heart disease. Epidural anesthesia is the preferred form of conduction anesthesia for cesarean section in women with most types of heart disease.

Bearing-down efforts raise intravascular pressure and increase the possibility of decompensation; consequently, they should be prevented by eliminating the perineal phase of labor as completely as possible. This can be accomplished by low forceps or vacuum extraction soon after the head begins to bulge the perineum and should be performed in most primigravidas. It is not necessary in multiparas, who usually will deliver with a few second-stage contractions. Epidural, spinal, or pudendal block anesthesia will obliterate the perineal sensation, thereby eliminating bearing-down efforts, and they do not interfere with oxygenation.

Ergonovine maleate (Ergotrate) sometimes produces

transient but severe hypertension and should not be used. If it is necessary to stimulate uterine contractions, oxytocin can be given safely.

Postpartum care. The heart is more likely to decompensate during the early puerperium than during labor, but the incidence can be kept low by meticulous care during pregnancy and labor. Those with cardiac symptoms should usually remain in bed until the symptoms have disappeared.

Ambulation for those in classes I and II usually need not be delayed. Antibiotics are continued until it seems certain that the danger from infection is past. Women with heart disease may nurse their babies if they have no cardiac symptoms and if nursing is not too tiring. The patient may be discharged whenever the physician is certain the danger from decompensation is past. Most patients should remain in the hospital longer than normal women, particularly if they must assume complete responsibility for care of the child and the home.

Reproduction in women with heart disease should usually be limited, the size of the family being determined by the functional capacity of the heart and the desires of the patient and her husband. The patient should be instructed about a reliable contraceptive method before she leaves the hospital. Tubal sterilization may be considered if the parents desire no more children and if the operation can be performed with only slight risk.

Coronary artery disease

Coronary occlusion or thrombosis does not occur often during pregnancy, but when it does, the mortality is high. Pregnancy usually is contraindicated in women who have had coronary occlusion, particularly if the blood pressure is elevated; therefore therapeutic abortion can justifiably be advised. Acute coronary occlusion in a gravid woman should be treated as though she were not pregnant. In most instances vaginal delivery is permissible if precautions are taken to prevent pain, unusual muscular activity, and hypoxia during labor and delivery.

Peripartum idiopathic cardiomyopathy

There is a clinical entity characterized by peripartum heart failure of obscure cause. Women

with this disease are more commonly older, multiparous, and black and have hypertension. In most patients the heart returns to normal size soon after delivery. Subsequent pregnancies for women with this disorder are inadvisable because it often recurs.

Congenital heart lesions

Most women with the milder forms of congenital heart disease have little difficulty during pregnancy, but the prognosis is less favorable for those with reduced cardiac function, particularly if they are cyanotic. The highest mortalities are associated with Marfan's syndrome (50%), Eisenmenger's syndrome (30% to 35%), uncorrected tetralogy of Fallot (10% to 15%), and coarctation of the aorta (10%). The mortality associated with these lesions is so high that therapeutic termination of early pregnancy often is justifiable. Abortion need not usually be considered for other congenital lesions unless the cardiac reserve is so limited that decompensation can be anticipated as pregnancy advances.

The most frequent causes of death are heart failure and, in women with septal defects and patent ductus arteriosus, bacterial endocarditis; rupture of the aorta is common in women with coarctation.

The basic principles of management are similar to those for women with other types of heart disease.

Most women with mild congenital heart lesions can be delivered vaginally unless cesarean section is indicated for obstetric reasons. Abdominal delivery frequently is safer for those with advanced coarctation because the changes in circulatory dynamics accompanying uterine contractions and bearing down are likely to rupture the defective or recently repaired aorta. Cesarean delivery may also be selected when women with more serious lesions must be delivered prematurely.

Pregnancy should offer less hazard if disturbed cardiac function has been corrected by surgical repair of the defect. In most instances, cardiac operations should be performed between pregnancies.

Congenital heart lesions in the mothers may be duplicated in their offspring. Infants born to mothers with congenital heart disease, particularly those with cyanosis, are likely to be small, presumably as a result of intrauterine growth retardation.

DISEASES OF THE BLOOD

Unlike the normal nonpregnant individual whose blood picture remains relatively stable, the blood of pregnant women undergoes both qualitative and quantitative alterations. The *plasma volume* increases, reaching its maximum during the third trimester. The *red blood cell mass* and, as a consequence, the *total blood volume* also increase. If iron intake is adequate, the *total hemoglobin* content increases; and serum iron, erythrocyte protoporphyrin, and iron-binding capacity remain normal.

The body of a normal woman contains about 4 g of iron; 60% to 70% of this is carried in hemoglobin; about 30% is stored in the liver, spleen, bone marrow, and other cells; and most of the rest is carried as transport iron in the iron–beta globulin complex. During pregnancy approximately an additional gram of iron is required: at least 400 mg for the expanded red cell mass, 300 or 400 mg for fetal hemoglobin, and at least 100 mg to replace that lost through bleeding during and after delivery. Although iron is absorbed from the intestinal tract more readily during pregnancy, the usual dietary intake provides less than that required; the estimated deficit averages about 400 mg.

The *white blood cell* count is slightly increased during pregnancy, but it seldom exceeds 12,000 in normal women. The differential cell count is unaltered except for a slight decrease in eosinophils.

Anemia

Anemia is associated with a hemoglobin (Hgb) value below the lower limits of normal. The value in normal adult women is 14.0 ± 2.0 g/dl. Using this level, 20% to 60% of the patients will be anemic. The clinical presentation includes symptoms of anemia such as fatigue, light-headedness,

weakness, and exertional dyspnea and symptoms of cardiovascular compensation, palpitations, and tachycardia. However, most commonly the diagnosis is made because of an abnormal value detected at the time of a routine blood count. Once the diagnosis is suspected, a careful history of underlying disease, the use of oxidant drugs, or the presence of gastrointestinal or genitourinary bleeding is sought.

Proper utilization of the complete blood count (CBC) is the next step. In addition to erythroid values, the CBC provides erythroid indices. The normal mean corpuscular volume (MCV) is 80 to 100 fl, and the mean corpuscular hemoglobin concentration (MCHC) is 31 to 36 g/dl. The red blood cell (RBC) morphology should be evaluated for anisocytosis, poikilocytosis, polychromatophilia, hypochromia, and the presence of specific cells such as sickle cells, spherocytes, and helmet cells. Evaluation of the white blood cell count, platelet count, and reticulocyte count provides additional information. The normal reticulocyte count is 48 to 152×10^9/L.

Anemia can be placed into one of three major groups based on the morphology. Coupled with information about the reticulocyte count, this approach allows a systematic definition of the precise diagnosis. Hypochromia reflects abnormal hemoglobin synthesis. The normocytic anemias represent a very diverse group, whereas macrocytosis implies either hemolysis or disordered maturation of the RBC. Additional studies useful in defining the diagnosis are listed in Table 22-1.

Iron deficiency. Iron deficiency is documented by demonstrating either low serum ferritin or low serum iron and elevated iron-binding capacity. Treatment consists of a 200-mg dose of oral elemental iron daily. Parenteral iron is rarely indicated and does not return the Hgb to normal any faster than does oral iron therapy.

Megaloblastic anemia. Folic acid is a water-soluble vitamin that is widely available in the diet. During pregnancy the minimum daily requirement increases from 50 to between 500 and 1,000 mg/day. Whereas 10% to 25% of women

TABLE 22-1 Laboratory studies useful in diagnosing the etiology of anemia.

Study	Normal value
Serum hemoglobin	<1 mg/dl
Serum haptoglobin	30-200 mg/dl
Total bilirubin	0.5-1.0 mg/dl
Stool guaiac	Negative
Direct Coombs'stest	Negative
G-6-PD	B+ (A+, A−, B−, 150 others)
Hemoglobin electrophoresis	97% A, <3.5%; A_2, <1.5% F
RBC enzymes	Multiple types, pyruvate kinase most common
Osmotic fragility	Normal curve
Bone marrow	Normal cellularity and maturation
RBC folate	165-760 µg/L
Serum B_{12}	190-950 ng/L
Plasma iron/iron-binding capacity	40-175/216-400 µg/dl
Serum ferritin	10-99 µg/L

who do not take supplements will have low RBC folate levels, very few will develop megaloblastic anemia. When presented with a macrocytic anemia with a low reticulocyte count, folate and B_{12} deficiencies are the most likely diagnoses. The specific deficiency is proven utilizing a serum B_{12} and RBC folate level.

Thalassemia. The thalassemia syndromes are a group of disorders in which a structurally normal globin chain is made at less than a normal rate. These disorders are most common in individuals of Mediterranean, African, or Asian ancestry and are characterized by a microcytosis and a low reticulocyte count. Diagnosis is made by demonstrating an elevated Hgb A_2 level in cases of beta-thalassemia. Alpha-thalassemia is diagnosed by excluding iron deficiency and beta-thalassemia in patients with microcytic RBCs.

Screening the partner of a woman with thalassemia is mandatory. If he is also found to have thalassemia, genetic counseling is important. In general, thalassemia has little effect on the course of pregnancy, and no treatment is necessary.

Structural hemoglobinopathies. In structural hemoglobinopathies, unlike thalassemias, the globin molecule is structurally abnormal because of one or more amino acid alterations in the globin chain. These alterations may or may not lead to altered function of the hemoglobin molecule or the red cell.

Sickle cell anemia (SCA) occurs in 1 of 1875 black adults and is associated with significant morbidity. Complications include anemia, megaloblastic crises, sequestration, painful crises, toxemia, pyelonephritis, pneumonia, pulmonary embolism, and antepartum hemorrhage. The maternal mortality has been reported to be 0 to 11%, and the perinatal mortality, 2% to 39%.

Sickle cell–hemoglobin C disease occurs in 1 of 1250 blacks and is similar to SCA in its presentation and complication. Although symptoms may be absent or mild in the nonpregnant woman, they frequently become much worse during pregnancy. The maternal mortality has been reported to be 0 to 33% with the perinatal mortality 0 to 67%.

Sickle cell–beta thalassemia occurs in 1 of 3333 blacks. Again the symptoms are milder in the nonpregnant state and worsen during pregnancy. The maternal mortality has been reported to be 0 to 3% and the perinatal mortality 0 to 19%.

Treatment for all of these disorders consists of careful observation during the prenatal course and periodic urine cultures. Therapeutic doses of folate should be given (1 mg/day), and painful crises are treated with prompt hospitalization for hydration, O_2 therapy, and analgesia. All infections should be treated promptly and vigorously. Partial exchange transfusion or prophylactic transfusion appears to be useful in improving both maternal and fetal outcome. The initial transfusion is performed at 20 to 24 weeks and repeated as needed to maintain the hematocrit (Hct) at >25% or if a painful crisis occurs. This approach is beneficial in cases of SCA and symptomatic cases of sickle cell–hemoglobin C disease and sickle cell–beta thalassemia.

Sickle cell trait occurs in about 10% to 12% of blacks. The fertility, abortion, maternal mortality, and perinatal mortality rates are not affected. There is an increased incidence of urinary tract infection.

Hemoglobin C trait and *disease* occur in 1 of 33 and 1 of 4444 blacks, respectively. Neither disorder is associated with reproductive consequences. Hemoglobin E trait produces a mild, microcytic anemia that requires no treatment. Individuals with homozygous disease have a mild to moderated microcytic anemia. Again, no treatment is required.

Leukemia

Patients with acute leukemia usually present with symptoms of hypermetabolism, anemia, infection, or bleeding. The diagnosis is suspected from the results of the CBC and is confirmed by examination of the bone marrow aspirate. Physical findings include fever, petechiae, splenomegaly, hepatomegaly, and lymphadenopathy. *Acute lymphocytic leukemia* (ALL) is predominantly a disease of children but can occur at any age. In contrast, the incidence of *acute nonlymphocytic leukemia* (ANLL) increases with age. Untreated, the mean survival is 2.5 months. Although advances in treatment of ANLL has led to a remission rate of 50% to 70%, the median duration of remission is only 1 year. The principle of treatment is to induce a hematologic remission with a combination of drugs and then to maintain remission by cyclic administration of additional agents. Drug combinations used for induction include cytosine arabinoside, 6-thioguanine, L-asparaginase, vincristine, doxorubicin, cyclophosphamide, and prednisone. Bone marrow transplantation after the initial remission may be useful in providing long-term survival.

There is extensive experience with treatment of acute leukemia during pregnancy with good maternal and fetal outcomes. When the diagnosis is made during the first trimester, chemotherapy should be begun and abortion performed (if it has not occurred spontaneously) after remission is achieved. When treatment is begun during the second and third trimesters, no fetuses have been found to be abnormal. Improvements in the area of supportive care have paralleled the advances in cytotoxic therapy. Most important have been aggressive and early use of antimicrobial antibiotics and transfusion therapy.

Chronic myelocytic leukemia (CML) is a disease of young and middle-aged adults. Typical symptoms include fatigue, weight loss, and abdominal fullness. Splenomegaly, hepatomegaly, and peripheral lymphadenopathy are common. The CBC demonstrates leukocytosis and anemia. Of the two phases of CML, one is chronic and the other an acute blast crisis. The chronic phase can last from months to years. The circulating granulocytes show maturation, and treatment is intermittent and aimed at reducing the white blood cell count to 8 to 10×10^9/L at which time it is stopped. Alkylating agents such as busulfan and hydroxyurea are used to control the white count and symptoms. A successful alternative during pregnancy has been the use of leukophoresis. Ideally, pregnancy should be undertaken during an inactive phase when no treatment is needed. Both maternal and fetal outcome have been reasonably good with the incidence of intrauterine growth retardation higher in fetuses exposed to alkylating agents.

Lymphoma

The lymphomas can broadly be grouped into *Hodgkin's disease* (HD) and *non-Hodgkin's lymphoma* (NHL). In HD the stage of the disease has far more effect on treatment and outcome than does histologic type. Thus careful and complete staging is essential. Treatment consists of radiation therapy for localized disease where a cure rate exceeding 90% can be anticipated. Advanced disease is usually treated with combined chemotherapy regimens that produce remission in 80% to 100% of patients and cure in 50%. Because the course of HD is typically slow, staging and treatment can usually be safely delayed. In early pregnancy, elective termination followed by complete staging and treatment is the ideal course. Although pregnancy clearly has no adverse effect on the course of HD, it seems prudent to advise a patient not to become pregnant for 2 years after treatment so that cure can be assured.

The NHLs tend to disseminate earlier in their course and commonly have extranodal involvement at the time of diagnosis. Staging principles are similar to HD. Radiation therapy is appropriate for only a small portion of patients with early disease. Combination chemotherapy is used for more advanced disease. The coexistence of pregnancy reflects the more advanced age typical for patients with NHL. Only small series are available in the literature. In the majority, therapeutic abortion, maternal death, and prematurity were the outcomes.

Thrombocytopenic purpura. *Idiopathic (autoimmune) thrombocytopenic purpura* is rarely encountered in gravid women. The bleeding tendency and the reduced platelet count are not affected by pregnancy. The infant may have a transient thrombocytopenia, which can usually be corrected by the administration of fresh blood or of adrenal corticosteroids. The mother is usually best treated with adrenal corticosteroids during pregnancy. If this medication does not correct the bleeding tendency, splenectomy is indicated. Some authors have suggested that delivery should always be by cesarean section. The operative route is chosen in the hope that avoiding labor and vaginal delivery will decrease the incidence of intracranial bleeding in those few infants who are profoundly thrombocytopenic. Because the available literature does not support this recommendation, the obstetric service at the University of California, San Francisco, allows labor and vaginal delivery unless there is an obstetric indication for cesarean section. An alternative is percutaneous umbilical blood sampling performed at term before the onset of labor. If the fetal platelet count is $\geq 50 \times 10^9/L$, there is not even a theoretical advantage to delivery by cesarean section. However, if the level is $<50 \times 10^9/L$, the risks and benefits of vaginal delivery versus cesarean section can be discussed with the patient.

Disseminated intravascular coagulation (DIC). A syndrome produced as part of an underlying disease process that in some way leads to activation of the coagulation mechanism, DIC is seen in association with placental abruption, gram-negative sepsis, amniotic fluid embolism, the dead fetus syndrome, and severe preeclampsia and eclampsia.

The signs and symptoms are basically those of the underlying disease plus hemorrhage and, on occasion, microvascular obstruction. The hemorrhage occurs because of consumption of procoagulants and the production of fibrin/fibrinogen split products that are themselves anticoagulants. The obstructive symptoms are produced by large numbers of microthrombi being formed faster than they are removed by the fibrinolytic system.

The diagnosis is confirmed by demonstrating a low level of platelets and fibrinogen, elevated levels of circulating fibrin/fibrinogen split products, and the presence of fragment red blood cells. The most important step in therapy is the recognition and treatment of the underlying disease process. If the levels of procoagulants are reduced and the patient is clinically bleeding, replacement therapy with cryoprecipitate and platelet concentrates is begun. In the rare circumstance of significant, clinically evident microvascular obstruction (acute cortical necrosis or gangrene of skin or digits), the patient should also be anticoagulated with heparin.

Thrombotic thrombocytopenic purpura is a rare and serious condition characterized by thrombocytopenia, microangiopathic hemolytic anemia, fever, central nervous system manifestations, and renal impairment. It can be confused with severe preeclampsia accompanied by hemolytic anemia and thrombocytopenia. The most effective treatment is plasma infusion, vincristine, corticosteroids, and oral antiplatelet agents. These modalities should be used sequentially, and, if a response is not achieved, splenectomy and PGI_2 infusion should be tried.

SUGGESTED READING

Alger LS, Golbus MS, and Laros RK Jr: Thalassemia and pregnancy: results of an antenatal screening program, Am J Obstet Gynecol 134:662, 1979.

Atkins JN: Maternal plasma concentration of pyridoxal phosphate during pregnancy: adequacy of vitamin B_6 supplementation during isoniazid therapy, Am Rev Respir Dis 126:714, 1982.

Benedetti TJ, Valle R, and Ledger WJ: Antepartum pneumonia in pregnancy, Am J Obstet Gynecol 144:413, 1982.

Bernard GR, Luce JM, Sprung GL, Rinaldo JE, Tate RM, and Sibbald WJ: High-dose corticosteroids in patients with the adult respiratory distress syndrome, N Engl J Med 317:1565, 1987.

Brown GC and Evans TN: Serologic evidence of Coxsackie virus etiology of congenital heart disease, JAMA 199:183, 1967.

Catanzarite VA and Ferguson JE: Acute leukemia and pregnancy: a review of management and outcome, 1972-1982, Obstet Gynecol Surv 39:663, 1984.

Cunningham FG, Pritchard JA, and Mason R: Pregnancy and sickle cell hemoglobinopathies: results with and without prophylactic transfusions, Obstet Gynecol 62:419, 1983.

Cutforth R and MacDonald CB: Heart sounds and murmurs during pregnancy, Am Heart J 71:741, 1966.

Fitzgerald D, Rowe JM, and Heal J: Leukophoresis for control of chronic myelogenous leukemia during pregnancy, Am J Hematol 22:213, 1986.

Fitzsimons R, Greenberger PA, and Patterson R: Outcome of pregnancy in women requiring corticosteroids for severe asthma, J Allergy Clin Immunol 78:349, 1986.

Garg A and Kochupillai V: Non-Hodgkin's lymphoma in pregnancy, South Med J 78:1263, 1985.

Gililland J and Weinstein L: The effects of cancer chemotherapeutic agents on the developing fetus, Obstet Gynecol Surv 38:6, 1983.

Greenberger PA and Patterson R: The management of asthma during pregnancy and lactation, Clin Rev Allergy 5:317, 1987.

Hiss RG: Evaluation of the anemic patient. In Laros RK, editor: Blood disorders in pregnancy, Philadelphia, Lea & Febiger, 1986.

Jacobs C, Donaldson SS, Rosenberg SA, and Kaplan HS: Management of the pregnant patient with Hodgkin's disease, Ann Intern Med 95:669, 1981.

Juarez S, Cuadrado PJM, Feliu J, Gonzalez Baron M, Ordonez A, and Montero JM: Association of leukemia and pregnancy: clinical and obstetric aspects, Am J Clin Oncol 11:159, 1988.

Kendig EL: The place of BCG in the management of infants born of tuberculous mothers, N Engl J Med 281:520, 1969

Laros RK: The hemoglobinopathies. In Laros RK, editor: Blood disorders in pregnancy, Philadelphia, 1986, Lea & Febiger.

Laros RK Jr: Acquired coagulation disorders. In Laros RK Jr, editor: Blood disorders in pregnancy, Philadelphia, 1986, Lea & Febiger.

Laros RK Jr, Hage ML, and Hayashi RH: Pregnancy and heart valve prostheses, Obstet Gynecol 35:241, 1970.

Lewis BJ and Laros RK: Leukemia and lymphoma. In Laros RK, editor: Blood disorders in pregnancy, Philadelphia, 1986, Lea & Febiger.

Milner PF, Jones BR, and Döbler J: Outcome of pregnancy in sickle cell anemia and sickle cell–hemoglobin C disease, Am J Obstet Gynecol 138:239, 1980.

Morrison JC, Schneider JM, and Whybrew WD: Prophylactic transfusion in pregnant patients with sickle hemoglobinopathies, Obstet Gynecol 48:274, 1980.

Mulvihill JJ, McKeen EA, Rosner F, and Zarrabi MH: Pregnancy outcome in cancer patients: experience in a large cooperative group, Cancer 60:1143, 1987.

Pitkin RM: Nutritional support in obstetrics and gynecology, Clin Obstet Gynecol 39:489, 1976.

Powars DR, Sandhu M, Niland-Weiss J, Johnson C, Bruce S, and Manning PR: Pregnancy in sickle cell disease, Obstet Gynecol 67:217, 1986.

Pritchard JA, Scott DE, Whalley PJ, Cunningham FG, and Mason RA: The effects of sickle cell hemoglobinopathies and sickle cell trait on reproductive performance, Am J Obstet Gynecol 117:662, 1973.

Reynoso EE, Shepherd FA, Messner HA, Farquharson HA, Garvey MB, and Baker MA: Acute leukemia during pregnancy: the Toronto Leukemia Study Group experience with long-term follow-up of children exposed in utero to chemotherapeutic agents, J Clin Oncol 5:1098, 1987.

Schaefer G, Zervoudakis IA, Fuchs FF, and David S: Pregnancy and pulmonary tuberculosis, Obstet Gynecol 46:706, 1975.

Schatz M, Zeiger RS, Harden KM, Hoffman CP, Forsythe AB, and Porreco RP: The safety of inhaled beta-agonist bronchodilators during pregnancy, J Allergy Clin Immunol 82:686, 1988.

Schenker JG, and Polishuk WZ: Pregnancy following mitral valvulotomy, Obstet Gynecol 32:214, 1968.

Snider D: Pregnancy and tuberculosis, Chest 86:10S, 1984.

Sullivan JM and Ramanathan KB: Management of medical problems in pregnancy—severe cardiac disease, N Engl J Med 313:304, 1985.

Ueland K, Akamatsu TJ, Eng M, Bonica JJ, and Hansen JM: Maternal cardiovascular dynamics, Am J Obstet Gynecol 114:775, 1972.

Ueland K and Hansen JM: Maternal cardiovascular dynamics, III. Labor and delivery under local and caudal analgesia, Am J Obstet Gynecol 103:8, 1969.

Ueland K, Novy MJ, and Metcalfe J: Hemodynamic responses of patients with heart disease to pregnancy and exercise, Am J Obstet Gynecol 113:47, 1972.

Whalley PJ, Pritchard JA, and Richards JR Jr: Sickle cell trait and pregnancy, JAMA 186:1132, 1963.

Whittemore R, Hobbins JC, and Engel MA: Pregnancy and its outcome in women with and without treatment of congenital heart disease, Am J Cardiol 50:641, 1982.

Russell K. Laros, Jr.

23

Digestive tract disorders during pregnancy

Objectives

RATIONALE: Gastrointestinal disorders occur relatively commonly during pregnancy. An understanding of their pathophysiology, diagnosis, and treatment are important for optimal prenatal care.

The student should be able to:
A. Explain the signs, symptoms, and diagnostic methods.
B. Demonstrate a knowledge of how to approach the patient with nausea and vomiting, jaundice, or inflammatory bowel disease.

The structural and functional changes that occur in the digestive organs during pregnancy may account for many disturbing symptoms. In the majority of gravid women the secretion of free hydrochloric acid and pepsin decreases, and gastric motility is reduced. The stomach is pushed upward and to the left by the enlarging uterus, and the tone of the entire intestinal tract is reduced.

CARE OF THE TEETH

Pregnancy does not induce or hasten tooth decay, but pregnant women should make regular visits to their dentists.

Dental operations do not cause abortion or other pregnancy complications. On the contrary, it is to the patient's advantage to have dental disorders corrected, regardless of the gestation period. Local anesthesia should be used when an anesthetic is necessary.

GINGIVITIS

In about 50% of pregnant women, the gums hypertrophy and become inflamed, spongy, and friable. The cause is not known, but it appears to be related to poor oral hygiene and the hormonal changes associated with pregnancy. The condition regresses spontaneously after delivery. Astringent mouthwashes may provide symptomatic relief for gingivitis.

PTYALISM

Excessive salivation is occasionally encountered. It usually corrects itself spontaneously by the middle of the second trimester, but during the peak of saliva production more than 1 L may be secreted daily. Although tincture of belladonna, atropine, and other drugs may be prescribed, they alter the salivary secretion only slightly.

NAUSEA AND VOMITING

The nausea and vomiting experienced by at least half of all women during the first trimester of pregnancy varies in degree from mild, transient morning nausea to severe, constant vomiting that endangers the life of the patient. The symptoms usually appear within 2 weeks after the period has been missed, reach a maximum in about 2 more weeks, and then begin to regress by the tenth to twelfth week of gestation. They usually disappear completely by the fourteenth week, but in a few women, nausea persists throughout the pregnancy. Nausea and vomiting usually reappear and, in fact, may become worse with each pregnancy.

Nausea and vomiting that begin after the tenth to twelfth week are more likely to be caused by a medical or surgical condition than by pregnancy alone.

The nausea is most likely to occur when the stomach is empty, on arising in the morning or before meals, and it may be precipitated by certain odors or foods. In many women, it is present on awakening and may persist until they have eaten breakfast. In others the symptoms are somewhat more pronounced; a few will be nauseated all day, and an occasional patient develops true *hyperemesis gravidarum*, with constant nausea and frequent vomiting that may seriously affect health.

Etiologic factors. The underlying causes responsible for nausea and vomiting during pregnancy are not completely clear, but it seems likely that the disturbance is caused by the addition of some substance new to the patient rather than by the sudden development of a deficiency of vita-

mins, hormones, or other substances. The symptoms appear at a time during which the trophoblastic tissue is actively invading and destroying the decidua and when the function of the endocrine organs and hormone production are being drastically altered.

The onset and severity of nausea and vomiting appear to parallel the rise of serum chorionic gonadotropin (hCG). In pregnancies where serum hCG levels are unusually high, nausea and vomiting tend to appear earlier and be more severe. Examples are multifetal gestations and trophoblastic disease.

It is not likely that nausea is initiated by an emotional disturbance, but women with such disturbances are more likely to vomit, and the nausea can certainly be aggravated by psychologic stimuli. In all probability most instances of severe nausea and vomiting (hyperemesis gravidarum) develop as a result of an emotionally stimulated increase of the "normal" pregnancy nausea. Psychiatric studies indicate that many women with hyperemesis unconsciously wish not to be pregnant, even though they may profess to want children. Some have even undergone extensive studies and treatment for infertility, whereas others have experienced orgasmic dysfunction, dyspareunia, and aversion to coitus.

Treatment. Because the basic cause for nausea and vomiting during pregnancy has not yet been established, treatment must of necessity be directed toward reducing the severity of the symptoms. Each patient should understand that the symptoms are temporary and that they not only can be improved but should disappear within a short time.

Nausea that appears in the morning when the stomach is empty can usually be eliminated by having the patient eat two or three soda crackers as soon as she awakens and before she gets out of bed. After 15 to 20 minutes she arises and eats a light breakfast, and, if there is no recurrence of the nausea during the day, no other treatment is necessary.

Nausea that is constant throughout the day often can be controlled by frequent small feedings, keeping something in the stomach at all times. The patient is directed to eat in small amounts at least every 2 hours from the time she awakens until bedtime. Dry foods such as crackers, toast, baked potato, white meat of chicken, and cereal are preferable because they are more likely to control the nausea. Hard candy frequently is effective. Liquids should be taken between feedings rather than with solid food; tea, ginger ale or other carbonated beverages, or anything else the patient can retain are permitted. It usually is not possible for these patients to adhere to a full pregnancy diet.

Many types of medication have been used in patients with nausea and vomiting during pregnancy, but none is uniformly effective. The mild symptoms can usually be controlled with diet alone, so drugs are unnecessary. If, however, the symptoms are more severe and do not respond to diet therapy, some sort of medication may be prescribed.

A combination of pyridoxine hydrochloride and doxylamine succinate was found to be very effective in alleviating symptoms. However, because of multiple lawsuits alleging a relationship with fetal anomalies, the fixed combination (Bendectin) was withdrawn from the market. This occurred in spite of overwhelming evidence against any teratogenic effects of these agents. As an alternative, 20 mg pyridoxine and 25 mg doxylamine (Unisom), can be given at bedtime.

The patient who has lost considerable weight and is dehydrated because of hyperemesis must be admitted to the hospital. The important factors in the treatment of hyperemesis are (1) to control the vomiting, (2) to replace the fluid, (3) to replace water-soluble vitamins, and (4) to restore electrolyte balance. Interruption of pregnancy, which has been resorted to frequently in the past, is almost never necessary.

The type and amount of *intravenous fluid* necessary to hydrate the patient and restore chemical balance will be determined by the urine volume and serum electrolyte and creatinine concentra-

tions, which should be repeated daily. Ascorbic acid and vitamin B complex should be administered in the parenteral fluids; a protein hydrolysate solution can also be given if the patient is seriously depleted. Parenteral administration of fluids is continued until the patient is able to retain food and fluids.

Prochlorperazine dimaleate (Compazine) can be administered intramuscularly in doses of 5 to 10 mg or by rectal suppository in a dose of 25 mg every 6 to 8 hours. If prochlorperazine alone does not control the vomiting, it may be necessary to reinforce its *sedative action* with intramuscular injections of amobarbital (Amytal) sodium, 0.4 to 0.6 g every 6 to 8 hours. It is seldom necessary to continue heavy sedation for longer than 48 to 72 hours.

The *diet* must be limited until the vomiting is controlled, after which small amounts of food can be ordered. One should proceed slowly with the addition of foods because the vomiting may recur if the progression toward a normal diet is too rapid.

Once the vomiting has been stopped and chemical balance has been restored, the pregnancy usually progresses without a recurrence of the symptoms. Occasionally, the vomiting does recur when the patient leaves the protective environment of the hospital, only to be easily controlled by readmittance. In such instances an emotional cause is likely, and an attempt should be made to identify the responsible factor in the patient's life situation.

HEARTBURN

Heartburn is a common complaint during pregnancy and varies in severity from occasional mild discomfort to constant incapacitating pain accompanied by nausea and vomiting. It is caused by regurgitation of stomach contents into the lower esophagus and is a result of changes in the pressure relationships in the stomach and in the esophagus at the level of the gastroesophageal sphincter. Reflux of acid stomach contents can occur if the pressure in the stomach is considerably higher than that in the esophagus.

In normal nonpregnant subjects the mean resting intragastric pressure was 12.1 cm H$_2$O, the sphincter pressure was 34.8 cm H$_2$O, and the stomach-to-sphincter gradient was 22.7 cm H$_2$O. In pregnant women without heartburn, the mean intragastric pressure was 17.2 cm H$_2$O, the maximum sphincter pressure was 44.8 cm H$_2$O, and the stomach-to-sphincter gradient was 27.6 cm H$_2$O, the latter being comparable to the control subjects. There was a striking difference in the pregnant women with heartburn; the intragastric pressure was unaltered, being 16.5 cm H$_2$O, but the maximal sphincter pressure was only 23.8 cm H$_2$O. The stomach-to-sphincter gradient of 7.3 cm H$_2$O was obviously not high enough to prevent reflex of stomach contents.

The management of heartburn is similar to that described for hiatus hernia.

HIATUS HERNIA

Hiatus hernia can be demonstrated in about 12% of women during the last half of pregnancy. It is more often present in multiparas than in primigravidas and may produce annoying or even serious symptoms. Heartburn, which usually begins before the middle of pregnancy, is almost always present with hiatus hernia. It is usually made worse by lying down; therefore it often is noted at night and may interfere with sleep. Belching, hiccoughing, and regurgitation of sour material into the mouth also occur, but nausea and vomiting are somewhat less characteristic.

Because the hernias almost always disappear after delivery, treatment should be directed toward controlling symptoms; surgical correction is almost never necessary. The regimen should include frequent small bland feedings and antacids such as aluminum hydroxide or magnesium hydroxide tablets taken whenever necessary. Elevation of the head on several pillows when the patient lies down will reduce regurgitation through the relaxed esophagogastric junction.

JAUNDICE

Although no definite histopathologic changes can be observed in liver cells by light microscopy, there are evidences of altered liver function during pregnancy. *Sodium sulfobromophthalein (BSP) excretion* is reduced; *serum alkaline phosphatase* may be doubled, probably from a source in the syncytiotrophoblast; and *plasma albumin concentrations* and *plasma cholinesterase activity* are reduced. *Serum cholesterol* is slightly increased, and *spider nevi* and *palmar erythema* may develop. The changes are thought to be caused by the increase in circulating estrogens. The usual liver function tests aspartate aminotransferase (AST, formerly serum glutamic-oxaloacetic transaminase [SGOT]) and alanine aminotransferase (ALT, formerly serum glutamic-pyruvic transaminase [SGPT]) are usually within the normal range. Jaundice develops in about one of 1500 pregnant women.

Cholestasis of pregnancy. Intrahepatic cholestasis presents as pruritus during the third trimester of pregnancy. It tends to recur in subsequent pregnancies and is most common in women of Scandinavian, Mediterranean, and Chilean ancestry. The pathophysiology remains unknown, and the histology is indistinguishable from other causes of cholestasis. Diagnosis is confirmed by demonstrating an increase in circulating bile acids (cholic acid and chenodeoxycholic acid). Additional changes include an increase in alkaline phosphatase (sevenfold to tenfold), total bilirubin (rarely to >5 mg/dl), ALT (usually <250 units), and AST. The prothrombin time is usually normal unless there is a significant degree of malabsorption.

Intrahepatic cholestasis is associated with an increased incidence of prematurity, fetal distress, and fetal loss with rates as high as 50%, 60%, and 9%, respectively, being reported. Although deposits of bile salts have been described in the placentas, the mechanism by which they adversely affect the fetus is unknown. However, once the diagnosis is confirmed, ongoing fetal surveillance is mandatory.

Symptomatic relief can be achieved in many patients with cornstarch baths, phenobarbital, or Benadryl. When these efforts are unsuccessful, cholestyramine can be expected to reduce symptoms in 50% of cases, but its use is associated with mild nausea, anorexia, and bloating. Additionally, cholestyramine therapy interferes with the absorption of many medications and fat-soluble vitamins. Thus, the prothrombin time should be monitored periodically when this regimen is used. Finally, high-dose s-adenosyl-L-methionine has been reported to be very effective in reducing both symptoms and abnormal liver function tests.

ACUTE FATTY LIVER OF PREGNANCY

In the past acute fatty liver of pregnancy had a reported maternal mortality rate approaching 90%. However, recent reports suggest that, with proper supportive care and early delivery, most patients survive. The disease presents most commonly during the third trimester in primigravidas and is also more commonly associated with multifetal gestations and preeclampsia/eclampsia. Initially the patient experiences nonspecific constitutional symptoms and epigastric or abdominal pain, which are followed in about a week with jaundice and neurologic symptoms. The serum amylase, creatinine, bilirubin (10 mg/dl), uric acid, ALT (300 to 500 units), and AST are all elevated. Evidence of coagulation abnormalities including hypofibrinogenemia, increased fibrin/fibrinogen degradation products, thrombocytopenia, and prolongation of the prothrombin and partial thromboplastin time are characteristic as the disease progresses. Anemia and leukocytosis are also seen, with the anemia being caused by microangiopathic destruction of red blood cells. Although liver biopsy demonstrating infiltration of hepatocytes with small droplets of fat remains the definitive diagnostic study, computerized tomography (CT) and magnetic resonance imaging (MRI) can be very helpful. The CT shows diffuse low density and the MRI an increased intensity image of the liver. The differential diagnoses include chemical hepatitis, cholangitis, hemolytic uremic syndrome, acute hepatitis, systemic lupus erythematosus, and preeclampsia/eclampsia.

Treatment of acute fatty liver should occur immediately after delivery. The route of delivery should depend on the clinical situation. Multiple system deterioration is common; special attention should be directed at combating infection and treatment of coagulation dysfunction. Use of a histamine H_2 receptor antagonist helps reduce the incidence of gastrointestinal bleeding. Although transaminase levels usually normalize promptly after delivery, other liver functions may remain abnormal for days to weeks.

To date no case of recurrent acute liver has been reported in the 20 or so women who have become pregnant again. However, one must still be cautious in counseling the woman contemplating another pregnancy.

TABLE 23-1   Features of viral hepatitis

Features	Hepatitis A	Hepatitis B	Non-A, Non-B hepatitis
Incubation period	15-50 days	30-180 days	30-160 days
Transmission	Fecal-oral	Parenteral or body fluids	Parenteral or waterborne
Vertical transmission to fetus	None	Common	Probable
Diagnosis	HA antibody	HB_SAg, HB_CAg, HB_E Ag, anti-HB_SAb, anti-HB_CAb, anti-HB_EAb	By exclusion
Maximum infectivity	Prodrome	Prodrome or HB_CAg+ and HB_SAg carriers	Prodrome and carriers
Carrier state	None	5-10%	10-40%
Acute form	Asymptomatic to fulminant	Asymptomatic to fulminant	Asymptomatic to fulminant

VIRAL HEPATITIS

Acute hepatitis during pregnancy is most commonly caused by a virus. Hepatitis A (HA), hepatitis B (HB), and non-A, non-B hepatitis are the three most common, but Epstein-Barr virus, cytomegalovirus, and herpes simplex can also be etiologic agents. Once a specific diagnosis is established by immunologic tests, proper isolation is indicated. Diet and activity are determined by patient tolerance. Corticosteroids are not indicated. Table 23-1 summarizes features of viral hepatitis.

In fulminant cases of viral hepatitis, the AST is usually elevated to 500 to 3000 units and the bilirubin to 20 to 30 mg/dl, and thrombocytopenia and DIC are rare. These findings differ from those in acute fatty liver of pregnancy, in which the transaminase and bilirubin values are lower and DIC is frequently present.

Prevention of vertical transmissions of HB is an important part of perinatal care. The first step is carrier identification in all gravidas. Selective screening is ineffective in that about 50% of carriers are missed. With a program of universal screening, all carriers can be identified and their newborns given passive and active immunization. Such programs have been shown to be highly cost-effective.

PEPTIC ULCER

The symptoms of peptic ulcer often subside during pregnancy, as gastric acidity and motility are reduced. Perforation and hemorrhage are rare, but either may occur. Medical treatment can be continued during pregnancy, but it may be necessary to alter the diet to meet the added nutritional requirements.

PANCREATITIS

Acute pancreatitis is rare in pregnant women, and, when it occurs, it often is not diagnosed. The clinical course is similar to that in nonpregnant women, but the presence of an advanced pregnancy may prejudice the medical attendants. The basic confirmatory study, elevated activity of serum amylase, is as valid during pregnancy as in nonpregnant women.

Pancreatitis may occur in pregnant women being treated with thiazide preparations and tetracycline and should be considered when a patient receiving treatment with these preparations develops abdominal pain, nausea, and vomiting.

The treatment is supportive, and operation is contraindicated if the diagnosis of pancreatitis is confirmed.

INFLAMMATORY BOWEL DISEASE

Inflammatory disease of the bowel is divided into ulcerative colitis, which involves only the colon and rectum, and Crohn's disease, which can involve any portion of the bowel. Both disorders present with abdominal pain, diarrhea, and weight loss, and, in 10% of cases, differentiation is impossible. Rectal bleeding is less common in Crohn's disease, and absence of rectal involvement essentially excludes ulcerative colitis. Extraintestinal manifestations of inflammatory bowel disease include arthritis, ocular inflammation, aphthous ulcers, hepatitis, and renal involvement with stones, fistula formation, and hydronephrosis.

Pregnancy has little if any influence on the course of inflammatory bowel disease. Because active disease appears to be associated with a slight increase in the abortion rate, women should delay conception until their disease is in remission.

Treatment is similar to that used in nonpregnant patients and includes oral sulfasalazine, oral or rectal corticosteroids, and immunosuppression. Each of these medications may be continued during pregnancy. Surgery may be required to treat fistulas, bowel obstruction, hemorrhage, abscess formation, perforation, malignancy, or the failure of medical management. Occasionally patients with active disease and perforation may require long periods of total parenteral nutrition.

Diseases requiring surgery

Acute surgical emergencies involving the gastrointestinal organs occur no less frequently in gravid than in nongravid women of a like age and must be treated in the same manner. With prompt diagnosis and surgical intervention, the operative risk is not increased because of the pregnancy; but complications develop rapidly, and the prognosis is more serious in the pregnant woman if a necessary operation is deferred.

Physiologic changes associated with pregnancy can increase the difficulty of early diagnosis. *"Physiologic" nausea and vomiting may be present during the early weeks, but they never begin after the first trimester and are not associated with abdominal pain.*

A leukocytosis of 12,000 or 14,000 is not uncommon during pregnancy, but granulocytosis with an increasing percentage of nonsegmented forms is abnormal. The *sedimentation rate* is increased in pregnancy and is of no value in differential diagnosis.

Pain must be distinguished from discomfort related to the enlarging uterus, the pelvic ligaments, the corpus luteum, or urinary tract disturbances.

The choice of anesthetic is the joint responsibility of the anesthesiologist and the obstetrician, with major considerations being freedom from pain, adequate relaxation, safety, and prevention of fetal hypoxia.

Antibiotic therapy is neither necessary nor desirable as a prophylactic measure simply because of the pregnancy. However, these drugs may be lifesaving when an operation must be performed in a contaminated field or when the problem is already complicated by infection. They should then be used in full amounts for a sufficient time and in accordance with the culture and sensitivity patterns.

Prevention of premature delivery should be considered after any intraabdominal operative procedure. The risk is particularly high if there has been heavy bacterial contamination of the peritoneal cavity. Careful electronic monitoring for increased uterine activity should be carried out during the first few postoperative days. If preterm labor is observed, tocolytic therapy with either a beta-mimetic agent or indomethacin suppositories should be started.

APPENDICITIS

Acute appendicitis occurs with the same frequency in pregnant as in nonpregnant women, but the diagnosis is more difficult, and delay in treatment is hazardous. The difficulty in diagnosis and delay in operative intervention increase with gestational age, as does maternal and fetal mortality. Today maternal mortality is low in cases of un-

complicated appendicitis but can be as high as 5% in cases associated with perforation.

The enlarged uterus may obscure the appendix, which tends to be displaced upward and laterally in the direction of the right iliac crest (Fig. 23-1). Its ultimate position, however, is variable.

Suppuration of the acutely inflamed appendix is rapid, and rupture occurs early. Diffuse spreading peritonitis results because the increased vascularity, reduced omental protection, and motion of the uterus hinder localization. Abortion or premature labor may occur if the infection involves the uterine serosa. Uterine contractions stimulated by the infection are frequently tetanic and predispose to fetal hypoxia and intrauterine fetal death.

Diagnosis. Nausea and vomiting, epigastric pain localizing in the right side of the abdomen, and tenderness anywhere from McBurney's point to the right flank are suggestive. Evidences of infection including elevated temperature and, more

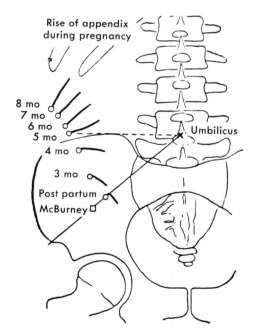

Fig. 23-1 Rise of appendix at various stages of pregnancy.

particularly, an increased pulse rate are usually present. A single white blood count is of doubtful value in the questionable case because a slight leukocytosis is physiologic during pregnancy. Serial studies at hourly intervals that reveal an increase in both total count and in young polymorphonuclear cells indicate the presence of an acute infectious process.

Differential diagnosis. Urinary tract infection or ureteral stone presents the greatest difficulty in the differential diagnosis. Examination of a catheterized urine sample is indicated in every case and should be repeated in an hour or two if the diagnosis is questionable. In the last trimester appendicitis must be differentiated from abruptio placentae or uncomplicated premature labor.

Treatment. Appendicitis complicating pregnancy requires surgery as soon as the diagnosis can be established.

A false-positive diagnosis during pregnancy is much more likely than in nonpregnant individuals. A rate of finding a normal appendix of 30% to 40% is quite acceptable, considering the morbidity and mortality of a delayed diagnosis in the face of perforation. If a normal appendix is found at laparotomy, it is preferable that it be removed. Microscopic appendiceal inflammation can be found in grossly normal appendices.

Technical difficulties are increased late in pregnancy because of the large uterus and the position of the appendix. Tilting of the patient to the left side is helpful. If leakage or perforation has occurred, the peritoneal cavity should be lavaged with large quantities of warm saline solution, and large dosages of broad-spectrum antibiotics should be administered parenterally. Because abortion or premature labor after appendectomy is not related to changes in hormone levels, the administration of progesterone after surgery is of little value.

If labor ensues soon after surgery and cannot be stopped, it should be conducted according to usual obstetric principles, but elimination of the second stage by low forceps delivery to prevent voluntary bearing-down efforts is advisable. Caudal or epidural anesthesia during labor and delivery can be a valuable aid in such circumstances.

Maternal mortality is no higher in gravid than in nongravid patients if there is no delay. After perforation the threat to the pregnant woman increases because a large uterus may prevent adequate localization of the infection. Fetal loss associated with peritonitis is high.

INTESTINAL OBSTRUCTION

Intestinal obstruction should be suspected in any pregnant woman with a history of previous abdominal surgery or infection in whom abdominal pain is accompanied by nausea, vomiting, and constipation. Changes in size and shape of the uterus, which then exerts tension on intraperitoneal adhesive bands, or kinking and constriction of adherent bowel are the usual causes. Volvulus accounts for 15 to 25% of all cases of intestinal obstruction.

Early in pregnancy, valuable time may be lost if the symptoms are regarded as physiologic nausea and vomiting, but examination of the patient should clarify this problem, as pain, tenderness, and distension are not characteristic of any physiologic process. *Vomiting that makes its first appearance after the first trimester must be considered to be caused by some condition other than pregnancy itself.* During late pregnancy, recurrent colicky pains must be differentiated from labor.

Decompression and correction of blood volume deficits with fluid, electrolytes, and plasma as indicated are essential first steps in management, but the necessary surgery should be performed as soon as possible thereafter. Operation should be aimed at removing the cause of obstruction without disturbing the pregnancy, even though labor ensues within a few hours; however, if exposure cannot be otherwise obtained, the uterus must be emptied irrespective of the gestation period.

RECTAL OPERATIONS

Hemorrhoids. Because of pressure from the enlarging uterus, the effect of pregnancy hormones, and the predisposition to constipation during pregnancy, the hemorrhoidal veins are frequently dilated. Medical treatment is preferable during the prenatal and puerperal periods, except for the acutely painful thrombotic hemorrhoid, which can be incised and the clot evacuated with local anesthesia. Hemorrhoidectomy is indicated only in the rare instance in which bleeding is persistent and depleting despite conservative therapy.

GALLBLADDER DISEASE

Physiologic changes during pregnancy alter gallbladder function. Real-time ultrasonographic studies reveal that after the first trimester the gallbladder volume, during fasting and after contraction, is twice that of nonpregnant control subjects. Delayed emptying time and incomplete evacuation permits the retention of cholesterol crystals. This may account for the increased incidence of cholelithiasis in parous women. Similar changes do not occur in women who are using oral contraceptives.

Symptoms usually appear in the latter half of pregnancy during the period corresponding to physiologic or gestational biliary stasis, but they may be encountered at any stage. In early pregnancy, pain and jaundice, if present, serve to differentiate cholecystitis and cholelithiasis from simple nausea and vomiting. In late pregnancy, gallbladder disease must be differentiated from severe preeclampsia, in which vomiting, upper abdominal pain, tenderness over the liver, and occasionally jaundice may be present. Gallstones can be demonstrated by ultrasonographic examination.

Medical management is preferred during pregnancy, and, in most cases, regulation of the diet and antispasmodic drugs provide adequate control. Operation should be performed if medical treatment fails or in patients with impacted common-duct stone or empyema.

HERNIA

Hernias may appear or increase in size during pregnancy. Inherently weak fascial structures are further weakened by the pressure of the enlarging uterus and by the effects of pregnancy hormones.

Inguinal or *femoral hernias* rarely give rise to serious complications. The enlarging uterus pushes the bowel upward and tends to occlude the defect.

Umbilical hernias are most common. If the ring is small, adherent omentum may fill the sac. Tension often produces pain, but obstruction is unusual. Large umbilical defects and ventral hernias are more likely to contain bowel, but these can be readily reduced. During labor the use of an abdominal support adds to the patient's comfort and prevents the uterus from protruding through a large ventral defect. Except in the rare instance in which strangulation occurs, herniorrhaphy should be delayed until after delivery.

PREGNANCY AFTER GI BYPASS

Following jejunoileal bypass, patients lose weight acutely and then either maintain a new lower weight or regain a small increment of the initial loss. Late complications of the procedure include diarrhea, diminished levels of folate or B_{12}, nephrolithiasis, cholelithiasis, and chronic liver dysfunction. Detailed studies of protein and amino acid metabolism in four women suggested little change from normal pregnancy. However, altered amino acid profiles were noted in one pregnancy patient still experiencing weight loss. Another report contrasted pregnancy outcome in women after bypass surgery with that experienced by morbidly obese women. The incidence of hypertension and babies who were large for gestational age was lower in the operated patients. Although there were no apparent adverse effects of the surgery, evaluation of glucose tolerance, liver function, and the levels of B_{12} and folate during early pregnancy is prudent.

SUGGESTED READING

Ahtone J and Maynard JE: Laboratory diagnosis of hepatitis B, JAMA 249:2067, 1983.

Arevalo JA and Washington AE: Cost-effectiveness of prenatal screening and immunization for hepatitis B virus, JAMA 259:365, 1988.

Braverman DZ, Johnson ML, and Kern F Jr: Effects of pregnancy and contraceptive steroids on gallbladder function, N Engl J Med 301:362, 1980.

Cordero JF, Oakley GP, Greenberg F, and others: Is bendectin a teratogen? JAMA 245:2307, 1981.

Cunningham FG and McCubbin JH: Appendicitis complicating pregnancy, Obstet Gynecol 45:415, 1975.

Donaldson RM Jr: Management of medical problems in pregnancy: inflammatory bowel disease, N Engl J Med 312:1616, 1985.

Douvas SG, Meeks GR, Phillips O, Morrison JC, and Walker LH: Liver disease in pregnancy, Obstet Gynecol Surv 38:531, 1983.

Fairweather DVI: Nausea and vomiting in pregnancy, Am J Obstet Gynecol 102:135, 1968.

Fisk NM and Storey GN: Fetal outcome in obstetric cholestasis, Br J Obstet Gynaecol 95:1137, 1988.

Frezza M, Pozzato G, Chiesa L, Stramentinoli G, and di Padova C: Reversal of intrahepatic cholestasis of pregnancy in women after high-dose S-adenosyl-L-methionine administration, Hepatology 4:274, 1984.

Goodacre RL, Hunter DJ, Millward S, Pirani M, and Riddle RH: The diagnosis of acute fatty liver of pregnancy by computed tomography, J Clin Gastroenterol 10:680, 1988.

Heikkinen J, Mäentausta O, Ylöstalo P, and Jänne O: Changes in serum bile acid concentrations during normal pregnancy, in patients with intrahepatic cholestasis of pregnancy, and in pregnant women with itching, Br J Obstet Gynaecol 88:240, 1981.

Johnston WG and Baskett MB: Obstetric cholestasis, Am J Obstet Gynecol 133:299, 1979.

Jonas MM, Schiff ER, O'Sullivan MJ, de Medina M, Reddy KR, Jeffers LJ, Fayne T, Roach KC, and Steele BW: Failure of Centers for Disease Control criteria to identify hepatitis B infection in a large municipal obstetrical population, Ann Intern Med 107:335, 1987.

Kaplan MM: Acute fatty liver in pregnancy, N Engl J Med 313:367, 1985.

Kauppila A, Huhtaniemi I, and Ylikorkala O: Raised serum human chorionic gonadotropin concentrations in hyperemesis gravidarum, Br Med J 1:1670, 1979.

Lind JF, Smith AM, McIver DK, Coopland AT, and Crispin JS: Heartburn in pregnancy: a manometric study, Can Med Assoc J 98:571, 1968.

Lunzer M, Barnes P, Byth H, O'Halloran M: Serum bile acid concentrations during pregnancy and their relationship to obstetric cholestasis, Gastroenterology 91(4):825, 1986.

Mabie WC, Dacus JV, Sibai BM, Morretti ML, and Gold RE: Computed tomography in acute fatty liver of pregnancy, Am J Obstet Gynecol 158(1):142, 1988.

Mixson JT and Woloshin HJ: Hiatus hernia in pregnancy, Obstet Gynecol 8:249, 1956.

Mogadam M, Dobbins WO III, Korelitz BI, and Ahmed SW: Pregnancy in inflammatory bowel disease: effect of sulfasalazine and corticosteroids on fetal outcome, Gastroenterology 80:72, 1981.

Nielsen OH, Andreasson B, Bondesen S, and Jarnum S: Pregnancy in ulcerative colitis, Scand J Gastroenterol 18:735, 1983.

Pesce AF, Crewe EB, and Cunningham AL: Should all pregnant women be screened for hepatitis B surface antigen? Med J Aust 150:19, 1989.

Porter RJ and Stirrat GM: The effects of inflammatory bowel disease on pregnancy: a case-controlled retrospective analysis, Br J Obstet Gynaecol 93:1124, 1989.

Purdie JM and Walters BN: Acute fatty liver of pregnancy: clinical features and diagnosis, Aust NZ J Obstet Gynaecol 28:62, 1988.

Richards DS, Miller DK, and Goodman GN: Pregnancy after gastric bypass for morbid obesity, J Reprod Med 32:172, 1987.

Riely CA, Latham PS, Romero R, and Duffy TP: Acute fatty liver of pregnancy. A reassessment based on observations in nine patients, Ann Intern Med 106:703, 1987.

Sorokin JJ and Levine SM: Pregnancy and inflammatory bowel disease: a review of the literature, Obstet Gynecol 62:247, 1983.

Soules MR, Hughes CL Jr, Garcia JA, Livingood CH, Prystowski MR, and Alexander E 3rd: Nausea and vomiting of pregnancy. Role of human chorionic gonadotropin and 17-hydroxy progesterone, Obstet Gynecol 55:696, 1980.

Stevens CE, Taylor PE, Tong MJ, and others: Yeast-recombinant hepatitis B vaccine. Efficacy with hepatitis B immune globulin in prevention of perinatal hepatitis B virus transmission, JAMA 257:2612, 1985.

Wilkinson EJ: Acute pancreatitis in pregnancy: a review of 98 cases and a report of 8 new cases, Obstet Gynecol Surv 28:281, 1973.

Wong VCW, Lee AKY, and Ip HMH: Transmission of hepatitis B antigens from symptom-free mothers to the fetus and infants, Br J Obstet Gynaecol 87:958, 1980.

Woods JR, Dandavino A, Brinkman CR, and Moore JG: Influence of jejunoileal bypass on protein metabolism during pregnancy, Am J Obstet Gynecol 130(1):9, 1978.

24

J. Robert Willson

Genitourinary tract disorders during pregnancy

Objectives

RATIONALE: Uterine and ovarian tumors and congenital anomalies of the reproductive organs can be responsible for infertility, early abortion, premature labor, and complications during labor. There are profound structural and functional changes in the urinary tract during pregnancy that may be interpreted as abnormal by physicians who are not aware of them. In addition, urinary infections are common and, if not treated properly, can result in permanent impairment.

The student should be able to:

A. Describe how ovarian and uterine tumors can complicate pregnancy and interfere with normal delivery.

B. Describe the common congenital anomalies of the uterus and how they may complicate pregnancy.

C. Outline structural changes in the kidney, ureters, and bladder during pregnancy.

D. Define changes in renal function during normal pregnancy and how they can affect tests for renal function.

E. Describe the background for urinary infections during pregnancy, appropriate treatment, and the long-range effects of inadequate treatment.

GENITAL TRACT

Pathologic conditions originating in the reproductive organs may complicate the course of pregnancy, labor, and delivery. Noninfectious conditions include (1) neoplasms, (2) uterine malpositions, and (3) congenital malformations of the uterus and vagina. Careful prepregnancy and early prenatal pelvic examination offers the best opportunity to diagnose genital tract disturbances and makes timely planning for their management possible.

Neoplastic growths

Various benign neoplasms involving the reproductive organs and occasional malignant growths are found in gravid women.

Cervical polyps. Cervical polyps tend to enlarge during pregnancy because of edema and increased vascularity. Most produce no symptoms and do not interfere with delivery. Those that are friable may bleed, particularly after intercourse. It usually is not necessary to remove polyps unless they are bleeding. Polypectomy during pregnancy may precipitate brisk local bleeding but will not induce abortion.

Cervical carcinoma. Screening cervical cytologic analysis is an essential part of the first prenatal examination. All suspicious or positive smears found during pregnancy require investigation. Colposcopic examination is a valuable aid in delineating abnormalities of visible areas of the cervix and vagina. The diagnosis and management of in situ and invasive carcinoma of the cervix complicating pregnancy are discussed in Chapter 44.

Uterine fibromyomas. The coexistence of uterine fibromyomas and pregnancy is relatively common. Small tumors are of little consequence unless their location is submucous, in which case the abortion rate is almost doubled. Although tumors of any size may produce symptoms of pain or pressure, surgical intervention is rarely necessary during pregnancy. Complications are principally related to the size and location of the tumors, to degenerative changes in the fibroid, or to torsion of a pedunculated tumor.

DIAGNOSIS. The main problem in diagnosis is the recognition of the existence of pregnancy in a fibroid uterus (Fig. 24-1). This is particularly difficult when implantation bleeding or threatened abortion complicates the early course. An accurate menstrual history is an important early guide. Delayed or abnormal bleeding, symptoms of early pregnancy, softening of the cervix, or recent increase in size of a fibroid uterus should suggest the possibility of pregnancy in every case. A pregnancy test or sonography should be done before an ill-advised laparotomy is performed.

COMPLICATIONS. Degenerative changes are likely to occur during pregnancy, the hemorrhagic variety *(red degeneration)* being the most common. Pain, local tenderness, and slight elevation of temperature are the usual symptoms. The pathologic process is ordinarily limited to the substance of the fibroid proper and tends to subside spontaneously in a few days. Hence conservative treatment with bed rest, local application of heat, and mild analgesics will control the symptoms in most instances.

Myomectomy is rarely necessary and is frequently followed by abortion if the uterine wall is incised. Occasionally a hysterectomy will be necessary to control bleeding. An exception is a *pedunculated subserous tumor,* which may twist and become necrotic as the uterus enlarges and rises out of the pelvis. If torsion occurs, laparotomy is imperative before gangrenous

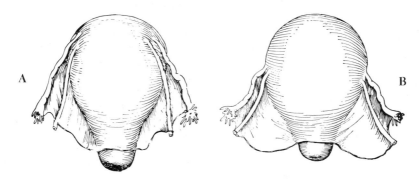

Fig. 24-1 Relationship of insertions of round ligaments and tubes to fundus gravid uterus (**A**) and nongravid uterus (**B**), with symmetric enlargement caused by fundal fibroid.

changes and peritonitis develop. Fortunately, this type of tumor can usually be removed with impunity if wedge incision through the pedicle and imbrication of the cut edges can be accomplished without invading the myometrium.

The major complications resulting from fibroids arise during labor and delivery: (1) obstruction of the birth canal, (2) an increased incidence of dysfunctional labor, (3) fetal malpositions, (4) faulty placental separation, and (5) hemorrhage following delivery.

Tumors blocking the inlet may make cesarean section necessary. Those situated low in the anterior wall are usually pulled up out of the pelvis as the lower uterine segment lengthens, but if the tumor is situated posteriorly in the hollow of the sacrum, elevation may be prevented by the promontory of the sacrum. Vaginal examination should be performed early in labor before deciding on the route of delivery. If the birth canal is not obstructed and the fetal position does not preclude vaginal delivery, a trial of labor should be given. Occasionally, the presence of fibroids alters uterine contractility and induces dysfunctional labor or hemorrhage following delivery. In rare instances the placenta is attached over a submucous or deep intramural fibroid, which may interfere with the normal process of separation and expulsion.

If cesarean section is necessary because of pelvic obstruction or abnormal labor, hysterectomy may or may not be indicated, but myomectomy should generally not be done. Except in the instance of the removal of a pedunculated tumor, cesarean section followed by myomectomy is attended by higher mortality and morbidity than cesarean section alone or cesarean section followed by hysterectomy.

During the puerperium the blood supply to uterine myomas may be reduced suddenly. Red degeneration is more common in the period following than at any other time. Laparotomy is indicated if symptoms of degeneration develop and persist during the stage of uterine involution.

Ovarian neoplasms. Ovarian neoplasms occur once in every 500 to 1000 pregnancies. Their existence may be unsuspected before the prenatal examination, at which time the finding of an ovarian enlargement may present considerable diagnostic and therapeutic difficulties.

DIAGNOSIS. The ovary containing the corpus luteum may be enlarged during the first trimester, but on reexamination at 2- or 3-week intervals it becomes progressively smaller after the eighth to tenth week of pregnancy. *True ovarian neoplasms* are usually larger than 5 cm in diameter and do not decrease in size on repeated examinations. *Theca-lutein cysts* and *leuteomas* develop during pregnancy in response to pregnancy hormones. They regress following delivery and need no treatment unless they undergo torsion (Chapter 46).

Discovery of an adnexal mass is much easier if the first prenatal pelvic examination is performed in the first trimester. As pregnancy advances, an ovarian cyst is displaced by the enlarged uterus. If it is displaced laterally or is trapped in the cul-de-sac, it is still palpable by bimanual examination, but frequently the cyst is carried upward above the uterus. In this case it is felt only by abdominal examination. In most instances the diagnosis can be made clinically, and the treatment is operative. Sonography may be helpful.

COMPLICATIONS AND MANAGEMENT. Ovarian tumors in pregnant women cannot be viewed with complacency because a small percentage of them are malignant. Small cysts found early in pregnancy should be reevaluated at 2- or 3-week intervals. Those larger than 5 cm that do not regress, those that increase in size, and all solid ovarian tumors require laparotomy. The most favorable time in pregnancy for their removal is during the early weeks of the second trimester for the following reasons: (1) nausea and vomiting of pregnancy are less likely to complicate the postoperative course, (2) the uterine size does not interfere with whatever surgery is necessary, (3) a corpus luteum cyst will have shown regression, and (4) placental hormone production is adequate to support the pregnancy. How long the corpus luteum is essential for maintenance of the pregnancy is debatable. There have been numerous instances of its removal in early pregnancy without abortion ensuing.

Immediate removal of the cyst is necessary, regardless of the stage of pregnancy if symptoms of torsion or hemorrhage arise or if rapid growth of the mass is detected. If the neoplasm is diagnosed late in pregnancy and the birth canal is not obstructed, vaginal delivery is preferable, but cystoophorectomy should be carried out in the immediate period following delivery. Torsion of the elongated pedicle is common as the uterine size decreases. If the cyst obstructs the pelvis (Fig. 24-2) it or

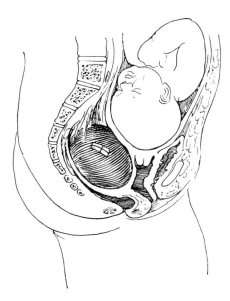

Fig. 24-2 Obstruction of birth canal by ovarian cyst.

the uterus may rupture during labor. No attempt should be made to evacuate the cyst by cul-de-sac aspiration or drainage, as leakage into the periotoneal cavity may result in widespread peritonitis, shock, or dissemination of malignant cells. Cesarean section and cystectomy are preferable. Because ovarian lesions are frequently bilateral, biopsy of the opposite ovary is indicated in every case in which it appears abnormal.

MALPOSITIONS OF THE UTERUS

Anterior displacement. Early in pregnancy the uterus is anteflexed, but it straightens as the uterus rises from the pelvis and meets the resistance of the anterior abdominal wall. Significant anterior displacement occurs during the last few weeks of pregnancy if the rectus abdominis muscles are widely separated or extremely lax. The uterus falls directly forward, producing sharp angulation at the cervicouterine junction.

Apart from the patient's discomfort, effects of anterior angulation on the pregnancy are minimal until labor begins. Dystocia is common if the position is uncorrected, as the force of uterine contractions is misdirected, driving the presenting part toward the sacrum rather than into the pelvis. In addition, the anterior portion of the cervix is compressed; hence retraction and dilation may be impaired. These difficulties can be overcome by application of a good support during pregnancy and a firm abdominal binder during labor.

Retrodisplacement. Some degree of uterine retroversion or retroflexion is observed in at least 30% of normal women. Ordinarily, fertility is not affected if the retroversion is uncomplicated. Spontaneous correction is the rule as the uterus gradually enlarges and rises out of the pelvis. This is true even in instances in which posterior adhesions resulting from previous infection or endometriosis are present. Adhesions of this type usually stretch or undergo dissolution, permitting spontaneous restitution by the twelfth week of pregnancy. Once the fundus rises above the sacral promontory, there is no danger of recurrence.

Occasionally, the retrodisplaced uterus fails to rise out of the pelvis and becomes impinged beneath the sacral promontory as it grows. Abortion occurs if the uterine circulation is significantly reduced by compression. Pressure symptoms may develop acutely if the condition is uncorrected by the thirteenth or fourteenth week, and the pregnant uterus becomes incarcerated in the pelvis. The rectum is compressed posteriorly, whereas the cervix is pulled sharply forward, exerting pressure against the urethra and vesicle neck. The patient may have difficulty urinating and may even develop urinary retention.

Manual replacement is indicated early in pregnancy if symptoms arise or after the twelfth week if spontaneous correction has not taken place. This is more easily accomplished with the patient in the knee-chest position. A pessary should then be inserted to maintain the correction. This can be removed by the sixteenth week. Anesthesia may be necessary to dislodge and elevate the uterus, but laparotomy is seldom indicated.

Prolapse. Descensus of the gravid uterus may be present before conception or may develop after pregnancy is established. Spontaneous correction will sometimes occur at about the sixteenth week when the uterus becomes too large to enter the pelvis, but mechanical replacement and the insertion of a pessary will provide earlier relief and prevent progressive elongation, edema, and congestion of the cervix. If the enlarging prolapsed uterus becomes incarcerated in the pelvis, abortion is likely to occur. Obviously, ulceration and infection increase the hazard of delivery, but, if treatment has been instituted beforehand, labor and delivery should be relatively uncomplicated.

CONGENITAL ANOMALIES

The müllerian ducts make their first appearance by the sixth week of embryonic life. Growth of the paired ducts and fusion of their lower portions forming the uterus and vagina should be complete by the sixteenth week. Failure of development on the one hand or failure of fusion on the other will result in absence or reduplication of related structures. Because of the close embryonic association, anomalies of the genital tract are frequently accompanied by malformations of the urinary apparatus. For example, when a double uterus is observed, absence of one kidney is common. Minor deviations may have no effect whatever on reproductive function, and, as a consequence, many remain undetected. On the contrary, the patient with pronounced uterine malformation is subject to many complications of pregnancy, labor, and delivery and consequently suffers a higher fetal loss. Early recognition, regardless of the gradation of the abnormality, is the best preventive measure.

Types. Various types of uterine malformations are demonstrated in Fig. 24-3.

Early complications. Genital malformations ordinarily do not reduce fertility. Although many pregnancies continue uneventfully, spontaneous abortions and premature labors are significantly increased. These accidents occur because the deformed uterus is less likely to provide a normal implantation site or to supply adequate nutrition for the early conceptus. In addition, the influence of underdeveloped uterine musculature may become apparent by lack of distensibility or accommodation, with premature contractions and early rupture of the membranes, or by ineffectual contractions after labor begins in women approaching term.

Pregnancy in one side of a double uterus is frequently associated with vaginal bleeding during the first trimester (Fig. 24-4). This bleeding can be associated with either a threatened abortion or with the casting off of decidua from the nonpregnant side. Recognition is important to avoid unnecessary medical treatment or surgical interference.

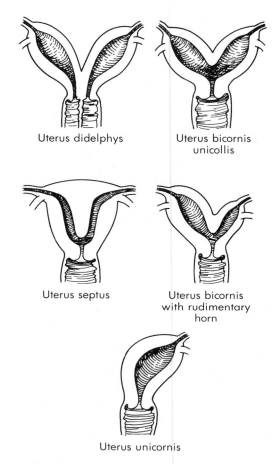

Uterus didelphys

Uterus bicornis unicollis

Uterus septus

Uterus bicornis with rudimentary horn

Uterus unicornis

Fig. 24-3 Different forms of anomalous uteri.

Late complications. Vaginal delivery can often be accomplished with little or no difficulty, and the opportunity should be afforded as long as conditions during labor remain satisfactory. Nevertheless, close observation is necessary because *malpositions,* particularly transverse lies, and *uterine inertia* are not uncommon complications. Occasionally, the birth canal becomes obstructed by the nonpregnant portion of a double uterus, and abdominal delivery is necessary. *Obstructed delivery* caused by vaginal septa requires nothing more than local excision. The third stage of labor is often complicated by *retained placenta* requiring manual removal.

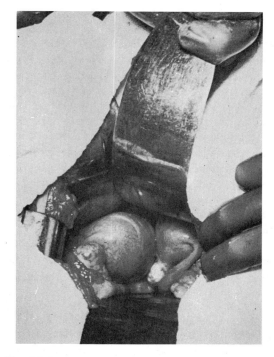

Fig. 24-4 Double uterus showing pregnancy in right uterus.

Diagnosis and management. Early diagnosis is difficult at best and becomes more so if the first prenatal examination is done after the fourteenth week of gestation. Discovery of a vaginal septum should arouse suspicion of other genital and urinary tract anomalies. Intravenous pyelography is indicated, except during pregnancy, whenever a malformation of the reproductive tract is discovered. Patients in whom preconception examination is suggestive and those with histories of repeated unexplained abortions, premature labors, or fetal deaths deserve further study by hysterosalpingography before another pregnancy is attempted.

Vaginal delivery can be expected if the fetal position is normal, if there is no obstruction from an accessory organ, and if the mechanism of labor is not faulty. Division of a vaginal septum is necessary only if descent of the presenting part is delayed. Manual removal of the placenta is frequently necessary, and as a result of defective musculature, poor uterine contractions after the third stage increase the likelihood of hemorrhage following delivery.

Delivery by cesarean section because of congenital malformations is necessary when vaginal delivery is impossible. Malformations of the uterus do not provide an indication for therapeutic abortions or sterilization.

A unification operation is highly effective in the treatment of double uterus, provided no other cause for pregnancy losses can be found. If these factors are normal, the occurrence of two or more consecutive abortions or pregnancy failures is ample indication for surgery.

Pregnancy in the rudimentary horn of uterus didelphys presents a rare but urgent problem in which early diagnosis is of utmost importance (Fig. 24-5). This condition differs from other uterine malformations in that the rudimentary horn may have an inadequate opening into the more developed uterine cavity. The clinical course resembles that of ectopic pregnancy except that the musculature, although defective, may permit a more advanced gestation than implantation in the fallopian tube. As a consequence, rupture may occur somewhat later and incite more profuse intraabdominal hemorrhage and shock.

Differential diagnosis usually rests between uterine myoma, ovarian cyst, and ectopic pregnancy. Treatment is surgical with complete removal of the rudimentary horn.

URINARY TRACT DISORDERS

The structure and function of the urinary organs are altered considerably during pregnancy, but unless the tissues are seriously damaged by infection or direct injury, they return to normal during the puerperium. Unless physicians are completely familiar with the changes that occur during normal pregnancy, they will be unable to assess the risks of pregnancy in women with chronic renal disease, and they may interpret normal physiologic alterations as abnormalities. These normal changes, which include pyeloureteral dilation and delayed urine transfer from kidney to bladder; increased glomerular filtration rate, renal plasma

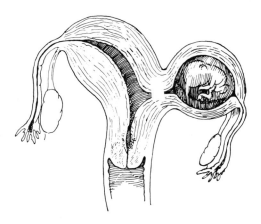

Fig. 24-5 Pregnancy in rudimentary horn.

flow, and filtration fraction; and increased clearance of endogenous creatinine are discussed in detail in Chapter 19.

The tests that are most helpful in evaluating renal function during pregnancy include *24-hour endogenous creatinine clearance* or *inulin clearance,* in which urinary excretion of insulin is measured while a constant serum level is maintained by continuous intravenous infusion. Clearance tests are much more informative than measurements of serum creatinine or urea. The blood levels of these substances may remain within normal ranges until clearances are considerably depressed. Because of the sustained increase in glomerular filtration, *the upper limit of serum creatinine is 0.5 mg/dl and that of urea 15 mg/dl.*

When performing 2- or 3-hour clearance studies, (1) the urine volume must be at least 2 ml/min, (2) the bladder must be emptied completely by catheter at the end of each accurately timed collection period, and (3) the patient must be in left lateral recumbent position, rather than supine. Although less accurate than well-controlled inulin clearance, *24-hour endogenous creatinine clearance* is adequate for clinical use.

The normal kidney does not permit the passage of more than *500 mg of protein* during a 24-hour period.

Concentration tests are unreliable during pregnancy because, in contrast to nonpregnant women, the volume of extravascular fluid is expanded during the day and the excess fluid is returned to the bloodstream and excreted during the night, when the woman is in a horizontal position. This accounts for both nocturia and the low specific gravity of early morning urine specimens.

Cystoscopy can be performed throughout pregnancy, but during the last 4 to 6 weeks it may be relatively uninformative. At this period of gestation, the bladder is pulled upward, and the presenting part descends, making insertion of the instrument and inspection of the interior of the bladder difficult.

Urinary tract x-ray film studies should rarely be performed because of possible ill effects on the fetus. Heavy exposure during the first few weeks may disturb embryonic development. If an x-ray film study is essential, it should be performed with the smallest amount of radiation that will provide the information needed and, if possible, delayed until after the twentieth gestational week. Urography can usually be delayed until after delivery.

INFECTION

Urinary tract infections occur frequently during pregnancy and after delivery, but almost all of them can be prevented. From 2% to 10% of all pregnant women have a significant but *asymptomatic bacteriuria* (more than 100,000 colonies/ml of a single organism in a catheterized or clean, voided urine specimen). A positive diagnosis can be made if the same organism is grown on repeat culture, even though the colony count is less than 100,000/ml. The diagnosis is in doubt if repeat culture is negative or if different bacteria are identified.

The probability that a woman will develop bacteriuria is determined by her parity, race, and socioeconomic status. The lowest incidence is in white, primigravid, private patients, and the highest is in black multiparas with sickle-cell trait.

The bacteria are usually present during the first

trimester, and there usually is no accompanying pyuria. The reason for the bacteriuria is not always obvious, but chronic pyelonephritis or lower tract infections can be demonstrated in some women, particularly those who have had repeated symptomatic urinary tract infections. *Escherichia coli* and *Enterobacter* species are the responsible organisms in most acute infections, but others may be present in women with chronic or recurring infections.

Because asymptomatic bacteriuria is so important in the genesis of symptomatic urinary tract infections during pregnancy or after delivery, it is advisable to screen all obstetric patients for the presence of bacteria. This is particularly important in patient populations in which urinary tract infections occur frequently.

An attempt should be made to eradicate asymptomatic bacteriuria because about 30% of those who are not treated will develop symptomatic infections later in pregnancy or after delivery. Few of those in whom the bacteriuria is treated successfully will develop clinically evident urinary tract infections. Most can be treated effectively with 100 mg nitrofurantoin (Macrodantin) daily, 1 g sulfisoxazole (Gantrisin) four times daily, or 1 g ampicillin daily for 10 days.

Repeat urine cultures should be obtained during pregnancy and after delivery in all women who have had either asymptomatic bacteriuria or symptomatic infections during pregnancy.

Urologic study, including pyelograms, is indicated for women who have had repeated infections or those in whom bacteriuria persists after delivery.

URETHROCYSTITIS

Acute lower urinary tract infections occur in 1 to 2% of women during pregnancy and more often after delivery. About one third of those who develop acute infections have had asymptomatic bacteriuria; detection and treatment of the latter would prevent most overt infections.

The principal symptoms are frequency, dysuria, and suprapubic pain and tenderness. The temperature may be normal. Many pus cells, red blood cells, and bacteria can be seen in the urine.

Sulfisoxazole, 1 g four times daily, nitrofurantoin, 100 mg once a day, or ampicillin, 500 mg every 6 hours, will eradicate most infections. Treatment should usually be continued for 10 days, although single-dose therapy with nitrofurantoin, 200 mg, sulfisoxazole, 2 grams, or ampicillin, 2 grams, with probenecid will eradicate bacteria in about 75% of patients. In addition to antibiotics, patients who have had urinary tract infections should be advised to void at least every 2 hours. Voluntary retention of urine and overdistension of the bladder predisposes to infection.

Pyelonephritis

Infection of the upper urinary tract may develop initially during pregnancy, or women with chronic pyelonephritis may conceive.

Acute pyelonephritis. Acute upper urinary tract infections usually develop late in the second trimester, early in the third, or after delivery. They occur in from 1% to 3% of all pregnant women, and even though they are treated intensively, they may recur in subsequent pregnancies. Approximately two thirds occur in women who have asymptomatic bacteriuria.

The usual symptoms are chills, fever, flank pain, dysuria, and nausea and vomiting. The temperature may swing from high levels of 40° to 41° C (104° to 106° F) to as low as 34° to 36° C (93° to 97° F). Patients with acute pyelonephritis look ill and usually are dehydrated. Palpation of the kidney area produces severe pain, and there may be tenderness along the course of the ureter and over the bladder. The right kidney is most often involved, but the infection frequently occurs bilaterally.

The diagnosis is confirmed by examination of a catheterized or clean, voided specimen of urine, which will contain many pus cells, red blood cells, and bacteria. At the peak of the infection, the white blood cell count may be as high as 20,000 to 30,000.

The *differential diagnosis* can be difficult, particularly in the recently delivered patient. The pain may begin in the right lower quadrant, and, because nausea and vomiting are frequently encountered in association with urinary tract infections, appendicitis may be suspected. Puerperal infection must also be ruled out as a cause in patients who have the symptoms following delivery.

TREATMENT. Undelivered patients with acute pyelonephritis are best treated in the hospital with parenteral antibiotics until the infection is brought under control. Most will respond to ampicillin given intravenously in doses of 1 g every 6 hours for from 48 to 72 hours, after which it can be given orally. The temperature usually returns to normal within 3 to 5 days, but the medication should be continued for at least 14 days. If there is no response, another antibiotic, as determined by sensitivity studies, should be ordered. A subsequent urine culture should be taken after the course of treatment is completed.

The patient should be encouraged to ingest at least 3000 ml of fluids daily unless she is vomiting, in which case an equivalent amount of 5% dextrose should be given intravenously. Urinary output should be checked carefully, because renal function is significantly reduced during the acute phase of the infection. Although septic shock is uncommon, it may develop during the first few days of the infection.

Recurrences usually mean that treatment has been discontinued before the infection is eradicated or that the fundamental cause of the infection is still present. If the infection recurs or if bacteriuria persists, an antibiotic or chemotherapeutic agent should be continued until after delivery.

It is seldom necessary to terminate pregnancy because of repeated episodes of pyelonephritis, but occasionally if the patient has several attacks in spite of adequate antibacterial treatment, the physician should consider the possibility of inducing labor as soon as it can be accomplished safely after the fetus has matured. This may prevent permanent damage to the kidney.

The urine should be examined for the presence of infection during the early puerperium and again after involution in all women who have had acute pyelonephritis during pregnancy. If the infection has been recurrent or if bacteriuria persists, pyelograms should be made 2 to 3 months after delivery in an attempt to demonstrate a lesion that could have caused the attacks or any damage that may have been produced by the infection.

Chronic pyelonephritis. If acute pyelonephritis is inadequately treated, the symptoms may subside, but the infection may never be completely eradicated. In time there may be enough tissue damage to impair kidney function and, occasionally, even to cause hypertension and renal insufficiency. However, at least half the women with chronic pyelonephritis have no history of antecedent urinary tract infections.

Chronic infection does not necessarily preclude pregnancy if kidney function is normal, but acute attacks are likely to occur. Women with chronic urinary tract infections can be treated prophylactically with small daily doses of medications throughout pregnancy to prevent acute recurrences. If renal function is impaired and the blood pressure is elevated, pregnancy may be contraindicated. The outcome depends on the ability of the kidney to respond to the demands of pregnancy.

Toxic effects of drugs

The physician must be aware that certain drugs used to treat urinary tract infections may cause undesirable reactions in either the mother or the fetus.

Tetracyclines. Several instances of acute toxic reactions and even death after the administration of tetracycline to pregnant women with pyelonephritis have been reported. In most of them, vomiting persisted, or it first appeared after treatment was started, and fatty metamorphosis of the liver, pancreatitis, azotemia, and jaundice developed. The toxicity may be a result of reduced renal function, allowing accumulation of high concentrations of tetracycline in the tissues. This can be prevented by using smaller doses and by stopping the medication if urinary output is reduced, if the blood urea nitrogen concentration increases progressively, or if there are other evidences of renal failure.

Tetracycline can also be deposited in the enamel of fetal teeth, giving them a permanent yellow, mottled, fluorescent appearance.

Sulfonamides. Sulfonamides enter the fetal circulation freely and are potentially dangerous if they accumulate in fetal tissues and are not eliminated promptly. Sulfonamides dissociate bilirubin from its binding to albumin, permitting bilirubin to circulate freely and to diffuse into fetal tissues. The most serious complication that may occur from high concentrations of unconjugated bilirubin is kernicterus, particularly in premature infants. This is not likely to occur while the fetus remains in the uterus, because the bilirubin is transferred across the placenta, but it is a problem in newborn infants.

Because of this possibility, only short-acting sulfonamides should be prescribed, and they should be used with caution in women who may deliver prematurely. They should not be used during labor.

Chloramphenicol. Chloramphenicol may depress maternal bone marrow; total white blood cell and differential counts should be obtained twice weekly in an attempt to detect the first evidence of depression. This drug probably does not harm the fetus in utero, but in large doses it causes the "gray syndrome" in newborn infants.

Nitrofurantoin. Nitrofurantoin may cause hemolysis of red blood cells and megaloblastic erythropoiesis in pregnant black women with glucose-6-phosphate dehydrogenase deficiency.

Renal tuberculosis

Tuberculosis of the kidney occurs rarely during pregnancy and may produce no symptoms unless the bladder is involved.

Antituberculosis drugs can be administered safely during pregnancy. Nephrectomy, when indicated, can be performed. It usually is not necessary to terminate pregnancy because of renal tuberculosis.

URINARY CALCULI

Calculi occur infrequently in pregnant women, the incidence of renal stones being about 0.04% and of ureteral stones about 0.08%, despite urinary stasis and infection, which occur regularly but transiently. Another factor is that calculous disease occurs most often in women older than 35 years of age, and most pregnancies occur in women younger than age 35.

Ureteral and renal calculi may produce fewer symptoms in pregnant than in nonpregnant women because of the decreased muscle tonus and dilation in the urinary tract. Small stones in the ureter may be passed spontaneously as the pregnancy changes develop.

Treatment depends on the size and position of the stones and the symptoms they cause. It may be necessary to remove obstructing calculi or those producing severe pain. It is rarely necessary to terminate pregnancy in women with stones.

HEMATURIA

Blood in the urine can come from a lesion at any level of the urinary tract. The possible causes of hematuria are severe infection, rupture of small varicosities of the bladder, calculi, acute glomerulonephritis, tuberculosis, tumors, and other rare lesions.

Although it is essential to attempt to determine the cause of hematuria, the usual urologic examination must be modified during pregnancy. Cystoscopy can be performed at any stage, but it is more difficult and less accurate during late pregnancy when the bladder is drawn upward and the presenting part is entering the pelvis. Usually x-ray film examination should be avoided; if it is essential, it should be modified to reduce the amount of radiation to the minimum necessary to make a diagnosis. The progression of ureteropelvic dilation can be monitored by ultrasound. In most instances, particularly when hematuria occurs late in pregnancy, complete examination can be deferred until after delivery.

NEPHRITIS
Acute glomerulonephritis

An initial attack of glomerulonephritis is uncommon in gravid women, but, when it occurs, the pregnancy adds a complicating factor. Urinary output is diminished or ceases completely; and the urine is smoky or bloody, is of high specific gravity, and contains large amounts of protein and many cellular casts. The blood pressure usually is elevated, there is generalized edema, and the patient feels and looks sick.

Spontaneous abortion, intrauterine fetal death, or premature delivery may occur during the acute phase. The place of therapeutic abortion is not clearly defined, but it is not often necessary, since the acute process usually subsides within 2 or 3 weeks.

Chronic glomerulonephritis

Fortunately, the combination of chronic glomerulonephritis and pregnancy is seldom encountered. The abnormal renal function and the accompanying changes in the cardiovascular system increase the hazards for both mother and baby considerably.

The prognosis depends in a large measure on whether the kidney is able to respond to the increasing demands as pregnancy advances. If the serum creatinine concentration is less than 1.5 mg/dl, the outlook is reasonably good, although in some women hypertension may increase and the placenta may separate prematurely. Conversely, when serum creatinine concentrations are above 1.6 mg/dl, the outlook for successful pregnancy is poor. Controlling hypertension may be difficult, and renal function may deteriorate rapidly. It often is necessary to terminate pregnancy prematurely.

If renal impairment is minimal and blood pressure is normal or only slightly elevated, pregnancy may be allowed to continue as long as the patient remains reasonably normal, but if the blood pressure rises progressively or if renal function diminishes as pregnancy advances, termination should be considered.

The *perinatal mortality* is much higher than that for normal pregnancy, the principal causes of death being abruptio placentae, growth retardation caused either by an unusually small placenta or extensive infarction—which is characteristic of hypertensive cardiovascular disease—and premature delivery. Because babies born of mothers with chronic glomerulonephritis are often smaller than the infants of normal women at a comparable stage of pregnancy, a relatively small uterus should not influence the physician to delay delivery if the vascular renal status is deteriorating. Unless the baby is delivered, it may die in utero.

Therapeutic termination of early pregnancy is advisable if renal function is significantly impaired. As the kidney lesions are irreparable, pregnancy will be no less hazardous in the future; consequently, sterilization should also be advised.

Abnormal menses and infertility, which occur frequently with chronic renal insufficiency, often are corrected by hemodialysis. Successful pregnancies have been reported in women who must rely on regular dialysis to survive, but as a general rule pregnancy should be prevented, and abortion should be made available to those who conceive.

CONGENITAL POLYCYSTIC KIDNEY DISEASE

Congenital polycystic kidneys are only rarely encountered in pregnant women. Landesman and Scherr reported that the diagnosis was made in 114 of 390,000 patients admitted to the New York Hospital. Only 28 were pregnant. The diagnosis is often overlooked in young women because clinical signs and symptoms usually do not appear until after the age period in which most women bear children.

Congenital polycystic kidney disease is an autosomal dominant trait, so 50% of the offspring of a parent with polycystic kidneys will inherit the gene. It is important that the diagnosis be made as early as possible so that young women with the disorder can consider the problems associated with childbearing. Milutinovic and colleagues, with the use of excretory urograms with nephrotomography and radionuclide imaging, diagnosed polycystic kidneys in about 50% of suspected cases in which the patient was older than 20 years (95% of those at risk) but in only 30% (60% of those at risk) between the ages of 15 and 19. Although the diagnosis should be made early, negative studies in young women may provide a false sense of security.

Unless renal function is depressed, women with polycystic kidneys usually do well during pregnancy. Blood pressure elevation alone does not contraindicate pregnancy, but if proteinuria is present and renal function is depressed, prompt termination usually is warranted.

SINGLE KIDNEY

The lack of a kidney is no contraindication to pregnancy if the function in the remaining one is normal. Renal function should be evaluated before pregnancy is contemplated, as soon as possible after conception, and periodically during pregnancy. Therapeutic abortion should be considered only if renal function is impaired, if there is a large calculus with infection, or if the patient has chronic pyelonephritis or repeated urinary tract infections that cannot be controlled.

KIDNEY TRANSPLANTS

A kidney transplant is not necessarily a contraindication to pregnancy if kidney function is normal, but the prognoses for both mother and infant must be guarded. The changes in renal function are like those that occur in normal women. As pregnancy advances, mothers with renal transplants are more prone to develop both bacterial and viral infections, particularly urinary tract infections, than are normal women because of the immunosuppressive drugs they must take. They also are likely to develop hypertension and reduced kidney function during late pregnancy. This may lead to kidney failure and eventually even death. Labor begins prematurely more often than in normal women, but the abortion rate is not increased significantly.

The disturbed menstrual function, which often occurs with chronic renal insufficiency, is usually corrected by kidney transplantation; hence women who were infertile before the operation are likely to conceive when normal menstrual function is resumed.

The prescription of a reliable contraceptive method is essential in the care of transplant patients. Pregnancy should be delayed until kidney function is normal and until the dosages of immunosuppressive drugs have been reduced to maintenance levels.

Women who are considering pregnancy after kidney transplantation, even when kidney function is normal, should be informed of the immediate hazards of pregnancy and of the long-term outlook. The life of a transplanted kidney is limited, so the mother may eventually need another operation or permanent dialysis. Her life expectancy also is limited, she may be chronically ill, and the chances of her leading a normal, healthy life until the child is grown are small.

Care during pregnancy is similar to that for normal women except that particular attention must be paid to monitoring kidney function and to detecting and treating asymptomatic bacteriuria and infections aggressively. Decreasing kidney function or the inability to eradicate infection are indications for termination. Sterilization following delivery should be considered even though kidney function has remained normal throughout pregnancy.

Women with transplanted kidneys can deliver normally unless the position of the kidney obstructs the pelvic inlet, in which event elective cesarean section is indicated.

SUGGESTED READING

Genital tract

Fenton AN and Singh BP: Pregnancy associated with congenital anomalies of the female reproductive tract, Am J Obstet Gynecol 63:744, 1952.

Golan A, Langer R, Bukovsky I, and Caspi E: Congenital anomalies of the Müllerian system, Fertil Steril 51:747, 1989.

Heinonen PK, Saarikoski S, and Pystynen P: Reproductive performance of women with uterine anomalies, Acta Obstet Gynecol Scand 61:157, 1982.

Jarco J: Malformations of the uterus, Am J Surg 71:106, 1946.

Rock JA and Schleff WD: The obstetric consequences of utero-vaginal anomalies, Fertil Steril 43:681, 1985.

Urinary tract

Baird D: Anatomy and physiology of the upper urinary tract in pregnancy: relation to pyelitis, J Obstet Gynecol Br Commonw 38:516, 1931.

Coe FL, Parks JH, and Lindheimer MD: Nephrolithiasis during pregnancy, N Engl J Med 298:324, 1978.

Davison JM: The kidney in pregnancy: a review, J R Soc Med 76:485, 1983.

Davison JM: The effect of pregnancy on kidney function in renal allograft recipients, Kidney Int 27:74, 1985.

Davison JM and Lindheimer MD: Pregnancy in renal transplant recipients, J Reprod Med 27:613, 1982.

Dunlop W: Serial changes in renal haemodynamics during normal human pregnancy, Br J Obstet Gynaecol 88:1, 1981.

Gabert HA, and Miller JM Jr: Renal disease in pregnancy, Obstet Gynecol Surv 40:449, 1985.

Gilstrap LG III, Cunningham FG, and Whalley PJ: Acute pyelonephritis in pregnancy: an anterospective study, Obstet Gynecol 57:409, 1981.

Harris RE: The significance of eradication of bacteriuria during pregnancy, Obstet Gynecol 53:71, 1979.

Harris RE, Gilstrap LC III and Pretty A: Single-dose antimicrobial therapy for asymptomatic bacteriuria during pregnancy, Obstet Gynecol 59:546, 1982.

Hou S: Pregnancy in women with chronic renal disease, N Engl J Med 312:836, 1985.

Kass EH: Bacteriuria and pyelonephritis of pregnancy, Arch Intern Med 105:194, 1960.

Kline AH, Blattner RJ, and Lunin M: Transplacental effect of tetracycline on teeth, JAMA 188:178, 1964.

Klein EA: Urologic problems of pregnancy, Obstet Gynecol Surv 39:605, 1984.

Kobayashi H and others: Successful pregnancy in a patient undergoing chronic hemodialysis, Obstet Gynecol 57:382, 1981.

Landesman R and Scherr L: Congenital polycystic kidney disease in pregnancy, Obstet Gynecol 8:673, 1956.

Milutinovic J, Fialkow PJ, Phillips LA, Agoda LY, Bryant JI, Denney JD, and Rudd TG: Autosomal dominant polycystic kidney disease: early diagnosis and data for genetic counseling, Lancet 1:1203, 1980.

Penn I, Makowski EL, and Harris P: Parenthood following renal transplant, Kidney Int 2:221, 1980.

Whalley PJ, Adams RH, and Combes B: Tetracycline toxicity in pregnancy, JAMA 189:357, 1964.

Whalley PJ and Cunningham FG: Short-term versus continous antimicrobial therapy for asymptomatic bacteriuria in pregnancy, Obstet Gynecol 49:262, 1977.

Whalley PJ, Martin FG, and Peters PG: Significance of asymptomatic bacteriuria detected during pregnancy, JAMA 193:879, 1965.

Whalley PJ, Martin FG, and Pritchard JA: Sickle cell trait and urinary tract infection during pregnancy, JAMA 189:903, 1964.

25

Russell K. Laros, Jr.

Disorders of the nervous system, the skin, and the bones and joints during pregnancy

Objectives

RATIONALE: Neurologic, skin, and orthopedic disorders may influence the course of pregnancy. Similarly, pregnancy may have an impact on the course of these disorders. An understanding of these relationships is necessary for optimal patient care.

The student should be able to:
A. Demonstrate a knowledge of the symptoms, physical findings and diagnostic methods.
B. Describe effects of the condition on pregnancy.
C. Outline effects of pregnancy on the condition.

With the exception of puerperal psychosis, disorders of the nervous system do not differ appreciably in pregnant and nonpregnant women from the standpoint of either their incidence or their prognosis. However, symptoms may be temporarily exaggerated when the mechanical and physiologic burdens of pregnancy are added to chronic disease of the nervous system. In general, skin diseases also affect gravid and nongravid women similarly. On the contrary, disturbances of the bones and joints are most frequently related to the physiologic changes of pregnancy that are responsible for separation and increased mobility especially affecting the pelvic joints.

DISORDERS OF THE NERVOUS SYSTEM
Seizure disorders

Among the various forms of epilepsy, only the idiopathic type poses a risk of *hereditary transmission,* which accounts for less than 2% of affected offspring.

Symptoms. Temporary effects of pregnancy are wholly unpredictable. In the majority of epileptic mothers, symptoms remain unchanged or become aggravated, but in some seizures are reduced throughout the prenatal period and return with their usual frequency after delivery. Rarely, grand mal attacks make their first appearance during pregnancy or in the puerperium and must be distinguished from eclampsia. Positive water balance associated with pregnancy can increase epileptic attacks, presumably as a result of cerebral edema.

Attacks during labor occur, but fortunately these are rare. Lactation does not increase convulsions, but nursing should be restricted or supervised to prevent injury to the baby if an attack occurs while it is at breast.

When a patient with epilepsy is contemplating pregnancy, the major consideration is continued control of seizures while minimizing teratogenesis for the fetus. In spite of multiple studies, a controversy continues with regard to the possible teratogenesis of many anticonvulsants. Phenytoin, phenobarbital, valproic acid, and trimethadone have all been cited as teratogens. The phenytoin syndrome with growth retardation, microcephaly, dysmorphic facies, and mental retardation is alleged to occur in 11% of fetuses exposed in utero. Valproic acid increases the incidence of neural tube defects, and trimethadone causes fetal malformations and mental retardation in a high percent of fetuses exposed.

When seizures first appear during pregnancy, careful evaluation including hematologic and metabolic screening studies, EEG, and a CT scan of the head are warranted. Prophylactic anticonvulsant therapy should be started if two or more seizures have occurred.

Treatment. The principle of therapy is to achieve optimal control by careful regulation of dosage. Trimethadone and valproic acid should be avoided. If the former has been used in early pregnancy, therapeutic abortion should be offered. If the latter has been used, screening for a neural tube defect is mandatory. Patients must be compliant in taking their medications, and blood levels should be monitored frequently. The agents most commonly used during pregnancy are carbamazepine, phenobarbital, primidone, ethosuximide, and clonazepam. Both phenobarbital and phenytoin can cause decreased levels of vitamin K in the newborn. This deficit should be dealt with by the use of an intramuscular injection of vitamin K_1 after delivery.

Status epilepticus. Repetitive seizures constitute a medical emergency. Slow intravenous injection of diazepam (Valium), 5 to 10 mg, and establishment of an airway are the first steps. Resuscitative measures may be necessary. In refractory cases intravenous diazepam may be repeated once in the first hour, and anticonvulsant therapy instituted with intravenous phenytoin given at the rate of 50 mg/min as a maximum for a total of 200 mg.

Sterilization should be considered for epileptic women who show progressive mental retardation and those with a history of status epilepticus.

Polyneuritis and polyradiculopathy (Guillain-Barré syndrome)

Polyneuritis as a result of dietary deficiencies has all but disappeared in the United States. It is occasionally found in connection with severe hyperemesis gravidarum. Deaths have occurred with polyneuritis as a result of cardiac or phrenic nerve involvement and respiratory failure.

Polyneuritis attributable to other causes such as diabetes, alcohol, drugs, and heavy metals must be differentiated from the foregoing, the cause removed, and substitution therapy instituted promptly.

Guillain-Barré syndrome, or polyradiculopathy, simulates poliomyelitis or polyneuritis with multiple peripheral and cranial nerve involvement, including bulbar paralysis, which is reported in one third of cases. The fetus in utero is not afflicted with the disorder per se but is at risk if maternal pulmonary support is inadequate. Diagnosis is made by examination of the cerebrospinal fluid in which there is a significant elevation of protein without pleocytosis. This is a temporary disorder, although remissions and exacerbations are known to occur. Recovery rate is high if appropriate supportive therapy is applied.

Myasthenia gravis

Myasthenia gravis is a neuromuscular disorder that is now recognized as an autoimmune disorder. An immunologic attack upon the acetylcholine receptors at the neuromuscular junction with resulting receptor loss is the basis of the symptoms. This loss, which produces interference or block of normal neuromuscular function, is responsible for the muscle weakness and fatigue characteristic of the disease.

Ptosis of the eyelids is usually an early symptom, with progressive weakness of skeletal muscles and difficulty in swallowing, in speaking, and in respiratory functions. The thymus gland may be enlarged, and thymomas have been found in 10% of cases. In these patients the disease is more serious, and the course more rapidly downhill. For this reason some authors advise that, in addition to anticholinesterase drugs, thymectomy is advisable early in the course of the disease, even before pregnancy is contemplated, because of its favorable effect on the overall course of the disease.

The clinical course of myasthenia is one of remissions and exacerbations. Although the effect of childbearing is not entirely predictable, in most instances the pregnancy is tolerated well, and normal vaginal delivery can be anticipated. The disease rarely provides an indication for abortion. The dosage of anticholinesterase medication frequently must be adjusted during pregnancy and the puerperium.

Ten to 20% of infants of mothers with this disease show evidence of neonatal myasthenia. Anticholinesterase drugs cross the placental barrier freely. The effects are usually transitory and tend to disappear within 2 to 4 weeks. Prompt treatment with neostigmine (Prostigmin) is essential for survival and should be continued for as long as muscle weakness persists. If there is doubt regarding the cause of respiratory difficulty in the newborn, parenteral injection of 0.05 ml edrophonium chloride (Tensilon) should be given. If the cause is transient myasthenia, improvement is evident immediately, and anticholinesterase drug therapy is required for at least a week or 10 days. Although the disease can be familial, congenital myasthenia gravis is exceedingly rare.

Multiple sclerosis

There is no evidence that exacerbations are increased or that the progress of multiple sclerosis is accelerated during pregnancy. The fetus is not affected.

Normal labor and delivery can usually be expected. Because this disease is progressive and ultimately incapacitating, childbearing should be limited.

Subarachnoid hemorrhage, cerebral aneurysm, and occlusive cerebral disorders

Subarachnoid hemorrhage is responsible for about 10% of maternal deaths. For women under 25 years of age, arteriovenous malformations are the most common cause of hemorrhage, whereas berry aneurysms are the common cause for bleeding in older women.

Diagnosis. The onset is generally sudden with severe headache, vomiting, paralysis, and eventually coma. The blood pressure may be elevated, but the character-istic findings of nuchal rigidity, increased intraspinal pressure, and grossly bloody spinal fluid differentiate this lesion from coma of intracerebral or metabolic origin. Cerebral arteriography and CT scanning are essential to clarify the diagnosis and guide therapy. The clinical course is determined by the size of the vessel involved and the extent of the hemorrhage. The mortality rate associated with spontaneous subarachnoid hemorrhage is high, amounting to almost 50%, whether the victim is pregnant or not. About half of fatalities occur within the first 24 hours.

Treatment. Initial treatment consists of bed rest, analgesia, and operative occlusion of the lesion if possible. Surgical treatment is aimed at preventing further bleeding. Although hypothermia and controlled hypotension have been used successfully during pregnancy, they should be avoided if possible. After successful surgery, patients can be allowed to proceed to labor and delivery without intervention. If the lesions are inoperable or incompletely ligated, elimination of the the Valsalva maneuver during the second stage of labor is mandatory. Whereas some authors have recommended delivery by elective cesarean section at 38 weeks of gestation, data supporting the necessity for this approach are lacking.

Nonhemorrhagic stroke. The occurrence of cerebral infarction and transient ischemic attacks is rare in young women but does increase about fivefold during pregnancy. The most frequent site of occlusion is the middle cerebral artery. Although atherosclerosis is the major cause of stroke in older patients, it is responsible for less than 25% of cases during pregnancy. Other causes such as mitral valve prolapse, atrial fibrillation, paradoxical embolism from leg vein thrombosis, and endocarditis should be sought.

Headache, seizures, and paralysis are the symptoms of vasoocclusive disease. The diagnosis is made with CT scanning and cerebral arteriography. Removal of the obstruction can be directly by surgery or angiographically. If the obstruction cannot be removed, anticoagulation or treatment with aspirin should be considered. Vaginal delivery unless obstetrically contraindicated is preferable to cesarean section.

Paraplegia-quadriplegia

Patients with spinal cord injuries are desirous of and able to successfully complete a pregnancy. If the patient has a cord transection above the T5-6 level, she is apt to develop a syndrome of autonomic hyperreflexia with excessive activity of viscus, including the uterus. The syndrome is characterized by headache, hypertension, reflex bradycardia, nasal congestion, and cutaneous vasodilation and piloerection above the level of the lesion and can be life-threatening during labor. The syndrome can be prevented by the use of lumbar epidural anesthesia. Additional complications include urinary tract infections, decubitus ulcers, anemia, and premature labor.

The uterus itself contracts normally during labor. Because patients with lesions above T10 will usually not feel their uterine contractions, the cervix should be examined at each visit after the twenty-fifth week. Also, the patient can be taught to monitor her uterine activity manually and by being cognizant of the symptoms of autonomic hyperreflexia. Delivery should be vaginal unless indicated by obstetric events. Most patients will not be able to push effectively, and the second stage must be terminated with forceps or vacuum.

Pseudotumor cerebri

This disorder, also referred to as *benign intracranial hypertension,* is characterized by papilledema, headache, and increased intracranial pressure. Cerebral edema is present, but there are no focal neurologic lesions. The CSF pressure is elevated, and, except for low protein levels, laboratory findings are normal. If pressure becomes high enough to cause loss of visual acuity, nausea and vomiting, and constant severe headache, lumbar puncture and removal of CSF fluid is necessary and may need to be repeated.

The cause is unknown but is presumed to be a hormone-related fluid retention process. Symptoms usually disappear after pregnancy although some loss of vision may persist. Recurrences in subsequent pregnancies are reported in about one third of cases.

Peripheral neuropathies

Neuritic disturbances of varying severity are observed during pregnancy. Manifestations range from sensory effects such as paresthesia and pain, which are common, to sensory and motor changes, which are rare.

Etiologic factors. Neuritis may be caused by:
1. Inadequate intake of vitamin B complex, which is responsible for most symptoms of numbness and tingling of the hands and feet and for the most severe form of polyneuritis

2. Mechanical factors, which are largely responsible for sciatic and traumatic neuritis

PARESTHESIAS. Paresthesias often persist throughout pregnancy despite therapy and disappear slowly thereafter.

Acrodysesthesia. Acrodysesthesia (brachialgia statica dysesthetica), or numbness, tingling, and stiffness of the upper extremities, may appear and persist during pregnancy. Symptoms are caused by stretching of or pressure on the brachial plexus when relaxation of the ligaments allows greater motion of the shoulder girdle in both forward and backward direction. Discomfort is greatest when steady traction is exerted, and for this reason the patient usually complains of numbness—sometimes almost complete anesthesia of the hands, particularly in the distribution of the ulnar nerve—on awakening from sleep. Relief can be obtained from this purely mechanical problem by supporting the shoulder in a favorable midposition by use of pillows at night and by assuming proper posture in the daytime. There is no permanent motor or sensory damage.

Carpal tunnel syndrome. Carpal tunnel syndrome is not an uncommon occurrence during pregnancy. Numbness, tingling, and sharp pain radiating up to the elbow region result from compression of the median nerve under the carpal ligament at the wrist. Edema of the perineural structures resulting from water retention during pregnancy is believed to be the cause. The symptoms can be severe. Diagnosis is confirmed by eliciting symptoms: with hyperextension and hyperflexion of the wrist or by the tourniquet test. Symptoms can be relieved by splinting the wrist or by local-steroid injection, but they disappear spontaneously after the pregnancy.

SCIATIC NEURITIS. Pain and tenderness over the sciatic and, occasionally, the femoral distribution result from relaxation of the sacroiliac joints and subsequent tension or trauma to the nerves involved. Immobilization of the sacroiliac joints by use of a firm back support and bed boards offers relief, but some discomfort may persist for several weeks after delivery.

TRAUMATIC NEURITIS OR MATERNAL OBSTETRIC PARALYSIS. Pain, paresthesia, or muscle weakness developing in the lower extremities during labor or soon afterward suggests the syndrome of traumatic neuritis or maternal obstetric paralysis. Dorsiflexors of the foot are most frequently affected. Compression of the lumbosacral trunk by the fetal skull is the usual cause. This may occur spontaneously with arrest of the fetal head at the pelvic brim, particularly in the platypelloid pelvis with reduced anteroposterior diameter, or as a result of a difficult forceps delivery. In some women, protrusion of a lumbar intervertebral disk is the cause.

The *peroneal nerve* can be injured by undue pressure against the stirrups during delivery. Footdrop is the result. Because the nerve is superficial as it passes laterally around the fibular neck, this area should be protected by padding when the patient is positioned and by avoiding pressure against the knee when the patient is anesthetized.

Treatment of traumatic neuritis consists of splinting, active and passive exercises, and galvanic stimulation of the affected muscles. Prognosis for recovery within several weeks after delivery is good.

The incidence of *Bell's palsy* is increased in pregnant women. Facial paralysis, pain, taste disturbance, and decreased tearing usually disappear gradually after delivery.

POLYNEURITIS. Fortunately, polyneuritis is a rare complication. Actual degenerative nerve changes that occur result in diminished sensation, paralysis, and muscular atrophy. The process may be limited to a single nerve but can become generalized and rapidly fatal with bulbar involvement. Manifestations are similar to those of Landry's ascending paralysis.

Treatment is preventive. Deficiency states developing in the course of severe hyperemesis or other depleting disorders should be prevented by early replacement of fluid, electrolytes, water-soluble vitamins, and carbohydrates. When nerve damage characteristic of polyneuritis develops, changes may be irreversible.

SKIN DISORDERS

With few exceptions, no cutaneous diseases occur only during pregnancy. Any of the *acute skin eruptions* can occur coincidentally, but their course and treatment are not appreciably altered in gravid women. *Chronic skin diseases,* however, are frequently influenced by pregnancy. Eczema, psoriasis, and various allergic skin manifestations may be improved in some patients and aggravated in others. Acne and hypertrichosis may be more apparent during pregnancy than otherwise.

Pruritus

Generalized pruritus is not an uncommon occurrence during pregnancy. Skin manifestations other than scratch marks are frequently absent, but occasionally urticarial reactions are visible. When there is no associated jaundice and no increase in blood bilirubin levels, a neurogenic cause is most likely. In some patients the itching is related to *idiopathic cholestasis* (see p. 293).

Symptoms range from mild discomfort to intolerable itching, restlessness, and fatigue. Treatment consists of antihistaminics, mild sedation, and local analgesic applications.

A relatively rare and intensely pruritic lesion is designated *pruritic folliculitis* or *papular dermatitis of pregnancy* and is characterized by the appearance of erythematous papules over the trunk and forearms. Lesions become excoriated with scratching. The cause is unknown, and treatment symptomatic. The disturbance disappears after delivery but tends to recur with subsequent pregnancies.

Pruritic urticarial papules and plaques of pregnancy (PUPPP) is a more common distinctive skin lesion of pregnancy. The incidence is underreported because of its relatively benign nature. The eruption appears first on the abdomen in late pregnancy as erythematous papules that blanch on pressure and urticarial plaques. Lesions spread, covering thighs, buttocks, and arms. Biopsy shows lymphocytic infiltration, edema, and local spongiosis. The cause is unknown, but immunofluorescent staining is negative for complement and immunoglobulins. There are no maternal or fetal complications. Treatment is symptomatic, and the eruption disappears after delivery.

Lupus erythematosus

Lupus erythematosus is of interest because it occurs most frequently in women during the reproductive years; although the spontaneous abortion rate is increased, particularly in those in whom *lupus anticoagulant factor* can be identified, it does not otherwise affect fertility. The disease is serious and unpredictable at best.

In preconception counseling, it is important to determine the status of organ involvement and the presence or absence of certain antibodies. *Lupus anticoagulant* (LAC) is not a single antibody but rather a group of substances that are associated with changes in the maternal coagulation system and repeated fetal loss. The presence of LAC is detected as an elevated cardiolipin antibody and/or a prolonged Russell Viper time or partial thromboplastin time. Women with LAC who are untreated have a rate of pregnancy loss approaching 90%. This rate can be lowered to 25% with aspirin and corticosteroid treatment.

Anti-Ro (anti-SSA) is specific for systemic lupus erythematosus (SLE) and correlates highly with neonatal lupus and congenital heart block.

The outcome in puerperal women depends more on the organ involved and severity of the disease than the existence of pregnancy. With the *discoid type,* neither mother nor baby is much affected. *Systemic lupus erythematosus* poses far greater risks for both mother and baby. Although patients with disseminated lupus experience remissions, those with renal involvement (which constitute over 50% of patients with systemic disease) are prone to exacerbations and progressive renal impairment. Maternal mortality is increased, and in survivors life expectancy is significantly shortened when active lupus glomerulonephritis is associated with pregnancy. Fetal death often occurs, particularly in the presence of lupus anticoagulant factor.

Because systemic lupus erythematosus can no longer be considered a rare disease, the diagnosis should be considered in otherwise unexplained proteinuria during pregnancy, especially in patients with fever, arthralgia, alopecia, or rashes.

Corticosteroid therapy provides the most effective form of treatment, and it can be administered during pregnancy without endangering the fetus. High dosages of corticosteroids continued during labor and after delivery in patients who have received prenatal therapy appear to reduce the possibility of postpartum exacerbation.

Abortion is of little value in improving the prognosis of severe systemic lupus. Mortality following abortion is in the range of 25%, and few instances of postoperative improvement have been reported.

Melanoma

Pigmented moles frequently become more obvious during pregnancy, just as increased pigmentation of other areas of the skin may be observed at that time. The question of which of these innumerable lesions, most of which are benign, should be removed often arises. Pigmented moles should be removed in the following circumstances: (1) those on the trunk that are subject to irritation and all those on the genitals and feet where true melanomas are disproportionately more common; (2) moles that are smooth and blue-black; and (3) those exhibiting growth, ulceration, or pain. These should be excised wide of the lesion and never removed by desiccation, as each specimen requires microscopic examination.

Malignant melanoma is a highly malignant tumor, whether associated with pregnancy or not. Overall 5-year survival rates are not significantly different, especially in the early stage when chance of surgical cure is likely. Endocrine manipulation, including termination of pregnancy, ovarian ablation, or administration of hormones has no benefits. Although not usual, placental metastasis and transmission to the fetus can occur.

Herpes gestationis

This vesicobullous disease of pregnancy, also termed *pemphigoid gestationis,* is an autoimmune process believed to be induced by certain hormones of pregnancy, as similar lesions have been encountered in patients with hydatidiform mole and choriocarcinoma. Eruptions, usually beginning in the periumbilical region, consist of superficial vesicobullous or pustular lesions with an erythematous base. These occur in patches that may be distributed over the entire body. An intense pruritus usually persists throughout pregnancy and disappears gradually after delivery. Blood counts show marked eosinophilia. Occasionally constitutional symptoms of chills and fever occur with periods of exacerbation.

Diagnosis can be established with certainty by direct immunofluorescence of lesional and normal skin.

Treatment with antihistaminics provides minimal relief of symptoms. Daily administration of corticosteroids has resulted in significant improvement of both symptoms and pregnancy outcome and is the mainstay of treatment of severe cases.

Maternal mortality is not increased. Risk to the fetus is debated. No increase in perinatal deaths in 33 cases was found, but a significant increase in low-birth-weight and "small for gestational age" infants occurred in the group. Only two newborns showed minor bullous eruptions, and they resolved within 1 week.

Impetigo herpetiformis

Impetigo herpetiformis is a rare inflammatory disease of the skin that occurs mainly in association with pregnancy but has also been found in patients with hypoparathyroidism. The cause is unknown, but lesions are so similar to those of psoriasis, both grossly and microscopically, that it may well be a form of that disease. Characteristic lesions are miliary pustules arranged in irregular or circinate clusters. The pustules spread peripherally as the centers undergo desiccation. Usual sites are the inner aspects of the thighs and genitocrural areas. Mucous membranes of the oral cavity may be involved with lesions that appear as grayish white plaques.

Symptoms include severe burning and itching of the skin, chills, fever, vomiting, diarrhea, and prostration. Mortality in reported cases has been high and often associated with septicemia. Antibiotic therapy, correction of dehydration, and corticosteroid therapy have greatly improved the outcome. Termination of pregnancy is rarely indicated.

BONE AND JOINT DISORDERS

The bones forming the pelvic girdle are solidly united in the adult woman except during preg-nancy, when hormonal effect on the sacroiliac joints and the symphysis pubis permits varying degrees of motion. Radiographic evidence of relaxation can be observed as early as the first trimester, becoming maximal by the beginning of the third trimester.

Sacroiliac relaxation

Sacroiliac relaxation is the most common cause of low back pain in pregnant women. Backache may be limited to the lower lumbar region or radiate down the back of the legs in the distribution of the sciatic nerve. Occasionally, pain follows the course of the femoral nerve over the anterior aspects of the lower abdomen and thighs. Although symptoms may be transitory, they frequently persist throughout pregnancy and for several weeks after delivery. Tenderness can be elicited by palpation over the posterior surface of the sacroiliac joint or by pelvic palpation below and lateral to the sacral promontory. X-ray film examination is generally contraindicated.

Complete immobilization is impractical, if not impossible, during pregnancy, and accordingly few persons are cured; however, relief can be obtained by the use of a firm sacroiliac support, bed boards, and increased periods of rest.

Symphyseal separation

Widening of the symphysis occurs regularly during pregnancy, and, although the increase is sometimes remarkable, symptoms arise less frequently than might be expected. It is likely that acute or chronic trauma to the periosteum is necessary before characteristic signs appear. These may occur during the course of pregnancy but are far more common after a difficult forceps delivery or the birth of a large baby.

The patient experiences severe pain over the pubic and lumbar regions on walking or in attempting to turn in bed. Efforts to reduce motion of the pelvic girdle result in a typical waddling gait. Motion of the pelvic bones can be demonstrated on direct palpation of the lower border of the symphysis while the patient transfers her weight from one extremity to the other. The degree of disability, however, is not necessarily related to the amount of separation.

Treatment. Immobilization of the pelvic girdle by an encircling elastic binder or tight maternity support will permit gradual ambulation. In most cases, symptoms disappear within 2 to 3 weeks after delivery, although some persist for months.

Spinal fusion

Patients who have had orthopedic problems involving the spinal column, particularly those requiring spinal fusion, need special management during pregnancy and delivery. A high proportion of patients who had fusion before pregnancy experience exacerbation of symptoms, and about half may require repeat fusion after delivery. This complication can usually be prevented by use of a support or brace that provides three-point fixation (symphysis pubis, lower sacrum, and upper lumbar–lower rib cage) and, often, hospitalization during the prenatal period.

Spondylolisthesis

The stress directed at the fifth lumbar and first sacral segments during late pregnancy may be a factor in the initiation or aggravation of spondylolisthesis in women. The lithotomy position can be detrimental. The use of human leg holders or delivery in the dorsal or lateral position is preferable in the conduct of vaginal delivery. Trial of labor should not be protracted. If progress is not satisfactory after 6 to 8 hours, operative delivery is advisable.

Ankylosis of the sacrococcygeal joint

Fusion or injury resulting in ankylosis of the sacrococcygeal joint may be suspected during prenatal pelvic examination if the configuration is unusual or the joint rigid. No difficulties arise until the patient is in labor and then only if the coccyx is angulated anteriorly. Descent of the presenting part is delayed, but fracture of the coccyx during forceps extraction usually permits vaginal delivery. In this event, pain during sitting or straining can be expected for several weeks.

Dislocation of the coccyx

Dislocation of the coccyx may cause excruciating pain that makes its appearance immediately after the parturient recovers from anesthesia. Replacement by rectal manipulation with the patient under morphine an-algesia or light anesthesia affords startling and prompt relief.

Osteogenesis imperfecta

Osteogenesis imperfecta has a strong hereditary tendency; it is transmitted by an autosomal dominant gene. The underlying process is a diffuse mesenchymal hypoplasia manifested by severe osteoporosis with fracture caused by minimal trauma, blue sclerae, and middle ear deafness. The disorder may be early in onset or latent. Neonatal osteogenesis imperfecta is often considered incompatible with life, but the outlook is not always so hopeless. We have delivered three infants of a family with paternal osteogenesis imperfecta. Fractures were demonstrable by x-ray film examination before delivery. All infants survived.

As ultrasound techniques have improved, accurate diagnosis is now possible in some, but not all, cases. This method should be used first, but, if findings are dubious, x-ray film examination is still warranted. The risk of fracture and hematoma formation is greater with vaginal delivery. Cesarean section is indicated if predelivery examination shows involvement of the fetus in utero.

SUGGESTED READING

Benson RC, and Inman VT: Brachialgia statica dysesthetica in pregnancy, West J Surg 64:115, 1956.

Birk K, Smeltzer SC, and Rudick R: Pregnancy and multiple sclerosis, Semin Neurol 8:205, 1988.

Branch DW, Scott JR, Kochenour NK, and Hershgold E: Obstetric complications associated with lupus anticoagulant, N Engl J Med 313:1322, 1985.

Bridge RG and Foley FE: Placental transmission of the lupus erythematosus factor, Am J Med Sci 227:1, 1954.

Cohn SL, Schrier R, and Feld D: Osteogenesis imperfecta and pregnancy, Obstet Gynecol 20:107, 1962.

Cross JN, Castro PO, and Jennett WB: Cerebral strokes associated with pregnancy and the puerperium, Br Med J 3:214, 1968.

Dalessio DJ: Seizure disorders and pregnancy, N Engl J Med 312:559, 1985.

Digre KB, Yarner MW, and Corbett JJ: Pseudotumor cerebri and pregnancy, Neurology 34:721, 1984.

Dumbroski RA: Autoimmune disease in pregnancy, Med Clin North Am 73:605, 1989.

Eden RD and Gall SA: Myasthenia gravis and pregnancy: a reappraisal of thymectomy, Obstet Gynecol 62:328, 1983.

Fennell DF and Ringel SP: Myasthenia gravis and pregnancy, Obstet Gynecol Surv 42:414, 1987.

Foldes FF and McNall PG: Myasthenia gravis: a guide for anesthesiologists, Anesthesiology 23:837, 1962.

Frith JA and McLeod JG. Pregnancy and multiple sclerosis, J Neurol Neurosurg Psychiatry 51:495, 1988;.

Greenspoon JS and Paul RH: Paraplegia and quadriplegia: special considerations during pregnancy and labor and delivery, Am J Obstet Gynecol 155:738, 1986.

Hertz KC, Katz SI, Maize J, and Ackerman AB: Herpes gestationis: a clinicopathologic study, Arch Dermatol 112:1543, 1976.

Hiilesmaa VK, Bardy A, and Teramo B: Obstetric outcome in women with epilepsy, Am J Obstet Gynecol 152:499, 1985.

Hill RM, Verniaud WM, Horning MG, McCulley LB, and Morgan NF: Infants exposed in utero to antiepileptic drugs: a prospective study, Am J Dis Child 127:645, 1974.

Holmes RC and Black MM: The fetal prognosis in pemphigoid (herpes) gestationis, Br J Dermatol 110:67, 1984.

Ip MS, So SY, Lam WK, Tang LC, and Mok TK: Thymectomy in myasthenia gravis during pregnancy, Postgrad Med J 62:473, 1986.

Lawley TJ, Hertz KC, Wade TR, Ackerman AB, and Katz SI: Pruritic urticarial papules and plaques of pregnancy, JAMA 241:1696, 1979.

Levine SE and Keesey JC: Successful plasmaphoresis for fulminant myasthenia gravis during pregnancy, Arch Neurol 43(2):1978, 1986.

Lookingbill DP and Chez RA: Herpes gestationis, Clin Obstet Gynecol 26:605, 1983.

Lubbe WF and Liggins GC: Lupus anticoagulant and pregnancy, Am J Obstet Gynecol 159:322, 1985.

Massey EW and Cefalo RC: Neuropathies of pregnancy: a review, Obstet Gynecol Surv 34:489, 1979.

Morrow CP and DiSaia PJ: Malignant melanoma of the female genitalia: a clinical analysis, Obstet Gynecol 31:233, 1976.

Nelson LM, Franklin GM, and Jones MC: Risk of multiple sclerosis exacerbation during pregnancy and breast-feeding, JAMA 259:3441, 1988.

Newman B and Lam AM: Induced hypotension for clipping of a cerebral aneurysm during pregnancy: a case report and brief review, Anesth Analg 65:675, 1986.

Singer JR, Hummelgard AB, and Martin EM: Ruptured aneurysm in pregnancy, J Neurosurg Nurs 17:230, 1985.

Thompson DS, Nelson LM, Burns A, Burks JS, and Franklin GM: The effects of pregnancy in multiple sclerosis: a retrospective study, Neurology 36:1097, 1986.

Trelford JD: Spondylolisthesis in pregnancy, Am J Obstet Gynecol 91:320, 1965.

Wiebers DO and Whisnant JP: The incidence of stroke among pregnant women in Rochester, Minn, 1955 through 1979, JAMA 254:3055, 1985.

Young DC, Leveno KJ, and Whalley PJ: Induced delivery prior to surgery for ruptured cerebral aneurysm, Obstet Gynecol 61:749, 1983;.

Zegart K and Schwartz R: Chorea gravidarum, Obstet Gynecol 32:24, 1968.

Zoberman E and Farmer ER: Pruritic folliculitis of pregnancy, Arch Dermatol 117:20, 1981.

26

Russell K. Laros, Jr.

Hypertensive disorders during pregnancy

Objectives

RATIONALE: Hypertensive disorders account for one sixth of all maternal deaths and a significant fraction of perinatal morbidity and mortality. Early diagnosis and treatment will virtually eliminate maternal mortality and markedly improve fetal outcome.

The student should be able to:

A. Classify and define the hypertensive disorders of pregnancy.

B. Explain the pathophysiology of hypertensive disorders during pregnancy.

C. Demonstrate a knowledge of the diagnosis and maternal and fetal complications of hypertensive disorders.

D. Devise a management plan for each of the hypertensive disorders.

Hypertensive disorders that occur during pregnancy are similar in that they are all characterized by elevated blood pressure. Some are specifically related to pregnancy and occur only when the uterus contains trophoblastic tissue. With others, pregnancy adds a complication to an already existing disease. Hypertensive disorders account for about one sixth of all maternal deaths and are significant factors in perinatal mortality. Many deaths can be prevented by early recognition of the condition and appropriate treatment.

CLASSIFICATION AND DIAGNOSIS

In the past, hypertensive disorders were designated by the nonspecific term *toxemia of pregnancy*. A more accurate classification, proposed by the Committee on Terminology of the American College of Obstetricians and Gynecologists, follows:

1. Preeclampsia
2. Eclampsia
3. Gestational hypertension
4. Gestational proteinuria
5. Gestational edema

6. Chronic hypertensive disease
7. Chronic hypertensive disease with superimposed preeclampsia

Hypertension indicates a rise in systolic blood pressure of at least 30 mm Hg and in diastolic pressure of at least 15 mm Hg or of a systolic pressure of at least 140 mm Hg and a diastolic pressure of at least 90 mm Hg. The levels must occur on two occasions at least 6 hours apart.

An alternative definition is an increase in mean arterial pressure (MAP) of 20 mm Hg or, if baseline values are not known, a pressure of 105 mm Hg. The mean arterial pressure is determined as:

$$\text{Mean arterial pressure (MAP)} = \frac{\text{Systolic BP} + (2 \times \text{Diastolic BP})}{3}$$

Proteinuria is defined as a concentration of protein greater than 0.3 g/L/24 hr or a concentration greater than 0.1 g/L (1+ or 2+) in two or more random urine samples obtained at least 6 hours apart. The specimens should be either clean catch or collected by catheterization.

Edema is the generalized accumulation of fluid that accounts for a weight gain of at least 2.4 kg (5 pounds) in a week or when there is 1 plus pitting edema after 12 hours of rest in bed.

The patient with *preeclampsia* appears normal during early pregnancy, but hypertension, proteinuria, and/or edema appear after the twentieth week. The exception is that certain women with hydatidiform moles can develop typical preeclampsia during the first half of pregnancy.

One can diagnose *eclampsia* when convulsions occur in a woman with preeclampsia if there is no other reason for the seizures.

Gestational hypertension refers to hypertension that develops during the last half of pregnancy or during the first 24 hours after delivery if there are no evidences of preeclampsia or of chronic hypertensive disease and if the blood pressure returns to normal within 10 days after delivery. Some of these women may have preeclampsia; in others the rise in blood pressure may be evidence of chronic hypertensive disease.

Gestational proteinuria is proteinuria occurring during pregnancy in women who have no evidence of acute or chronic hypertension or of renal disease.

Gestational edema is edema that fits the criteria for the diagnosis of edema, which have already been listed.

Chronic hypertensive disease is diagnosed if hypertension was present when the patient became pregnant, is found before the twentieth week of gestation, or persists beyond the forty-second day after delivery.

In some patients with chronic hypertensive disease the blood pressure will rise at least 30/15 mm Hg during the second half of pregnancy, and the rise will be accompanied by proteinuria, edema, or both. Alternatively, the MAP may rise by 20 mm Hg and be accompanied by proteinuria and/or edema. This is *chronic hypertension with superimposed preeclampsia*.

INCIDENCE

About 5% of all pregnancies are complicated by preeclampsia. The incidence may be as high as 10% in indigent women and as low as 2% in those who are more affluent.

PREECLAMPSIA-ECLAMPSIA

Because preeclampsia and eclampsia are phases of a single disorder and differ only in severity, they will be discussed as a single progressive process, preeclampsia-eclampsia.

Preeclampsia-eclampsia occurs only in pregnant human beings; it has no exact counterpart in the hypertensive states in nonpregnant persons. The signs appear after the twentieth week of pregnancy except in the rare instances in which it is associated with hydatidiform mole. It is more common in both young and older primigravidas than in multiparas and is characterized by *edema, proteinuria,* and *hypertension.*

Clinical course. The first evidence of an abnormality is usually an excessive gain in weight, more than 1 kg (2 pounds) a week. After a period of abnormal weight gain, the other signs appear together or one slightly in advance of the other. If the condition is untreated, it may progress until the patient develops eclampsia, which is the most advanced stage of acute pregnancy-induced hypertension.

EDEMA. Total body water is increased by 6 to 8 L during normal pregnancy. This requires the retention of enough sodium and other electrolytes to maintain an isotonic concentration.

The physiologic high levels of both total body water and exchangeable sodium are increased even more when a pregnant woman develops preeclampsia-eclampsia. Whether this represents an exaggeration of the normal mechanism or is a new process has not yet been determined. Nonetheless, a rapid increase in body weight usually precedes the other clinical signs of preeclampsia by days or weeks.

Fluid and sodium are retained by normal pregnant women despite changes that favor increased sodium excretion: (1) the remarkable increase in glomerular filtration; (2) a high concentration of circulating progesterone, which favors natriuresis; (3) reduced resistance in renal blood vessels; and (4) decreased plasma oncotic pressure. Obviously, sodium depletion would occur rapidly if tubular reabsorption were not increased enough to compensate for these changes. The result is retention of fluids and electrolytes, which is responsible for the expanded plasma volume and for the accumulation of fluid in the extravascular compartments. During most of pregnancy there is a positive sodium balance that reaches at least 20 to 25 mEq/week during the last weeks. The total excess is about 1000 mEq, or 60 g, of sodium chloride for the entire pregnancy.

The pathophysiologic changes with preeclampsia that may favor excessive sodium and fluid retention are (1) decreased glomerular filtration, (2) increased renal vascular resistance, and (3) reduced plasma volume. Because of decreased glomerular filtration, a smaller sodium load reaches the tubules. In addition, altered rates of secretion of aldosterone, deoxycorticosterone, and other substances may be important factors, but their roles have not yet been clearly defined. The changes in fluid and electrolyte exchange and in renal function are results, not the cause, of preeclampsia. The disorder is not induced by the ingestion of salt, but an excessive sodium intake can exaggerate the pathophysiologic changes.

The end result of this alteration in salt metabolism can be demonstrated by injecting hypertonic saline solution intravenously and measuring the urinary output of sodium and chloride. The excess electrolytes and water are eliminated less rapidly in normal pregnant women than in nonpregnant women, but there is a further delay in those with preeclampsia. In normal pregnant women the sodium excretion during the first 2 hours after the administration of 1000 ml of 2.5% salt solution averaged 267 mEq/L. Of the normal women, 88% eliminated the excess fluid rapidly, returning to the pretest weight within 48 hours; 70% of those with preeclampsia had not returned to the pretest weight within 96 hours.

HYPERTENSION. The most important pathophysiologic change with preeclampsia-eclampsia is widespread arteriolar spasm, which is the direct cause of hypertension that characterizes preeclampsia-eclampsia. Hypertension is seldom the initial sign of the disorder. The height of the blood pressure in itself does not indicate the overall severity, the average systolic blood pressure in preeclampsia being only about 160 mm Hg. The rise in diastolic pressure may be disproportionate to that of the systolic pressure, thereby *narrowing the pulse pressure*. Diastolic pressures of 110 to 120 mm Hg are not unusual.

Although any blood pressure over 140/90 or MAP over 105 mm Hg is considered to be abnormal, the physician should not wait for the blood pressure to reach this level before suspecting that something is wrong. Because the blood pressure during normal pregnancy usually is below the prepregnancy level, a gradual but persistent rise should arouse one's suspicions. An increase of more than 30 mm Hg in systolic pressure or of more than 15 mm Hg in diastolic pressure or in MAP of more than 20, even if they remain within the limits of normal, is suggestive that preeclampsia is developing.

The vascular changes can be seen in the retinal and conjunctival vessels and can be measured in the kidney and in the brain. *Renal blood flow* becomes progressively more reduced as preeclampsia progresses. The alteration is a result of increased resistance in the afferent glomerular arterioles and narrowing of the lumina of the glomerular capillaries. *Increased vascular resistance in cerebral vessels* occurs, although blood flow and cerebral oxygen consumption remained normal. *Uterine blood flow* also is reduced.

The mechanism by which arteriolar spasm is initiated and maintained is not as yet clearly understood, but it probably has no relationship to changes in the autonomic nervous system. The blood pressure in pregnant women with essential hypertension will fall, sometimes precipitously, in response to ganglionic blocking agents. These drugs have little effect on the hypertension associated with preeclampsia.

The arteries in women with preeclampsia are much more responsive to pressor substances, such as norepinephrine and angiotensin, than are those of normal pregnant women. This may be, at least in part, a result of the increased sodium concentration in the arteriolar walls, which increases vascular reactivity in isolated vessels. *Prostaglandins,* or prostaglandin-like substances, may play a role in this reaction. Prostaglandin, which is synthesized in the vascular wall, may prevent the vessel from responding to the stimulus of angiotensin. This reaction can be eliminated by prostaglandin inhibitors.

PROTEINURIA. The third important sign of preeclampsia is the excretion of protein in the urine. This makes its appearance at about the same time as the hypertension and increases in severity as the disease progresses.

The examination of the urine in patients with early preeclampsia reveals no abnormality except for the presence of protein. The amount increases with the severity of the condition, and eventually more than 10 g may be excreted daily.

One of the important prognostic signs is the amount of urinary protein. A qualitative measurement of protein is likely to be misleading because a given amount of protein diluted in a large amount of urine may be read 1 plus, whereas the same amount in a small quantity of urine may give a 3 or 4 plus reaction. By measuring the total excretion in successive 24-hour periods, the physician has an accurate means of evaluating changes in renal function. This simple test should be part of the study of every pregnant woman with hypertension.

URINE MICROSCOPY. As the disease progresses, the urinary findings increase; in the severe case, red blood cells, white blood cells, and all kinds of casts may be found. At this stage the urine examination is of little value in the differential diagnosis of the condition.

RENAL FUNCTION. The renal function in early preeclampsia is slightly reduced as shown by insulin, creatinine, and uric acid clearances that are below those for normal pregnancy. *A pregnant woman must always be in the lateral recumbent position during clearance studies to obtain an accurate result.* Glomerular filtration and sodium excretion are significantly lower in the upright and dorsal positions than in the lateral.

As the disease becomes severe, there is progressive diminution both in renal function, as shown by a further depression in the excretion of the various testing substances, and in urine volume. Women with severe preeclampsia and eclampsia may excrete only 100 to 200 ml of urine in a 24-hour period or may even be completely anuric.

That the decreased function is not directly related to the elevated blood pressure is suggested by the fact that after delivery the renal function is reestablished, with the blood pressure at a level that usually is at least as high as in the predelivery period.

PLASMA VOLUME. A progressive *hemoconcentration,* the result of the abnormal flow of fluid from the bloodstream into the tissue spaces and cells, accompanies severe preeclampsia. As the blood volume decreases, so does the amount of urine excreted; the patient with severe preeclampsia or eclampsia may be anuric. There can be no diuresis without a reversal of the flow of fluid back into the bloodstream from the tissue spaces and reestablishment of blood flow through the glomerular capillaries.

HEMODYNAMIC PROFILE. The cardiovascular alterations characteristic of preeclampsia/eclampsia have been studied by right heart catheterization.

Most patients had hyperdynamic left ventricular function and high-normal to elevated mean systemic vascular resistance. Pulmonary vascular resistance and colloid osmotic pressure are normal in most cases.

Stroke volume and cardiac indices are also normal when normalized for body surface area. In the absence of myocardial dysfunction or valvular disease, capillary wedge pressure can be used to estimate left ventricular end-diastolic pressure. The wedge pressure is normal to high in the majority of patients; however, the central venous pressure is low in more than 50%. This decrease probably reflects the contracted intravascular volume previously discussed.

URIC ACID. Uric acid metabolism also is disturbed. As preeclampsia becomes more severe, the renal clearance of uric acid becomes progressively more reduced, and subsequently the serum concentration rises. The maximum normal serum uric acid concentration is 6 mg/dl, and the minimum normal uric acid clearance is 10 mg/min. The increase in serum uric acid is probably a result of decreased renal excretion.

SEVERE PREECLAMPSIA. Progression of the pathophysiologic changes is reflected in changes in physiologic functions and physical findings. Severe preeclampsia can be diagnosed when any of the following develop:

1. Systolic blood pressure of at least 160 mm Hg or diastolic pressure of at least 110 mm Hg on two or more occasions at least 6 hours apart with the patient resting in bed
2. At least 5 g of protein in a 24-hour urine specimen (qualitative 3 or 4 plus)
3. Less than 400 ml urinary output in 24 hours
4. Cerebral or visual symptoms
5. Pulmonary edema or cyanosis
6. Epigastric pain
7. Abnormalities in liver function or coagulation

ECLAMPSIA. Eclampsia represents a progression of preeclampsia with the addition of convulsions or coma or both.

The physiologic changes are simply a continuation of those found in severe preeclampsia. There is a further increase in blood pressure, but this need not be to exceedingly high levels; the systolic blood pressure is often below 200 mm Hg except during the actual convulsions, but the diastolic pressure may be 120 to 130 mm Hg. The oliguria increases to anuria, and there is a further increase in the hemoconcentration, the hematocrit at times reaching 45 to 50. A retention of nitrogenous material accompanies the depression of kidney function, and for the first time a rise in blood urea nitrogen may be observed.

Eclampsia may develop before the onset of labor, during labor, or within the first 24 hours after delivery.

Etiologic factors. The cause of preeclampsia-eclampsia has not been clearly established, but it is evident that the condition can develop only in women with active trophoblastic tissue. One important factor appears to be the amount of placental tissue. Preeclampsia occurs more often during pregnancies with multiple fetuses and with hydatidiform mole; in both there is a greater volume of trophoblastic tissue than with a single fetus. The incidence is increased in patients with chronic cardiovascular renal disease, diabetes mellitus, fetal hydrops, and severe anemia.

The role of *dietary deficiency* in the development of preeclampsia-eclampsia is not clearly defined, but it is presumed to be an important factor. Pregnancy-induced hypertension develops more often in women of the lower socioeconomic classes than in middle- and upper-class women. This has been attributed to chronic malnutrition, particularly to an inadequate intake of protein, but the precise role of diet is not clear. If malnutrition were the sole cause of preeclampsia-eclampsia, the disease would occur in multiparas, particularly those who had been affected in previous pregnancies, as often as in primigavidas, but it does not. It is unlikely that dietary, economic, and environmental conditions will change enough between pregnancies to account for the reduction in incidence in parous women.

The possibility of an *immunologic factor* being

responsible for the development of preeclampsia has been proposed. This is an intriguing suggestion because the development of the disorder during the first exposure to trophoblast appears to provide protection against its recurrence in subsequent pregnancies. Much more information is necessary before such a mechanism can be confirmed.

Many attempts have been made to correlate geographic and climatic conditions with its development. So far no convincing evidence has been advanced.

The most tenable current theory is that of *uterine ischemia*. A reduction in blood flow to the choriodecidual space could alter placental function, permitting the trophoblast or the decidua to produce thromboplastin or thromboplastin-like material, pressor polypeptides, or other substances that might initiate the characteristic vascular changes. The basic theory has much in its favor. Preeclampsia-eclampsia occurs most often in young primigravidas, particularly those with twins, and in women with hydatidiform moles, particularly those in whom the uterus is larger than that expected for the duration of pregnancy. In each of these the uterus tends to be either tense or more distended than usual. This could cause a reduction in blood flow through the smaller vessels. The incidence in women with preexisting hypertensive disorders and with diabetes, particularly those with vascular degeneration, also is high. In these women, too, uterine blood flow is reduced.

Several primate models have been developed. Relative uterine ischemia is produced by constriction of the aorta below the level of the renal vessels. The animals develop hypertension, a decrease in plasma renin activity, an increase in renal resistance, an increase in serum uric acid and glomerular changes consistent with those seen in human preeclampsia.

Clinically significant disseminated intravascular coagulation (DIC) is rare, occurring in only 10% of patients with severe preeclampsia or eclampsia. One report demonstrated thrombocytopenia in 29% and a prolonged thrombin time (an indicator of circulating fibrin/fibrinogen split products) in 50% of 95 eclamptic women. Directly measured fibrin/fibrinogen degradation products were only elevated in 3%, and circulating fibrin monimer in 5% of the cases. However, if sensitive tests of procoagulant consumption are used, such as the ratio of factor VIII activity/factor VIII antigen or beta thromboglobulin, changes are almost always found. Deposits of fibrin have been reported by some, but not all investigators in liver, kidneys and other organs. Fibrin deposition is invariably present in the intravillous space. This suggests that focal deposition at the placental site rather than generalized DIC may be the pathophysiology of procoagulant consumption.

The more severe the toxemia, the more pronounced the changes. Some women with advanced preeclampsia-eclampsia develop a full-blown coagulation defect.

Several authors have presented data that define a unique group of preeclamptic women. These individuals develop hemolysis, elevated liver enzymes, and thrombocytopenia; the so-called HELLP syndrome. This is probably not a unique syndrome but rather a variant of severe preeclampsia that may develop either before or after delivery.

In one study the incidence of first-pregnancy toxemia in the daughters of women who had had preeclampsia was 26% and of toxemia in subsequent pregnancies, 22%. The incidence of first-pregnancy toxemia in daughters-in-law of the same women was 8%. Daughters-in-law were selected as control subjects because their ages and social status were comparable to those of the study group.

Prediction. One can always anticipate that preeclampsia may develop in primigravid women who have diabetes or chronic cardiovascular renal disease, those who are poor and malnourished, and those with multifetal pregnancies. It is more difficult to predict that it will occur in presumably normal women.

The *rollover test* may be useful in predicting

gravidas at risk of developing preeclampsia. Blood pressures are recorded between 28 and 32 weeks after stabilization first in the lateral recumbent position and then in the supine position. In the study a rise in diastolic pressure of more than 20 mm Hg occurred on assuming the supine position in 93% of normotensive multiparas who later developed pregnancy-induced hypertension. In addition, most of the same women demonstrated a rise in blood pressure in response to angiotensin. Conversely, 91% of those with minimal blood pressure elevation with a change in position and with little response to angiotensin remained normal throughout pregnancy. Although not absolutely accurate, this simple test may indicate most women who are in danger of developing preeclampsia.

Prophylaxis. It will not be possible to prevent the development of acute pregnancy-induced hypertension until more is known about its basic cause. The serious advanced stages with their high perinatal and maternal mortality can be prevented if the alert physician detects the earliest evidence of preeclampsia and institutes appropriate treatment.

Because of the theoretical role of prostaglandins and DIC in the pathophysiology of preeclampsia, several investigators have tried treatment and/or prophylaxis with both anticoagulants and antiprostaglandins. A large prospective study selected patients based on clinical risk factors and a positive rollover test. Study patients were given 100 mg of aspirin daily, and the controls received inert placebo. The rate of preeclampsia was 35.5% in the placebo-treated group, as compared to 11.8% of those taking aspirin. Although this difference is statistically significant, confirmatory studies are needed before aspirin prophylaxis becomes a standard mode of care.

Primigravid women and those who have conditions that predispose them to the development of preeclampsia-eclampsia should be seen more often than normal multiparas during the last half of pregnancy. The signs of developing preeclampsia can be detected in almost every instance if the patient is examined every other week between the twenty-eighth and thirty-fifth weeks of pregnancy and weekly thereafter.

Treatment. The signs and symptoms of preeclampsia can be divided into groups that indicate progressive severity of the condition. The list has been expanded to include laboratory changes and may be used as an aid in guiding treatment.

Group A
Edema (weight), hypertension, proteinuria

Group B	
Cerebral	*Visual*
Headache	Diplopia
Dizziness	Scotomas
Tinnitus	Blurred vision
Tachypnea	Amaurosis
Tachycardia	*Renal*
Fever	Oliguria
Gastrointestinal	Anuria
Nausea	*Laboratory*
Vomiting	Evidence of DIC
Epigastric pain	Evidence of hepatocellular
Hematemesis	disease
	Hematuria
	Hemoglobinuria
	Advancing hyperuricemia

The only evidences of preeclampsia before its immediate preconvulsive stage are those in group A, which the physician must recognize. The patient usually has no symptoms as the condition is developing; in fact, she may have none with severe preeclampsia. The presence of group B signs and symptoms suggests that eclampsia is imminent.

OFFICE TREATMENT OF PREECLAMPSIA. The earliest evidence of pregnancy-induced hypertension can be recognized by an alert observer, but whether treatment influences the course of preeclampsia is questionable.

Excessive weight gain associated with exaggerated fluid retention is often the earliest warning that preeclampsia may be developing. A diagnosis cannot be made on the basis of weight gain or edema alone, however, because most women have dependent edema during the last weeks of pregnancy and few develop preeclampsia. The other signs, hypertension and proteinuria, will appear in those whose edema is caused by early preeclampsia.

Women who gain weight suddenly, those who gain more than 1 kg (2 pounds) per week, and those with obvious edema must be seen more often than patients who gain at an anticipated rate. In those with preeclampsia, the blood pressure will rise and proteinuria will appear. These changes will not occur in the others.

Because blood pressure generally rises slowly as preeclampsia is becoming evident, examinations approximately every 3 days are adequate to recognize the changes. Abrupt blood pressure rises, which sometimes occur, will also be detected promptly with this schedule.

The only *laboratory studies* that may be helpful in differentiating early preeclampsia from excessive fluid retention are uric acid and creatinine clearances, which may be reduced slightly in women with early preeclampsia. Serum uric acid concentrations, which rise as clearance is reduced, may be in the normal range at this stage.

There is no *treatment* that will effectively reverse the pathologic processes of preeclampsia. It has been customary to recommend low-sodium diets for edematous women and for those with preeclampsia, but this is not appropriate. Sodium is necessary, even in women with preeclampsia, to supply tissue needs and to prevent contraction of plasma volume and the fluid volume in the extravascular compartments. Bed rest in the lateral recumbent position will enhance excretion of excess fluid, but diuretics are contraindicated. Of course, adequate nutrition is essential, but improving an inadequate diet at this late stage will not solve the immediate problem.

Because the placental site is one of the target organs in preeclampsia, less than optimal placental function should be anticipated. This can be evidenced by intrauterine fetal growth and evidence of diminished placental reserve. When preeclampsia is mild, fetal well-being should be assured with biweekly nonstress tests (NSTs) and/or contraction stress tests (CSTs) and biweekly ultrasonic evaluation of fetal growth and amniotic fluid volume. If the preeclampsia is severe, the NSTs or CSTs should be performed daily.

If the blood pressure rises and proteinuria appears during the period of observation, a diagnosis of preeclampsia can be made, and the patient should be admitted to the hospital or observed very closely as outpatients.

HOSPITAL TREATMENT OF PREECLAMPSIA. The initial hospital treatment of preeclampsia concerns itself primarily with the classification of severity of the condition and the initiation of a regimen designed to control the signs and symptoms. With the exception of an evaluation of the duration of pregnancy, the size and position of the fetus, and the adequacy of the pelvis, the pregnancy is, at the onset, ignored.

The *blood pressure* should be checked four times daily, and the patient *weighed* each morning at the same time. The *fluid intake* and *urine output* are carefully measured and recorded daily, and the amount of edema is evaluated. Daily quantitative determination of the *total urinary protein excretion* likewise is of prognostic significance. A steady increase or a constant excretion of more than 3 to 5 g daily is a grave sign. Daily protein excretion greater than 5 g is associated with a definite increase in intrauterine fetal death. The *serum uric acid, coagulation function, liver function,* and *creatinine clearances* should be checked twice a week. The *retinal vessels* should be examined at regular intervals for evidence of increasing spasm and alterations in the vessel walls.

Women with preeclampsia should remain in bed much of the day, as bed rest enhances sodium and water excretion. The lateral recumbent position is preferable to the supine because renal function is further reduced in the dorsal position. A *regular diet* can usually be ordered, unless there is a reason other than preeclampsia for a special diet. There is no need to limit *fluid intake.*

Success is determined by stabilization or reversal of the abnormal signs (weight, blood pressure, and proteinuria) and by the absence of symptoms. If the response to this regimen is favorable, that is, if an adequate urine output (at least 1500 ml) is maintained, the proteinuria does not increase, the clearances do not fall to dangerous levels, coagulation and liver function remain normal, the blood pressure is controlled, and the weight is stabilized, the regimen may be continued until the cervix is "ripe," at which time labor can be induced.

Advance in severity of the condition is characterized by increasing weight and edema, a progressive diminution in urinary output with an increase in total protein, an increase in serum uric acid and creatinine, a decrease in uric acid and creatinine clearances, further elevation of blood pressure, evidence of liver or coagulation disfunction, hemoconcentration as indicated by an increase in hemoglobin and hematocrit, progressive change in the retinal arterioles, and, in many cases, the appearance of symptoms that become progressively more pronounced.

It is important to recognize that weight loss and regression of edema can occur, even though the other signs indicate an increasingly severe process; hence evaluation on the basis of a change in one sign alone is inappropriate.

Stimulation of renal function. The maintenance or promotion of urinary output is desirable in treating severe preeclampsia, but it cannot always be achieved. It is essential that the patient not be overloaded with fluid that she cannot excrete. Reduction of vasospasm may be helpful, but diuretics are usually contraindicated because they are ineffective in stimulating urine output.

Anticonvulsant therapy. Magnesium sulfate can be given intramuscularly as a 50% solution or intravenously in a 20% or 25% solution. Intramuscular injection has the disadvantages of being painful and of the unpredictable absorption rate because of vascular spasm. When given intravenously, an initial dose of 4 to 6 g is administered during a period of 4 to 5 minutes. The maintenance dosage is about 1 g/hr using an infusion pump. Calcium gluconate, which counteracts the effect of magnesium promptly, should be kept at the bedside where it will be readily available if needed.

Magnesium intoxication is possible but is unlikely to occur if the patient is being observed properly. Magnesium is excreted in the urine; consequently, an adequate urinary output is essential. If the urine volume decreases below 30 ml/hr, the dosage of magnesium sulfate must be reduced. Magnesium sulfate also decreases hyperactive reflexes, thereby decreasing the possibility of convulsions. The reflexes can be used to monitor dosage; as long as the patellar reflexes are present, there is no immediate danger of magnesium toxicity. Reflexes should be checked about every 30 minutes.

TABLE 26-1 Clinical effects of various magnesium levels

Clinical condition	Serum magnesium level	
	(mg/dL)	(mEq/L)
Normal	1.8-3	1.5-2.5
Therapeutic	6-8	5-6.7
Loss of patellar reflex	12	10
Respiratory depression	18	15
Cardiac arrest	36	30

In many institutions serum magnesium levels are monitored. Certainly they are required if one is to administer magnesium in cases in which the patellar reflexes initially are depressed or in which the patient is oliguric. Table 26-1 shows the clinical effects anticipated at various magnesium levels.

Control of blood pressure. Unless the blood pressure is greatly elevated, hypotensive drugs ordinarily are unnecessary in the treatment of severe preeclampsia because the magnesium sulfate will usually depress the blood pressure to a reasonably safe level. If the pressure falls to an unusually low level or sometimes even to the normal range, the output of urine may be greatly reduced.

If the systolic blood pressure is rising rapidly or is over 160 to 180 mm Hg or if the diastolic pressure is higher than 110 mm Hg, a definite effort should be made to control it. *Hydralazine (Apresoline),* 10 to 20 mg diluted to 20 ml and slowly given intravenously, will often lower the blood pressure and maintain it at a safe level for several hours. This is particularly effective during labor. The effect of hydralazine on cerebral blood vessels and blood flow is similar to that of magnesium sulfate but more pronounced. When given by mouth, the drug has much less effect.

In severe hypertensive crisis, nitroprusside or nitroglycerin can be used. Sodium *nitroprusside* is an extremely rapid-acting agent that acts on both arterial and venous smooth muscle. Central monitoring with a pulmonary artery catheter is essential for the safe use of this agent. The objective is to lower systemic vascular resistance while maintaining venous return and cardiac output.

The drug is started at an infusion rate of 0.25 μg/ kg/min and increased by the same amount every 5 minutes until blood pressure control is achieved. In experimental animals, toxic levels of serum cyanide have been reported in the fetus but only after long periods of infusion. This complication has not been noted in humans; however, caution is warranted. An alternate drug is *nitroglycerin*. The initial infusion rate is 10 μg/min, which is doubled every 5 minutes until an adequate response is achieved.

Termination of pregnancy. The decisive cure for preeclampsia-eclampsia is termination of pregnancy at a carefully chosen time. In most women with severe preeclampsia any response to medical treatment is temporary, and the progression of the disease cannot be halted. Delivery after a preliminary period, during which attempts are made to stabilize the process, is the only way to prevent eclampsia with its increased maternal and perinatal mortality. Women with mild preeclampsia that progresses despite treatment and those with severe preeclampsia, even though it responds to medical therapy, should usually be delivered regardless of the duration of pregnancy. Delaying delivery in an attempt to increase infant survival by permitting the fetus to become more mature is usually ineffective. This is particularly true when the pregnancy has advanced to at least 30 to 32 weeks and facilities for intensive neonatal care are available. As discussed above, fetal growth retardation is common with severe preeclampsia because of compromised uteroplacental circulation, and the fetus may die in utero.

Labor can often be induced in these women, even though the cervix may feel unfavorable; hence in most instances the membranes should be ruptured and oxytocin given as an initial procedure. Cesarean section can be performed if labor has not begun within 6 to 12 hours.

HOSPITAL TREATMENT OF ECLAMPSIA. If the patient develops convulsions, the prognosis at once becomes grave.

Unless the natural tendency to overtreat the patient with eclampsia is curbed, the mortality may be increased by the treatment administered. Before any medication is ordered for a convulsing patient, she must be examined to be certain that she actually has eclampsia and to evaluate her general condition. If she is comatose, as most women with eclampsia are, large doses of sedative drugs may be harmful.

The aims in the treatment of eclampsia are (1) to control convulsions, (2) to lower blood pressure, and (3) to terminate pregnancy.

General treatment. The patient is placed in a dimly lighted, quiet room with an attendant constantly present. A *mouth gag,* prepared by wrapping gauze around a tongue blade, should be available to insert between the teeth during convulsions to prevent injury to the tongue. Facilities for *aspiration of mucus* from the pharynx and trachea should be available. Recordings of *blood pressure, urine volume, temperature, pulse, respirations,* and *response to treatment* should be made every 30 minutes. Nothing is given by mouth until after delivery, and the stomach should be aspirated if the patient is vomiting. An *intravenous infusion of 5% dextrose* is run at a rate of about 100 ml/hr.

Because hypoxia always is associated with hemoconcentration, the administration of *oxygen* is a valuable aid in therapy. Copious pulmonary secretions may fill the bronchi and lower trachea, thereby obstructing the airway. Oxygenation can be improved by performing *endotracheal intubation* whenever pulmonary edema is diagnosed, when respirations are labored, or when there is a suggestion of cyanosis.

Renal function. An indwelling catheter is inserted into the bladder, and hourly urine outputs are recorded. The ordinary diuretic preparations are completely valueless, because the anuria is a result of decreased glomerular filtration and most diuretics act at a tubular level. Because the decrease in glomerular filtration is at least in part a result of glomerular arteriolar spasm, the most important part of the treatment is to decrease peripheral vasospasm, which can best be accomplished with magnesium sulfate and other antihypertensive agents.

Control of convulsions. Control of convulsions is an important step in treatment. Magnesium sulfate, administered as described for severe preeclampsia, will usually provide adequate sedation and control the convulsions. If the convulsions continue, one should suspect that the dose of magnesium sulfate is inadequate. Sibai and colleagues, studying women who continued to convulse despite what was considered to be adequate doses of the drug, found that blood levels often were below those that usually are effective (6 to 8 mg/dl).

Convulsions that continue despite adequate magnesium sulfate therapy can often be controlled by the intravenous administration of diazepam (Valium), 1 mg, or amobarbital sodium (Amytal), 300 mg. These drugs should not be necessary often and should be used with caution, as they are powerful cerebral depressants.

Control of blood pressure. It is not necessary to lower the blood pressure to a normal level; in fact, in some patients even a moderate fall in blood pressure will reduce the renal output of urine. If the diastolic pressure remains above 100 mm Hg, an antihypertensive agent should be administered. *Hydralazine,* 10 to 20 mg diluted to 20 ml, can be given slowly intravenously. The blood pressure should be checked several times as the drug is being injected to detect the precipitate drops that sometimes occur. If the diastolic pressure remains above 110 mm Hg, an additional dose can be given in about 20 minutes. Hydralazine can be repeated if a significant rise in diastolic blood pressure occurs.

Cardiovascular monitoring. Pulmonary edema occurs in patients with severe preeclampsia or eclampsia because of increased intravascular pressure, decreased oncotic pressure, increased capillary permeability, or a combination of the three. Because of the threat of pulmonary edema and the difficulty of its management without continuous evaluation of cardiopulmonary function, many clinicians advise the placement of a pulmonary artery (Swan-Ganz) and radial artery catheter in all cases of eclampsia and in many cases of severe preeclampsia. Minute-to-minute monitoring allows appropriate and timely use of preload and afterload reduction and inotropic stimulation. Our approach has been to insert a central venous pressure (CVP) line that can be converted to a pulmonary artery catheter in all patients with severe preeclampsia or eclampsia. If the CVP is low, we proceed with intravascular volume expansion and the other modalities of treatment. However, if the CVP is *normal or high,* the central line is converted to a Swan-Ganz type catheter.

Termination of pregnancy. Termination of the pregnancy is the decisive step in the treatment of both preeclampsia and eclampsia, but ill-advised attempts at delivery at an inopportune time may result in the death of a patient who otherwise might have survived. Initial treatment by delivery by any method without a preliminary period of medical treatment of the disease is accompanied by an alarming maternal mortality; hence control of convulsions and hypertension must precede delivery. Ordinarily, patients with eclampsia should be delivered soon after convulsions are controlled.

Vaginal delivery is preferred if there are no contraindications. Cesarean section is to be considered only for those in whom there is a contraindication to vaginal delivery or for those in whom labor cannot be induced by rupturing membranes and administering oxytocin.

Care following delivery. Any patient with severe preeclampsia may develop eclampsia during the first 24 hours after delivery. During this time, diuresis should begin; if this occurs, it is unlikely that the condition will progress. Should the anuria continue, however, the patient is in danger of convulsing. The same careful observations and the same treatment given the undelivered, severely preeclamptic patient are continued after delivery until the disease process has reversed itself. The urine output is carefully measured at hourly intervals. Anticonvulsant therapy should be continued for about 48 hours after delivery but in diminishing amounts. These patients should not be allowed out of bed until the process has definitely reversed itself.

Pathologic changes. The morphologic changes are mostly the result of the characteristic circulatory changes. Fibrin emboli and the acute degenerative changes that can be observed in the small vessels and the hemoconcentration of eclampsia certainly disturb the blood flow through the tissues and may lead to local anoxia and functional or anatomic disruption.

KIDNEY. Acute degenerative changes and fibrin deposition may be observed in the smaller vessels. The size of the glomerular capillary lumina is reduced by swelling of the endothelial cells, by the deposition of amorphous material beneath the normal basement membrane of the capillaries, and by proliferation of the intercapillary cells that lie between the vascular loops. These changes, called *glomerular endotheliosis,* which formerly were thought to be from thickening of the capillary basement membrane, have been clarified by electron microscopy. The tubular cells appear to be degenerated, but the changes probably are caused by excessive absorption of protein. *Cortical necrosis* may occur in women with severe abruptio placentae.

Histologic identification of the precise kidney lesion

will establish the diagnosis more accurately than will the clinical signs alone. In one study the changes characteristic of chronic renal disease were found in renal biopsies from 16 of 62 primigravidas in whom a diagnosis of preeclampsia had been made and in 32 of 152 multiparas diagnosed as having chronic hypertension with superimposed preeclampsia.

ADRENAL GLANDS. Adrenal hemorrhage and necrosis may occur, particularly in patients who die in a state of vascular collapse.

LIVER. Fibrin thrombi in the vessels and exudates and hemorrhage or actual tissue necrosis in the periportal areas may be found with severe preeclampsia-eclampsia. Extensive subcapsular hemorrhage often occurs when a coagulation defect develops. Liver involvement is minimal or absent with mild preeclampsia.

BRAIN. The same vascular changes may be observed in the brain as elsewhere. Hemorrhage from the rupture of large cerebral vessels is the cause of death in about 15% of women with eclampsia. Cerebral edema may be a postmortem change.

RETINAL VESSELS. Narrowing of the vessels and retinal edema may be observed relatively early. As the toxemia advances, hemorrhages and complete retinal detachment may occur. Recovery usually is complete.

Mortality. The maternal mortality for preeclampsia is low in general, and in the early stages there should be no mortality from the disease itself. As it progresses in severity, there may be mortality from the disease and also from the treatment. The maternal mortality for properly treated eclampsia should be less than 5%.

Principal causes of death are congestive heart failure, cerebral hemorrhage, and liver necrosis. Others are infection and adrenocortical necrosis with vascular collapse. Hemorrhage is even more lethal than with normal delivery because of hemoconcentration, which is so characteristic of eclampsia; much more hemoglobin is lost in concentrated than in an equal amount of normal blood.

The perinatal mortality also is high, averaging 20% to 25%. The principal causes of death are intrauterine anoxia, the complications of prematurity, toxemia, and infection.

Relationship of eclampsia/preeclampsia to chronic hypertension. There has been much discussion concerning the relationship between eclampsia and the subsequent development of chronic vascular disease. Most studies have suggested no direct relationship, but the numbers of women who could be included in such studies are small because so frequently the immediate prepregnancy blood pressure is unknown. In a classic study of 270 women who had been treated for eclampsia between 1931 and 1951, women who had eclampsia in the first pregnancy carried to viability had the same prevalence of hypertension more than 20 years later as did an unselected control group of the same ages. The remote mortality for white women who had eclampsia in the first pregnancy carried to viability was like that of the control group, but death rates were increased two to five times in all black women who had eclampsia and in white women whose eclampsia occurred after the first pregnancy. The authors suggest that this represents an increased basic tendency to the development of vascular disease rather than an effect of eclampsia and conclude that there is no relationship between eclampsia and the subsequent development of chronic vascular disease.

An unexpected finding in this study was that diabetes was increased two and one-half times in women who had eclampsia during the first pregnancy and four times if eclampsia developed in multiparous women.

CHRONIC HYPERTENSIVE DISEASE IN PREGNANCY

Essential hypertension may be present in a woman who becomes pregnant or may first manifest itself during pregnancy. It may become a serious complication jeopardizing the lives of both mother and infant.

Diagnosis. If the patient has a history of hypertension either between pregnancies or repeatedly during pregnancy, it is likely that the present episode is a chronic vascular disease. The blood pressure elevation usually is present before the twentieth week of pregnancy, and there may be other evidences of chronicity of the condition such as organic changes in the retinal vessels. Cardiac enlargement and serious renal pathologic findings are seldom encountered in hypertensive pregnant patients because they are usually young women who have not had severe hypertension long enough to produce these changes. If the elevation in blood pressure is not accompanied by edema (abnormal weight gain) and proteinuria, a diagnosis of essential hypertension is likely.

Effect of pregnancy on hypertension. Pregnancy often has no effect on the hypertension, but this cannot be relied on. In about a third of all pregnant women with essential hypertension, acute preeclampsia is superimposed on the chronic condition. This presents a much more serious problem than preeclampsia in the otherwise normal patient, and the incidence of both fetal and maternal death is increased. In another third of patients with chronic hypertension the blood pressure falls during the second trimester; it may reach normal levels, but this is the exception rather than the rule. Generally, it rises to at least its prepregnancy level during the last few weeks. In the remaining patients the blood pressure is unchanged throughout the entire pregnancy.

Effect of hypertension on pregnancy. In most women with essential hypertension, the pregnancy progresses uneventfully, but the complications that can develop are severe.

The principal danger from essential hypertension during pregnancy is to the fetus, but the mother's life may also be endangered. The infant almost always weighs less than do those born after normal pregnancies of the same duration. The cause of the *growth retardation* is altered placental function. The placenta usually is smaller than expected, and its functional capacity may be further reduced by *multiple small infarcts* as a result of hemorrhage into the decidua from maternal arterioles supplying the choriodecidual space. The placental tissue overlying the area of hemorrhage

separates. If enough placental tissue is involved, the placenta's ability to maintain normal function is reduced; fetal growth may be compromised, or the fetus may even die in utero. *Early abortion,* which occurs frequently, adds to the fetal loss. A patient who begins pregnancy with a systolic blood pressure higher than 200 mm Hg and a corresponding rise in diastolic pressure has no more than a 50% chance of delivering a normal baby.

ABRUPTIO PLACENTAE. About half of all cases of severe premature separation of the placenta occur in women with vascular disease. This is associated with a high fetal and an increased maternal mortality.

ACUTE PREECLAMPSIA. Of all women with vascular disease, 30 to 40% will develop signs characteristic of preeclampsia during pregnancy. The complication usually appears late in the second trimester at about the period of viability and is associated with a high fetal and maternal mortality. The signs appear earlier, and the disease progresses more rapidly than does the similar process in normal women. The blood pressure may rise to alarming heights in a few days, and renal function deteriorates rapidly. The condition is even less responsive to treatment than is preeclampsia in women with normal vascular function.

CEREBRAL HEMORRHAGE. Intracranial hemorrhage is a more common cause of death in chronic hypertensive disease than in preeclampsia because the vessels may have undergone an organic degenerative change and because the arterial blood pressure usually is much higher.

RENAL CORTICAL NECROSIS. Renal cortical necrosis is sometimes encountered in women with hypertension and premature placental separation.

Treatment. Patients with severe hypertension should be quickly and completely evaluated when first seen. The examination should include (1) general physical examination; (2) frequent blood pressure recordings; (3) eye examination for evidence of retinitis; (4) renal function studies such as fluid intake and urine output measurements, creatinine and uric acid clearances, quantitative protein determinations, and microscopic urine examination; (5) blood urea nitrogen determination; and (6) cardiac evaluation. A baseline is thus established for repeat examinations during pregnancy, and a decision can be made as to whether pregnancy should continue.

INTERRUPTION OF PREGNANCY. Pregnancy is dangerous, and interruption should be recommended if the systolic blood pressure is higher than 180 to 200 mm Hg or the diastolic pressure is 110 mm Hg or more and remains elevated after a period of bed rest, if there are degenerative changes in the retinal arterioles, if the patient has had a previous cerebral hemorrhage or preeclampsia during a previous pregnancy, or if renal function is reduced.

TEST OF PREGNANCY. If the pregnancy is allowed to continue, the patient is informed of her condition and advised of the possibilities. She is told to be prepared to enter the hospital at any time and to remain in the hospital for a long period. As long as the pregnancy remains uneventful, it is to be allowed to continue, but should the patient develop superimposed preeclampsia that does not respond to treatment, interruption must be considered.

PRENATAL CARE. Patients with chronic hypertension should be examined at least every 2 weeks and often more frequently. They should rest every morning and afternoon and spend at least 10 hours in bed each night.

Antihypertensive drugs may serve a useful purpose, particularly if the blood pressure is already being maintained at a normal level when conception occurs. If treatment is started during pregnancy, the initial drug should be a thiazide diuretic. If adequate control is not achieved, additional agents are added in a stepwise manner. Table 26-2 summarizes the effects of various antihypertensive agents.

Any prenatal patient with hypertension should be admitted to the hospital at once if (1) the blood pressure rises, (2) protein appears in the urine, (3) weight gain is abnormal or edema develops, or (4) symptoms appear.

TERMINATION OF PREGNANCY. If the patient with hypertension develops superimposed preeclampsia that cannot be controlled with medical treatment, the pregnancy must be terminated even though the infant is not yet viable. Indications for termination of pregnancy are (1) rising blood pressure that fails to respond to treatment, (2) increasing evidence of retinal vascular damage, or (3) decreasing renal function. Because these

women usually are multiparas, labor often can be induced by amniotomy if the cervix is effaced; otherwise, cesarean section may be necessary.

If the blood pressure remains stable throughout the pregnancy or falls slightly and if preeclampsia does not develop, the prognosis is reasonably good. It usually is advisable to induce labor as soon as conditions for induction are favorable and if amniotic fluid examination indicates fetal maturity because the fetal death rate increases after approximately 39 weeks.

CARE DURING LABOR. Hydralazine may be given if the blood pressure is unusually high or rises during labor. Nitroglycerin or nitroprusside can be used for acute hypertensive crisis as described previously.

POSTPARTUM CARE. During the immediate period after delivery the blood pressure must be taken at regular intervals because it may either rise rapidly or fall precipitously, and the output of urine must be recorded every hour until diuresis has been established.

Special problems. Special problems involve fetal death, abruptio placentae, and future pregnancies.

PREVIOUS FETAL DEATH. Some of the women may have had previous intrauterine fetal deaths at about the same time in each pregnancy. If the infant can be delivered either vaginally or by cesarean section while it is still alive, it may survive, even though it is premature. Tests for fetal well-being and continuing growth (indicating adequate placental function) are *periodic fetal activity, contraction stress tests, nonstress tests,* and *periodic sonographic measurement of various fetal diameters* to determine if they are increasing (Chapter 32).

ABRUPTIO PLACENTAE. Placental separation usually is severe and may be associated with a high mortality. The prompt transfusion and delivery of such patients will reduce the maternal mortality.

FUTURE PREGNANCIES. Tubal sterilization should be considered for any patient with essential hypertension who has evidence of degenerative vascular changes in the retinal vessels, decreased renal function, or cardiac enlargement. Those whose blood pressure is higher after each pregnancy and those who have had repeated intrauterine fetal deaths and premature placental separation also are poor risks for further pregnancy. If more pregnancies are not contraindicated, the deliveries

TABLE 26-2 Antihypertensive agents in pregnancy

Drug	Mechanism of action	Cardiac output	Renal blood flow	Side effects
Thiazide	*Initial:* Decreased plasma volume	Decreased	Decreased	*Maternal:* Electrolyte depletion, increased uric acid, thrombocytopenia, pancreatitis
	Later: Decreased peripheral vascular resistance	Unchanged	Unchanged	*Neonatal:* Thrombocytopenia
Methyldopa	False neurotransmitter	Unchanged	Unchanged	*Maternal:* Lethargy, fever, hepatitis, hemolysis, positive Coombs's test
Reserpine	Depletes norepinephrine from sympathetic nerve	Unchanged	Unchanged	*Maternal:* Nasal stuffiness, depression *Neonatal:* Nasal congestion, increased respiratory tract secretions, cyanosis
Hydralazine	Direct peripheral vasodilator	Increased	Unchanged	*Maternal:* Flushing, headache, tachycardia, palpitations, lupus syndrome
Beta-blockers	Beta-adrenergic blockade	Decreased	Decreased	*Maternal:* Increased uterine tone with possible decreased placental perfusion *Neonatal:* Depressed respirations
Prazosin	Direct peripheral	Unchanged	Unchanged	*Maternal:* Hypotension with initial dose; little data on use in pregnancy
Clonidine	CNS effect	Unchanged	Unchanged	*Maternal:* Rebound hypertension; little data on use in pregnancy
Ganglionic blockers	Decrease in peripheral resistance by adrenergic ganglionic blockade	Decreased	Decreased	*Maternal:* Marked sensitivity with secondary hypotension *Neonatal:* Meconium ileus

should be spaced about 18 months apart to complete childbearing while the patient is young and before the degenerative vascular changes appear.

Mortality. The maternal mortality is increased ten to twenty times over that of the normal patient, and the fetal loss is as high as 30 to 40%. The principal causes of death are abruptio placentae, eclampsia, cerebral hemorrhage, postpartum collapse, renal cortical necrosis, and infection. The mortality can be reduced by recognition of the fact that hypertension is a serious complication of pregnancy requiring special attention. Careful prenatal care and interruption of pregnancy at any time the vascular signs progress and fail to respond to treatment will contribute most to this reduction in deaths.

SUGGESTED READING

Benedetti TJ, Kates R, and Williams V: Hemodynamic observations in severe preeclampsia complicated by pulmonary edema, Am J Obstet Gynecol 152:330, 1985.

Cavanagh D, Papineni SR, Knuppel RA, Desai U, and Balis JU: Pregnancy-induced hypertension: development of a model in the pregnant primate, Am J Obstet Gynecol 151:987, 1985.

Chesley LC: Diagnosis of preeclampsia, Obstet Gynecol 65:423, 1985.

Chesley LC, Annitto JE, and Cosgrove RA: The familial factor in toxemia of pregnancy, Obstet Gynecol 32:303, 1968.

Chesley LC, Annitto JE, and Cosgrove RA: The remote prognosis of eclamptic women, Am J Obstet Gynecol 124:446, 1976.

Cotton DB, Lee W, Huhta CJ, and Dorman KF: Hemodynamic profile of severe pregnancy-induced hypertension, Am J Obstet Gynecol 158:523, 1988.

Easterling TR and Benedetti TJ: Preeclampsia: a hyperdynamic disease model, Am J Obstet Gynecol 160:1447, 1989.

Friedman SA: Preeclampsia: a review of the role of prostaglandins, Obstet Gynecol 71:122, 1988.

Gant NF, Chand S, Worley RJ, Whalley PJ, Crosby UD, and MacDonald PC: A clinical test useful for predicting the development of acute hypertension in pregnancy, Am J Obstet Gynecol 120:1, 1974.

Hughes EC, editor: Obstetric-gynecologic terminology, Philadelphia, 1972, FA Davis Co.

Lindheimer MD and Katz AI: Hypertension in pregnancy, N Engl J Med 313:675, 1985.

Pritchard JA, Cunningham FG, and Pritchard SA: The Parkland Memorial Hospital protocol for treatment of eclampsia: evaluation of 245 cases, Am J Obstet Gynecol 148:951, 1984.

Roberts JM: Pregnancy-related hypertension. In Creasy RK and Resnik R, editors: Maternal fetal medicine: principles and practice, Philadelphia, 1989, WB Saunders Co.

Rubin PC: Beta-blockers in pregnancy, N Engl J Med 305:1323, 1981.

Saleh AA, Bottoms SF, Welch RA, Ali AM, Mariona FG, and Mammen EF: Preeclampsia, delivery and the hemostatic mechanism, Am J Obstet Gynecol 157:331, 1987.

Schiff E, Peleg E, Goldenberg M, Rosenthal T, Ruppin E, and Tamarkin M: The use of aspirin to prevent pregnancy-induced hypertension and lower the ratio of thromboxane A2 to prostacyclin in relatively high risk pregnancies, N Engl J Med 321:351, 1989.

Sibai BM, Lipshitz J, Anderson GD, and Dilts PV Jr: Reassessment of intravenous MgSO$_4$ therapy in preeclampsia-eclampsia, Obstet Gynecol 57:199, 1981.

Spargo B, McCartney CP, and Winemiller R: Glomerular capillary endotheliosis in pregnancy, Arch Pathol 68:593, 1959.

Sutherland A, Cooper DW, Howie PW, Liston WA, and MacGillivray I: The incidence of severe pre-eclampsia amongst mothers and mothers-in-law of pre-eclamptics and controls, Br J Obstet Gynecol 88:785, 1981.

Weinstein L: Preeclampsia/eclampsia with hemolysis, elevated liver enzymes, and thrombocytopenia, Obstet Gynecol 66:657, 1985.

27

Russell K. Laros, Jr.

Bleeding during late pregnancy

Objectives

RATIONALE: Third-trimester bleeding may represent an obstetrical emergency. Prompt, logical evaluation and treatment are necessary to minimize the threat to mother and fetus.

The student should be able to:

A. Develop an approach to the diagnosis
and treatment of third-trimester bleeding.

B. List the signs and symptoms of placental abruption.

C. List the signs and symptoms of placenta previa.

At least half of the women who bleed from the vagina during late pregnancy do not have a serious lesion, but, because bleeding of any type is abnormal, the physician should attempt to determine its source whenever it occurs.

PLACENTA PREVIA

About once in every 200 deliveries (0.4%), the entire placenta or part of it is implanted in the lower portion of the uterus rather than in the upper active segment. This is called *placenta previa*.

Types (Fig. 27-1). The types of placenta previa are determined by the relationship of the placenta to the internal cervical os. In *complete placenta previa* the entire cervical os is covered by placen-

tal tissue; in *incomplete placenta previa* the os is only partially covered. *Marginal placenta previa* is one in which the edge of the placenta extends to the margin of the cervical opening. With a *low-lying placenta,* a portion of the placenta is implanted in the lower uterine segment, but the placental edge may be several centimeters above the internal os.

The classification is made on the basis of findings at the initial examination and may change as labor advances. For example, the placenta may encroach only slightly on the cervical opening when the cervix is dilated no more than 2 to 3 cm. As labor progresses and as the lower segment retracts, the inferior portion of the placenta will be separated from the uterine wall. When the cer-

338

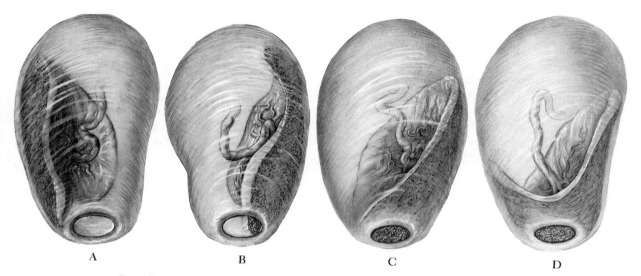

Fig. 27-1 Types of placenta previa. **A**, Marginal. **B**, Incomplete. **C** and **D**, Total.

vix is 6 to 8 cm dilated, as much as half of the opening may be covered by placenta. Conversely, if the border of the placenta extends just across the opening when labor begins, one cannot feel the edge, and complete placenta previa is diagnosed. As the cervix dilates, the placenta will be drawn upward with the retracting lower uterine segment; late in labor the placenta covers only part of the opening. If the first examination is made at this time, the diagnosis will be incomplete placenta previa.

Etiologic factors. The reasons that the ovum implants in the lower segment are not always obvious. Placenta previa occurs more often in multiparas than in primigravidas, in women who are pregnant late in their reproductive lives, and in those who have been delivered previously by cesarean section. The group at greatest risk are women with multiple prior cesarean sections. The risk rises linearly, with the number of prior sections reaching 10% with four or more cesarean deliveries.

Signs and symptoms. Bleeding is the most reliable single sign of placenta previa. Characteristi-

cally, the bleeding is painless, and the blood bright red because it flows directly into the vagina from the open sinuses just above the internal cervical os. The first bleeding occurs late in the second trimester or early in the third, usually before the thirty-second week. A few patients may have had bleeding, suggesting threatened abortion during the first half of pregnancy; others will have aborted. The initial episode usually consists of spotting or a gush of bright red blood. Overwhelming hemorrhage rarely occurs at the onset, unless the placental edge is separated from the uterine wall by digital examination or during coitus.

Each bleeding episode generally subsides, only to recur in a few days or at the most after a week or two. Subsequent bleedings are likely to become progressively heavier until, finally, profuse hemorrhage may occur. Occasionally, placenta previa produces no symptoms until late in pregnancy or even until labor begins.

The source of bleeding is maternal blood from the choriodecidual spaces, and the cause is the mechanical separation of a portion of the placenta from its uterine attachment as the lower segment lengthens during late pregnancy.

Diagnosis. Placenta previa can be suspected from a history of painless bleeding that begins during the last part of pregnancy.

EXAMINATION. The reason for bleeding can be determined only by examining the patient.

Abdominal examination. An exact diagnosis cannot be made by abdominal examination alone, but it may provide suggestive information. *Transverse lie and breech positions occur frequently with placenta previa. If the presenting part is high above the inlet and deviated anteriorly or laterally and cannot be pushed into the pelvic inlet, the placenta may be preventing its descent.* The location of the placental souffle is of little value in determining placental site.

Vaginal examination. A digital examination must be made at some time on almost every patient suspected of having placenta previa to confirm the diagnosis and to determine the degree of involvement. If the patient is bleeding profusely, vaginal examination should be performed as soon as arrangements can be made in the operating room because it undoubtedly will be necessary to deliver her regardless of the stage of the pregnancy.

Immediate vaginal examination for those who are several weeks from term and are bleeding only slightly is usually contraindicated. The manipulations necessary to make an accurate diagnosis may separate enough placenta to cause an alarming hemorrhage and force the delivery of a premature baby who may not live. Under such circumstances it is preferable to obtain a placental localization study and to withhold digital examination until the baby has matured enough to survive outside the uterus. A sterile speculum examination should be performed to eliminate a cervical lesion as the source of the bleeding, but the cervix should not be manipulated.

Vaginal examination should be performed when it is appropriate to terminate pregnancy, either because of hemorrhage or when pulmonary maturity has been documented. The following precautions are necessary:

1. The examination must be performed in an operating room that is ready for any type of treatment necessary to control the bleeding and deliver the patient.
2. Compatible blood, 1000 ml, should be available before the examination is made.
3. An operating team of obstetricians, anesthesiologists, and nurses must be available.
4. A pediatrician, an anesthesiologist, or an obstetrician should be available to resuscitate the infant if its respirations are depressed.

If the cervix is soft and patulous, the index finger is carefully introduced in an attempt to feel the cotyledons of a complete placenta previa covering the opening or the edge of an incomplete variety. If the fetal membranes and the presenting part are felt directly above the cervical os, the examining finger is swept gently around the lower segment in an attempt to reach the edge of the placenta. The finger is withdrawn as soon as the placenta is felt; vigorous manipulation will certainly separate more of it and initiate bleeding.

If the cervix is closed, no attempt should be made to force the finger through it.

Placental localization. If the implantation site can be located, one can either implicate or eliminate placenta previa as a likely cause of bleeding.

Placental localization studies are usually contraindicated if bleeding is profuse because it probably will be necessary to deliver the patient, and a decision as to the most appropriate method for delivery can only be made after the patient has been examined. Placental localization studies are also unnecessary after the thirty-seventh week of pregnancy. Women who bleed at this stage should generally be delivered promptly; hence diagnostic vaginal examination is appropriate.

Ultrasonography is the most accurate (95%) of all the methods of placental localization. It can be performed any time after the end of the first trimester, when the placenta can first be identified. The entire placenta and its relationship to the uterine wall and the cervical os can be seen in the sonogram (Fig. 27-2); hence the degree of placenta previa can be estimated. In contrast to other methods, posterior wall implantation can usually be seen clearly.

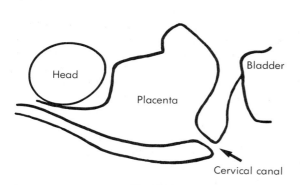 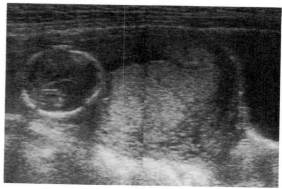

Fig. 27-2 Sonogram of complete placenta previa, longitudinal view.

The concept of "placental migration" must be considered in ultrasonic evaluation. During the second trimester, the placenta may cover as much as half the surface of the uterine cavity, and before the thirtieth week it often appears to be implanted near or over the cervix. As pregnancy advances, the lower uterine segment lengthens, and the placenta is drawn upward with the enlarging uterus. The placenta will be normally situated at term in almost all patients in whom an ultrasonic diagnosis of placenta previa is made during the early part of pregnancy. This is true even when the first study was made because of bleeding.

The rate of spontaneous resolution of placenta previa detected in the second trimester is about 90%. At 26 to 28 weeks, the sonogram should be repeated. If the condition is still present, it is more likely to persist to term. However, even when present at 26 weeks, asymptomatic placenta previa still has approximately a 75% chance of resolution by the time of delivery. Thus another sonogram should be performed at 36 weeks.

Differential diagnosis. Bleeding like that resulting from placenta previa can also be produced by benign or malignant lesions of the cervix, rupture of placental vessels, premature labor, premature separation of the normally implanted placenta (abruptio placentae), bladder or bowel lesions, and other causes. These can be excluded during the course of the examination.

Treatment. To maintain a low maternal and in-fant mortality, the treatment of placenta previa must be planned individually for each patient.

DELAYED TREATMENT. Under certain circumstances, termination of the pregnancy may be delayed in the interests of the fetus. Because placenta previa may manifest itself while the fetus is quite immature, immediate delivery is associated with a high fetal loss. This can be reduced if the pregnancy is allowed to continue until a later date. It is seldom appropriate to delay termination if the fetus is mature.

A placental localization study is obtained, and the cervix is inspected with a sterile speculum. No digital examinations are performed: the examining finger can separate the placental edge and precipitate bleeding profuse enough to require immediate delivery. If a lower segment implantation site is identified and the bleeding ceases or is slight, active treatment can be delayed until it is made necessary by a progressive increase in bleeding or by the onset of labor. When the pregnancy reaches the thirty-seventh week, the patient should usually be delivered if evaluation of the amniotic fluid ratio indicates that the fetus is mature.

Delayed treatment is feasible only if the bleeding is slight and if compatible blood and facilities for rapid treatment of hemorrhage are constantly available. Blood transfusions can be given if the hematocrit falls significantly after repeated small bleeds. Delay is contraindicated if the bleeding is profuse, if the fetus is dead or abnormal, or if the fetus is mature. If treatment facilities are inadequate, the patient should be transferred to a perinatal center for care.

Patients whose placenta previa is still present at 36 weeks and who are not anemic should be encouraged to donate two units of autologous blood. These donations should be made during the thirty-sixth week and be available at the time of delivery.

ACTIVE TREATMENT. When the patient is to be delivered, vaginal examination, performed with the precautions outlined previously, will indicate the condition of the cervix and type of placenta previa so that the proper method for delivery can be selected.

Incomplete placenta previa. Cesarean section is the best method for terminating pregnancy in most women with placenta previa.

If the fetus is dead, the cervix is soft and patulous, only an edge of placenta can be felt, and bleeding is minimal, vaginal delivery may be possible. This is particularly true if labor has already started. Induction of labor is hazardous but occasionally is a logical choice. Cesarean section is justifiable, even though the baby is dead, if bleeding is profuse and cannot be controlled.

Vaginal delivery may also be possible in an occasional multipara with a soft, effaced, and partially dilated cervix and a minor degree of anterior placenta previa. If the membranes are ruptured, the fetal head will descend, exert pressure against the placenta, and compress the bleeding uterine sinuses beneath it. *Vaginal delivery usually increases the hazard for the infant because compression of the placenta by the presenting part obstructs fetal vessels. If a large enough area of fetal circulation is eliminated, the infant will die of anoxia. Electronic fetal monitoring is essential in patients who are allowed to labor.*

Vaginal delivery is most appropriate before the twenty-eighth week, when the baby has little chance of surviving. Under these circumstances, if labor can be induced and bleeding controlled until the infant is de-

livered, the potential problems of a uterine scar during subsequent pregnancies will be prevented.

When vaginal delivery is selected, there are several possible methods for reducing maternal blood loss, but all are appropriate only when the baby is dead or has little chance of surviving. *Scalp traction* with a long Allis forceps or a tenaculum may be used if simple rupture of the membranes does not suffice. The force necessary to compress the maternal sinuses is supplied by manual traction on the forceps or a weight. When the breech presents and the cervix is partially dilated, one or both legs can be pulled down, permitting the *buttocks to tamponade the placenta.*

Whenever the placenta is implanted in the lower segment, the tissues in that part of the uterus and in the cervix are far more vascular and friable than in normal pregnancy. They are easily torn by manipulations designed to control bleeding from the placental site, and many deaths have occurred as a result of ill-advised attempts to effect delivery through the vagina simply to avoid cesarean section.

Complete placenta previa. The patient with complete placenta previa should be delivered by cesarean section, even though the fetus is dead.

SUPPORTIVE TREATMENT. Lost blood must be replaced with blood. No other fluid will do. Maternal mortality will be high if blood is not replaced promptly and adequately. Plasma, glucose, or saline solution may be used only as a temporary measure while blood is being obtained.

The steps in the diagnosis and management of women suspected of having placenta previa are shown in Fig. 27-3.

Effect of placenta previa on mother and infant. Low implantation of the placenta can be responsible for *early abortion. Postpartum hemorrhage* occurs more often because the lower segment does not contract and control bleeding as well as the upper part of the uterus.

Maternal deaths are mostly from blood loss and should be rare with adequate fluid therapy and blood replacement. The *perinatal death rates* in the Collaborative Perinatal Study were 176.06 for 142 white women and 190.91 for 110 black women with placenta previa. In the group of

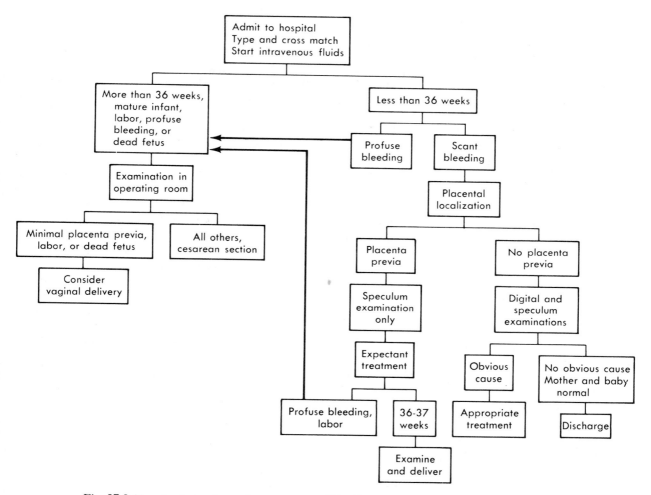

Fig. 27-3 Steps in diagnosing and management of bleeding during late pregnancy placenta previa.

white women the stillbirth rate was 70.42 and the neonatal death rate, 113.64. For black women the stillbirth rate was 63.64 and the neonatal death rate, 135.92. Comparable perinatal death rates for pregnancies not complicated by placenta previa were 26.17 for white women and 33.20 for black women.

The principal causes of perinatal mortality are *prematurity, intrauterine anoxia* as a result of placental separation and prolapsed cord, *respiratory distress syndrome, injury,* and occasionally *exsanguination from placental injury. Developmental anomalies* are more common with placenta previa.

Complications. *Placenta accreta* is frequently associated with placenta previa, especially if the patient has delivered previously by cesarean section. The coexistence of placenta previa and accreta was 67% in one series of women who had had multiple prior cesarean deliveries. In almost all cases, total abdominal hysterectomy is required to control hemorrhage.

Vasa previa is uncommon, occurring in only one in 3000 deliveries. It is the presence of a velamentous insertion of the umbilical cord such that the cord vessels course through the membranes over the cervical os. These unsupported fetal vessels are prone to rupture, especially at the time of rupture of the membranes. Fetal mortality has been reported to be 50% to 75% as a result of both fetal exsanguination and hypoxia caused by compression of the vessels by the presenting part. In order to make a diagnosis of vasa previa in time to save the fetus, a high degree of suspicion is required. The onset of bleeding with rupture of the membranes should prompt testing of the blood to differentiate between maternal and fetal blood. Immediate delivery by cesarean section is usually the only way to save the fetus.

ABRUPTIO PLACENTAE

The term *abruptio placentae,* or *premature separation of the normally implanted placenta,* indicates a complication of late pregnancy in which the placenta separates from its normal implantation site in the upper segment of the uterus before the birth of the baby. The mild types that ordinarily occur during labor are at least as common as placenta previa. The more severe ones, however, usually occur before the onset of labor and are encountered approximately once in 500 deliveries. If the placenta is completely detached from the uterine wall, *complete separation* can be diagnosed, but, if a portion of it retains its connection, it is termed *partial separation.*

Etiologic factors. The cause of placental separation is not always obvious, but *trauma* and *short umbilical cord* play a minor role in its production.

Premature separation occurs more often in woman of *high parity* than in those who have had no more than five children.

Hypertension is often associated with abruption placentae, the reported incidence varying from about 11% to about 65%. Elevated blood pressure is more likely to be present in women with complete placental separation than in those with minor degrees.

The *supine hypotensive syndrome,* in which the vena cava is compressed by the weight of the uterus, has been suggested as a cause of premature placental separation. The increased venous pressure below the block may produce bleeding in the choriodecidual space and placental separation. Although this may occur, it probably does not do so often. Vena caval ligation during pregnancy does not necessarily interfere with uterine circulation.

Severe abruptio placentae *recurs* in about 10% of patients, probably because the factors causing the initial separation are still present. Submucous fibroids and uterine anomalies are the most common recurring causes.

Cigarette smoking has been reported to be associated with decidual necrosis. There is an increased incidence of abruption in women who smoke more than 10 cigarettes per day during pregnancy.

Cocaine abuse is also associated with an increased incidence of placental abruption. Most likely this association is related to the vasoactive properties of cocaine. At our county hospital, 5% of women who use cocaine during the last trimester of pregnancy have pregnancies that terminate with an abruption.

ACCIDENTS OF LABOR. Any sudden decrease in size of a uterus overdistended by hydramnios or multiple pregnancies may produce partial placental separation.

Mechanism of separation and clinical course. Bleeding into the decidua basalis from disruption of an abnormal blood vessel separates an area of placenta from its attachment to the uterus. The extent of placental separation is determined by the amount of decidual bleeding. If the area is small and the bleeding is readily controlled by the pressure from the surrounding tissues, a small infarct may develop. If the bleeding is more extensive, part or all of the placenta may be dissected off the uterine wall.

As the bleeding continues, the blood may remain in the retroplacental area, gradually dissecting the placenta off the uterine wall without any visible hemorrhage at the onset. This is known as *concealed bleeding.* The blood may also remain concealed if it dissects upward between the membranes and the uterus rather than downward toward the cervix and if the fetal head occludes the internal os so completely that the blood cannot escape into the vagina. In most instances, the blood escapes from beneath the placenta, dissects the membranes off the uterine wall, and flows through the cervix, producing *external hemorrhage.*

The physiologic effects of hemorrhage are directly related to the volume of blood lost, but the signs may not correlate with the amount of *visible* bleeding. This occurs in part because a large volume of blood may be retained within the uterine cavity *(concealed hemorrhage),* but there are other reasons. Blood is also lost through hemorrhage into the uterine wall *(Couvelaire uterus or uteroplacental apoplexy),* through extrauterine hematoma formation, and through bleeding beneath serosal surfaces and mucous membranes if a *clotting defect* develops. An overt clotting defect is most likely to occur with complete placental separation, but alterations in the clotting mechanism may develop with less serious varieties.

The clotting defect is caused by activation of the normal coagulation mechanism. Thromboplastin from abnormal subplacental decidua, the disrupted placenta, and serum in the subplacental clot enters the bloodstream through the open vessels at the placental site and initiates an exaggerated intravascular clotting process. Fibrinogen is converted to fibrin, which may occlude small vessels throughout the body, producing local tissue anoxia. As more thromboplastin is introduced into the circulation, more fibrinogen and consumable clotting factors are used and become seriously depleted. The blood then becomes incoagulable, and abnormal bleeding is evident.

Because the coagulation defect is a *consumption coagulopathy,* or *disseminated intravascular coagulation,* factors other than fibrinogen are involved. Factors V, VIII, and XIII and platelets are consumed. A fibrinolytic process that disintegrates the fibrin emboli is initiated; as a consequence, *fibrin degradation (split) products* form.

They inhibit platelet aggregation and have a direct antithrombin effect that interferes with fibrin conversion and the production of normal fibrin threads in the clot.

Patients with severe abruptio placentae may develop anuria because of *acute tubular necrosis* or *bilateral renal cortical necrosis.* Those with tubular necrosis will recover if the damage is not too extensive, but they may need renal dialysis. Most patients with cortical necrosis die. These lesions seem to develop because of intrarenal vasospasm, and their severity is probably determined by the amount of blood lost and the depth and duration of hypovolemic shock. The outcome appears to be related directly to how rapidly and completely blood is replaced.

The less severe types of placental separation usually occur during labor and may be the result of mechanical separation of a portion of placenta. This can be suspected if the patient develops more pain than she has been experiencing, particularly if the fetal heart tones become a bit irregular, the vaginal bleeding increases, and the labor becomes tumultuous. This type of separation ordinarily does not affect maternal or infant mortality.

Signs and symptoms. *Bleeding* associated with *pain* that varies in severity is characteristic of premature separation of a normally implanted placenta. In one large series, vaginal bleeding occurred in 78% of 59 cases, uterine tenderness or back pain in 66%, fetal distress in 60%, high-frequency contractions in 17%, uterine hypertonus in 17%, premature labor in 22%, and dead fetus in 15%.

The pain may come on suddenly and be severe and constant when there is a major separation or milder and intermittent with a less severe lesion.

The blood may be dark or even clotted if it is retained within the uterine cavity for a time before it is discharged into the vagina. This is in contrast to the bright red blood with placenta previa, which comes from the placental site just within the cervical opening. Discharge may consist only of blood-stained serum, which is squeezed out of the retroplacental clot. If there is a considerable amount of concealed bleeding, the pain will increase in severity as the uterus becomes distended and the muscular wall is infiltrated with blood.

Diagnosis. Ordinarily, it is not difficult to recognize the severe forms of abruptio placentae, but milder degrees may be less obvious.

CLINICAL EXAMINATION. In most instances the diagnosis can be made by history and clinical examination of the patient.

Abdominal examination. The abdominal findings change as the condition progresses in severity, but, in general, the *uterus feels firm and is tender to the touch*. At the onset the tenderness may be confined to a small area of the uterine wall, but eventually the gentlest palpation at any point produces pain.

If there is a considerable amount of concealed bleeding, the uterus will gradually enlarge as the blood collects within its cavity and infiltrates the muscular wall.

At the onset, intermittent uterine contractions can usually be palpated, but eventually they may no longer be discernible. The uterus is hard and tetanically contracted, and one may not be able to outline fetal parts because of tenderness and the contracted uterus. Uterine contractions are usually of higher frequency but lower amplitude than in normal labor. Because the baseline tonus is frequently elevated, contractions may be difficult to palpate and may not be recorded by an external tocodynamometer.

Fetal heart rate. The fetal heart tones may be normal if only a small amount of placenta is separated, or they may be completely absent in the more severe forms. Slow and irregular fetal heart tones suggest severe intrauterine hypoxia.

Vaginal examination. Vaginal examination should usually be performed in the delivery or operating room as an aid in diagnosis and to determine how delivery will be effected. In contrast to placenta previa, placental tissue will not be felt within the cervical canal, and the presenting part may be deep in the pelvis rather than high, as it is with an abnormally implanted placenta.

Ultrasound examination. A subplacental blood clot can sometimes be detected, but failure to identify a clot does not eliminate abruptio placentae. Sonography is appropriate only for minor degrees of separation as an aid in clinical diagnosis.

Laboratory examinations. The hemoglobin may be reduced, the level depending on the amount of bleeding. The white blood cell count often is elevated to 20,000 or 30,000, whereas in placenta previa it is more likely to be within the normal range.

A *clotting defect* is present in 10% of cases of abruption and is more common in severe abruption associated with either fetal death or brisk hemorrhage. The proposed mechanism is disseminated intravascular coagulation (DIC) initiated by an infusion of serum from the retroplacental clot into the maternal vascular compartment. Serum is a potent stimulant of intravascular clotting and leads to rather prompt consumption of fibrinogen, factor V, and factor VIII and stimulation of fibrinolysis. To a lesser degree, platelets are also consumed. Whenever the diagnosis of placental abruption is entertained, coagulation studies (platelet count, prothrombin time, partial thromboplastin time, fibrinogen, and a test for fibrin split products) should be ordered promptly and repeated at regular intervals. While awaiting the results of formal coagulation studies, information can be gathered by observing a tube of whole blood allowed to stand undisturbed *(clot observation test)*. If a clot fails to form or forms and is promptly lysed, a coagulation abnormality can be assumed.

Differential diagnosis. Abruptio placentae can be confused with placenta previa, but in most instances it is possible to differentiate between them (see box on p. 347).

Treatment. Each patient must be carefully evaluated before a plan for treatment is evolved.

COMPLETE PLACENTAL SEPARATION. Complete placental separation usually occurs before the onset of labor. The infant often is dead, and the patient is in poor condition from blood loss. The first step in treatment is to improve the general condition by treating shock with

ABRUPTIO PLACENTAE VS. PLACENTA PREVIA

Abruptio placentae

1. The bleeding usually is accompanied by pain.
2. The blood usually is dark.
3. Signs of shock may be out of proportion to visible bleeding.
4. The first bleeding often is profuse.
5. The uterus may be firm, tender, and tetanically contracted.
6. The fetus may be difficult to feel, and fetal heart tones may be absent or irregular.
7. The placenta cannot be felt.
8. The patient may have acute or chronic hypertensive disease, but the blood pressure may be low because of excessive bleeding.
9. The urine may contain protein, or the patient may be anuric.
10. A clotting defect may be present.

Placenta previa

1. The bleeding is painless unless labor has started.
2. The blood is bright red.
3. Observed bleeding and signs of shock usually are comparable.
4. The bleeding is usually slight at the onset.
5. The uterus is soft, not tender, and may be contracting if labor has started.
6. The fetus can be felt easily, and fetal heart tones usually are present.
7. The placenta may be felt.
8. There usually is no hypertensive disease.

9. The urine usually is normal.

10. The blood usually clots normally.

oxygen and intravenous fluid, followed as rapidly as possible by an appropriate volume of red blood cells.

Whenever the diagnosis of abruptio placentae is suspected, blood is drawn for a *clot observation test* and for *basic coagulation studies*. If the blood fails to clot or if an unstable clot forms and disintegrates, a clotting defect can be diagnosed, and treatment should be started. The clot observation test does not detect falling levels of fibrinogen. The normal concentrations of plasma fibrinogen during pregnancy range between 300 and 700 mg/dl, and the clotting test does not change until the concentration is less than 100 mg/dl. The actual concentration of fibrinogen and numbers of platelets should be measured at intervals in women with abruptio placentae who do not have an overt coagulation defect.

Transfusion with appropriate blood product is tailored to the individual patient's needs. Red cells are appropriate when bleeding is ongoing and the patient has lost $\geq 25\%$ of her blood volume or when the hemoglobin falls below 7 g/dl. A combination of *fresh frozen plasma* and *cryoprecipitate* will replace the deficient plasma factors. If the platelet count is below 50×10^9/L or below 100×10^9/L and cesarean section is planned, *platelet concentrates* are also indicated.

Many patients with placental separation are given inadequate amounts of blood. This may contribute to the development of renal failure and delay reversal of the abnormal coagulation mechanism. Some patients may need as much as 6 L or more to replenish the blood adequately. The amount of blood and fluid required to correct hypovolemia and to maintain a normal volume is best determined by continuous *central venous pressure* or *pulmonary wedge pressure measurement*.

DELIVERY. Patients with severe abruptio placentae should be delivered as soon as possible. Prompt delivery will prevent the development of abnormal clotting if the mechanism has not already been disturbed. If a coagulation defect is present, delivery will remove the source of thromboplastin, which initiates clotting, and the abnormal mechanism will reverse itself promptly. In addition, delivery will allow the uterus to contract and control bleeding.

Even though the cervix is uneffaced, vaginal delivery may be possible. Therefore a sterile vaginal examination should be performed *to rupture the membranes* soon after emergency treatment has been started. Dilute *oxytocin* solution can also be administered intravenously to stimulate uterine contractions. Oxytocin solution must be given with even more than the usual care because the uterus can rupture if it is infiltrated with blood.

Vaginal delivery is more often possible in multiparas than in primigravidas, but one may be surprised by the rapidity with which many primigravidas deliver. If labor has already begun, amniotomy may hasten its progress. Electronic fetal monitoring is essential, and cesarean section should be performed promptly if evidence of fetal distress is detected.

Cesarean section, in the interest of the fetus, should be considered with the milder forms of abruptio placentae if bleeding and uterine tenderness are increasing and delivery is not imminent. Conversely, cesarean section performed solely in the interest of the fetus is contraindicated if the fetal heart monitor tracing indicates irreversible damage. In cases in which profuse bleeding continues even though the fetus has died, cesarean section should be performed if early vaginal delivery cannot be anticipated.

Uteroplacental apoplexy is caused by the coagulation defect, and the bleeding into the uterine wall and from serous surfaces should respond to its treatment. Hysterectomy should seldom be necessary to control bleeding.

INCOMPLETE PLACENTAL SEPARATION. Incomplete placental separation usually occurs during labor and is much less severe than the complete variety. The only treatment usually necessary is to hasten labor by rupturing the membranes, to administer oxygen to the mother, and to complete the delivery as soon as it can be done safely. Fetal heart rate should be monitored continuously. If the fetal heart pattern remains normal, no particular haste is necessary, but, if the infant shows signs of hypoxia, delivery as soon as it can be accomplished safely usually is advised. The uterus almost always contracts well, and bleeding is not excessive because clotting defects rarely, if ever, occur with milder types of premature separation.

Perinatal mortality. The perinatal mortality reported by the Collaborative Perinatal Study was 144.61 in 408 white women and 295.73 in 328 black women with partial abruptio placentae. The rates for complete separation were 862.07 in 29 white women and 826.09 in 46 black women. Perinatal mortality rates in white women without abruptio placentae was 23.88 and in black women, 28.94.

In a more recent series of 59 cases, a fetal mortality of 17% and neonatal mortality of 14% was reported. The perinatal mortality of infants alive on admission was 18%. Mortality for those delivered vaginally was 20%, and for those delivered by cesarean section it was 15%. The principal causes of death are anoxia from placental separation, the complications of prematurity, and maternal toxemia.

Maternal mortality. The maternal death rate should be about 1%. It has been suggested that results with vaginal delivery are better than those with cesarean section, but this is not borne out by experience in most clinics. Most patients with more serious abruptio placentae are delivered by section, whereas those with the less severe forms are delivered vaginally, thus weighing the statistics in favor of vaginal delivery. Patients who are given liberal blood volume replacement and in whom coagulation defects are recognized and corrected are most likely to survive.

Anuria may follow abruptio placentae. This occurs most often in association with the severe lesions occurring in hypertensive patients. Failure to produce urine may result from renal cortical necrosis, in which event treatment appears to be valueless, or from *tubular necrosis,* the course of which may be influenced by adequate care. It may be possible to prevent renal complications by prompt recognition and treatment of coagulation defects and by early and adequate blood replacement.

OTHER CAUSES OF BLEEDING

Cervical lesions. Benign or malignant lesions of the cervix may bleed during late pregnancy, particularly if the cervix is manipulated. The cervix should be inspected as part of the examination of any pregnant woman with bleeding. Tissue should be taken for biopsy from any suspicious-looking cervical lesion. Lesions other than carcinoma ordinarily need not be treated.

Bladder and bowel lesions. The source of the bleeding may not always be obvious to the patient and may come from bladder or bowel lesions. Hemorrhoids often bleed during pregnancy, and occasionally a pregnant woman will bleed from benign or malignant rectal lesions. Bladder hemorrhage can be detected by examining a catheterized specimen of urine.

SUGGESTED READING

Abdella TN, Sibai BM, Hays JM, and Anderson GD: Relationship of hypertensive disease to abruptio placentae, Obstet Gynecol 63:365, 1984.

Chervenak FA, Lee Y, Hendler MA, Monoson RF, and Berkowitz RL: Role of attempted vaginal delivery in the management of placenta previa, Obstet Gynecol 64:798, 1984.

Clark SL, Koonings PP, and Phelan JP: Placenta previa/accreta and prior cesarean section, Obstet Gynecol 66:89, 1985.

Comeau J, Shaw L, Marcell CC, and Lavery JR: Early placenta previa and delivery outcome, Obstet Gynecol 61:577, 1983.

Cotton DB, Read JA, Paul RH, and others: The conservative aggressive management of placenta previa, Am J Obstet Gynecol 137:687, 1980.

Crenshaw C Jr, Jones D, and Parker RT: Placenta previa: a survey of twenty years' experience with improved perinatal survival by expectant therapy and cesarean delivery, Obstet Gynecol Surv 28:461, 1973.

Hurd WW, Miodovnik M, Hertzberg V, and Lavin JP: Selective management of abruptio placentae: a prospective study, Obstet Gynecol 61:467, 1983.

Knab DR: Abruptio placentae: an assessment of the time and method of delivery, Obstet Gynecol 52:625, 1978.

McShane PM, Heyl PS, and Epstein MF: Maternal and perinatal mortality resulting from placenta previa, Obstet Gynecol 65:176, 1985.

Niswander KR, and Gordon M: The women and their pregnancies: The Collaborative Perinatal Study of the National Institute of Neurological Diseases and Stroke, Philadelphia, 1972, WB Saunders Co.

Odendal HJ: Uterine contraction patterns in patients with severe abruptio placentae, S Afr Med J 57:908, 1980.

Pritchard JA and Brekken AL: Clinical and laboratory studies on severe abruptio placentae, Am J Obstet Gynecol 97:681, 1967.

Pritchard JA, Mason R, Corley M, and Pritchard S: Genesis of severe placental abruption, Am J Obstet Gynecol 108:22, 1970.

Sher G and Statland BE: Abruptio placentae with coagulopathy: a rational basis for management, Clin Obstet Gynecol 28:15, 1985.

Silver R, Depp R, Sabbagha RE, Dooley SL, Socol ML, and Tamura RK: Placenta previa: aggressive expectant management, Am J Obstet Gynecol 150:15, 1984.

Tatum HJ and Mulé JG: Placenta previa: a functional classification and a report on 408 cases, Am J Obstet Gynecol 93:767, 1965.

28

J. Robert Willson

Determination of position and lie

Objectives

RATIONALE: Exact identification of fetal presentation and position are essential in determining whether normal labor and delivery are likely to occur.

The student should be able to:
A. Define the terms *lie, presentation, position,* and *fetal attitude.*
B. Describe the possible fetal presentations.
C. Describe how the clinical diagnoses of presentation and position are made.

The position of the fetus within the uterine cavity is of no importance during pregnancy, but it must be favorably situated if labor and delivery are to progress normally.

The term *lie* refers to the relationship between the long axis of the mother and the long axis of the infant. In a *transverse lie* the infant's spine crosses that of the mother at a right angle, whereas in a *longitudinal lie* the fetal and maternal spines are parallel. In an *oblique lie* the baby's spine crosses the mother's at an acute angle.

The *presenting part* is the portion of the fetus that descends first through the birth canal. It is therefore the part that can be palpated through the cervix with the examining finger. *Presentation,* which has been used as a synonym of *lie,* is now generally used to indicate the intrauterine situa-

tion of the fetus somewhat more accurately and simply. For example, the terms *face* and *breech presentation* are used to indicate longitudinal lies in which the face or the breech is the presenting part.

The exact fetal *position* is determined by the relationship of some definite part of the baby (the presenting part) to a fixed area of the maternal pelvis. The presenting part may be directed anteriorly toward the symphysis, posteriorly toward the sacrum, laterally toward the acetabula, obliquely anteriorly toward the area between the symphysis and the acetabula, or obliquely posteriorly toward the area between the sacrum and the acetabula. The possible positions clockwise around the pelvis are therefore direct anterior (A), left anterior (LA), left transverse (LT), left posterior (LP), direct posterior (P), right posterior (RP), right transverse (RT), and right anterior (RA) (Fig. 28-1).

Attitude refers to the relationship of the parts of the fetus to each other. This, ordinarily, is one of complete flexion with the chin resting on the chest, the spine flexed in a smooth curve, the arms folded across the chest, and the hips and knees flexed. With the *deflexed attitude* the head is extended, and the curve of the spine is reduced (Fig. 28-2).

The position and presentation vary considerably

during pregnancy because the fetus can move freely within the amniotic cavity, particularly when there is a relatively large amount of fluid. During the last 8 weeks of pregnancy, the fetal mass expands rapidly, and the volume of amniotic fluid is relatively decreased. As a consequence, the fetus fills the uterine cavity more completely, it can no longer move freely, and its position becomes more stable. Some portion of the fetal head is the presenting part in about 96% of women at term, but this is not true during the earlier weeks. Breech presentation can be diagnosed in about a third of all women at the middle of pregnancy, but the incidence gradually decreases to about 3.5% at delivery. Transverse lies are encountered in only 0.25% to 0.5% of deliveries at term, but the total incidence at some time during pregnancy is far greater.

Of all the reasons that have been advanced to account for the preponderance of vertex positions, the most logical is that the infant can accommodate itself most comfortably to the shape of the uterine cavity with its head down. The buttocks, thighs, and feet are more bulky than the head and fit better in the comparatively wide uterine fundus than in the lower segment.

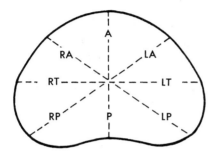

Fig. 28-1 Directions of fetal position in maternal pelvis from below.

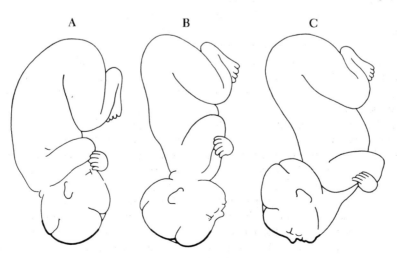

Fig. 28-2 Degrees of deflexion of head. **A,** Flexed (occiput position). **B,** Partially deflexed (brow position). **C,** Completely deflexed (face position).

DIAGNOSIS OF FETAL POSITION

The physician can usually determine position by clinical examination alone, particularly if the pregnancy is well advanced. Until about the thirtieth week, however, diagnosis is less accurate because the fetus is small and there may be a relatively large amount of amniotic fluid. Fortunately, precise diagnosis of position is of little importance before the last 8 weeks because it changes frequently and because abnormalities in presentation are far less formidable complications of labor during early pregnancy than they are later, when the infant is much larger.

Abdominal palpation. A reasonably accurate diagnosis of the position of the infant can be made by abdominal palpation unless the abdominal wall is unusually thick or resistant, the uterus is tender or irritable, or there is an excessive amount of amniotic fluid. Any of these may prevent the physician from outlining the fetal structures.

Abdominal examination should be performed systematically and gently with the patient in the dorsal position on the examining table (Fig. 28-3). The examiner first determines which fetal pole occupies the fundus of the uterus. The head is round, firm, and smooth and can be ballotted between the fingers if there is enough fluid; the breech is softer, less regular, more pointed, and not ballottable. The back is located by palpating through the sides of the uterus with the palmar surfaces of the fingers of each hand. The fetal spine presents a smooth convex curve in contrast to the ventral surface, which is concave, soft, and irregular; the motion of the extremities can be felt on the side opposite the back.

The fetal pole that lies over the inlet should be felt next to identify the presenting part; the fetal pole is easier to identify if it has not yet entered the pelvic inlet than if it is deeply engaged. If the vertex is presenting, one can usually palpate the *cephalic prominence,* which is, as the name implies, the part of the fetal head that is most readily felt. This area, which is opposite the back if the head is flexed and on the same side as the

back in deflexed attitudes, can usually be felt without difficulty unless the face is pointed almost directly posteriorly (Fig. 28-3, *C*). The examiner can tell how deeply the head has descended through the inlet by grasping it between the fingers of one or both hands and attempting to move it back and forth or by palpating the anterior shoulder to determine how far it has descended toward the pubis.

Auscultation of the fetal heart. This method is not accurate for determining position, although the heart is usually heard best above the level of the umbilicus with breech positions and in the lower quadrants when the head presents. The heart sounds are transmitted through the area of the fetal chest wall that lies in contact with the uterine wall and are usually loudest about a third of the distance from the mother's umbilicus to the anterior superior iliac spine in occipitoanterior positions and more laterally in the occipitoposterior positions. The heart may be inaudible in obese women or those with hydramnios or if the infant's position is unfavorable.

Vaginal examination. Identification of the presenting part by direct digital palpation will aid in establishing position. For greatest accuracy the cervix must be open enough to permit the insertion of the finger; consequently, this method is more often used during labor than earlier in pregnancy. The landmarks on the presenting part may be obscured by edema or intact membranes, and if there has been little descent, the physician may be unable to insert the finger deeply enough to reach it.

The principal identifying structures on the fetal skull are the diamond-shaped *anterior fontanel (bregma),* the triangular *posterior fontanel,* and the *sagittal suture,* which connects the two (Fig. 28-4).

The posterior fontanel is located at the juncture of the sagittal suture and the two lambdoidal sutures. The anterior fontanel is located at the juncture of the sagittal suture, the frontal suture, and the two coronal sutures.

The anterior fontanel is usually the larger of the

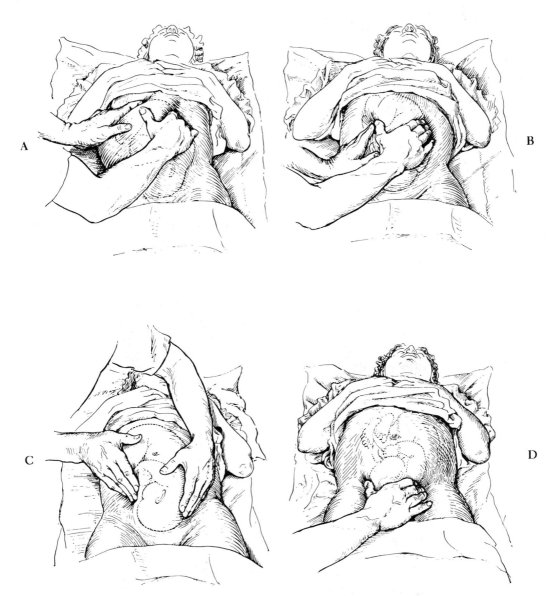

Fig. 28-3 Diagnosis of fetal position. **A,** Palpation of superior pole. **B,** Palpation of fetal back and small parts. **C,** Palpation of cephalic prominence. **D,** Ballottement of presenting part.

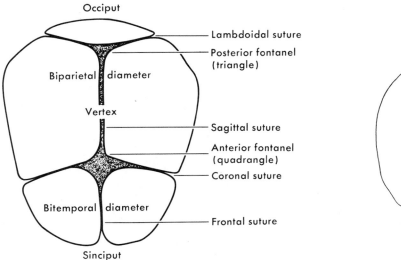

Fig. 28-4 Landmarks on fetal skull.

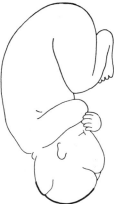

Fig. 28-5 Occiput position. Note smooth curve of flexed spine and head. Cephalic prominence (forehead) is on same side as fetal small parts.

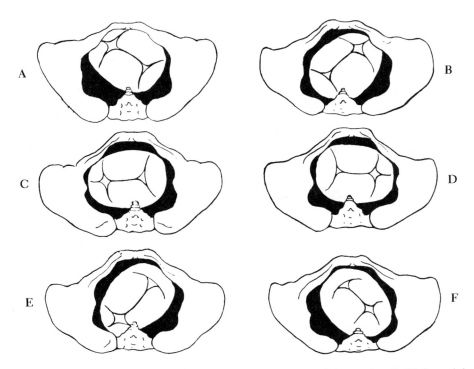

Fig. 28-6 Landmarks on fetal skull in various occiput positions. **A,** Left occipitoanterior. **B,** Right occipitoposterior. **C,** Left occipitotransverse. **D,** Right occipitotransverse. **E,** Left occipitoanterior. **F,** Right occipitoanterior.

two, but, if the head is molded, the differences in size and shape may not be appreciable. It usually is possible to identify a fontanel by sweeping the examining finger around it and counting the sutures that enter it, four anteriorly and three posteriorly.

Sonography. If the presentation and position cannot be determined by physical examination, the presentation can be identified by an ultrasonographic study.

LONGITUDINAL LIE

In longitudinal lies, some portion of the head is almost always the presenting part.

Occiput positions. In the occiput positions, which comprise about 96% of all vertex presenta-

tions, the fetal head is flexed, and its occipital portion becomes the presenting part (Fig. 28-5). On abdominal examination, the breech is felt in the fundus, the back on the right or left side of the uterus, and the head in the inlet in a flexed attitude, with the cephalic prominence on the side opposite the back. The landmarks on the fetal skull and their relationships to the bony pelvis as they would feel on vaginal examination are illustrated in Fig. 28-6.

The possible occiput positions are also shown in Fig. 28-7. Their abbreviations are as follows:

Occipitoanterior	OA
Left occipitoanterior	LOA
Left occipitotransverse	LOT
Left occipitoposterior	LOP

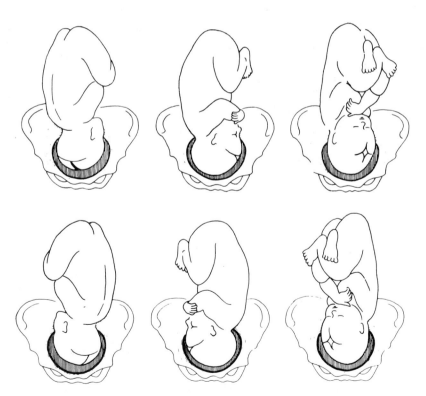

Fig. 28-7 Varieties of occiput positions. *Left to right: above,* right occipitoanterior, right occipitotransverse, and right occipitoposterior; *below,* left occipitoanterior, left occipitotransverse, and left occipitoposterior.

Occipitoposterior   OP
Right occipitoposterior   ROP
Right occipitotransverse   ROT
Right occipitoanterior   ROA

Of these, approximately 60% are occipitotransverse, 15% to 20% are oblique anterior or posterior, and the rest are direct anterior or posterior positions when labor begins. The position is determined by the shape of the bony pelvic canal. The long anteroposterior axis of the oval fetal skull tends to accommodate itself to the long axis of the pelvic inlet, which is most often the transverse, thus accounting for the predominance of occipitotransverse positions. In the direct occipitoanterior or posterior positions the anteroposterior axis of the bony pelvis is usually longer than the transverse.

Brow positions. If the head is partially extended, some part of the vertex anterior to the occiput becomes the presenting part (Fig. 28-8). The position is designated as a brow or frontum when the area of the head between the anterior fontanel and the supraorbital ridges descends first through the cervix. The possible brow positions and their abbreviations are as follows:

Frontoanterior   FA
Left frontoanterior   LFA

Left frontotransverse   LFT
Left frontoposterior   LFP
Frontoposterior   FP
Right frontoposterior   RFP
Right frontotransverse   RFT
Right frontoanterior   RFA

Face positions. If the head is completely deflexed to a point at which its occipital region lies in contact with the infant's back, the face descends through the birth canal first, and the chin (mentum) becomes the presenting part (Fig. 28-9). The possible face positions and their abbreviations are as follows:

Mentoanterior   MA
Left mentoanterior   LMA
Left mentotransverse   LMT
Left mentoposterior   LMP
Mentoposterior   MP
Right mentoposterior   RMP
Right mentotransverse   RMT
Right mentoanterior   RMA

Breech positions. If the breech or buttocks present at the pelvic inlet, the sacrum becomes the guiding point, and the possible positions and their abbreviations are as follows:

Sacroanterior   SA
Left sacroanterior   LSA

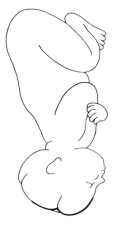

Fig. 28-8 Brow position. Note deflexion of head, extension of spine, and cephalic prominence on each side.

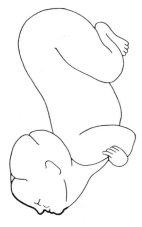

Fig. 28-9 Face position. Note extension of spine and complete deflexion of head with cephalic prominence on same side as fetal back.

Left sacrotransverse	LST
Left sacroposterior	LSP
Sacroposterior	SP
Right sacroposterior	RSP
Right sacrotransverse	RST
Right sacroanterior	RSA

TRANSVERSE LIE

A transverse lie or shoulder presentation is one in which the long axis of the fetus lies at a right angle to that of the mother. The position is designated according to the quadrant of the pelvis toward which the scapula is directed. The possible positions and their designated abbreviations are as follows:

Left scapuloanterior	LScA
Left scapuloposterior	LScP
Right scapuloposterior	RScP
Right scapuloanterior	RScA

SUGGESTED READING

Hughey MJ: Fetal position during pregnancy, Am J Obstet Gynecol 153:885, 1985.

Scheer K and Nubar J: Variation of fetal presentation with gestational age, Am J Obstet Gynecol 125:269, 1975.

29

J. Robert Willson

Labor and delivery

B. Describe the principles of managing patients whose membranes have ruptured prematurely.

Postdates Pregnancy

RATIONALE: Perinatal mortality and morbidity are increased significantly with postdates pregnancy. These can be reduced by early diagnosis and appropriate management.

The student should be able to:
A. Define postdate pregnancy.
B. Describe the risks for the fetus.
C. Describe methods of diagnosis and the principles of management.

Labor is the mechanism by which the products of conception are expelled from the uterus and vagina and the beginning regression of the pelvic organs is initiated. This is accomplished almost entirely by the activity of the uterine muscles.

Certain definitions that are essential to an understanding of labor and delivery are based on the duration of pregnancy. Pregnancies are dated from the first day of the last normal menstrual period, even though fertilization does not occur until later. *Abortion* is the expulsion of the products of conception before 20 completed weeks. Termination between the beginning of the twenty-first week and the end of the twenty-seventh week is called *immature labor*. Delivery between the beginning of the twenty-eighth week and the end of the thirty-sixth week when the infant weighs about 2500 g is called *premature labor*. The difference between prematurity based on weight and on duration of pregnancy is discussed later. *Delivery at term* occurs between the beginning of the thirty-seventh week and the end of the forty-second week. *Postterm birth* occurs after the forty-second week.

A woman is a *parturient* when she is in labor and a *puerpera* after delivery. The term *gravida* refers to the total number of pregnancies, regardless of their type, location, and time or method of termination. For example, a woman who has had two normal intrauterine pregnancies, one tubal pregnancy, one abortion, and one hydatidiform mole is a gravida 5. A *primigravida* is pregnant for the first time, and a *nulligravida* has never been pregnant.

Parity refers to the number of deliveries of viable infants. In the past a *viable infant* was considered to be one weighing 1000 g, which corresponds to about the twenty-eighth week of pregnancy. However, because of obstetrical and neonatal advances, infants weighing less than 1000 g survive. The survival rate for infants above 800 g is significant, and obstetricians intervene with a cesarean section if it is necessary to avoid the stress of labor and vaginal delivery in infants estimated to be this weight or greater.

A fetus weighing 400 g can theoretically live an independent existence; this corresponds to a pregnancy of about 20 weeks. *Para* therefore indicates the number of pregnancies, regardless of the method of delivery, which terminate after the twentieth week. A *nullipara* has never carried a pregnancy beyond the twentieth week, a *primipara* has carried one pregnancy beyond the twentieth week, and a *multipara* has carried more than one. Parity refers to the number of deliveries, not the number of babies born; for example, the delivery of quadruplets at the thirty-fourth week by a primigravida makes her a para 1. A woman who has had five pregnancies, including one abortion, one ectopic pregnancy, one infant delivered normally at 26 weeks, one set of twins delivered normally at 36 weeks, and a single infant delivered by cesarean section at 41 weeks, is a gravida 5 para 3.

A more complete description of past pregnancies can be indicated by summarizing their outcomes by a series of numbers indicating, in order, term deliveries, premature deliveries, abortions, and presently living children. For example, 4-2-0-

1 means four term deliveries, two premature deliveries, no abortions, and one living child.

CHANGES PRECEDING THE ONSET OF LABOR

According to Reynolds, the growth of the uterus during pregnancy is divided into three phases.

1. The first is a short period of preparation during which the progestational changes necessary for nidation develop.
2. The second phase is a period of uterine enlargement characterized by hypertrophy of muscular and connective tissue elements, producing a rapid increase in the weight of the uterus. During this phase, which ends at about 20 weeks, the uterus is spherical in shape.
3. This is followed by a period of uterine stretching during which the rate of growth,

as indicated by a slower increase in weight, is much less rapid. The progressive enlargement of the cavity to accommodate the rapidly growing fetus is accomplished primarily by longitudinal stretching and thinning of the muscular walls so that the uterus becomes elongated rather than spherical. The uterus also becomes wider as the infant grows, but the lateral expansion is less than the longitudinal (Fig. 29-1).

Uterine weight increases from 60 to 80 g at conception to about 800 g by the twentieth week and about 1000 g at term (Fig. 29-2).

Certain other changes take place in the uterus during pregnancy. These consist of the demarcation of the uterus into two separate divisions: the *upper uterine segment,* which is composed of the active contracting muscle tissue that supplies the force necessary to complete delivery; and the thin, passive *lower uterine segment,* through

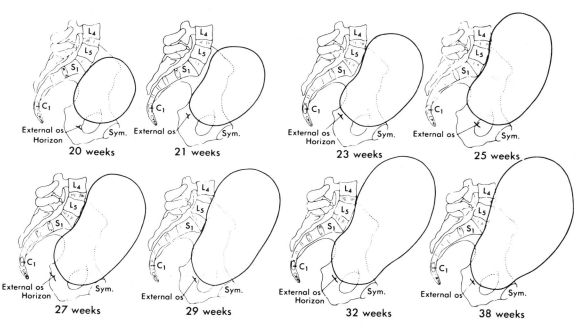

Fig. 29-1 Change in shape of uterus during pregnancy. (From Gillespie EC: Am J Obstet Gynecol 59:949, 1950.)

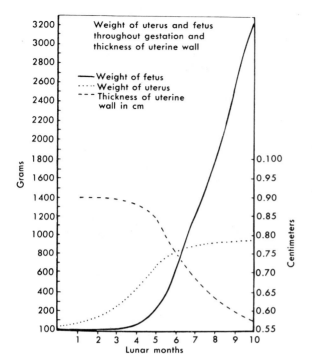

Fig. 29-2 Composite graph expression certain weights and measurements. Around the twentieth week uterine growth diminishes; myometrium therefore begins to thin and fetus begins to increase rapidly in weight. (From Gillespie EC: Am J Obstet Gynecol 59:949, 1950.)

which the presenting part passes into the pelvic cavity.

The lower uterine segment is derived principally from the isthmus of the uterus—the area of the muscular corpus that is situated immediately superior to the histologic internal os of the cervix. The muscle tissue of the isthmus is indistinguishable from that of the rest of the body of the uterus, which is a predominantly muscular organ. In contrast, the stroma of the cervix contains fibrous connective tissue with some elastic tissue and only a few smooth muscle cells. Less than 15% of total mass is muscular.

Until about the sixteenth week of pregnancy, identifying the isthmus as a distinct entity is almost impossible, but at about that time the area of the isthmus begins to lengthen, or *unfold,* as an aid in providing room to accommodate the rapidly growing fetus. The entire fibrous portion of the cervix below the isthmus remains closed (Fig. 29-3).

Uterine muscle fibers have certain characteristics that are essential for normal pregnancy and successful delivery. They must be able gradually to *elongate* to permit the progressive increase in uterine size necessary to accommodate the growing fetus. As pregnancy advances, the length of individual muscle cells increases from an original 50 μm to about 500 μm. They must be *elastic* so they can return to their normal length after periods of uterine distension. Because labor and delivery are accomplished by the force generated by uterine muscle activity, they must be able to *contract* and force the products of conception from the uterus. It is evident that unless the uterus remains closely approximated to the fetus as it is gradually expelled from the cavity, the effect of each successive contraction will be diminished. As labor advances and the fetus descends through the birth canal, the uterine cavity gradually becomes smaller so that effective force is maintained. This is accomplished by *brachystasis,* the unique ability of uterine muscle fibers to become progressively shorter and thicker while they retain their power to contract forcibly.

Muscular activity, which is present throughout pregnancy, has been studied extensively by recording the effects of the contractions on amniotic fluid pressure. The *uterine tonus,* the amniotic fluid pressure between contractions, is from 3 to 8 mm Hg during normal pregnancy. *Two types of spontaneous contractions can be identified:* small contractions that occur in localized areas of the uterine wall and that increase the pressure by 2 to 4 mm Hg, and *Braxton Hicks contractions,* which involve more uterine muscle and increase pressure by 10 to 15 mm Hg. Both are painless, and only the latter can be felt by the pregnant woman. Braxton Hicks contractions occur irregularly dur-

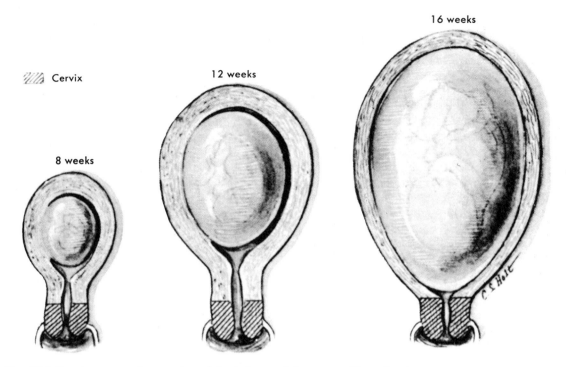

Fig. 29-3 Development and expansion of the isthmus of the uterus. (From Danforth DN: Am J Obstet Gynecol 53:541, 1947.)

ing early pregnancy but become stronger and closer together as pregnancy advances.

Uterine activity increases during the last 8 to 10 weeks of pregnancy. The Braxton Hicks contractions gradually become stronger, and the small contractions can no longer be identified. By the time labor begins, the intrauterine pressure during a contraction averages 28 mm Hg. *The increased muscle activity is responsible for the characteristic prelabor changes in the uterine corpus and cervix.*

Because the fibers in the active upper segment shorten during each contraction, it is obvious that this portion of the uterine wall must become shorter and thicker during periods of muscle activity. Such a change would reduce the capacity of the uterine cavity unless a compensatory expansion of some other area of the uterus occurred

during a contraction. This is in fact what happens. As the muscle fibers of the upper active segment shorten during a contraction, the inferior border of this portion of the uterus is drawn upward, exerting tension on the lower uterine segment. In response, the relatively passive fibers in the wall of the isthmus elongate as they are pulled upward because the relatively firm cervix remains closed. The wall of the lower part of the uterus therefore becomes thinner during each contraction.

As the muscle of the upper segment relaxes at the end of the contraction, the individual fibers lengthen, the lower border of the upper segment returns almost to its original position, and the isthmus shortens and its wall thickens. Each individual contraction produces no perceptible permanent change, but the upper segment gradually becomes shorter and shorter and its wall thicker and thicker from progressive retraction of individual muscle fibers. Simultaneously, the lower segment gradually becomes longer and thinner.

During this initial period of preparation for labor, the increased length of the lower segment is almost entirely a result of elongation of the isthmus; the cervix remains closed until the last 2 to 3 weeks and in many cases remains closed until labor begins. Eventually, however, the cervix is *effaced*, or *taken up*, by a process similar to that by which the isthmus is lengthened. As the isthmus is stretched by the contraction and retraction of the muscle fibers in the active segment, the internal cervical os begins to open, being gradually pulled upward around the membranes and the presenting part and incorporated with the isthmus in the lower segment.

As a result of the upward traction on the internal os against the resistance of the presenting part of the fetus, the cervical component of this cervical uterine complex lengthens, becomes thinner (this becomes apparent on vaginal examination), and assumes a funnel shape; as effacement continues and the internal os is pulled higher and higher, the cervical canal becomes shorter and shorter, until finally it is completely obliterated.

The completely developed lower uterine segment is about 10 cm long; the thinned-out, elongated isthmus and the effaced cervix each make up approximately half its length. The area of demarcation between the thick, upper, contractile portion of the uterus and the thinner, passive, lower segment has been called the *retraction ring*. The junction can be appreciated by palpating the interior of the uterus, but it is not visible on the external surface.

In primigravidas the cervix is usually well effaced before the contractions of true labor begin (Fig. 29-4), but preparation of the cervix in multiparas differs slightly. In multiparas the cervix may be incompletely effaced when labor starts. The isthmus of the uterus elongates, and the internal os is retracted and opened. The cervical canal is wide, patulous, and considerably shortened; it

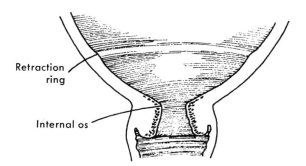

Fig. 29-4 Ripe cervix in multipara. Retraction ring is at junction of isthmus and active upper segment.

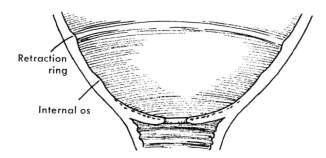

Fig. 29-5 Ripe cervix in primigravida.

usually is possible to insert two fingers through it without difficulty. In many multiparas, however, the cervical canal is completely obliterated when labor begins (Fig. 29-5).

The changes in the cervix can be felt most accurately by vaginal palpation, and the physician should become thoroughly familiar with them to be able to recognize the *prepared*, or *ripe, cervix*.

FORCES IN LABOR

Labor occurs as a result of the force of muscular contractions. The *primary force*, produced by the involuntary contractions of uterine muscle, is more important than the *secondary force*, produced by voluntary increase in intraabdominal pressure. Labor can often be completed by the primary forces alone, but the secondary powers are effective only during the second stage. The secondary forces play no part in dilating the cervix.

Primary force. Uterine muscle contractions during labor have certain distinctive characteristics. They are *involuntary* and *recur intermittently* and *rhythmically,* and they usually *produce discomfort.*

During the prelabor period, Braxton Hicks contractions recur more often and become progressively stronger. They involve more and more uterine muscle as term approaches. Uterine contractions during labor are presumed to be initiated by one of two *pacemakers* situated in the cornual areas of the fundus. One predominates, and during normal labor each contraction is initiated by a single pacemaker. The contraction is propagated downward from its site of origin at a speed of about 2 cm/sec; in about 15 seconds the entire uterus is contracting. The contraction mechanism is so well coordinated that the peak of contraction is reached in all parts of the uterus simultaneously. This means that the systolic phase of the contraction is longest in the region of the pacemaker and that it becomes progressively shorter in areas more distant from the fundus of the uterus. There is more muscle in the fundus than in the lower part of the uterus; hence the intensity of the contraction in this area is approximately twice that in the isthmus.

At the onset of labor contractions may come irregularly and last only a few seconds, but they soon recur at shorter and shorter intervals, last longer, and produce more discomfort. During advanced normal labor, the contractions recur at intervals of 2 to 4 minutes and generate an intrauterine pressure of 35 to 55 mm Hg at their peak. The resting *intrauterine tonus* between contractions is from 4 to 12 mm Hg.

Each uterine contraction is slight at its onset but can be palpated or recorded several seconds before the patient is aware of it; the intensity gradually increases until the uterus becomes hard and cannot be indented with finger pressure applied through the abdominal wall to the fundus. At this time the patient feels pain, which probably

is caused by pressure of the presenting part against the cervix and the other structures in the pelvis. After reaching its acme, the force of the contraction gradually subsides. Between contractions the uterus in normal labors is soft and relaxed.

The exact duration of each contraction is difficult to determine without using precise recording devices. The uterus can be felt to contract after an increase in amniotic fluid pressure to about 20 mm Hg, but the patient will feel no discomfort until the pressure rises to about 25 mm Hg. The uterine fundus can usually be indented until the pressure has increased to about 50 mm Hg, after which it is too firm to depress. After reaching its acme, the force of the contraction gradually diminishes, and the uterus softens. By clinical observation a normal contraction may last 90 seconds, but the pressure changes can last as long as 200 seconds (Fig. 29-6).

The ultimate effect of the three principal characteristics of a normal labor contraction—propagation of the wave downward from a fundal source, a prolonged fundal systolic phase, and a maximal fundal intensity—is a gradient of force directed from the fundus to the least active and weakest area of the uterus, the cervix. This is called *fundal dominance.* The force generated by each contraction is applied to the amniotic fluid and directly against the pole of the infant that occupies the upper segment. Therefore each time the muscle contracts the uterine cavity becomes smaller, and the presenting part of the infant or the forebag of waters lying ahead of it is pushed downward into the cervix. This tends to force it to open, or *dilate* it.

A more potent factor in cervical dilation, however, is the *retraction of the upper segment.* As this area of the uterus becomes shorter and thicker, it pulls the lower segment and the dilating cervix upward around the presenting part at the same time the uterus contracting directly against the infant tends to push it through the cervical opening (Fig. 29-7). The cervix opens or is dilated by a combination of these two factors, but

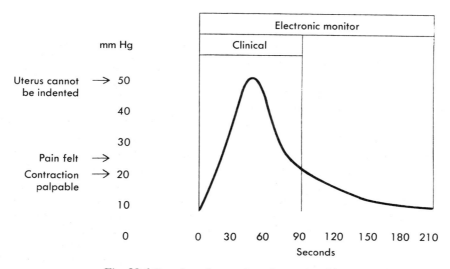

Fig. 29-6 Duration of normal uterine contraction.

retraction is probably more important than the pressure of the presenting part, since dilation will occur even though the presenting part does not descend into it. This can be observed with a transverse lie, with which the cervix may dilate completely even though the presenting part, the shoulder, cannot enter the pelvis. A *completely dilated cervix* that will permit a term infant to pass through it has a diameter of about 10 cm.

Secondary force. Voluntary contractions of the abdominal muscles with the diaphragm fixed after forced inspiration increase intraabdominal and, secondarily, intrauterine pressure. *The secondary forces have no effect on cervical dilation, but they are of considerable importance in aiding the expulsion of the infant from the uterus and vagina after the cervix is completely dilated.* Contractions of the abdominal muscles can begin involuntarily when the patient feels the presenting part pressing on the rectum and distending the perineum. When the pressure sensation is eliminated by analgesic drugs or by anesthesia, the *bearing-down* efforts cease, and the second stage may be prolonged indefinitely if the primary forces are not strong enough to expel the infant.

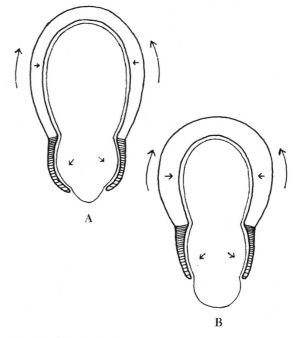

Fig. 29-7 **A,** Cervix is partially dilated and has not yet retracted around presenting part. **B,** Cervical dilation is complete, and cervix is being pulled upward as presenting part descends.

CAUSE OF LABOR

Why labor begins is not definitely known, but changes in the amniotic fluid, placenta, fetus, myometrium, cervix, and pituitary gland all seem to be important.

The uterus is active throughout pregnancy, but during the last 8 to 10 weeks the contractions increase in frequency and duration and in the immediate prelabor period are similar to those of the normal first stage. The effects of changing concentrations of estrogen, progesterone, oxytocin, and prostaglandins on uterine muscle activity have not been clearly defined, but it seems likely that altered concentrations of these substances are important factors in muscle contraction.

Endogenous prostaglandins probably are responsible for the biochemical changes in the cervix during pregnancy that permit the cervical tissues to stretch. *Myometrial oxytocin receptors* increase progressively as pregnancy advances, and a sharp rise occurs with the onset of labor to permit the uterine muscle to respond to low levels of oxytocin. Plasma *prostaglandin levels* change little until after labor begins, but they increase as the cervix dilates. The increase in prostaglandin synthesis may be stimulated by oxytocin. The propagation of muscle contractions is facilitated by the development of *intercellular gap junctions* that permit a rapid multicellular response after a contraction is initiated. Much more study is necessary before the precise mechanism by which contractions are initiated can be established.

The role of the *fetus* in initiating labor is not clear, but many animal studies suggest that biochemical or hormonal stimuli from a mature fetus and placenta are an important factor in initiating labor at an appropriate time.

Destruction or removal of the hypothalamus, pituitary, or both adrenal glands of a single sheep fetus will prolong pregnancy indefinitely. If the operation is performed on only one of twins, labor will begin at the usual time. The operations prevent the increased fetal cortisol secretion that precedes the onset of labor in sheep and goats. The increasing concentration of cortisol presumably causes decreased progesterone and increased estrogen secretion and a consequent stimulation of prostaglandin synthesis, which results in uterine contraction.

A similar reaction occurs in human pregnancies with anencephalic fetuses. The hypothalamus fails to develop; hence the anterior pituitary is hypoplastic and produces no hormones. The absence of ACTH results in fetal adrenal hypoplasia and reduced cortisol secretion. Pregnancy is likely to be prolonged unless there is associated hydramnios.

MECHANISM OF NORMAL LABOR

The *mechanism of labor* is a term applied to the series of changes in the attitude and position of the fetus that permits it to progress through the irregularly shaped pelvic cavity. A complete understanding of how this is accomplished is fundamental to the practice of intelligent obstetrics and is an absolute necessity for safe operative delivery, as the normal mechanism must be followed as closely as possible. Physicians who have a clear understanding of the basic concepts of the mechanism of normal labor for the occiput positions can determine what to expect during any labor and what the probable mechanism will be for any position the fetus can assume.

The steps in the mechanism of labor for the occiput positions are *descent, flexion, internal rotation, extension, restitution,* and *external rotation.* These do not occur as separate processes but are combined. For example, descent through the pelvis, flexion, and internal rotation may all occur more or less simultaneously.

The progress of labor is the result of the tendency for each uterine contraction to push the fetus downward through the pelvis, of the resistance of the soft tissue and the bony pelvis to its descent, and of the shape of the fetal head, which must conform to the different shapes of the pelvic cavity at its various levels. The infant itself is entirely passive. With each uterine contraction the fetus is pushed lower into the pelvic cavity, and its position gradually is altered to accommodate it to the shape of the part of the pelvis through which it must pass.

Descent. In occiput positions the longest diameter of the infant's head, the anteroposterior, enters the normal pelvis in the longest diameter of the inlet, the transverse, in almost every instance.

If the sagittal suture is equidistant from the symphysis and the sacral promontory, the head is said to be entering the inlet in a *synclitic* manner. Some degree of *asynclitism* generally is present (Fig. 29-8). If the sagittal suture lies closer to the sacrum than to the pubis and the anterior parietal bone lies over the inlet, an *anterior parietal bone presentation* can be diagnosed. If the sagittal suture lies closer to the pubis and the posterior parietal bone lies over the inlet, it is a *posterior parietal bone presentation*. The latter is usually present at the onset of normal labor.

When labor begins, the area of the infant's head just below the parietal eminence rests on the sacral promontory, the opposite parietal eminence lies above the superior border of the pubis anteriorly, and the sagittal suture is in the transverse diameter of the inlet, closer to the pubis than to the sacrum (Fig. 29-8, *C*). As uterine contractions become more effective, the anterior parietal bone is slowly forced downward behind the pubis. During this process the sagittal suture gradually moves posteriorly as the head assumes a synclitic position in the inlet. The head *descends* through the inlet with its biparietal diameter approximately parallel to the plane of the inlet (Fig. 29-8, *B*).

Generally, some degree of *molding of the fetal head* is correlated with descent through the inlet. The term *molding* describes the changes in the shape of the head that are necessary to permit it to

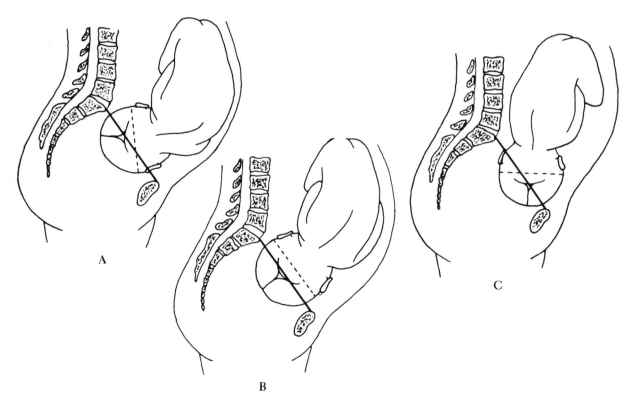

Fig. 29-8 Descent through inlet. **A,** Anterior parietal bone presentation. Sagittal suture is in posterior segment of inlet. **B,** Synclitism. Sagittal suture is equidistant from sacrum and pubis. **C,** Posterior parietal bone presentation. Sagittal suture is in anterior segment of inlet.

adapt itself to the size and shape of the maternal pelvis through which it must pass. Molding is accomplished by gradual elevation or depression of the parietal, frontal, and occipital skull plates made possible by the mobility of these bones, which are not yet fused to each other. Rearrangement of the relationships between the skull plates alters the transverse, anteroposterior, and vertical measurement of the fetal skull. Molding is a dynamic process: the shape of the head changes constantly throughout labor. Little molding is necessary to permit a normal-sized fetus to pass through a normal pelvis; however, if pelvic diameters are reduced, considerable change in the shape of the head may be necessary to permit vaginal delivery.

The head is said to be *engaged* after the widest transverse diameter, the biparietal, has passed the plane of the inlet. In the normal unmolded head, the distance between the occiput and the plane of the biparietal diameter is less than the distance between the ischial spines and the inlet; hence, if the occiput is the presenting part, engagement occurs as the head passes the level of the spines. *However, the fact that the lowest portion of the head is at the level of the spines does not always mean that engagement has occurred.* If there has been considerable molding and elongation of the head to permit it to pass an inlet with reduced measurements, the biparietal diameter may still not have entered the true pelvis when the lowest portion reaches the level of the spines. When the head is completely deflexed, as in face positions, the biparietal diameter does not pass the pelvic inlet until the presenting part reaches the pelvic floor.

Descent can be delayed by an incompletely dilated cervix; resistant soft tissues; disproportion between the size of the head and the size or shape of the pelvic cavity; and weak, ineffective uterine contractions. Descent usually occurs more gradually in primigravidas than in multiparas because the cervix dilates more slowly and the soft-tissue resistance is greater.

The degree of descent is gauged by the *station*

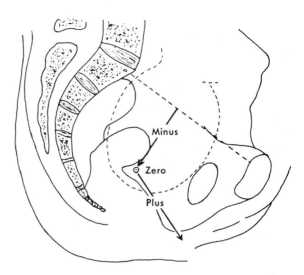

Fig. 29-9 Stations of birth canal. Presenting part *(dotted lines)* is just below station 0. Biparietal diameter has passed plane of inlet.

of the presenting part (Fig. 29-9), which is its relationship to the plane of the ischial spines. If the lowest point of the presenting part is at the level of the spines, it is at station 0; if it is one third of the distance between the spines and the pelvic inlet, at station minus 1 if two thirds of the distance to the inlet it is at station minus 2, and if it is at the inlet it is at station minus 3. If the lowest level of the presenting part is above the plane of the pelvic inlet, it is said to be *floating*. The distance between the plane of the ischial spines and the pelvic floor is also divided into thirds. A station plus 1, therefore, indicates that the lowest level of the head is one third of the distance between the spines and the pelvic floor. When the presenting part reaches station plus 3, it usually has just reached the pelvic floor.

Flexion. The head usually lies in the pelvic inlet during late pregnancy in a partially flexed attitude. The degree of flexion increases during descent, particularly if the pelvis is small. The

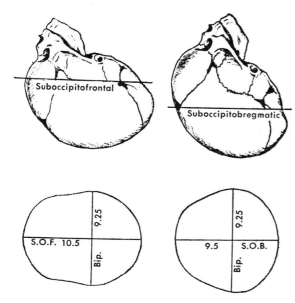

Fig. 29-10 As flexion increases, anteroposterior diameter of head, which must pass through pelvis, becomes shorter. (From Beck AC: Obstetrical practice, Baltimore, 1955, The Williams & Wilkins Co.)

purpose of flexion is to substitute the suboccipitobregmatic diameter of 9.5 cm for the occipitofrontal diameter, which measures 10.5 to 11 cm (Fig. 29-10). Descent of the head through the inlet and upper pelvis is illustrated in Fig. 29-11.

Flexion occurs because the force applied by the resistance of the maternal bone and soft tissues to the anterior portion of the head is greater than that applied to the posterior portion. If the anteroposterior diameter of the infant's head is considered as a lever with its fulcrum at the foramen magnum, where the spinal column joins the skull, one can see how this might occur. The anterior arm of the lever is longer than the posterior arm; consequently, when equal force is applied to each, the resultant force anteriorly is greater, and the head flexes (see Fig. 29-10). The smaller the pelvis, the greater the resistance and the more complete the flexion. The head may flex only slightly if the pelvis is large and the baby is small.

Internal rotation. Rotation of the long axis of the fetal head from the transverse diameter in which it descended through the upper pelvis to the anteroposterior diameter at the outlet is essential. The transverse diameters of the normal middle and lower pelvis are too short to permit the head of a normal-sized infant to descend further without rotating. Rotation begins at the level of the ischial spines but is not completed until the presenting part reaches the lower pelvis.

The bispinous diameter is too short to permit a normal-sized head to pass in the transverse diameter; consequently, it is rotated slightly by simple pressure from one of the protruding spines. In an occiput left transverse position, for example, the occiput is directed to the left as it descends through the upper pelvis. As flexion increases, the occiput is lower than the frontal portion of the head and will reach the spine first. The spine lies slightly posterior and therefore will contact the posterior portion of the occipital area. Each time the uterus contracts and the head descends slightly, the occiput will be pushed anteriorly a bit more by the pressure of the ischial spine. As the occiput rotates anteriorly, the face rotates posteriorly. When the anteroposterior diameter of the head coincides with a diameter of the pelvis in which it can descend, the head will pass the midpelvis (Fig. 29-11, *D* and *E*).

Rotation is completed because the bony side walls of the lower pelvis slope anteriorly and slightly inward and because the levator ani muscles form a double-included plane, the resultant slope of which is anterior. As the flexed head descends, its presenting part, the occipital portion that already has been rotated slightly anteriorly by the spine, strikes the bony pelvis and the levator sling anteriorly and with each uterine contraction slides further up the muscle plane until it lies in the midline beneath the pubic arch (Fig. 29-11, *F* and *G*).

Both the levators and the bony pelvis are important for anterior rotation. This is illustrated in

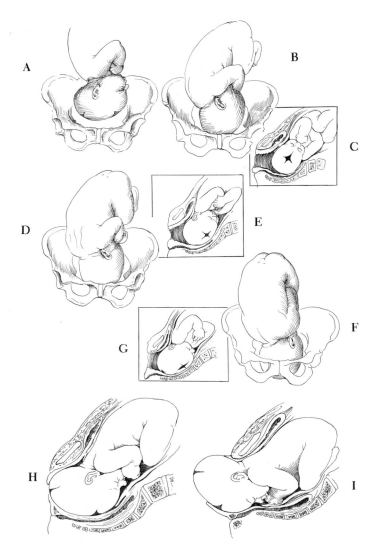

Fig. 29-11 A, Position of head in inlet when labor begins. **B,** Flexion as head descends. **C,** Head descends to mid-pelvis in transverse position. **D** and **E,** Partial anterior rotation as head passes spines. **F** and **G,** Further anterior rotation as occiput reaches lower pelvis. **H** and **I,** Complete anterior rotation and extension of head.

a negative sense in multiparas in whom the head fails to turn anteriorly when muscular support has been compromised by previous childbirth injury and in women with normal levator slings that have been paralyzed by continuous regional anesthesia. In a few women the shape of the bony pelvis is so altered or the diameters are so shortened that they present a mechanical obstruction to rotation.

Extension. The upper half of the pelvic canal is directed posteriorly toward the sacrum and the lower half anteriorly, making the canal a curved rather than a straight tube. The course of descent of the presenting part must therefore change to conform to the pelvic architecture. After the occiput has rotated to an anterior position, the suboccipital area impinges beneath the pubis, and the parietal bossae impinge on the levators and the descending pubic rami, where they remain while the forehead slides up the inclined plane formed by the perineum as the head extends. The forehead, face, and chin progressively emerge from the introitus, and the face then falls posteriorly, freeing the occiput. At this stage of labor the fetal spine is no longer flexed but is extended to conform to the contour of the birth canal (Fig. 29-11, *H* and *I*).

Restitution. After the head is free from the introitus, it rotates 45 degrees to the right or left of the midline to assume its normal relationship to the back and shoulders. If the fetal back is on the left, the occiput rotates in that direction; and if on the right, it rotates to that side.

External rotation. As the shoulders descend and rotate within the pelvis, the occiput rotates further externally; thus external rotation of the head actually indicates a change in position of the undelivered body of the fetus.

With an occiput left position the shoulders pass the inlet after the head is delivered and descend with the long bisacromial diameter in the left oblique diameter of the pelvis. The anterior shoulder, the right one, meets the levator sling first as descent continues and, like the occiput, is rotated 45 degrees anteriorly to a position beneath the pu-

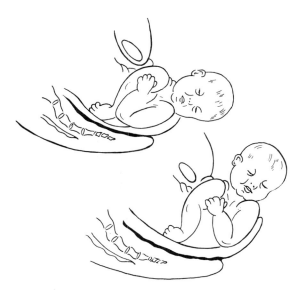

Fig. 29-12 Anterior shoulder remains beneath pubic arch, as posterior shoulder is forced anteriorly over distended perineum.

bic arch. The left shoulder then lies directly over the sacrum in the muscular gutter formed by the two levator muscles. The anterior shoulder remains impinged beneath the pubic arch, and the fetal spine bends laterally as the posterior shoulder is forced up over the perineum. When the posterior shoulder is free, it falls backward, and the opposite one is pushed out from beneath the pubic arch. The body of the infant is delivered without any particular mechanism (Fig. 29-12).

The mechanisms for occiput right and occiput left positions are identical except that in the former the occiput and back descend down the right side of the pelvis and rotate from right to left.

CLINICAL COURSE OF LABOR

Prodromes. Certain symptoms and objective signs precede the onset of labor.

ENGAGEMENT. In primigravidas the fetal head begins to settle into the upper pelvis from 2 to 3 weeks before labor begins. This coincides with the period of elongation of the lower segment and the progressive effacement of the cervix, which permits the head to descend. In multiparas, development of the lower segment and effacement is less complete, and the head usually remains high until early in labor. If engagement fails to occur with the first pregnancy, the physician should consider the possibility of a contraction of the bony pelvis, placenta previa, a pelvic tumor, abnormal fetal position, or anything else that might prevent the head from descending.

As the infant "drops," the pressure on the diaphragm is reduced; consequently, the patient breathes more easily, but she experiences more pelvic pressure, frequency of urination, and discomfort as the presenting part presses on the pelvic organs.

VAGINAL DISCHARGE. As the cervix effaces and the pressure on it increases, the patient may note more mucous discharge. Labor often begins a few days after this is observed.

PASSAGE OF MUCOUS PLUG. The thick mucus in the canal, the *mucous plug,* and portions of the hypertrophied crypts are expelled from the obliterated cervix. This often is blood streaked and is called the *show*.

Onset and diagnosis of labor. The contractions of labor produce discomfort and thus differ from the Braxton Hicks contractions during pregnancy. They occur irregularly at the onset of labor but usually increase until they recur every 2 to 3 minutes and last from 60 to 90 seconds. *The contractions of true labor produce progress such as thinning of the cervix, dilation of the cervical opening, or descent of the presenting part.*

The principal criterion necessary for the diagnosis and evaluation of labor therefore is progress rather than the character of the contractions. In some patients, labor progresses rapidly, although the contractions recur irregularly and feel weak. In others no progress can be detected despite contractions that are regular, feel forceful, and are painful. This is called *false labor*. The contractions of false labor usually stop after a few hours

and can almost always be controlled by the administration of a barbiturate. False labor can be diagnosed, therefore, if no progress is made and if the contractions cease spontaneously or with medication.

Stages of labor. *Labor begins when the patient first experiences recurring painful uterine contractions, which terminate in delivery.*

FIRST STAGE. The first stage of labor lasts from its onset until the cervix is completely dilated. The membranes usually rupture during the latter part of the first stage. They may remain intact until delivery.

SECOND STAGE. The second stage begins when the cervix is completely dilated and ends with the delivery of the baby.

Neither the first nor the second stage can be timed accurately unless the patient is examined frequently; during normal labor the exact duration of each of the two stages is not particularly important.

THIRD STAGE. The third stage begins when the baby leaves the uterus and ends with the delivery of the placenta.

COURSE AND DURATION OF LABOR

One of the most critical of several variables that influence the calculated length of labor is the decision as to when labor began. The progression of uterine activity from prelabor to real labor, when recognizable changes in the cervix occur, is difficult to pinpoint, even though the contractions are monitored continuously. A record of the time at which the patient first became aware of the contractions and the time at which changes in the cervix are first appreciated is helpful in deciding how to manage abnormal labor.

The decision as to when labor began is made by the physician who admits the patient to the labor-delivery unit and is recorded on the labor graph. If this is not done, the time of onset may be modified if subsequent progress is not normal. Cesarean section for an "arrest" in the active phase of cervical dilation may be justified if the hours of prelabor are included; this can be inter-

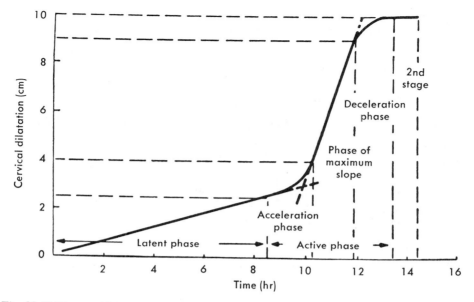

Fig. 29-13 Phases of labor in primigravida. (From Friedman EA: Obstet Gynecol 6:567, 1955.)

preted as an abnormally prolonged total labor. Conversely, one can justify permitting the labor to continue in the hope that the fetus can be delivered vaginally if the latent phase is not considered to be an integral part of the entire process. *Such arbitrary modifications can be avoided if the time at which the patient first felt uterine contractions, even though they may have been irregular and short at the beginning, is considered to be the time at which labor began and is recorded in the labor record when the patient is admitted.* Errors are inevitable. Some women thought to be in early labor will be discharged later with a diagnosis of false labor, whereas cervical dilation in others thought not to be in labor will progress rapidly.

Friedman made a major contribution to the understanding of labor by graphing the progress of cervical dilation against time (Fig. 29-13). He divided the first stage of labor into the *latent phase*, during which effacement is completed and cervical dilation begins, and the *active phase*, during

which cervical dilation is completed. His *deceleration phase*, if it occurs, is difficult to detect.

There are no absolute values for the normal length of the first stage of labor. "Normal" lengths in four separate groups of women are depicted in Fig. 29-14. These statistical evaluations show variations that may reflect differences in the patient populations or in clinical practice.

The second stage can be evaluated more closely. Calkins states that the second stage is concluded with no more than 20 contractions in primigravidas and with 10 or fewer in multiparas. This corresponds well with a median duration of 50 minutes for primigravidas and of 20 minutes for multiparas reported by Hellman and Prystowsky.

The duration of labor in any individual is determined by parity, the size and position of the fetus, the shape and capacity of the pelvis, the consistency of the cervix, the efficiency of the uterine contractions, and the patient's attitude toward pregnancy and motherhood.

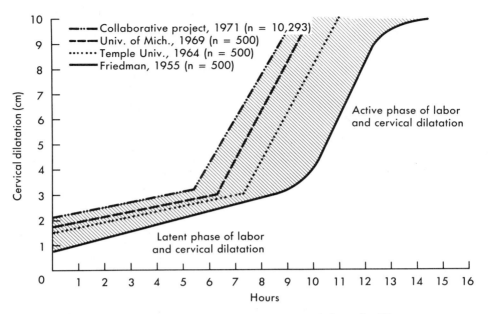

Fig. 29-14 Cervical dilation graphs from four populations of nulliparas.

PREPARATION FOR LABOR

During the prenatal period, physicians and their associates should make every effort to eliminate misunderstandings and fears and to instill confidence in their patients. The primigravida, who has not yet experienced labor, is certain to be apprehensive, particularly if she has acquired a considerable amount of misinformation from her friends and relatives. As the weeks go by, much can be learned about the patient's attitudes by simple questions, and many of her fears can be allayed.

The principal concerns are about the length of labor, how much pain there will be and how it will be relieved, anesthesia, the welfare of the baby, what happens in the hospital, and who will be responsible for her care. It often is helpful to take the patient and her partner on a tour of the maternity unit during the last weeks of pregnancy. This will give them an opportunity to learn about admitting procedures, to see the labor-delivery area, to meet some of the personnel, and to ask questions.

The parents should have an opportunity to participate in childbirth education courses if they are interested. Those that concentrate on the complications of pregnancy and how they are recognized and on the mechanics of delivery are not particularly helpful. The most effective childbirth education courses are designed to provide couples with an understanding of what actually will happen physiologically during labor and delivery and of the part each can play to make childbirth safe and satisfying.

Instructions to the patient. Some time during the last month the patient must be instructed as to how to recognize the onset of labor and what to do when the contractions begin.

WHEN TO ENTER THE HOSPITAL. The normal primigravida should usually enter the hospital when the contractions are recurring regularly at about 5-minute intervals, but multiparas must come in earlier because so many have rapid labors.

RUPTURE OF MEMBRANES. Rupture of the membranes should be reported because the physician will usually want to examine the patient to be certain that a serious complication such as prolapse of the umbilical cord has not occurred.

BLEEDING. Any vaginal bleeding, no matter how slight, should be reported.

FOOD. The gastric emptying time is prolonged during labor, and food may be vomited and aspirated during delivery. *Patients should be warned against ingesting either solid food or liquids after the contractions begin or the membranes rupture.*

Each patient should be examined as soon as she arrives at the hospital. Her prenatal record should be available for review. A brief interval history is recorded, and a physical examination is made. The fetal position and presentation, the location, rate, and regularity of the fetal heart tones, the height of the fundus, and the frequency and the duration of the uterine contractions are determined by *abdominal palpation* and *ausculation*. Unless there is bleeding a *vaginal examination* is next made to confirm fetal position and to determine the amount of cervical dilation and the station. The *blood pressure* is recorded, a *urine specimen* is examined for protein and glucose, and a *hemoglobin* or *hematocrit* determination is made.

Unless the patient is about to deliver, an external recording device should be applied to the maternal abdomen, and a 30-minute recording of fetal heart rate made. More intensive monitoring will be required if baseline fetal heart rate is flat, if decelerations are observed, if labor appears to be abnormal, or if the patient is classified as "high risk."

CARE DURING LABOR

Patients in labor, even though they are multiparas, are usually apprehensive and uncomfortable, and every effort must be made to allay fear and to make the entire experience as rewarding as possible. The attendants must refrain from laughing, joking, and loud conversation near the labor rooms because these are all annoying to the patients. The discussion of other patients and particularly of obstetric problems must be strictly

avoided if there is any chance that the conversation can be overheard.

Under ideal conditions, an experienced labor nurse or a physician should remain with each patient throughout her labor, but practically this is not always possible. As an alternative, nurses and physicians should visit each patient every few minutes to make certain that labor is progressing normally. No laboring patient, particularly one who is unusually apprehensive, should be left alone for any appreciable period of time.

The father may remain in the room if he and the patient so desire. He may be particularly helpful and supportive if he and the patient have had a childbirth education course. His presence should not influence close observation of the patient by professional attendants. If the father is not present, the mother should be able to have some person with her during labor to offer support.

Observations during labor. The following observations will indicate the condition of the mother and her infant and the progress of labor.

FETAL HEART. In term pregnancies the fetal heart sounds are an index of the condition of the fetus and should be counted and recorded at least every 15 minutes during the first stage and more often during the second stage of normal labor. More complete evaluation can be done with an external recording of fetal heart sounds made during labor. This technique is of great help in identifying fetuses at risk. Even though the preliminary monitor strip is normal, observations of the fetal heart must be continued throughout the labor. One can either continue using the external monitor or follow the heart sounds with a stethoscope. If the latter is used, the heart rate is checked during or immediately after a contraction as well as in the interval between contractions because changes caused by interference with fetal oxygenation are usually heard first during the period of uterine activity.

Electronic monitoring of the fetal heart is indicated during premature labor and whenever the pregnancy is complicated. This provides a more accurate assessment of heart rate and permits continuous rather than intermittent evaluation. Fetal heart monitoring is discussed in detail in Chapter 32.

BLOOD PRESSURE. The blood pressure is recorded at 30-minute intervals because it may rise to alarming levels during labor.

CONTRACTIONS. The length, duration, and intensity of uterine contractions and the interval between them are recorded at 30-minute intervals. The length is determined by palpation rather than by the patient's statements because she cannot feel the contraction until several seconds after it has begun and the discomfort disappears before the uterus is relaxed. Intensity is estimated by the firmness with which the muscle contracts.

Electronic monitoring of uterine contractions is probably not necessary during normal labor at term if there are no fetal heart rate abnormalities. The equipment and someone familiar with its use and with the interpretation of the tracings should be available in the labor-delivery area of hospitals that provide obstetric services. Monitoring of the uterine contraction pattern and of the fetal heart rate is essential during abnormal labor, if fetal heart rate abnormalities are present and whenever labor is induced or stimulated.

Examinations. The progress of labor is determined by various examinations.

ABDOMINAL EXAMINATION. Abdominal examinations are performed to evaluate the uterine contractions and to follow the descent of the presenting part into the pelvis. As descent occurs, the cephalic prominence and the anterior shoulder, which can be palpated above the pubis, move downward. When the head is deep in the pelvis, the cephalic prominence can no longer be felt, and the shoulder lies just above the pubis.

PERINEAL PALPATION. The presenting part can be palpated through the perineum after it has reached the pelvic floor. A bit later, perineal bulging and crowning can be seen.

VAGINAL EXAMINATION. The progress of cervical dilation and of descent can be determined by vaginal palpation. Because bacteria inevitably are carried on the fingertips from the introitus and the vagina to the interior of the uterus, it is essential that vaginal examinations be performed properly and that they be limited in number. As a general rule no more than three or four are necessary during a normal primigravid labor: one when the patient is admitted, one when it appears that she may need sedation, and one or two more as labor advances.

Examinations made simply to determine position, station, and cervical dilation can be performed in the labor bed with the patient in dorsal position. The examiner wears sterile gloves, and an antiseptic solution is used to cleanse the vulva and act as a lubricant. The labia are separated with the fingers of one hand, and the index and second fingers of the other are inserted into the vagina, palpating the fetal head and the cervical rim. If more information must be obtained, for example, if there is a question of cephalopelvic disproportion or of placenta previa or if an abnormal presentation is suspected, the examination must be performed with the patient in the lithotomy position.

It is essential that physicians' examinations and nurses' observations and treatment be recorded accurately in the labor record. The progress of labor is best appreciated if cervical dilation, descent, and position are plotted on a labor graph (Fig. 29-14). On such a graph, deviations from the normal are obvious and can be appreciated much earlier than by other recording methods.

General care. General nursing care during labor is directed toward making the patient as comfortable as possible and protecting her from infection and injury.

POSITION. Patients in early labor may be out of bed if they wish, but they usually prefer to lie down when labor is advanced. Most are more comfortable on their sides than on their backs, and in fact the lateral position has many advantages, the most important of which are that the force of uterine contractions, uterine perfusion, and fetal gas exchange are greater in the lateral position. Presumably this is a result of enhancing vena caval blood flow, which may be impeded by pressure from the uterus in the dorsal position. Those who have been sedated should be confined to bed.

FOOD. The gastric emptying time is delayed during normal labor, and the administration of analgesic and sedative drugs decreases it even more. Fluids and food should not be ingested orally during labor. Glucose solution can be administered intravenously if labor is prolonged.

BLADDER. As the lower segment lengthens and the cervix is retracted, the bladder is pulled upward. This and the pressure from the descending presenting part may make spontaneous voiding impossible. The distended bladder can be seen and felt as a fluctuant mass in the lower abdomen. If the patient cannot void during labor, she should be catheterized at intervals.

Transfer to delivery room. Patients should be taken to the delivery room in their beds in time to prepare them properly for delivery. Primigravidas are moved when the presenting part begins to distend the perineum, and multiparas are moved when they are 8 to 9 cm dilated.

The recent action to make the atmosphere of the hospital obstetric unit more homelike has led to the development of beds that can be used both during labor and for delivery. Such beds eliminate the need to transfer the patient to the delivery room and to a delivery table (Chapter 1).

As the presenting part descends deep into the pelvis during the second stage and begins to exert pressure on the pelvic floor, the patient will feel as though she needs to evacuate her rectum and will ask for a bedpan. Soon after this she will begin to hold her breath, tense her abdominal muscles, and strain or *bear down* in an attempt to expel the baby each time the uterus contracts. As this occurs, the relatively high-pitched cry at the time of the contraction changes to a sustained grunt, which can be recognized as indicating the second stage whenever it is heard. Bearing down during the first stage serves no useful purpose and should not be permitted because it will only tire the patient. The bloody vaginal discharge usually increases as cervical dilation is completed, and

the pressure of the presenting part may force small amounts of fecal material from the rectum.

NORMAL DELIVERY

Everyone in the delivery room should wear a cap that covers the hair completely and a face mask that covers both the nose and the mouth, and those participating directly in the delivery should wear sterile surgical gowns and gloves. Others wear clean surgical dresses or suits, and no one is admitted in street clothes.

An undelivered patient should never be left alone in the delivery room. She needs attention and support during the expulsive stage; in addition, she may deliver while the attendants are out of the room.

Fetal heart monitoring, either electronic or auscultatory, should be continued in the delivery room, which should have the capability of electronic recording. If the heart is being checked by stethoscope, the rate should be counted during and after almost every contraction.

When the patient is ready to deliver, she is placed in a suitable position. For spontaneous delivery, particularly of multiparas, the *dorsal recumbent position* is satisfactory. There is less stretch on the perineum than in the lithotomy position; hence perineal lacerations occur less often. Episiotomy can be performed, if necessary, but it is difficult to repair adequately in this position. Forceps delivery cannot be performed properly in dorsal recumbent position.

The *lithotomy position* is less comfortable for patients, but it provides better exposure of the perineum, making delivery easier with less likelihood of contamination. The lithotomy position is essential for any operative delivery and for adequate repair of more than a shallow episiotomy. A significant advantage is that the entire birth canal can be examined for injury after the placenta has been delivered; this is not possible in the recumbent position.

The vulva and anus, the upper portions of the thighs, and the skin over the pubis and lower abdomen are cleansed with an antiseptic solution, preferably one containing iodine, wiping from anterior to posterior and discarding the cotton sponge after each stroke. No attempt is made to cleanse the vagina; the constant discharge of amniotic fluid serves to keep it clean. Sterile leggings are placed over the feet and legs, and the ab-

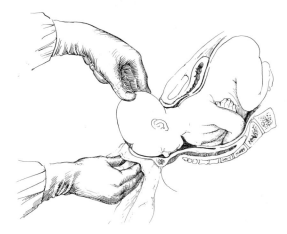

Fig. 29-15 Modified Ritgen's maneuver.

domen is covered with a sterile sheet. In many hospitals a sterile sheet is also placed posteriorly covering the anus, but this is usually promptly saturated with blood and amniotic fluid and contaminated by fecal material expressed from the rectum. It is seldom necessary to catheterize the patient before spontaneous delivery because the bladder has been pulled up entirely out of the pelvis. The bladder should be emptied before forceps extraction.

Episiotomy, when necessary, is performed after the perineum has been flattened out well by the crowning head, and it should be deep enough to sever the fascia covering the lower surface of the levator muscles.

With each contraction, the head will extend, and more of the scalp will be visible through the dilated introitus. Delivery of the head can be controlled by *Ritgen's maneuver* (Fig. 29-15), with which upward pressure is applied through a sterile towel with the thumb and forefinger of the pronated right hand, or the first and second fingers with the hand supinated, first to the supraorbital ridges and later to the chin through the distended perineal body. The upward pressure, which increases extension and prevents the head from slipping back between contractions, is counteracted by downward pressure on the occiput with the fingertips of the

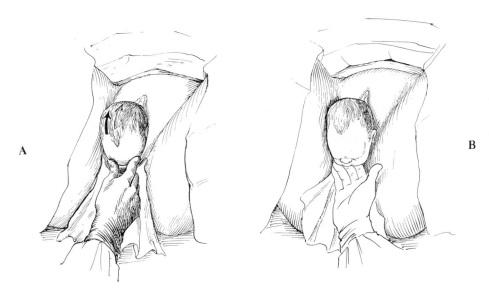

A   B

Fig. 29-16 Completion of delivery of head. **A,** Forehead is supported to maintain extension. **B,** Face is freed from perineum.

other hand; this tends to prevent extension. With this maneuver, the delivery of the head can be readily controlled, and its rapid expulsion, which causes perineal tearing, can be prevented. As the head descends further, the perineum is pushed backward over the face and chin (Fig. 29-16).

As soon as the head is delivered, the physician feels for a loop of cord around the neck. If a long, loose loop is present, it can be slipped over the head; a shorter, tighter one can be slipped over the advancing shoulder. If there are several tight loops, it may be impossible to slip them either way, in which event the cord is doubly clamped, cut, and unwound.

After the head is delivered, the anterior shoulder descends and rotates to a position beneath the pubic arch. At this point the shoulder is said to be *impinged* beneath the pubis, but actually it can be considered to be delivered, since it and the upper humerus are visible. Impingement of the anterior shoulder can be aided by

downward traction on the head (Fig. 29-17); little force should be applied to accomplish this because the brachial plexus may be stretched and injured by the maneuvers. After the shoulder is visible, the physician waits for about 30 seconds to permit the muscle fibers in the fundus to retract and reduce the size of the uterine cavity, from which part of the baby has been delivered. During the wait mucus is aspirated from the nasopharynx. The head is then elevated toward the ceiling, and traction is applied to deliver the posterior shoulder over the perineum (Fig. 29-18). After another 30-second wait, the remainder of the body is slowly extracted by traction on the shoulders (Fig. 29-19).

Some delay in clamping and cutting the umbilical cord probably is beneficial to the infant. If the newborn infant is held below the level of the introitus, blood will be infused from the placental vessels to the baby. The amount is determined by the time interval between delivery and cord clamping, but as much as a 75- to

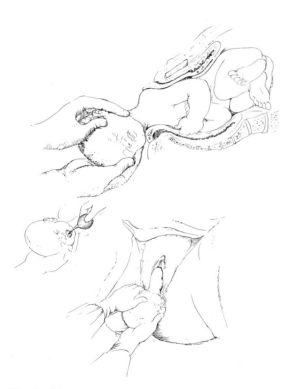

Fig. 29-17 Delivery of anterior shoulder and aspiration of nasopharynx.

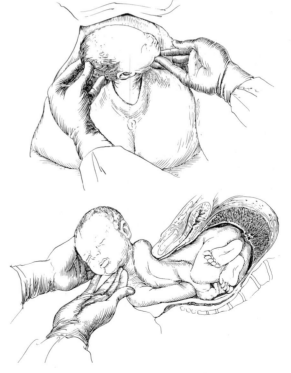

Fig. 29-18 Delivery of posterior shoulder.

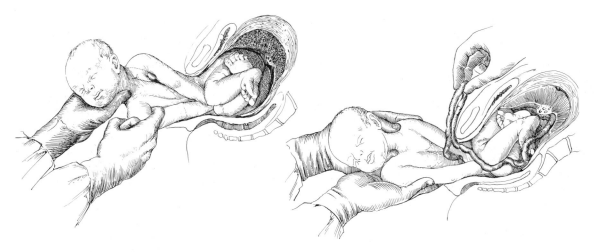

Fig. 29-19 Delivery of body.

100-ml increase in blood volume can be anticipated. Conversely, there is no transfer of blood if the infant is held above the level of the mother's abdomen.

The infant is placed in a heated crib with its head slightly lower than its body. The head-down position should not be too deep, neither should the infant be held upside down for any period of time because the pressure of the abdominal viscera against the diaphragm interferes with normal respiratory efforts.

PREMATURE LABOR AND DELIVERY

The term *premature delivery* indicates the termination of pregnancy before the end of the thirty-sixth week. In the past a diagnosis of premature or term delivery was made on the basis of the birth weight of the infant. If the baby weighed less than 2500 g (the average for white infants at the end of the thirty-sixth completed week), a diagnosis of prematurity was made automatically. The terms *low-birth-weight infant, small for gestational age,* or *growth retardation* may be more accurate because many infants weighing less than 2500 g actually are not premature by date; their low weight is the result of some other factor.

The fact that an infant weighs more than 2500 g at birth is no guarantee of maturity. The babies of mothers with diabetes are excellent examples; some may weigh 3500 to 4000 g at 35 or 36 weeks, but their development is comparable to that of infants of similar gestational age.

About 7% of all pregnancies terminate in the delivery of low-birth-weight infants; this occurs in from 3% to 5% of private and in about 15% of clinic patients. Low-weight infants are born more often to black than to white women.

It is not always possible to distinguish true premature delivery, in which pregnancy terminates before the thirty-seventh week, from delivery of growth-retarded infants, whose weight is less than that anticipated at any given week of pregnancy. This is particularly true in women who are first examined during the last weeks of pregnancy. If a patient is seen early and if uterine and fetal growth conform to the normal pattern, one can logically make a diagnosis of premature labor after the delivery of a small infant whose development is appropriate for the stage of gestation. Conversely, one can suspect growth retardation if fetal and uterine growth are behind those anticipated at specific periods of pregnancy and if the development of the infant at delivery corresponds to the dates, even though the baby weighs less than anticipated.

Etiologic factors. The reasons for premature labor are not completely understood, but it may occur in women with *placenta previa, abruptio placentae, multifetal pregnancy,* and *hypertensive cardiovascular disease.* It may also be necessary to induce labor prematurely in the treatment of these as well as other conditions, notably preeclampsia. The *membranes often rupture prematurely,* after which labor begins.

Bacterial contamination may play an important role in initiating premature labor. Bobitt and Ledger have demonstrated high bacterial counts in the amniotic fluid of women in premature labor. In the genital tract bacteria that often are cultured from amniotic fluid, Bejar and associates found an enzyme that releases prostaglandins. Naeye has found microscopic evidence of infection in the placenta and fetal membranes after the spontaneous onset of premature labor.

The infants of *women who smoke excessively* and *those addicted to heroin and other drugs* weigh less at birth than the babies of nonusers. Low-birth-weight infants are born more often to *women at extremes of the reproductive years,* that is, to the young teenager and the woman over age 35, than to those between the ages of 18 and 30. The part played by *anemia, malnutrition, infection, general poor health,* and *inadequate medical supervision,* all so characteristic of women of the *lowest socioeconomic levels* who have the highest rates of low-birth-weight delivery, has not been completely assessed. Many of these are examples of growth retardation rather than premature labor.

Premature delivery, with its consequently increased perinatal mortality, can also occur because of inappropriate early *elective induction of labor* or *elective repeat cesarean section.* These can be prevented by carefully documenting the relationships between presumed duration of pregnancy, uterine size, and fetal development during the prenatal period and by proving fetal maturity before elective delivery.

Prevention. Because the causes of premature labor are not always obvious, and because labor may begin early without warning, it is not always possible to prevent it. Under certain circumstances, however, the birth of premature infants can be prevented.

Delivery can usually be delayed until the fetus is mature when there is a minor degree of placenta previa with slight bleeding, with stabilized maternal hypertension, with well-controlled maternal diabetes, and with other medical problems. The delivery of premature infants after elective induction of labor or elective repeat cesarean section can be prevented by confirming fetal maturity before setting a date for delivery.

Ritodrine hydrochloride, a beta-mimetic agent, has an inhibitory effect on uterine activity. When given in early labor, ritodrine may prevent labor from progressing. The actions of this drug are not limited to the myometrium; there usually is an increase in maternal heart rate and an increase in systolic and a decrease in diastolic blood pressure. Tachycardia occurs in the fetus and in the mother. Metabolic effects include an increase in maternal glucose and insulin levels and a drop in serum potassium. If these effects adversely influence the medical status of the mother, the use of the drug is contraindicated.

Another agent that may reduce uterine activity is *magnesium sulfate* given intravenously. This drug is widely used during labor and is safe when the patient can be carefully monitored.

Aspirin and *indomethacin* appear to decrease the intensity of uterine contractions and delay the onset of labor. The action presumably is from interference with prostaglandin synthesis. Prostaglandin inhibitors may produce premature closure of the ductus arteriosis in some animals, but not in the human.

The only reason to consider stopping premature labor is in the interest of the fetus. *Attempts to arrest premature labor are contraindicated* if (1) the pregnancy is of at least 37 weeks' duration, (2) the membranes are ruptured, (3) the cervix is 4 or 5 cm dilated, (4) the infant is abnormal, or (5) there is maternal disease such as hypertension, abruptio placentae, or another serious condition for which delivery is indicated.

Management. If premature labor cannot be prevented, one must do everything possible to protect the infant during labor and delivery.

Bed rest in the lateral position and *intravenous fluids*

may inhibit uterine contractions and usually should be tried before drugs are prescribed.

Sedative and analgesic drugs should be administered in small amounts and only when there is no other alternative for pain relief. They depress fetal cerebral function, and if the infant is born during the period of depression, it may be unable to establish its vital functions. Morphine and meperidine often are given in an attempt to stop premature labor, but they should not be used because they have little effect on uterine contractions.

The fetus that weighs less than 1500 g does not tolerate the stress of labor well. For this reason, electronic monitoring is indicated during every premature labor. *Cesarean section* should be performed if persistent late decelerations or moderate-to-severe variable decelerations are recognized. As a general rule, cesarean section is preferred over vaginal delivery for stressed infants without obvious anomalies if their estimated weight is at least 800 g and if the labor is being conducted in a prenatal center with an intensive care neonatal nursery.

FETAL GROWTH RETARDATION

Fetal growth retardation is most likely to occur when the fetus develops abnormally because of congenital anomalies, intrauterine infection, or maternal disease or when there are abnormalities of placental development or function. The latter is probably the most common cause. For example, growth retardation, which is characteristic of severe chronic cardiovascular renal disease, probably begins because the placenta is usually smaller in women with vascular disorders than in normal women. Placental function is further compromised by infarction and by diminished uterine blood flow. The end result is that the reduced functional area of placenta is unable to meet all the requirements of the fetus and its growth is delayed. The fetus grows to the maximum size the placenta can support at any stage of pregnancy. Cessation of placental growth is followed by cessation of fetal growth and death if the fetus is not delivered. Although growth is delayed, development occurs at a reasonably normal rate.

Other causes of growth retardation are *chronic hypoxia* related to sickle cell disease or maternal disease, *cigarette smoking, alcoholism, use of cocaine, heroin,* and other hard drugs, *prolonged pregnancy, growth retardation in previous pregnancies, fetal infections,* and *fetal malformations*.

Growth retardation can be anticipated in any high-risk pregnancy, particularly when the mother is very young, over age 40, malnourished, or chronically ill or has chronic vascular or renal disease. *Sonographic measurement* of the biparietal diameter of the fetal skull at 20 to 22 weeks provides baseline information to which growth of the head during the last weeks of pregnancy can be related.

If growth retardation is suspected, measurements of the biparietal diameter and abdominal circumference at 2-week intervals will indicate the rate at which the head and body are growing. As long as the biparietal diameter, abdominal circumference, and total intrauterine volume increase progressively, one can be reasonably certain that placental function is adequate. Conversely, if growth ceases, one can suspect that maximal functional capacity of the placenta has been reached and that the fetus is in jeopardy.

Growth retardation is of two types: *symmetric* if the fetal head and body grow at the same rate and *asymmetric* if there is a disparity between growth of the head and that of the body. In the latter the head often is spared; abdominal circumference and total volume are below those anticipated from the biparietal diameter. Differentiation of a symmetrically growth-retarded fetus from one that is normal but smaller than the average may be difficult.

Additional information concerning the status of the fetus can be obtained by *biophysical evaluation*. If fetal activity and heart rate tests are normal, the fetus probably has not reached the functional capacity of the placenta. If the fetus ceases to grow, and the biophysical tests become abnormal, prompt delivery is necessary to prevent fetal death.

One of the best indicators of the duration of pregnancy is accurate dating of the day of the onset of the last normal menstrual period. When this is combined with early examinations that substantiate the information provided by the menstrual history, there should be little confusion about the date of delivery (Chapter 20). If such information is available, one should not revise the anticipated delivery date solely because the fetus seems too small. Rather, one should assume that its growth is retarded and initiate the studies that will determine its status. When growth retardation is suspected but the dates are uncertain, the preceding suggested studies should be obtained.

As a general rule, the growth-retarded fetus should be delivered whenever there is evidence that it has outgrown the capacity of the placenta or when maturity can be established, even though there is no clear evidence of fetal deterioration. Ultrasonic evidence of a diminution or absence of amniotic fluid is an indication that the fetus is in jeopardy; it usually should be delivered promptly. Cesarean section often is the most appropriate method for delivery.

PROLONGED PREGNANCY

Sometimes pregnancy is prolonged for several weeks past the due date, during which time the fetus may die. This is most often observed in primigravidas, and according to some authorities, it is more frequently a cause of perinatal mortality with the first pregnancy than is prematurity.

The causes of true prolongation of pregnancy have not been established, but the fetus may play an important part in determining when labor begins. Pregnancy is prolonged by several weeks in certain animals if the fetal pituitary gland is absent or abnormal, and prolongation is associated with adrenal hypoplasia. This also occurs in humans, for example, with anencephaly without hydramnios.

After the forty-second week of gestation the amount of amniotic fluid decreases and vernix disappears; in affected infants the skin appears dry and cracked. Meconium, passed because of hypoxia, stains the placental surface, the umbilical cord, and the remaining vernix yellow-green. In more advanced cases the fingernails and toenails of the infant are also stained. The babies weigh less than the usual term infant and appear to have lost weight.

The cause of the abnormality in the infant is chronic hypoxia from placental dysfunction. The placenta can maintain the requirements of the infant only until it reaches a certain size, which is determined by the amount of functioning chorionic tissue. If the placenta is small or a portion of it has been destroyed, as occurs with chronic hypertensive disease, the baby will be smaller than usual; it often dies in utero before term and shows the same changes as the so-called postmature infant. *Placental deficiency syndrome* is therefore a better term than postmaturity.

Because of the danger to the infants in pregnancies that have gone beyond the calculated due date, induction of labor or even cesarean section has been advised at the forty-second week. These recommendations should not be accepted without reservation; in most instances of presumed postterm pregnancy the baby is normal, and the due date probably was miscalculated. This is particularly true in multiparas.

However, if the dating of the pregnancy is accurate, the cervix favorable, and the fetus mature, an attempt can be made to induce labor after 42 weeks. If the induction fails and if the biophysical tests suggest that the fetus is compromised, cesarean section may be indicated.

If there is a question as to the actual duration of pregnancy, the management is determined by the maturity and condition of the fetus. If pregnancy extends past what is presumed to be 40 weeks, one should begin *biophysical testing*. If the biophysical tests indicate that the fetus is normal, nothing need be done. If placental function is normal, the fetus will continue to grow, but growth will stop when the maximum capacity of the placenta to support the fetus is reached.

Cesarean section is not often necessary in prolonged pregnancy, but it should be performed without hesitation when one establishes the need for delivery and when induction is unsuccessful or contraindicated.

PREGNANCY AND LABOR IN YOUNG PRIMIGRAVIDAS

Labor usually is normal in girls less than 16 years of age, and vaginal delivery can almost always be anticipated; but rates for maternal complications, low-birth-weight infants, and perinatal mortality are all increased.

The reported incidence of *preeclampsia-eclampsia* varies from 4.3% to 23.5%. Semmens, studying 12,857 pregnancies in teenagers, found a toxemia rate of 5.9% for the entire group but 17.7% in those less than 15 years of age. *Infections,* particularly *gonorrhea* and *syphilis, anemia,* and *malnutrition* are common. The figures collected by the Collaborative Perinatal Study indicate an increased rate of low-birth-weight infants born to teenagers. The rates for white girls and women are as follows: ages 10 to 15 years, 97.4; ages 16 to 17 years, 79.29; ages 18 to 19 years, 66.35; and ages 20 to 24 years, 67.04. Comparable figures for black girls and women are 172.92, 157.47, 149.53, and 130.47. The rates for children neurologically abnormal at 1 year of age delivered of white teenagers and women are as follows: ages 10 to 15 years, 35.40; ages 16 to 17 years, 19.7; ages 18 to 19 years, 10.97; and ages 20 to 24 years, 14.92. Comparable figures for black teenagers and women are 9.76, 13.86, 14.62, and 16.67.

Labor generally is of normal duration and terminates in spontaneous or low forceps vaginal delivery. In Semmens's study, labor was prolonged in 8%, and only 1.4% were delivered by cesarean section.

The fact that normal labor and delivery can be anticipated for almost all pregnant teenagers does not justify a complacent attitude. Pregnancy in a teenage girl is a high-risk pregnancy, and patients should be treated accordingly. Many are unmarried and of lower socioeconomic classes, and all need social counseling, in addition to medical care. If the number of pregnant teenagers justifies a special session, a "teenage clinic" should be established. Such a clinic is appropriately staffed by physicians, nurses, social workers, and psychiatrists who are familiar with the problems of teenage pregnancy. A major educational objective of such a clinic is to help patients develop the motivation necessary to prevent recurring pregnancies.

PREGNANCY AND LABOR AFTER AGE 35

Almost all women more than 35 years of age and pregnant for the first time will deliver without difficulty, but cesarean section is necessary more often than in younger patients. The incidence of essential hypertension, preeclampsia-eclampsia, heart disease, uterine fibroids, and other conditions that appear during the fourth decade is higher than in younger women. *Perinatal mortality* was increased two to three times, but, if the mother is healthy and the pregnancy is normal, a favorable outcome can be anticipated. The incidence of chromosomal abnormalities, particularly trisomies, increases after age 35. Genetic amniocentesis should be offered each patient (Chapter 2). First pregnancies in this age group will be encountered more often in the future as more and more women are delaying pregnancy until after age 30.

LABOR IN MULTIPARAS

Physicians tend to direct less attention toward multiparous women, particularly those who have had several children. This attitude cannot be justified, because both maternal and perinatal mortalities are increased. Disproportion, prolonged and obstructed labor, and ruptured uterus and fetal death may occur because babies tend to become progressively larger with each succeeding pregnancy, and the uterine mechanism becomes less effective. The impaired uterine mechanism also is responsible for a high incidence of postpartum hemorrhage. Hypertension and degenerative vascular disease are most common in multiparas because they are often in the older age groups.

PRECIPITATE LABOR AND DELIVERY

Precipitate labors, those lasting less than 3 hours, occur in only about 10% of all deliveries and are encountered more often in multiparas than in primigravidas. The baby may be injured during rapid, uncontrolled labor.

Patients who have delivered rapidly in previous pregnancies should enter the hospital at once if the membranes rupture or when contractions begin. Elective induction is indicated for those who live some distance from the hospital.

The physician should remain with the patient during her labor. It usually is wise to move her to the delivery room when she is about half dilated. If labor progresses so rapidly that it seems unlikely that she can be moved, it is safer to deliver her in bed than to risk the trip to the delivery room. Under no circumstances should the head be restrained forcibly or an anesthetic administered in an attempt to prevent delivery.

INDUCTION OF LABOR

Labor may be induced artificially by amniotomy or by the administration of oxytocic drugs.

In some patients, particularly those with conditions that might be aggravated by continuing pregnancy, induction serves an important purpose, but it is contraindicated if the pregnancy is normal.

Selection of patients. It is difficult to induce labor safely unless it is about to begin spontaneously. Many complications associated with induction occur because it is attempted in women who actually are not yet ready to start. In most instances the condition of the cervix is the best indication of whether attempted induction is likely to be successful. If the cervix is firm, uneffaced, and occupies a position in the posterior part of the vagina, attempts at induction are likely to be unsuccessful. If immediate delivery is necessary, cesarean section should be considered. On the other hand, it usually is possible to initiate labor when the cervix is soft, effaced, partially dilated, and situated in the middle of the vagina (Table 29-1).

Indications. Most indicated inductions are performed for preeclampsia-eclampsia or chronic hypertension, bleeding complications, and premature rupture of membranes.

PREMATURE RUPTURE OF THE MEMBRANES. Premature rupture of membranes (that is, spontaneous rupture before labor begins) occurs in about 10% to 12% of all pregnant women. The principal complication associated with premature rupture of the membranes is infection, causing fetal and neonatal death.

TABLE 29-1 Method for predicting success of induction of labor

Physical findings	Rating			
	0	1	2	3
Cervix				
Position	Posterior	Midposition	Anterior	
Consistency	Firm	Medium	Soft	
Effacement (%)	0-30	40-50	60-70	≥80
Dilation (cm)	0	1-2	3-4	≥5
Fetal head station	−3	−2	−1	

The *latent period* is the interval between rupture and the onset of labor. The latent period usually is short when the membranes rupture near term, but the less advanced the pregnancy, the longer the latent period.

The principal clinical concern when the membranes rupture prematurely is for intrauterine infection and its consequences for both the fetus and the mother. The amniotic cavity may already have been invaded by bacteria when the membranes rupture; if not, the infection may develop afterward. The decision as to when to terminate the pregnancy is based on weighing the possibility of serious fetal and maternal infection against the risks of prematurity. The latter may be a greater hazard than is infection, particularly if neonatal intensive care is not available.

The patient should be examined to confirm rupture of the membranes and to determine fetal position and the degree of cervical effacement and dilation. Occasionally, the sudden discharge of urine or of thin vaginal or cervical secretions may simulate the gush of fluid that occurs when the membranes rupture. If the cervix is exposed with a sterile speculum, one can determine the character of the fluid in the vagina. If *vernix caseosa* can be seen, the membranes clearly have ruptured. Amniotic fluid that is uncontaminated with blood, meconium, or vaginal secretions will produce a *fern pattern* when allowed to dry on a glass slide. The *pH of amniotic fluid* is alkaline. Because of the possibility of introducing bacteria, no more examinations should be performed after rupture of the membranes has been confirmed.

Premature rupture of the membranes is usually an indication for delivery if the pregnancy is of at least 36 weeks' duration and the fetus is mature. The longer the membranes have been ruptured before the infant is delivered, the greater is the possibility of chorioamnionitis and fetal infection. Bacteria enter the fetus either by aspiration of infected amniotic fluid and exudates or through the fetal bloodstream from foci of infection in the placenta.

To help determine whether prompt delivery is necessary, samples of amniotic fluid can be obtained by transabdominal aspiration from isolated pockets identified by ultrasound. If the fluid is not infected, the risk for the fetus is low, and pregnancy can be allowed to continue. Conversely, if the amniotic cavity already is heavily contaminated, the pregnancy should usually be terminated, particularly if the infant is mature enough to have a good chance of surviving and of developing normally. There is no reason to delay in the hope that survival will be better if the fetus is stressed; evidence that this is effective is not available.

The pregnancy should also be terminated if the mother becomes febrile or begins labor. *Chorioamnionitis* can be diagnosed when the temperature rises and the uterus becomes tender. Cefoxitin or cefotetan should be administered, and electronic fetal monitoring started. If labor has already begun, it should be allowed to continue. There are no arbitrary time limits within which the fetus must be delivered, but labor should be terminated promptly if the fetus becomes distressed. If labor has not already started when chorioamnionitis is diagnosed, an oxytocin induction is appropriate.

Cesarean section is often necessary if labor does not progress or if fetal distress is recognized. Cesarean section is also appropriate if breech or another abnormal position is diagnosed or if any other abnormality such as prolapsed cord is detected.

Other indications. Other indications for induction include certain patients with *diabetes mellitus, prediabetes, Rh sensitization, recurrent pyelonephritis,* and *repeated intrauterine fetal death.*

Technique. Labor can be induced by *artificial rupture of the membranes,* by the infusion of *1:1000 oxytocin solution* intravenously, by a combination of both, or with *prostaglandins.*

Labor will usually begin promptly after *amniotomy* if the head is well engaged and the cervix is soft, effaced, partially dilated, and in an anterior position. Oxytocin supplementation is appropriate if labor has not yet begun within 6 hours after amniotomy.

The principal dangers from amniotomy to induce labor are prolapse of the cord, which may occur even though the head is well fixed in the pelvis, and failure. Unless contractions can be stimulated with oxytocin if amniotomy alone does not induce them, risks from infection are increased. Amniotomy should not often be performed unless the head is engaged.

Oxytocin must be administered with great caution, since the physician cannot determine in advance how responsive the uterus will be. An excessive dose may produce tumultuous contractions, which may injure the baby or even rupture the uterus of a multiparous patient. An intravenous infusion of 5% dextrose is started, and the needle is secured in the vein. The needle from a second 1-L bottle of 5% dextrose to which 1 ml (10 U) of oxytocin has been added is connected through an infusion pump to the tubing of the first intravenous infusion set. The flow from the bottle of plain 5% dextrose solution is adjusted to about 5 drops/min, just enough to maintain a constant flow.

The dosage of oxytocin is calculated in milliunits (mU). If 1 ml of oxytocin (10 IU or 10,000 mU) is added to 1000 ml of 5% dextrose, each milliliter of the resultant solution contains 10 mU of oxytocin. The dosage necessary to stimulate contractions varies, but it may be as low as 0.5 mU/min; consequently, the constant infusion pump is set to deliver this dosage. If the uterus fails to respond within 20 to 30 minutes, the dosage can be increased to 1 mU/min. The dosage is gradually increased by 1-mU increments at 20- to 30-minute intervals until the contractions are similar to those of normal labor.

It is important that someone remain with the patient during an induction, recording the duration of each contraction and checking the patient's pulse and blood pressure frequently. During the early phase of the induction, the uterine contractions and the fetal heart rate can be recorded from external monitors. As soon as is possible, these should be replaced by an intrauterine pressure recording system and a fetal scalp monitor. If the contractions become tetanic, recur too frequently, or last too long, the infusion rate must be reduced.

The total dosage of oxytocin in any uninterrupted period should be limited. Large dosages of oxytocin administered in electrolyte-free fluids over long periods of time are contraindicated because oxytocin may have an antidiuretic effect. This combination may produce edema or even water intoxication and convulsions.

Uterine contractions can also be initiated by the intravenous, intraamniotic, vaginal, or extraovular administration of *prostaglandin F_2* or *F_2 alpha.* Although these substances appear to be as effective as oxytocin in inducing labor, much more study is necessary before they can be used clinically. They seem to be particularly effective in ripening the cervix before induction.

Contraindications. Any condition that makes labor hazardous for the mother or the fetus is a contraindication to induction. These include *abnormal fetal positions and presentations, obvious* *fetopelvic disproportion, uterine scars from previous cesarean sections,* or *uterine operations.* Oxytocin should be used with caution in *women of high parity* because of the increased risk of uterine rupture. *Elective induction* is contraindicated.

SUGGESTED READING

Anderson ABM, Laurence KM, Davies K, Campbell H, and Turnbull AC: Fetal adrenal weight and the cause of premature delivery in human pregnancy, J Obstet Gynaecol Br. Commonw 78:481, 1971.

Anderson GA: Postmaturity: a review, Obstet Gynecol Surv 27:65, 1972.

Bejar R, Curbelo V, Davis C, and Gluck L: Premature labor. II. Bacterial sources of phospholipase, Obstet Gynecol 57:479, 1981.

Bishop EH: Pelvic scoring for elective induction, Obstet Gynecol 24:266, 1964.

Bobitt JR and Ledger WJ: Amniotic fluid analysis: its role in maternal and neonatal infection, Obstet Gynecol 51:56, 1978.

Brook CGD: Consequencies of intrauterine growth retardation, Br Med J 286:164, 1983.

Caldeyro-Barcia R, Noriega-Guerra L, Cibils LA, Alvarez H, Poseiro JJ, Pose SV, Sica-Blanco Y, Mendez-Bauer C, Fielitz C, and Gonzalez-Panizza VH: Effect of position changes on the intensity and frequency of uterine contractions during labor, Am J Obstet Gynecol 80:284, 1960.

Caldeyro-Barcia R and Poseiro JJ: Oxytocin and contractility of the pregnant human uterus, Ann NY Acad Sci 75:813, 1959.

Calkins LA: The second stage of labor: the descent phase, Am J Obstet Gynecol 48:798, 1944.

Cibils LA and Hendricks CH: Normal labor in vertex presentation, Am J Obstet Gynecol 91:385, 1965.

Cotton DB and others: Comparison between magnesium sulfate, terbutaline and a placebo for inhibition of premature labor, J Repro Med 29:92, 1984.

Danforth DN: The fibrous nature of the human cervix, and its relation to the isthmic segment in gravid and nongravid uteri, Am J Obstet Gynecol 53:541, 1947.

Danforth DN, Graham RJ, and Ivy AC: Functional anatomy of labor as revealed by frozen sagittal sections in Macacus rhesus monkeys, Surg Gynecol Obstet 74:188, 1942.

Danforth DN and Ivy AC: The lower uterine segment: its derivation and physiologic behavior, Am J Obstet Gynecol 57:188, 1942.

Friedman EA: Primigravid labor: a graphicostatistical analysis, Obstet Gynecol 6:567, 1955.

Fuchs AR and others: Oxytocin receptors and human parturition: a dual role for oxytocin in the initiation of labor, Science 215:1386, 1982.

Gillespie EC: Principles of uterine growth in pregnancy, Am J Obstet Gynecol 59:949, 1950.

Hellman LM and Prystowsky H: The duration of the second stage of labor, Am J Obstet Gynecol 63:1223, 1952.

Husslein P, Fuchs AR, and Fuchs F: Oxytocin and the initiation of human parturition, Am J Obstet Gynecol 141:688, 1981.

Koh KS, Chan FH, Monfared AH, Ledger WJ, and Paul RH: The changing perinatal and maternal outcome in chorioamnionitis, Obstet Gynecol 53:730, 1979.

Ledger WJ: Monitoring of labor by graphs, Obstet Gynecol 34:174, 1969.

Ledger WJ and Witting WC: The use of a cervical dilatation graph in the management of primigravidae in labour, J Obstet Gynaecol Br Commonw 79:710, 1972.

Munsick RA: Renal hemodynamic effects of oxytocin in antepartal and postpartal women, Am J Obstet Gynecol 108:729, 1970.

Naeye RL: Causes of perinatal mortality in the U.S. Collaborative Perinatal Project, JAMA 238:228, 1977.

Niebyl JR, Blake DA, Johnson JWC, and King TM: The pharmacologic inhibition of premature labor, Obstet Gynecol Surv 33:507, 1978.

Reynolds SRM: Physiology of the uterus with clinical correlations, New York, 1949, Paul B Hoeber, Inc, Medical Book Department, Harper & Brothers.

Schulman H and Ledger WJ: Practical applications of the graphic protrayal of labor, Obstet Gynecol 23:442, 1964.

Seitchik J and Castillo M: Oxytocin augmentation of dysfunctional labor, Am J Obstet Gynecol 144:289, 1982.

Semmens JP: Implications of teenage pregnancy, Obstet Gynecol 26:77, 1965.

30

Russell K. Laros, Jr.

Obstetric analgesia and anesthesia

Objectives

RATIONALE: Proper use of analgesia and anesthesia during labor and delivery are very beneficial components of optimal obstetric care. However, misuse of the potent agents available can turn benefit into increased morbidity and even mortality for both mother and fetus.

The student should be able to:

A. Demonstrate a knowledge of the approach to the use of systemic analgesia during labor.

B. Describe principles of the use of conduction analgesia and anesthesia.
C. List the principles of the use of general anesthesia for delivery.
D. Describe the technique of administering local and pudendal anesthesia for delivery.

In 1847 the Scottish obstetrician James Y. Simpson reported to the Edinburgh Medical-Chirurgical Society that he had been able to abolish pain of delivery with chloroform and thereby initiated a new era in obstetrics. Among those most bitterly opposed to the use of anesthesia were some of the members of the clergy. They argued that according to the Bible women were meant to bring forth their children in "sorrow." Simpson countered with the point that anesthesia must be acceptable to God because He himself had put Adam to sleep to remove the rib from which Eve was created. Despite the controversy, chloroform was readily accepted by women in labor who were not particularly impressed by the theoretical arguments of the clergymen. The opposition was substantially reduced by Queen Victoria's acceptance of chloroform for the delivery of her eighth child in 1853.

Many drugs have been given to make labor and delivery less painful, but unfortunately all have disadvantages that limit their usefulness. The "perfect" agent must provide relief from pain while it neither interferes with the progress of labor nor adds to the maternal or fetal risk. Such an agent has not yet been discovered.

An important concept to remember is that anesthesia for delivery often is emergency anesthesia. There may be no time to prepare patients as there is before a planned surgical procedure. They may have eaten recently or have acute respiratory infections or other disorders that increase the anesthetic hazards.

CONTROL OF PAIN DURING LABOR

Our concept of a *normal childbirth* is one in which labor progresses at a regular rate and terminates in the birth of a healthy infant. This does not preclude the use of analgesia during labor and anesthetic for delivery, as long as neither increases the risk for the mother or the fetus.

Painless labors do occur, but even in primitive societies they are exceptional. The amount of pain experienced is determined in part by the patient's attitude toward pregnancy, labor, and delivery and in part by the length of labor and delivery process. However, other factors may also be very important. In a study of the pain threshold in rats, a gradual increase was observed throughout pregnancy with a marked rise just before the onset of labor. This increased threshold could be abolished by the administration of a narcotic antagonist. These observations suggested that there may be an increase in endogenous beta-endorphine secretion. Studies in humans found that beta-endorphine concentration in peripheral plasma was fairly stable during pregnancy but increased significantly during labor and then decreased within the first hour postpartum. Patients who were delivered by cesarean section without labor did not demonstrate this rise, whereas those operated on after a period of labor did. Finally, intrathecal administration of human beta-endorphine to women in labor abolished the pain associated with labor without affecting the course of labor.

Fetal endorphins are less affected by labor than are maternal concentrations, except that, after the fetus has been stressed in utero, they are increased. The difference suggests that fetal endorphin secretion is unrelated to maternal changes.

As a general rule, women who approach delivery with a maximum of understanding and a minimum of apprehension require the least medication. A normal woman can achieve this state with the help of childbirth education classes designed to provide an understanding of labor as a normal and emotionally satisfying experience and of empathetic attendants who are willing to devote time and thought to meeting individual needs for prenatal education. The results of a similar program in women who are emotionally less well oriented toward pregnancy and motherhood often are unsatisfactory.

Women who have attended predelivery educational courses such as those in which the Lamaze and similar methods are taught often can proceed through labor and delivery with a minimum of discomfort. In many instances the labor progresses more rapidly than is anticipated.

It is essential that attendants understand that their principal role is supportive and that there is no need to interfere as long as labor is progressing normally and the mother is reasonably comfortable. However, it is equally important that the patient and her attendant reach an understanding of the goals before labor begins. The attendant must never force the patient to take an analgesic drug or anesthetic; neither must the patient think that she cannot have one simply because she has chosen one of the psychoprophylactic methods. On the other hand, they must agree that should the labor not progress normally, the attendant automatically has the prerogative of ordering whatever medication is necessary for the procedure required to correct the abnormality.

The understanding, participation, and support of the attendant, the nursing staff, and the father are essential factors in a successful outcome.

There are many methods for providing analgesia during labor, no one of which is suitable for every individual. No "routine" method is possible because some women neither want nor need medication, and in others it may be contraindicated. Each dose should be ordered individually after the attendant is satisfied that it will benefit the patient.

Because no single method can be applied to all women, it is necessary that the attendant be familiar with more than one type. The techniques, however, must be ones that are safe in a particular environment. Certain methods that are permissible in large, well-staffed maternity hospitals may be too dangerous to use in smaller institutions or at home.

Systemic analgesia

The ability to reduce pain during labor with meperidine, fentanyl, and other narcotics is limited by their effects on the newly born infant. Because these drugs cross the placenta, they exert a cerebral depressant effect on the fetus as well as on the mother. This is not particularly important while the fetus is in the uterus, as long as the exchange of respiratory gases across the placenta is maintained at the usual rate. At birth the infant must breathe for itself; the onset of respiration may be delayed many minutes if the infant's respiratory center is depressed by the drugs administered to the mother. The effects of oversedation may last for several days.

Systemic analgesics should be used to reduce the discomfort to a tolerable level and to relax the patient enough to permit her to rest during the pain-free interval between contractions rather than to eliminate pain completely. This can be accomplished without increasing the risk for the infant.

Drugs used to provide systemic analgesia should be injected intravenously or intramuscularly because gastric motility and emptying time are considerably reduced during labor, thus making absorption of oral medications uncertain.

The most important factors to be considered when one prescribes a systemic analgesic are the *amount of the drug and the stage of labor at which it is administered*. Most women do not need analgesia during early labor when the contractions are relatively far apart and of short duration. An ataractic drug, such as promethazine (Phenergan), 50 mg, will usually relax them enough to permit them to rest, or even sleep, until labor is well established. For primigravidas the first injection of analgesic drugs should usually be delayed until the contractions are recurring at 2- to 3-minute intervals and the cervix is 4 to 5 cm dilated. Conversely, if the medication is given too late, the infant will be born during the period of its maximal effect and may well be depressed. Sedation should usually not be administered within 3 hours of delivery.

Meperidine. Meperidine relieves pain as well as morphine, and the usual doses do not alter the course of labor significantly. It does cross the placenta, and if too much is given or if it is administered too late in labor, the newborn infant may be depressed.

A combination of promethazine, 25 to 50 mg, and meperidine, 50 to 100 mg, injected intramuscularly provides excellent analgesia and relaxation without untoward effect on the infant. A maximal analgesic effect is reached in about 45 minutes. Subsequent doses of meperidine when necessary vary between 25 and 50 mg. A second injection of the phenothiazine can be given in 4 to 6 hours if the patient is restless or uncomfortable.

The drugs can be administered intravenously when a more rapid effect is desired. The usual initial dose by this route is no more than 50 mg meperidine and 25 mg promethazine.

Fentanyl. Fentanyl is a rapid-acting narcotic with properties similar to morphine. Analgesia is almost instantaneous following intravenous administration. The peak effect occurs within 3 to 5 minutes, and the duration of action is usually 30 to 60 minutes. When administered intramuscularly, the onset is 7 to 8 minutes, the peak at about 30 minutes, and the duration of action 1 to 2 hours. Usual doses are 25 to 50 μg intravenously and 50 to 100 μg intramuscularly.

Barbituric acid derivatives. These have no analgesic properties and therefore are not used for pain relief during labor. They exert a more profound depressant effect on the fetal respiratory center than do the narcotics, and they may produce considerable excitement in certain individuals.

Complications. The most important complication accompanying the use of systemic analgesics is *depression of the infant's respiratory center* and subsequent apnea neonatorum, which is particularly likely to occur if general anesthesia is also administered. This can be prevented by using small doses of the drugs and by attempting to time the last injection to precede delivery by at least 3 hours.

If the infant is narcotized by meperidine, fentanyl, or similar substances, the effect of the drugs can be neutralized by injecting naloxone (Narcan), 10 μg/kg, into an umbilical vein. Unlike nalorphine (Nalline), which is antagonistic only to morphinelike drugs and may increase the depression produced by barbiturates and inhalation anesthetics, naloxone has no other obvious pharmacologic effect.

The *heavily medicated patient cannot cooperate during the second stage;* thus the number of required operative deliveries is increased by excessive sedation.

Inhalation analgesia

Almost all the volatile anesthetic agents have been used to relieve pain during labor, but none is entirely satisfactory. The most often used is a mixture of *nitrous oxide (50%) and oxygen (50%),* which, when inhaled during each uterine contraction, will reduce the discomfort considerably. Somewhat higher concentrations of nitrous oxide can be used if necessary, but if the concentration of oxygen is reduced much below 30%, the fetus may become hypoxic.

This method is most valuable at the end of the first stage in multiparas and during the second stage in both multiparas and primigravidas. The gas can be inhaled intermittently for some time without interfering with uterine contractions or compromising the infant.

Regional analgesia

The transmission of pain impulses can be controlled by nerve block. With this type of analgesia, the mother is awake and comfortable, and the baby rarely is depressed. Major nerve block techniques require an experienced individual to administer the anesthetic and supervise the patient during the rest of her labor and delivery; as a consequence, some of these forms of analgesia are usually available only in large institutions.

Pain sensations from the uterus, the cervix, and the upper vagina are transmitted to Frankenhäuser's ganglions, which lie just lateral to the cervix; then through the inferior and superior hypogastric plexuses, and by way of the lumbar and lower thoracic sympathetic chains, to the spinal cord through nerves arising from T10, 11, and 12 and L1.

The major pain sensations from the lower vagina and posterior vulva and perineum, which are the principal sources of discomfort as the presenting part distends the lower vagina and delivers, are transmitted through the pudendal nerves, which are derived from the ventral branches of S2, 3, and 4.

Epidural (peridural) block. The injection of an anesthetic drug into the extradural space controls pain by blocking the transmission of painful stimuli without interfering with the muscular activity of the uterus. Control of the voluntary muscles in the legs is maintained, but the pelvic muscles are relaxed, making delivery easier for both the mother and her infant. Because peridural block does not alter oxygenation unless the maternal blood pressure falls, it is particularly valuable during premature labor and in women with heart disease, diabetes, and pulmonary diseases.

The block is established by injecting an anesthetic agent into the peridural space between two lumbar vertebrae *(epidural block)* or through the sacral hiatus *(caudal block).* The injection is made after labor is well established and is progressing normally and when the patient is uncomfortable enough to desire relief. Because the duration of pain relief from an injection is limited, *continuous caudal and epidural techniques* have generally replaced single injections. A polyethylene catheter is threaded through the needle and is left in place as the needle is withdrawn over it. Subsequent injections are made as needed to keep the patient comfortable until the infant is delivered.

Epidural anesthesia is *contraindicated* in patients with a skin infection near the proposed puncture site, in those with any disease of the spine or central nervous system, in those who are bleeding or in shock, and in those with hypertension. It is far more suitable for the delivery of primigravidas than of multiparas, particularly those who have had rapid easy labors in the past. Epidural block should not be attempted unless an experienced individual can supervise the insertion of the needle and catheter and the injections of the anesthetic agent throughout the labor.

The *complications,* some of which are potentially lethal, can be kept at a minimum by strict observation of the necessary precautions. The most serious complications are *massive spinal anesthesia* following the inadvertent injection of the agent into the subarachnoid space, *meningitis, epidural abscess, intravenous injection,* and *breakage of the needle or catheter.* Less serious complications are *hypotension,* which is minimal in normal women, and *anesthetic failure.*

The agents most commonly used for epidural block are chloroprocaine, bupivacaine, and lidocaine. The concentration and volume of the agent is varied to achieve different levels and degrees of sensory and motor block. The agents vary in their potency, rapidity of onset, and duration of action.

Because sympathetic block is a common complication of any type of regional anesthesia, several measures aimed at reducing the incidence are appropriate, including administration of a fluid bolus prior to placement of the block, left uterine displacement, and prophylactic administration of ephedrine. If hypotension still occurs, additional left uterine displacement should be applied, the patient should be placed in Trendelenburg's position, and intravenous fluid administered rapidly. If these maneuvers are not successful, additional ephedrine, 10 to 15 mg, should be given intravenously and O_2 administered. When recognized and properly treated, transient maternal hypotension does not lead to maternal or fetal morbidity.

Although there may be a temporary depression of uterine activity after the injection, epidural block does not usually affect cervical dilation. The second stage may be prolonged because the loss of pain sensation in the vagina and on the perineum eliminates involuntary expulsive efforts and interferes with voluntary attempts to use the secondary forces to expel the baby.

Epidural narcotics are now widely used after cesarean section. The principle is that long-lasting analgesia can be produced by a minimal dose of narcotic when it is applied almost directly to the dorsal horn of the spinal column. Following delivery of the infant, 5 mg of preservative-free morphine sulfate is administered through the epidural catheter. This will generally provide satisfactory analgesia for 24 to 36 hours. The most common side effects are pruritus seen in almost 70% of patients. The most serious side effect is delayed respiratory depression. To avoid this risk, a precise monitoring schedule and very cautious administration of any systemic narcotics are required. Urinary retention and nausea and vomiting are also minor but annoying side effects.

Paracervical (uterosacral) block. The pain during the first stage of labor arises from the dilating cervix and upper vagina and generally can be controlled by blocking the sensory and autonomic nerves that supply these areas. To accomplish this an anesthetic agent is injected at about the junction of the uterosacral ligaments, through which the nerve fibers pass, and the cervix. The block usually is administered when painful contractions are recurring regularly and the cervix is dilated 5 to 6 cm in primigravidas and slightly earlier in multiparas.

A hollow metal guide, such as an Iowa trumpet, is inserted along the fingers into the vagina until its tip rests against the lateral fornix at about the 4 o'clock position. A 15-cm, 20-gauge needle is passed through the guide until its point punctures the vaginal epithelium. The tip of the needle is inserted to a depth of about 0.5 cm, and, after aspiration to make certain that it has not punctured a blood vessel, 5 or 10 ml of 0.5% lidocaine (Xylocaine) is injected into the tissue. The procedure is repeated on the opposite side at the 8 o'clock position. The anesthetic agent must be injected superficially to avoid introducing it into a blood vessel, the uterus, or even directly into the fetus.

Paracervical block provides prompt and effective pain relief in at least 75% of patients. The duration of action varies, but it often lasts an hour or more; the injection can be repeated if pain recurs and the cervix is still incompletely dilated.

In some patients, *uterine contractions stop* for a short time after the injection; however, when the contractions begin again, labor progresses normally. *Fetal bradycardia,* which has been observed frequently, is probably caused by absorption of the anesthetic agent into the fetal circulation or because of hypoxia resulting from spasm of the arteries in uterine muscle. If the concentration of the drug in fetal tissues is high enough, the infant may be depressed at birth or even die. Paracervical block should not be used if there is any suggestion of placental insufficiency or when uterine blood flow is reduced by hypertension.

The incidence of fetal bradycardia can be substantially reduced by decreasing the dose of the drug used and by injecting it superficially in the vaginal wall rather than deep. If the needle is inserted too far, the anesthetic may be injected into the myometrium or into one of the large blood vessels in the broad ligament, thereby increasing the possibility that a large amount will reach the fetus.

This technique does not anesthetize the lower vagina or the perineal structures; consequently, pudendal block or local infiltration is necessary for delivery.

ANESTHESIA FOR DELIVERY

Relief of pain during the actual delivery of the infant plays an important part in modern obstetrics. Pain relief is not an important enough reason to justify an increase in maternal or fetal morbidity or mortality, but such an increase is not necessary if the physician selects the anesthetic most suitable for each patient and provides for its safe administration.

Inhalation anesthetic

Apprehensive women may demand inhalation anesthesia to obliterate all consciousness of what is happening during delivery. Although this can be accomplished with relative safety by the proper selection and administration of the agent, certain hazards accompany the use of inhalation anesthesia. *Vomiting* and *aspiration* are serious complications and a major cause of maternal deaths. Patients should be cautioned against eating after the contractions begin and not allowed anything by mouth during labor. Regional anesthesia should be used for women who have eaten recently, or if this is not available, the stomach should be emptied, and the patient should be given 30 ml of milk of magnesia or an antacid shortly before delivery to neutralize the remaining stomach contents. If she vomits and aspirates, there will be less pulmonary damage if acidity of the vomitus is reduced.

Prolonged deep anesthesia may *interfere with uterine contractions,* thereby increasing the incidence of bleeding during the third stage. Because the inhalation anesthetic agents cross the placenta, *the infant may be anesthetized and apneic at birth* if deep anesthesia has been induced. This need not occur during normal delivery, but prolonged anesthesia is a distinct hazard when the uterus must be relaxed with inhalation anesthesia.

This method generally is preferred over spinal or epidural anesthesia for women with hypotension from bleeding or other causes, for those with disorders of the spine or nervous system, or for emergency cesarean section when it is important to deliver the baby rapidly. Inhalation anesthesia is essential whenever it is necessary to abolish uterine contractions and relax the uterine muscle to complete delivery.

Inhalation techniques are being used less often for normal or forceps delivery as more obstetricians and their patients become aware of the advantages of conduction anesthesia. Many women want to be awake during the birth of their babies, and obstetricians are concerned over the potential dangers that are inherent with inhalation anesthesia. Fortunately, the variety of available conduction techniques permits the selection of one that is suitable under almost any circumstance.

When general anesthesia is required, a rapid sequence induction technique is preferred. The patient should be premedicated with antacid and preoxygenated for 3 minutes if possible with high flow rates (greater than 6 L per minute). Atropine, 0.4 mg, or glycopyrrolate, 0.2 mg, and curare, 3 mg, are given intravenously. Induction of anesthesia is achieved with thiopental, 4 mg/kg, and succinylcholine 1.5 mg/kg. An assistant should apply cricoid pressure to lessen the chance of vomiting until intubation is completed. If uterine relaxation is not required, N_2O, 5 L per minute, and O_2, 5 L per minute, are given by mask and succinylcholine administered as needed for muscle relaxation. If uterine relaxation is required, 1% halothane and 99% O_2 are used. Methoxyflurane and enflurane are inhalation anesthetic agents that can also be used effectively for obstetrical anesthesia.

Conduction anesthesia

Some form of nerve block anesthesia usually is preferable to inhalation types because it permits the mother to be awake and it relieves pain without disturbing fetal oxygenation. Some methods, however, have a high potential mortality, but all must be administered with the greatest caution. The two principal types of regional anesthetic agents are those that produce loss of pain sensation by blocking the nerve roots and those that block the nerves peripherally.

Nerve root block. For the most part these techniques relieve pain completely but do not interfere with the uterine contractions. There is an associated vasodilation below the anesthetic level that may be responsible for a fall in blood pressure. These anesthetic techniques do not depress the respiratory center and therefore are beneficial to the fetus unless the maternal blood pressure falls enough to interfere with uterine blood flow, thus decreasing the amount of oxygen available to the fetus. Relaxation of the voluntary pelvic and perineal muscles decreases the pressure on the fetal head, but this loss of resistance may interfere with the normal mechanism of labor, particularly rotation. The relaxation makes forceps delivery easier and less traumatic, but the fact that uterine contractions are not altered makes nerve root block unsuitable for intrauterine manipulation.

Epidural anesthetic may be used for analgesia during labor and anesthesia for delivery and is particularly advantageous for women in whom the usual methods for relieving pain during labor and delivery are contraindicated. It can be administered only by trained and experienced individuals.

Epidural anesthesia may be unsatisfactory when given only for delivery when labor is progressing rapidly. It may take 20 to 30 minutes to insert the catheter and to obtain an adequate anesthetic level. If one starts too late, the patient may deliver before the anesthetic has become effective. This is particularly true in multiparas.

Spinal anesthesia has rightly been considered a dangerous method for producing anesthesia because the mortality is high if it is improperly used. The dangers that are inherent with this technique can be obviated by being aware of them and attempting to avoid them. The vasomotor system is unstable in gravid women, and shock may follow ordinary doses of medication given intraspinally.

Spinal anesthesia is of greatest value in primigravidas, to whom it is administered when the head is bulging the perineum. If given to multiparas too early, descent of the head often is prevented, even though uterine contractions continue, because the patient no longer has an urge to bear down. It should usually be administered to multiparas when the cervix is 8 to 9 cm dilated and the heat well below the ischial spines. It is only to be used in carefully selected patients in hospitals where there is sufficient help to treat the fall in blood pressure and other complications that may be associated with its administration.

Low spinal or *saddle block,* the type of spinal anesthesia most often used for delivery, is given with the patient sitting up. It is better used as a terminal anesthetic for delivery than to provide analgesia during labor. Appropriate doses are tetracaine, 3 to 5 mg in 10% dextrose, or lidocaine, 25 to 40 mg, for vaginal delivery. The smaller doses will achieve an S1 to S5 level; the larger ones will raise the level of block to T10. For cesarean section an anesthetic level to T6 is desirable, and the doses of tetracaine and lidocaine are 8 mg and 50 to 75 mg, respectively.

Headache often follows the administration of spinal or saddle block anesthesia for delivery. The incidence can be reduced substantially by the use of a 26-gauge needle rather than the standard larger sizes. The loss of spinal fluid through the dural defect, which is thought to be a major factor in the production of headache, is minimized when the small needle is used. Other more important complications of spinal anesthesia include *arachnoiditis, nerve root injury* from chemical or direct trauma, and an *overdose of the drug*—any one of which may result in disability or death. Complications can be kept at a minimum by exercising every possible precaution during the preparation of the solution and its administration.

Peripheral nerve block. Local injection of anesthetic agents to block the peripheral nerve endings affords the same advantages to the fetus that nerve root blocks do, but they are less effective in relieving pain and providing muscle relaxation. They do not require unusual equipment or the presence of an anesthesiologist.

Simple infiltration of the perineum or injection along the line of the proposed episiotomy with 0.5% to 1% procaine or lidocaine is often sufficient for normal delivery but is usually inadequate for forceps delivery.

Pudendal nerve block by injection of 10 ml of 0.5% to 1% lidocaine around each perineal nerve trunk as it

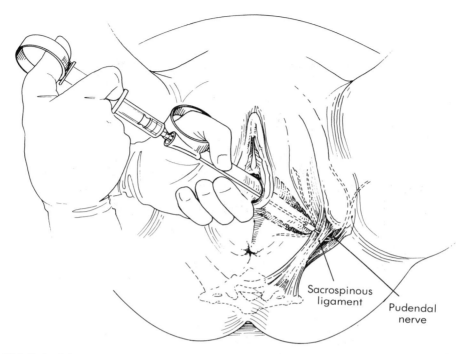

Fig. 30-1 Pudendal nerve block. Needle point is directed behind inferior tip of ischial spine by fingertip.

passes behind the ischial spine provides excellent pelvic anesthesia for normal or low forceps delivery and for episiotomy and repair. It provides inadequate anesthesia for most manual or forceps rotations. It is safe, easy to learn, and requires no anesthesiologist or expensive equipment. This procedure should be suitable for almost all normal deliveries (Figs. 30-1 and 30-2).

A hollow metal guide such as an Iowa trumpet is passed along the palmar surface of the index or second finger toward the ischial spine. The tip of the guide is directed to a position just beneath the tip of the spine and is held firmly in place. A 15-cm, 20-gauge needle attached to a syringe containing lidocaine is inserted through the guide until its tip reaches the vaginal wall. With further pressure, the needle is pushed through the triangle formed by the sacrospinous and sacrotuberous ligaments and the obturator internus muscles until the tip is in Alcock's canal, through which the pudendal nerve trunk runs. If the needle is properly placed, it can be moved back and forth without resistance. Blood can be aspirated if the pudendal artery or vein has been punctured; in this event the needle should be withdrawn slightly before the anesthetic agent is injected.

A 10-ml deposit of the lidocaine solution is made in the pudendal canal behind each ischial spine, where it is in direct contact with the pudendal nerve trunk. The anesthetic effect will be evident within 2 to 3 minutes. Muscular relaxation as well as anesthesia is effected and will last as long as an hour.

SPECIAL PROCEDURES

The judicious use of analgesics and anesthetics does not affect the outcome of normal labor adversely, but when complications are present, the choice of an inappropriate agent or method can add significantly to the risk for the mother or her baby. For instance, a combination of systemic analgesics and inhalation anesthesia for the *delivery of a premature infant* is generally contraindicated. A small infant is likely to be seriously depressed by these agents, whereas they have less effect on a mature fetus. Epidural or spinal anesthesia is generally contraindicated in women with *hypertension,*

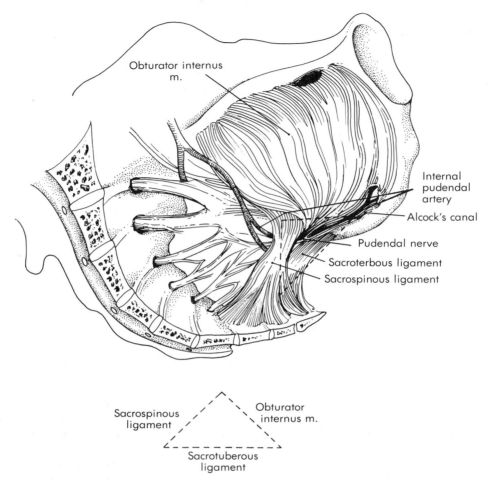

Fig. 30-2 Pudendal nerve block. Localizing landmarks in region of ischial spine and relationship of pudendal nerve to pudendal and inferior gluteal vessels.

particularly when the blood pressure is labile, and for those who are bleeding from *placenta previa* or *abruptio placentae*. Conversely, conduction anesthesia is preferable for patients with *heart disease, pulmonary disease, diabetes (if the blood pressure is normal),* and *conditions that predispose to uterine relaxation and bleeding following delivery.* These are discussed elsewhere in the text with consideration of the specific complications.

SUGGESTED READING

Arnolds CW, Anderson CJ, and Sherline DM: Prepared childbirth, Clin Obstet Gynecol 24:575, 1981.

Chestnut D, editor: Obstetric analgesia and anesthesia, Clin Obstet Gynecol 30:485, 1987.

Cohen SE: The aspiration syndrome, Clin Obstet Gynecol 9:235, 1982.

Facchinetti F, Bagnoli F, Petraglia F, Parrini D, Sardelli S, and Genazzani AR: Fetomaternal opioid levels and parturition, Obstet Gynecol 62:764, 1983.

Gintzler AR: Endorphine-mediated increases in pain threshold during pregnancy, Science 210:193, 1980.

Hoffman DI, Abdoud TK, Haase HR, Hung TT, and Goebelsmann V: Plasma β-endorphine concentrations prior to and during pregnancy, in labor, and after delivery, Am J Obstet Gynecol 150:492, 1984.

King JC and Sherline DM: Paracervical and pudendal block, Clin Obstet Gynecol 24:587, 1981.

Oyama T, Matsuki A, Taneichi T, Ling N, and Guillemin R: Beta-endorphine in obstetric analgesia, Am J Obstet Gynecol 137:613, 1980.

Riss PA and Bieglmayer C: Obstetric analgesia and immunoreactive endorphin peptides in maternal plasma during labor, Gynecol Obstet Invest 17:127, 1984.

Scanlon J: Effects of obstetric anesthesia and analgesia on the newborn: a select and annotated bibliography for the clinician, Clin Obstet Gynecol 24:649, 1981.

Shnider SM, and Levinson G: Anesthesia for obstetrics, Baltimore, 1987, The Williams & Wilkins Co.

31

J. Robert Willson

Third stage of labor and postpartum hemorrhage

Objectives

RATIONALE: Postpartum hemorrhage continues to be a major cause of maternal mortality and morbidity, in spite of the fact that excess bleeding and its complications can usually be prevented.

The student should be able to:

A. Describe the normal mechanism for placental separation and expulsion.

B. Describe the management of the third stage of labor.

C. Define *postpartum hemorrhage,* list the causes, and indicate how each can be recognized.

D. Describe the principles involved in preventing and treating postpartum hemorrhage.

The third stage, the interval between the delivery of the infant and the delivery of the placenta, is the most dangerous part of the entire labor. Abnormalities of placental separation and expulsion are often accompanied by profuse bleeding that may end in death. At least 15% of maternal deaths result from postpartum hemorrhage, but most can be prevented if the attendant recognizes that blood loss is excessive, determines the cause, controls the bleeding, and replaces the lost blood promptly. Few postpartum hemorrhages occur so rapidly that there is no time for appropriate treatment. In most instances death occurs several hours after delivery when the pa-

tient has been exsanguinated by a steady trickle of blood rather than by a sudden overwhelming hemorrhage.

Blood loss during the third stage varies considerably. Newton reported the average measured blood loss during the first 24 hours after vaginal delivery to be about 650 ml. Pritchard and colleagues reported a similar figure and also observed that 5% of women who delivered vaginally lost more than 1000 ml of blood. Ueland measured a blood volume loss of 610 ml 60 minutes after vaginal delivery. The highest measurements of blood loss are those of Quinlivan and Brock, who calculated the decrease in blood volume after delivery to be 1115 and 1023 ml by the two methods used. This corresponded to their measured loss of 1106 ml.

It has been customary to diagnose *postpartum hemorrhage* when the total blood loss with delivery and during the first 24 hours after delivery is *estimated* to exceed 500 ml. It is obvious from the studies in which blood loss was measured accurately, rather than estimated, that 500 ml is far too low a figure to accept as the upper limit of normal. A more logical maximum is 1000 ml.

NORMAL THIRD STAGE

Placental separation. Under normal circumstances the placenta is relatively noncontractile and has only limited ability to alter its size and shape to compensate for changes in the area of the uterine wall over which it is attached. As the uterus becomes smaller during expulsion of the infant, the surface area of its cavity must of necessity diminish. As the area of the placental site is reduced, the placenta thickens, and its diameter decreases. Because placental size cannot be altered enough to equal the change in the muscular

uterine wall beneath it, the placenta is at least partially sheared off as the uterus contracts during the expulsion of the fetus. The completeness with which the placenta is separated is determined by how much the subplacental area of the uterine wall is reduced (Fig. 31-1).

The separation occurs in the spongy portion of the decidua basalis; a thin layer of decidua remains on the uterine wall, and the remainder covers the cotyledons of the maternal surface of the placenta.

After the birth of the baby, the uterus continues to contract regularly. At this stage the uterine muscle may be even more active than it was during late labor. The uterus is diskoid, being wide transversely but relatively flattened in its anteroposterior diameter, and lies in the midline with its superior surface below the level of the umbilicus. The placenta has already been partially or completely separated during the expulsion of the baby, but it still is in the upper part of the cavity. The continuing uterine contractions complete the separation of the placenta and force it downward into the flaccid, distended lower segment.

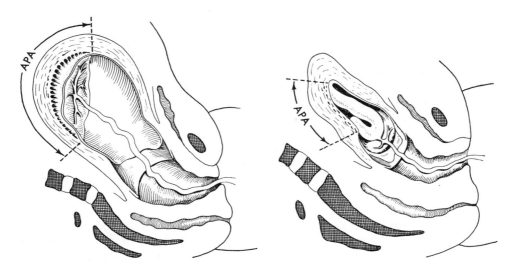

Fig. 31-1 Reduction in size of area of placental attachment *(APA)* as upper segment contracts, separates placenta, and expels it into lower uterine segment.

As the placenta is expelled from the upper segment, this portion of the uterus becomes globular, its cavity is almost obliterated, and the thickness of the wall increases to as much as 5 cm. The bulky placenta distending the relaxed lower segment forces the globular fundus upward and to the right; the superior surface of the uterus can often be felt above the level of the umbilicus.

The placenta ultimately is forced from the lower segment and vagina by voluntary bearing-down efforts of the mother or, as is more often the case, is expressed by the attendant.

The duration of the third stage will be from 15 to 30 minutes or even longer if the physician waits for the mother to expel the placenta herself. When the placental phase of labor is managed actively by the medical attendant, its duration can be less than 5 minutes in almost every instance.

Control of bleeding. The branches of the uterine arteries wind between the interlacing smooth-muscle bundles as they traverse the uterine wall, and they eventually open into the large sinuses in the decidua basalis at the placental site. *The source of the blood loss after delivery, except that caused by soft-tissue injury, is the sinuses that are left open by separation of the placenta.* Excess bleeding is prevented by firm contraction of the uterine muscle bundles, which kink and compress the vessels passing between them. This is followed by clot formation and retraction in the sinuses, the usual method by which bleeding from open vessels is controlled.

Placental expulsion. The so-called signs of separation of the placenta are more accurately evidences of its expulsion from the firmly contracted uterine fundus into the lower segment and vagina and indicate that it can be delivered. The signs consist of the following:

1. A *show of blood* appears as the uterus contracts and the placenta is forced downward. If the placenta is separated completely as the infant is delivered, it usually folds on itself like an inverted umbrella with the fetal surface preceding the periphery through the cervix. With this type of expulsion, the *Schultze mechanism,* the placenta occludes the cervical opening; and there is little obvious bleeding until it is expelled, at which time the blood retained within the uterus gushes out. With the less common *Duncan mechanism,* there is a constant trickle of blood because an edge of the placenta, rather than an inverted surface, appears in the cervical opening and the blood can leave the uterus freely.

2. *The cord advances.* The length of cord visible outside the introitus is increased as the placenta descends into the lower segment and vagina.

3. *The fundus rises* and is deviated toward the right as the placenta, distending the lower segment, elevates the contracted upper portion.

4. *The shape of the uterus changes.* The uterus becomes globular rather than wide and flat after the placenta has been expelled into the lower segment.

5. *Nontransmission of impulse occurs.* As slight traction is made on the cord while the uterus is pushed downward by pressure on the fundus, the amount of cord outside the vagina increases. If the placenta is still in the upper segment, the cord is withdrawn into the vagina when the suprapubic pressure is released and the uterus is allowed to rise. If the placenta is detached and in the lower segment, the cord retracts very little when the uterus rises.

Management. During the second stage the physician should attempt to empty the uterus slowly, thereby permitting the muscle fibers to retract and decrease the size of the cavity gradually as the infant is being delivered. This encourages prompt and forceful contraction and more complete placental separation.

After the head has been born, the anterior shoulder is delivered beneath the pubic arch, where it is allowed to remain for 15 to 30 seconds to permit retraction of the muscle fibers in the fundus. The head is then elevated, and traction is

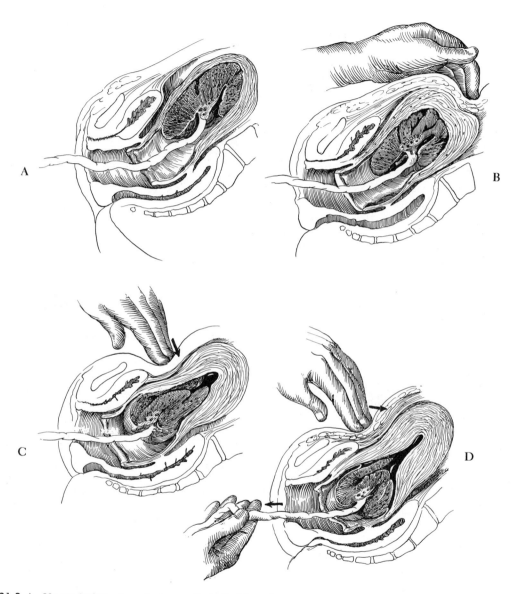

Fig. 31-2 A, Uterus before placenta is expelled. **B,** Manual pressure on fundus as uterus begins to contract aids expulsion of placenta into lower segment **(C),** from where it can be expressed by upward pressure on contracted fundus and tension on cord **(D).**

exerted until the posterior shoulder has cleared the perineum. After another wait to permit further readjustment of the uterine muscle fibers, the rest of the body is slowly and deliberately extracted. The physician should not try to restrain delivery if the spontaneous uterine contractions are forcing the baby through the birth canal, but the mother should be urged not to bear down lest the baby be expelled so rapidly that the soft tissues are torn.

After the cord has been clamped and cut, the uterus is gently palpated through the sterile drapes while the cord is held taut but without undue traction. The uterus should not be massaged and manipulated, and no attempt should be made to express the placenta until the uterus contracts. As the fundus becomes firm and globular, placental expulsion can be aided by downward pressure over the superior surface of the uterus with the palmar surfaces of the fingers; it should not be squeezed (Fig. 31-2). Downward pressure is no longer necessary after the placenta enters the lower segment; therefore, at the moment placental descent can be detected, the pressure is transferred from the fundus to the suprapubic area directly over the lower segment. As the contracted uterine fundus is pushed *upward* away from the placenta by firm pressure with the fingertips, the afterbirth, which by now should be visible at the introitus, can be delivered by applying slight traction on the cord.

After the placenta has been delivered, the contracted fundus is kept from dropping back into the pelvis by maintaining upward pressure on it through the abdominal wall; this will promote muscular contraction and reduce bleeding. While a nurse or an assistant applies the pressure necessary to hold the uterus up, the physician examines the placenta to make certain it is intact and that none of its cotyledons has been left in the uterine cavity. An oxytocic drug is usually given at this time to stimulate uterine muscle contraction.

Uterotonic (oxytocic) drugs stimulate firm uterine contraction and when properly used will reduce the blood loss accompanying placental separation and de-

livery. It generally is preferable to withhold uterotonic drugs until the placenta has been delivered.

The purified ergot derivative *ergonovine maleate (Ergotrate),* when administered intravenously or intramuscularly in 0.5 to 1 ml (0.1 to 0.2 mg) doses, produces a sustained tetanic contraction of the uterine muscles that reduces the blood loss from the vessels at the placental site. Ordinarily, it is given intravenously as soon as the placenta has been delivered. *Methylergonovine maleate (Methergine),* a synthetic preparation, is equally effective in the same doses.

Ergonovine maleate, and to a lesser degree methylergonovine maleate, may produce vasoconstriction and an alarming rise in blood pressure in susceptible women. Neither should be given to women with hypertension or to those with labile blood pressures.

Oxytocin from which almost all the vasopressor factor has been removed can be administered instead of ergot preparations as an aid in managing the third stage. It is preferred over either ergonovine maleate or methylergonovine maleate for women with hypertensive disorders because it is less likely to produce alarming blood pressure elevations. The dosage is 0.1 to 0.2 ml (1 to 2 U) intravenously, 0.5 ml (5 U) intramuscularly, or 2 ml (20 U) dissolved in 1000 ml of 5% dextrose solution as an intravenous drip. The latter method is preferred if an intravenous infusion already is running.

One potentially serious side effect of oxytocin is its cardiovascular action. The rapid intravenous injection of a bolus of 0.5 ml (5 U) of oxytocin may be followed by a profound decrease in blood pressure. This is less likely to occur with the small amounts administered in dilute solution and with intramuscular injection.

Manual removal of the placenta. Some obstetricians separate and remove the placenta and explore the interior of the uterus as a routine procedure. Although the risk is not great, it is usually unnecessary if normal placenta separation and expulsion can be anticipated. Conversely, manual removal is indicated when the placenta fails to separate within a reasonable time and as part of the treatment of postpartum hemorrhage.

Fetomaternal transfusion. A small amount of fetal blood probably enters the maternal circulation during almost every delivery. This accounts for some instances of Rh isoimmunization. The danger of immunization can be reduced by using a method of placental delivery that minimizes fetomaternal transfusion.

Simple expression of the placenta after spontaneous separation probably provides the smallest infusion of fetal blood from the placenta into the maternal blood in the choriodecidual spaces. Infusion may be increased by the injudicious use of oxytocic agents before the completion of the third stage and by manual removal of the placenta.

POSTPARTUM HEMORRHAGE

Postpartum hemorrhage should occur in less than 5% of all deliveries. In almost every instance, excessive bleeding can be controlled, and the blood can be replaced so rapidly that no woman should die as a result of postpartum bleeding.

Etiologic factors. The most important causes of excessive bleeding at delivery or during the early puerperium are *uterine atony* and *soft-tissue injury*. Of these, the first is by far the more common.

The source of the bleeding is either the sinuses of the placental site that remain open after the placenta has separated because the uterus fails to contract properly or blood vessels of the birth canal that are torn during delivery. In either event the amount of bleeding is determined by the size of the involved vessels and the length of time before the blood loss is checked.

Predisposing factors. Certain factors increase the possibility that excessive bleeding will occur after delivery. Most of these interfere with the normal mechanism for controlling bleeding.

OVERDISTENSION OF THE UTERUS. If the uterus has been overdistended by twins, a large infant, or hydramnios, the muscle fibers have been stretched to a point from which they may not be able to retract rapidly enough and contract firmly enough to occlude the open vessels promptly after delivery. Delayed contraction also is likely to occur if the uterus is emptied rapidly.

ANESTHESIA. Deep inhalation anesthesia reduces the force of uterine muscle contraction and may inhibit uterine activity completely. Deep anesthesia therefore can eliminate the normal mechanism by which bleeding after delivery is controlled.

DYSFUNCTIONAL OR PROLONGED LABOR. Ineffective uterine contractions often continue into the third stage.

IMPROPER MANAGEMENT OF THE THIRD STAGE. Manipulation and massage in an attempt to express the placenta before it has separated completely may interfere with the normal mechanism and increase bleeding.

INJURY. A considerable amount of blood may be lost from vaginal lacerations, uterine rupture, or even the episiotomy. Odell and Seski state that the average blood loss from a mediolateral episiotomy is about 250 ml.

RETAINED PLACENTA. Excessive bleeding occurs if the uterus cannot expel a partially separated placenta or if a large fragment of placenta, for example, a succenturiate lobe, is retained.

HISTORY. Postpartum hemorrhage can be anticipated in multiparous women who have had excessive bleeding after other deliveries. The cause may not be obvious.

Clinical course. Deaths from postpartum bleeding are rarely caused by sudden overwhelming hemorrhage. Excessive blood loss is usually the result of a prolonged trickle of blood rather than a single massive hemorrhage, but unless the flow is checked the end result is the same. Pregnant women, because of the expanded blood volume, withstand hemorrhage better than do nonpregnant women, but the amount any individual woman will tolerate cannot be determined in advance. *Those with anemia or chronic debilitating disease and those whose blood volume is decreased because of prolonged labor and dehydration or severe preeclampsia-eclampsia may go into shock with relatively minimal bleeding.*

Prevention. Most postpartum hemorrhages can be prevented, but some cannot, and all pregnant women should be considered potential candidates for excessive bleeding. Predisposing causes should be eliminated, and anemia and nutritional inadequacies should be corrected whenever possible.

Abnormal labor should be shortened by recognizing inadequate contractions early and instituting measures that will be helpful in preventing prolonged labor. Regional anesthetic should be used whenever possible, and the second as well as the third stage should be managed in a manner calculated to encourage retraction and firm contraction of uterine muscle fibers.

Treatment. The most important factors in preventing deaths from postpartum hemorrhage are to recognize abnormal bleeding before the blood loss has been excessive, to determine the source of the bleeding, to control it as rapidly as possible, and to replace lost blood promptly.

Before the delivery of women with conditions that predispose to excessive bleeding, an intravenous infusion of saline solution should be started through a 15-gauge needle. Blood should be administered to all in whom clinical evidence of blood loss can be detected, even though the amount of bleeding does not seem excessive.

Severe bleeding after the birth of the baby is more often the result of inadequate uterine muscle contraction than of injury. The first step in determining the cause therefore is to palpate the uterine fundus rather than to search for lacerations in the birth canal. If the uterus is soft and boggy, it is almost always the source of bleeding; this is particularly true if the placenta has not yet been delivered.

AT END OF SECOND STAGE. The placenta is expressed if possible or removed manually, and the uterus is pushed upward out of the pelvis and massaged between one hand inserted in the vagina and the other palpating through the abdominal wall to stimulate contraction. Oxytocin is added to the infusion fluid, or 1 or 2 U can be given intravenously while the uterus is being stimulated. If the uterus does not contract under the influence of oxytocin, methylergonovine, 0.5 ml (0.1 mg), can be given intravenously unless there is a contraindication to using it. If the uterus remains relaxed despite these measures, manual exploration to search for an injury or retained placental tissue should be performed promptly.

A prostaglandin F_2-alpha analogue, (15S)-15-methyl prostaglandin F_2-alpha tromethamine, injected intramuscularly or directly into the uterine wall, has been used with some success in treating postpartum hemorrhage when the uterus fails to contract after the administration of oxytocin and ergot compounds. Prostaglandin preparations have not yet been approved for use in managing postpartum hemorrhage.

If bleeding continues, the physician must consider the possibility of a clotting defect and test for it.

Hysterectomy may be indicated if all other methods have failed to control bleeding. It should not be delayed until the patient is dying.

AT END OF THIRD STAGE. If abnormal bleeding begins after the placenta has been delivered, the physician should explore the uterus to make certain that it is intact and empty and then stimulate it by manual massage and oxytocics as described previously.

Postpartum hemorrhage from injury. Unless the vagina is extensively lacerated or there are deep cervical tears extending upward into the lower segment, bleeding from injury is less severe than that from atony. The usual cervical lacerations seldom bleed profusely. *Injury should be suspected and sought whenever vaginal bleeding continues despite a firmly contracted fundus.*

Bleeding from vaginal lacerations can usually be controlled with sutures, which must be placed precisely to make certain that they approximate the entire length of the injured area. An assistant to expose the laceration is essential if bleeding is excessive or if the upper vagina is involved. Continued oozing after the placement of sutures can usually be checked with pressure from a tight vaginal pack.

Cervical lacerations should be repaired regardless of whether they are bleeding. Deep lacerations that extend upward into the lower uterine segment will often bleed profusely; unless the upper end of the laceration can be identified and sutured, a laparotomy is necessary for adequate repair. Hysterectomy is usually necessary to control hemorrhage from ruptured uterus.

Delayed hemorrhage. Hemorrhage may occur at any time during the first 24 hours after delivery *(early delayed hemorrhage)* or several days later *(late delayed hemorrhage).*

EARLY. Hemorrhage during the first 24 hours is most often the result of atony, retained placental fragments, or relaxation of the uterus, but it may be from the episiotomy or a laceration.

If the uterus is soft and distended with blood, it will

contract with manual stimulation and the administration of an oxytocic. If the distension is a result of simple atony, it will usually stay contracted after these simple measures have been used.

If atony and bleeding recur, one must consider the possibility of retained placental fragments or of bleeding from a vaginal or cervical injury. If the patient is lying in bed, blood from a vaginal tear can flow upward into the uterus, distending it and giving the appearance of atony.

If bleeding and relaxation recur after an oxytocic has been given, the vagina and uterine cavity must be explored.

LATE. Bleeding that begins or becomes profuse several days after delivery is most often caused by retained portions of placenta, although occasionally an injury may be responsible. In most instances the uterovaginal canal should be explored promptly. Placental tissue can be removed with a large curet.

Another form of late postpartum hemorrhage is that designated *placental site bleeding.* This usually begins suddenly between the twelfth and twenty-first days and may be profuse. It is presumably the result of separation of the crust of organized fibrin and hyalinized vessels covering the placental site and can usually be controlled by curettage. Blood transfusion may be necessary.

RETAINED PLACENTA

Occasionally, the third stage is prolonged because the placenta fails to separate or because the uterus cannot expel the placenta even though it is partially or completely detached. If the placenta is still completely attached, there can be no bleeding, but if it is partially separated the blood loss from the open placental site sinuses can be profuse. This is a common cause of excessive third-stage bleeding.

Failure of placental separation may be mechanical or a result of abnormal penetration of the trophoblast into the uterine wall *(abnormally adherent placenta).* With a mechanical failure, the uterine muscle at the placental site may be relaxed and boggy, even though that of the rest of the upper segment is fairly firmly contracted. Because of failure of the muscle at the placental site to contract, the usual mechanism for placental separation does not come into play.

With abnormally adherent placenta, all or part of the decidua basalis is absent, and the chorionic tissue grows directly into the muscle, thereby eliminating the normal cleavage plane. The term *placenta accreta* indicates a relatively superficial penetration of the muscle. Deeper penetration is called *placenta increta; placenta percreta* indicates that the trophoblast has grown to or completely through the serosa.

Placenta accreta occurs more often in women of high than of low parity, in those who have delivered previously by cesarean section, after the uterus has been curetted, and in association with placenta previa. In these patients the placenta implants over a scar or in an area is which the decidua is so poorly formed that the trophoblast invades the myometrium directly.

Placenta accreta can be *partial,* if only a portion of the placenta is abnormally adherent, or *complete.* With the partial type, bleeding can be profuse when the normal portion of the placenta separates because the uterus cannot complete the separation of the placenta and expel it. Bleeding cannot occur with complete placenta accreta because none of the placenta can separate from its abnormal attachment in the uterine muscle.

Management. If bleeding is active and the placenta cannot be expressed in the usual manner, it must be removed immediately by inserting the hand into the uterus, completing the separation, and extracting it (Fig. 31-3).

In the absence of bleeding it is safe to wait longer for spontaneous separation and expulsion, but there is no reason to delay more than 5 to 10 minutes.

Hysterectomy usually is necessary for placenta accreta unless the abnormally adherent portion of the placenta involves only a small area. The uterus may be perforated, or profuse bleeding may be produced by attempts to dig the cotyledons out of the uterine wall.

INVERSION OF THE UTERUS

Inversion of the uterus occurs rarely; when it does, the mortality is high unless it is recognized and treated promptly. The inversion may be *partial* or *complete;* those discovered at delivery are *acute,* and those not detected until days or weeks later are *chronic.*

In most instances the uterine muscles near the placental site, which frequently is in the fundus, are relaxed, permitting the upper part of the uterus to prolapse through the dilated cervix. Vigorous attempts to deliver the placenta by suprapubic pressure or by cord traction are probably important factors in inverting the fundus.

In most instances, shock develops promptly when

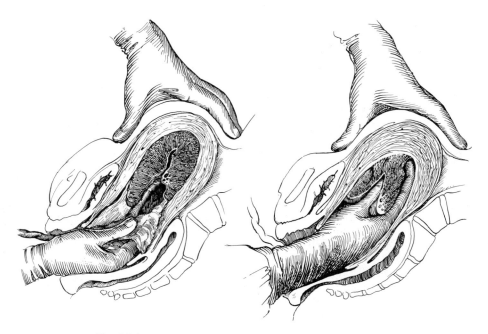

Fig. 31-3 Technique of manual removal of retained placenta.

the inversion occurs. The diagnosis can be suspected if the fundus is indented (incomplete inversion) or cannot be felt above the pubis (complete inversion). It can be confirmed by palpating the inverted fundus within the lower uterine segment or in the vagina.

The uterus can usually be replaced without difficulty if the diagnosis is made promptly. The entire hand is inserted into the vagina, with the fingertips exerting equal pressure around the collar of uterus just within the cervical opening and the fundus resting on the palmar surface of the hand. The fundus is gradually replaced, and oxytocin or a prostaglandin F_2-alpha analog is administered.

POSTPARTUM PITUITARY NECROSIS

Partial or complete necrosis of the anterior pituitary gland may follow excessive bleeding during pregnancy. This condition, *Sheehan's syndrome,* usually cannot be detected in women who die soon after delivery because necrotic changes have not had time to develop. The entire anterior lobe or portions of it may be destroyed.

In the typical patient with severe damage the breasts remain flaccid, and no milk is secreted. Pubic and axillary hair may fall out. The genital organs atrophy, and the menses do not return. The endocrine glands that are under the control of the anterior pituitary cease to function. Complete pituitary necrosis is rarely seen, but the less severe states may be encountered occasionally. There may be enough tissue to carry on normal function, the deficiency only becoming obvious when the gland is subjected to unusual stress, such as another pregnancy, a surgical operation, or a serious infection.

Although the exact cause of pituitary necrosis is not known, prevention of excessive bleeding and the prompt replacement of blood may reduce the severity of pituitary damage.

AMNIOTIC FLUID INFUSION

Amniotic fluid can enter the bloodstream through the vessels at the placental site or those opened by injury. The membranes must be ruptured to permit the escape of amniotic fluid, and the intrauterine pressure must be increased. Rupture of the membranes and the administration of an oxytocic to induce labor increases the possibility of amniotic fluid infusion, as does placenta previa. Amniotic infusion is most likely to occur in women in labor at or near term, and many patients have been given oxytocin to induce or stimulate labor. Parous women are more often affected than are primigravidas.

The symptoms occur suddenly, and the first evidence of the abnormality may be dyspnea and cyanosis or sudden shock. Death may occur promptly or be delayed for several hours. If a coagulation defect occurs, vaginal bleeding usually is evident.

The pathophysiologic changes, which result from sudden obstruction of the pulmonary capillaries by the particulate matter in the infused amniotic fluid, include acute cor pulmonale, decreased left atrial pressure, decreased cardiac output, and peripheral vascular collapse.

Treatment consists basically of cardiopulmonary resuscitation and insertion of a Swan-Ganz catheter and an intraarterial catheter for the administration of fluids and to measure blood pressure. Blood must be administered if the patient is bleeding excessively, and the coagulation defect corrected by appropriate treatment.

Amniotic fluid infusion can be diagnosed with certainty only by demonstrating the presence of fetal epithelial cells and amniotic debris in the lung capillaries. It can be suspected, however, in a patient in whom a state of collapse develops late in labor or immediately after delivery, and it is essential that treatment be instituted promptly.

SUGGESTED READING

Breen JL, Neubecker R, Gregori CA, and others: Placenta accreta, increta and percreta, Obstet Gynecol 49:43, 1977.

Hayashi RH, Costillo MS, and Noah ML: Management of severe postpartum hemorrhage with a prostaglandin F_2-alpha analogue, Obstet Gynecol 63:806, 1984.

Hendricks CH and Brenner WE: Cardiovascular effects of oxytocic drugs used post partum, Am J Obstet Gynecol 108:751, 1970.

Hendricks CH, Eskes TKAB, and Saameli K: Uterine contractility at delivery and in the puerperium, Am J Obstet Gynecol 83:890, 1962.

Magil B: PGF$_2$-alpha for postpartum hemorrhage—how well does it work? Contemp Obstet Gynecol p 111, 1984.

Newton M: Postpartum hemorrhage, Am J Obstet Gynecol 94:711, 1966.

Odell LD and Seski A: Episiotomy blood loss, Am J Obstet Gynecol 54:51, 1947.

Platt LD and Druzin ML: Acute puerperal inversion of the uterus, Am J Obstet Gynecol 141:187, 1981.

Price TM, Baker VV, and Cefalo RC: Amniotic fluid embolism. Three case reports with a review of the literature, Obstet Gynecol Surv 40:462, 1985.

Prichard JA, Baldwin RM, Dickey JC, and Wiggins KM: Blood volume changes in pregnancy and the puerperium. II. Red blood cell loss and changes during and following vaginal delivery, cesarean section and cesarean section plus total hysterectomy, Am J Obstet Gynecol 84:1271, 1962.

Quinlivan WL and Brock JA: Blood volume changes and blood loss associated with labor, Am J Obstet Gynecol 106:843, 1970.

Read JA, Cotton DB, and Miller FC: Placenta accreta: changing clinical aspects and outcome, Obstet Gynecol 56:31, 1980.

Reid DE, Weiner AE, and Roby CC: Intravascular clotting and afibrinogenemia, the presumptive lethal factors in the syndrome of amniotic fluid embolism, Am J Obstet Gynecol 66:465, 1953.

Schneeberg NG, Perloff WH, and Israel SL: Incidence of unsuspected "Sheehan's syndrome": hypopituitarism after postpartum hemorrhage and/or shock: clinical and laboratory study, JAMA 172:20, 1960.

Secher NJ, Arnsbo P, and Wallin L: Haemodynamic effects of oxytocin (Syntocinon) and methylergometrine (Methergin) on the systemic and pulmonary circulations of pregnant anaesthetized women, Acta Obstet Gynecol Scand 57:97, 1978.

Sheehan HL: Simmonds' disease due to postpartum necrosis of the anterior pituitary, J Obstet Gynaecol Br Commonw 50:27, 1943.

Steiner PE and Lushbaugh CC: Maternal pulmonary embolism by amniotic fluid as cause of obstetric shock and unexpected death in obstetrics, JAMA 117:1245, 1941.

Ueland K: Maternal cardiovascular dynamics. VII. Intrapartum blood volume changes, Am J Obstet Gynecol 126:671, 1976.

32

Russell K. Laros, Jr.

Care of the infant during pregnancy and labor and after delivery

Objectives

RATIONALE: The goals of antepartum and intrapartum care as far as the fetus is concerned are maintenance of fetal health, growth, and well-being.

The student should be able to:

A. Demonstrate a knowledge of the definitions, etiologies, and methods of diagnosis and treatment of fetal macrosomia and intrauterine growth retardation.

B. Explain circumstances in which isoimmunization is likely to occur and the methods of diagnosis and treatment.

C. Describe techniques of electronic fetal heart rate monitoring and of normal and abnormal fetal heart rate patterns.

During its intrauterine life the fetus is completely dependent on the transfer of respiratory gases and the materials essential for its growth from the maternal bloodstream. At birth, however, it must assume responsibility for maintaining all its functions. The highest mortality occurs during the first 24 hours of life while the infant is attempting to make this change.

The fetus in utero swallows amniotic fluid, which is absorbed from the intestinal tract and ultimately is excreted by the kidneys and returned to the amniotic sac. There is little peristaltic activity in the intestine of the normal infant until birth; the passage of meconium by the unborn infant usually indicates intrauterine hypoxia. Respiratory efforts that move amniotic fluid in and out of the nasopharynx and trachea and into the alveoli have been demonstrated in human fetuses and in experimental animals. The infant responds to tactile and auditory stimuli while it is still in the uterus. It is important that all the necessary functions be developed and in operation by the time the infant is born. Abnormally formed infants may be unable to survive outside the uterus. Those born before 25 weeks' gestation usually cannot cope with an independent existence, even though they are otherwise normal.

To survive, the infant must have developed

normally and be born alive and uninjured. The hazards of labor and delivery are increased for the premature infant whose delicate structures may be injured easily and for the excessively large infant who may be damaged during attempts to deliver it.

The goals of antepartum care, as far as the fetus is concerned, are the prevention of intrauterine death and the delivery of a healthy infant at term. This requires that the obstetrician recognize potential risk factors and treat them properly. There is a tendency to equate the effectiveness of antepartum care only with improved infant survival, but this is too limited a view. Four fetal deaths occur between the twentieth week of pregnancy and the onset of labor for every intrapartum death. Furthermore, the leading cause of neonatal death is prematurity. Thus any interventions that reduce fetal deaths and/or premature labor will have a significant effect on perinatal mortality.

Antepartum evaluation of the fetus is difficult because it must be done indirectly. We cannot ask it, "How do you feel today?" The methods by which we can evaluate the condition of the fetus in utero will be discussed in this chapter.

PRENATAL INFLUENCES ON THE FETUS

From time immemorial people have assumed that the growth of the fetus could be altered by maternal emotional experiences. We know now that most specific episodes cannot be correlated with congenital defects because they rarely occur at a time when the involved structure is developing, but we are learning more and more about the influence of drugs, chemicals, nutrition, infection, hypoxia, endocrine imbalance, and physical and even emotional stimuli on fetal growth and development.

The periods during which organs and tissues develop vary in length and occur at different stages of pregnancy. For each there exists an early stage during which the primordial tissue begins to differentiate; this is followed by a period of cellular growth and beginning development of the structure, and finally the period during which development is completed. Subsequent change is almost entirely one of growth. To produce an anomaly, a stimulus must be applied before development is completed; it will have little effect except to interfere with growth if it is applied after differentiation is completed. Almost all important organ systems are developed by the end of the twelfth week, but some take longer.

Most pregnant women are regularly exposed to stimuli of one kind or another that may alter fetal development. Fortunately, these stimuli are generally either too slight to affect the tissue, or they occur after the structure already has been formed. Physicians prescribe many medications for their pregnant patients, often with too little thought of their potential effect on the fetus. Most of these drugs have been thoroughly tested on experimental animals, but, unfortunately (thalidomide is an outstanding example), they may be toxic only to human fetal tissue. No animal model currently available accurately predicts damage to the human fetus.

Physicians and their patients are now aware of the possibilities of disturbing embryonic development and are becoming more reasonable about drug therapy during pregnancy—the physician about prescribing it and the patient about demanding it. *As a general rule no medication, no matter how innocuous it is presumed to be, should be prescribed during pregnancy unless there is a specific indication for its use and unless the patient may be harmed if it is not used.* The various infectious agents, drugs, and environmental agents that can adversely affect the fetus are discussed in Chapters 13 and 40.

ERYTHROBLASTOSIS FETALIS RESULTING FROM BLOOD GROUP INCOMPATIBILITY

If the fetus's blood group is different from that of its mother, and if the mother has been sensitized to an antigen in the fetal blood cells, her blood will contain an antibody that can cross the placenta and hemolyze fetal red blood cells.

Erythroblastosis is most often a result of Rh incompatibility, but differences in the ABO and other blood factors can also cause the disorder.

The fetus is more seriously affected by Rh incompatibilities than by most of the other types. The characteristic fetal manifestations, each of which is related to the hemolytic process, are (1) anemia; (2) erythroblastic hyperplasia of bone marrow; (3) extramedullary centers of erythropoiesis in the liver, spleen, kidneys, and other tissues; (4) erythroblastemia; (5) jaundice, particularly hemolytic but also hepatocellular, appearing soon after birth and with possible resulting kernicterus; (6) tissue damage from anoxia; (7) edema from cardiac failure and hypoproteinemia; and (8) purpura from complete bone marrow suppression.

Etiologic factors. The blood of about 85% of white people contains the Rh antigen; these are Rh_0 (D)–positive. If Rh_0 (D)–positive fetal red blood cells enter the maternal circulation of an Rh_0 (D)–negative woman, an antibody against them may be formed. Fetal blood cells may mix with the mother's blood in the intervillous spaces if placental blood vessels are torn during abortion or delivery, intact cells may cross the undamaged placenta by pinocytosis, or the products of disintegrated cells containing the antigen may enter the maternal circulation. Probably the most common method by which fetal red blood cells enter the maternal circulation is by disruption of the fetal placental vessels during the third stage of labor. Maternal antibodies of an IgG group will also be produced in response to blood transfusion with Rh_0 (D)–positive donor blood.

The Rh_0 (D) factor is the one most often responsible for sensitization, but others that may have the same effect are hr' (c), rh' (C), rh" (E), and hr" (e).

The maternal antibody crosses the placenta and enters the fetal circulation without difficulty; it hemolyzes fetal blood cells and produces the changes characteristic of erythroblastosis.

Although the first infant born of an Rh-incompatible pregnancy almost always is normal, the second or subsequent ones may be affected. After a woman has borne one infant with erythroblastosis, the rest of her children are almost certain to have a similar condition if the father is homozygous Rh_0 (D)–positive. If he is heterozygous, half the spermatozoa will contain Rh factor, and half will contain none. As a general rule the disease in the first affected infant is mild, but one cannot predict what will happen during subsequent pregnancies. In some all the babies are only slightly affected, whereas in others the second and all subsequent fetuses develop hydrops or die in utero because of the severity of the hemolytic process.

Management. An antibody screen should be performed on the serum of a pregnant woman during the first trimester. If the woman is Rh-negative, the antibody screen should be repeated at 16 to 18 weeks and every 4 to 6 weeks thereafter. If the initial antibody screen is positive, the exact antibody must be identified, and a determination made as to whether it is of the IgG or IgM type.

Unfortunately, changes in antibody titer may not accurately reflect the condition. Fetal hydrops and intrauterine death have been observed with relatively low titers, and slightly affected or even Rh-negative babies have occurred when the titer had risen to astronomically high levels. As a consequence one cannot base treatment on Rh antibody titer alone.

A much more accurate evaluation of fetal conditions can be made by *spectrophotometric analysis of amniotic fluid*. The spectral absorption curves for amniotic fluid are determined for visible light-spectrum wavelengths between 350 and 700 nm. Optical density is then plotted as the ordinate, and wavelength as the abscissa. A normal curve will be fairly smooth, but the bilirubin in the amniotic fluid of fetuses affected by erythroblastosis alters the optical density and produces a deviation at about 450 nm.

The exact peak of this deviation from linearity is expressed as the difference between the expected and observed optical density at 450 nm as measured from a tangent line drawn between 365 and 550 nm on semilogarithmic paper. The optical density difference (ΔOD) correlates well with the degree of fetal anemia from 26 weeks on. At earlier gestational ages, a preferable method is directly sampling of the fetal circulation and determining the degree of anemia by measuring the hemoglobin and hematocrit.

Treatment is based on the level of anemia and the gestational age of the fetus. If the anemia is so severe that hydrops is a risk and the gestational age is greater than 32 weeks, preterm delivery is carried out (usually by cesarean section) and the newborn is treated as discussed below. Before 32 weeks, the fetus is transfused in utero. Fetal transfusion can be accomplished either by the direct intravascular route or by placing the donor blood into the fetal peritoneal cavity. In the former instance, a needle is placed directly into the umbilical vein with ultrasonic visualization of the fetal structures. An appropriate amount of Rh-negative, packed RBCs compatible with the mother's serum is infused. If intravascular access is difficult, the donor cells are placed into the fetal peritoneal cavity via a polyethylene catheter. In the absence of hydrops, complete absorption occurs over a period of 3 to 5 days. If hydrops is present, the intravascular route is far more effective. Formulas based on the estimated fetal weight and the degree of anemia are available for calculating the correct volume of donor cells required for each route of transfusion. The need for repeat transfusion will depend on the fetal age and anticipated life span of the transfused cells.

Based on extensive experience, the risk of traumatic fetal death from intraperitoneal transfusion is 3.7% per transfusion. The risk is probably similar for intravascular transfusion; however, the published experience to date is far smaller. Other hazards of both techniques include premature rupture of the membranes, intrauterine infection, premature labor, and overtransfusion. Intrauterine transfusion undoubtedly saves fetal lives. Results from different centers indicate survival rates from 50% to 85%. The variation depends on whether hydropic fetuses are included and the gestation age at which transfusion is begun.

Treatment of the infant. Whenever a patient who probably has an erythroblastotic baby is in labor or her delivery is planned, preparations should be made to examine and treat the baby as soon as it is born. A pediatrician experienced with exchange transfusion should be present at the delivery. A specimen of cord blood is obtained for blood typing, hematocrit, reticulocyte count, bilirubin, and a direct Coombs test. Exchange transfusion should be performed promptly if the baby has erythroblastosis and the hematocrit is low. Kernicterus, a major cause of death and disability in premature infants with erythroblastosis, can be almost completely prevented by exchange transfusions.

Prevention. Our present management of erythroblastosis is crude and ineffective when compared with what can be achieved by prevention. The Rh_0 (D) hyperimmune human gamma globulin (RhIG), when injected intramuscularly into unsensitized Rh_0 (D)–negative individuals, prevents the development of an antigen against Rh_0 (D)–positive red blood cells. In a large cooperative study, only one of 1081 unsensitized Rh_0 (D)–negative women who were treated with this material after the delivery of an Rh_0 (D)–positive infant became sensitized, whereas 51 of 726 control women developed antibodies.

We now give RhIG to all unsensitized Rh_0 (Du)–negative women during the first 72 hours after they have delivered an Rh_0 (D)–positive infant. Those selected for treatment must be Rh_0 (Du)–negative without identifiable antibodies, and the baby must be Rh_0 (D)–positive with a negative direct antiglobulin (Coombs) test on cord blood. Because fetal cells pass into the maternal circulation during the course of pregnancy, approximately 2% of sensitizations occur before delivery. This sensitization can be largely prevented by the administration of RhIG at 28 weeks' gestation to all Rh-negative mothers with Rh-positive partners.

An Rh_0 (D)–negative patient who has aborted a pregnancy more than 8 weeks after the onset of the last menstrual period should also be treated if her husband is positive, even though the blood type of the embryo cannot be determined. Unsensitized women should be treated after each delivery. In addition, all Rh-negative unsensitized women requiring amniocentesis should be given RhIG after the amniocentesis has been performed.

ERYTHROBLASTOSIS FETALIS RESULTING FROM ABO INCOMPATIBILITY

A fetus of blood group A, AB, or B may develop hemolytic disease from maternal antibodies against any of the antigens not already present in the mother's blood. For example, if the mother is blood type O, she may become sensitized to either A or B, or if she is A and her fetus is B or AB, she may become sensitized to B.

This situation is similar to Rh sensitization in several ways, but there are differences. Rh sensitization always occurs because of a transfusion of Rh_0 (D)–positive red blood cells into the maternal blood; ABO sensitization may develop in this manner, but there are naturally occurring antibodies that may already be present when the patient becomes pregnant for the first time. The antigen responsible for ABO sensitization is secreted in body fluids, as well as being contained in red blood cells. Thus a mother can become sensitized by the antigen "secreted" by the fetus into amniotic fluid from which it is absorbed into the maternal circulation.

There is no reliable way to prognosticate the development of ABO incompatibility during the prenatal period as there is with Rh erythroblastosis fetalis, but it can be anticipated by comparing the blood group of the mother with that of the child's father. If the mother's blood group is O and the father's A, B, or AB, the infant is a candidate for ABO incompatibility, and a direct antiglobulin (Coombs) test should be performed on cord blood. Fortunately, the process is almost never as severe as that caused by Rh sensitization and does not cause intrauterine fetal death. The treatment is exchange transfusion.

EVALUATION OF FETAL CONDITION DURING PREGNANCY

In the past, one could only assume that the fetus was healthy if it continued to grow and was active because the only valid assessment of fetal well-being was the heart rate. There are now several reasonably accurate ways to assess fetal maturity (Chapter 20) and to determine the condition of the fetus before labor begins and while the membranes are still intact. The information gained by these tests frequently is helpful in making a decision as to the most appropriate time to terminate pregnancy.

These tests are of greatest value when *intrauterine growth retardation* on the basis of small or abnormal placenta is suspected, for example, in women with chronic hypertensive cardiovascular disease and cyanotic heart disease, or when the possibility of postmaturity exists. The tests also may be of value in patients with *diabetes* and other metabolic disorders that may affect the development of the fetus and whenever the *expected date of confinement cannot be determined accurately.*

Sonography. It is possible to measure the biparietal diameter of the fetal skull and femoral length with reasonable accuracy during pregnancy. If the size of the uterus at 16 and 20 weeks does not correspond to the date of the onset of the last menstrual period, an initial study should be obtained without delay. If the patient is not examined until late in the second trimester and the uterus is smaller than anticipated, ultrasonic fetal measurements should be obtained promptly.

Between the thirtieth and the fortieth weeks of pregnancy the biparietal diameter increases at a rate of about 2 mm/wk. The biparietal diameter will be greater than 8.7 cm in almost 100% of infants after the thirty-sixth week of pregnancy.

Sonographic measurement of the biparietal diameter and body size should be obtained at biweekly intervals whenever growth retardation is suspected. These studies will identify both symmetrical and asymmetrical growth retardation.

A steady normal increase in the various measurements provides good evidence that the placenta is capable of supplying the metabolic needs of the fetus and that the baby is growing at the usual rate. A less than normal increase or failure to increase at all is indicative of growth retardation and suggests that the fetus has outgrown the ability of the placenta to meet its needs.

Counting of fetal movements. Fetal movements can be quantified by the mother. She is instructed to recline comfortably after a meal and then to count the number of "kicks" occurring during a 10-minute period. "Kick counts" for 10 minutes range between 5 and 20 in a healthy fetus. Generally, fetal movements decline rapidly over a day or two and are then absent for another 1 to 2 days before intrauterine death occurs.

Biophysical evaluation. New noninvasive techniques for recording fetal heart rate and uterine contractions and refined ultrasonic equipment have expanded our capabilities for evaluating the status of the fetus in utero. These techniques are almost 100% accurate in predicting a healthy fetus—that is, a normal test connotes a normal fetus—but they are less accurate in predicting an unhealthy fetus. There are many more abnormal tests than abnormal newborns. Because of this, a need exists for more than one test when an abnormal biophysical evaluation occurs.

The *nonstress test* (NST) is designed to evaluate the reactivity of the fetus during the antepartum period. It is called nonstress because the mother is not given oxytocin to induce contrac-

tions. The great advantage of the test is that it is easy to do and requires no drug administration to the mother. Nonstress tests are most appropriate for women suspected of having placental dysfunction or insufficiency; for example, those with chronic hypertension or diabetes or with fetuses suspected of growth retardation or postmaturity.

A continuous record of fetal heart rate is made with Doppler or electrocardiographic equipment while the mother is resting in a lateral supine position. She is asked to report each fetal movement that she feels, and the effect of fetal movement on the heart rate is determined. A normal reaction to fetal movement is an acceleration in fetal heart rate of 15 beats/min or more above the baseline for 15 seconds or more (Fig. 32-1). If at least four such accelerations are seen in a 20-minute interval, the test is reactive, and the fetus is presumed to be healthy.

If only one or no accelerations occur during a 20-minute period, the fetus may be unhealthy or simply resting. It is important to recognize the resting state because there are many more nonreactive tests than there are unhealthy fetuses. If no accelerations occur during an additional 20-

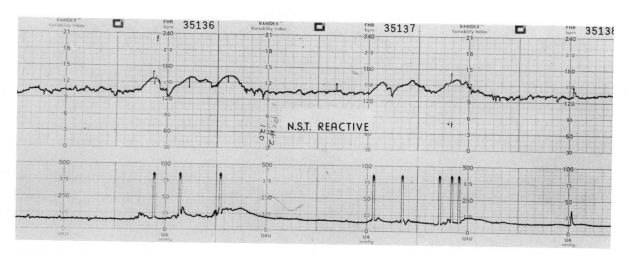

Fig. 32-1 Reactive nonstress test *(NST)*. *Arrows* on lower panel document timing of fetal movement. Strip has 12 minutes of observation, and accelerations are clearly evident.

minute observation period, a *contraction stress test* (CST) should be performed promptly.

The most ominous sign in nonstress testing is prolonged bradycardia, lasting for more than a minute (Fig. 32-2), which indicates incipient intrauterine fetal death. When bradycardia is recognized, fetal heart rate monitoring should be con-

tinued while the mother is moved to the labor and delivery area. Delivery by carefully monitored induction or by cesarean section is indicated if the bradycardia recurs. Fortunately, these serious patterns are rarely seen. The more usual problem is dealing with the patient with a nonreactive test.

The *CST, oxytocin challenge test, or nipple*

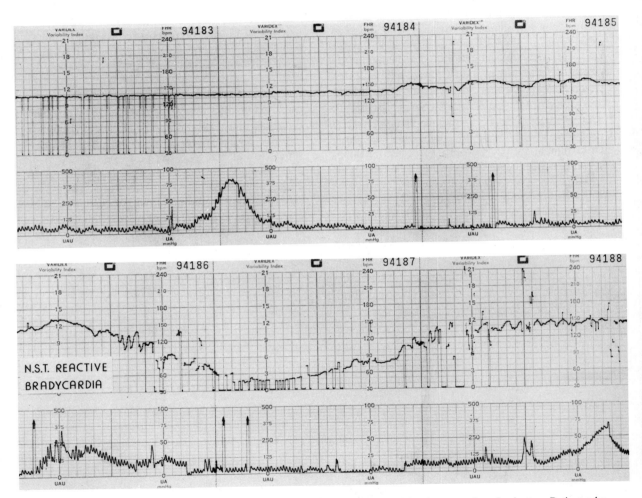

Fig. 32-2 Reactive nonstress test *(NST)* involving prolonged bradycardia, that is, more than 5 minutes. Patient who was beyond term was immediately transferred to labor and delivery area, where a carefully monitored induction was performed. Another prolonged bradycardia occurred, emergency cesarean section was performed, and an infant with tight nuchal cord and thick meconium was delivered. Infant was resuscitated at birth and had an uncomplicated course after birth.

stimulation test is designed to stress the fetoplacental unit and test the reserve of the fetus. Oxytocin is administered intravenously in a dosage that will produce three contractions in 10-minute intervals, and the effect of the contractions on heart rate is observed (Schifrin's "10-minute window"). Similarly, nipple stimulation, which induces the secretion of maternal oxytocin, can be used to cause uterine contractions. If late decelerations are seen with each contraction, the test is positive, and the patient should usually be delivered. If no decelerations occur during the 10-minute period, the test is normal (Fig. 32-3). This categorization is particularly important because it sharply reduces the number of equivocal tests, in which a late deceleration is occasionally seen.

A decision as to whether the patient should be delivered by cesarean section or vaginally cannot always be made on the basis of the test alone. The actual force of the uterine contractions cannot be measured by external recordings. Nearly half of women with a positive contraction stress test will go through labor without late decelerations.

Biophysical profile. Some authors have advocated use of a biophysical scoring system. The fetus is evaluated sonographically for fetal breathing movements, gross body movements, muscle tone, and the quantity of amniotic fluid, and an NST is performed. The fetus is given a score of "2" or "0" for each of these five parameters. Fetuses having a score of "8" or more are at low risk for chronic asphyxia. Those scoring "0" or "2" are strongly suspected of being chronically asphyxiated; and the remainder form an intermediate, "suspicious" group.

Doppler ultrasound fetal velocimetry. Doppler flow technique allows measurement of the umbilical artery systolic and diastolic flow. Because the fetal heart rate can affect the waveform and the systolic/diastolic ratio is minimally affected by rate, the ratio rather than flow rate is used to evaluate fetal well-being. Abnormal ratios are associated with less favorable outcomes, especially in cases of intrauterine growth retardation. Reverse diastolic flow is a rare outcome and is almost always associated with poor fetal outcome. However, the precise place of Doppler velocimetry in clinical practice is not yet clear. Certainly, an abnormal systolic/diastolic ratio warrants the use of the conventional method of fetal surveillance but should not be used by itself to dictate management decisions.

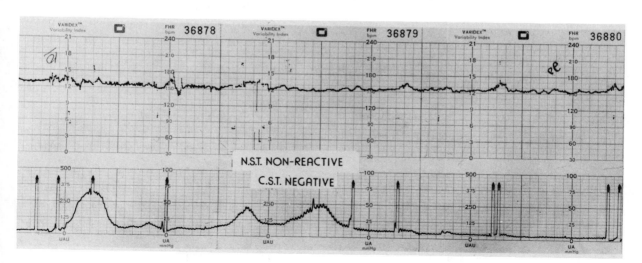

Fig. 32-3 Normal contraction stress test *(CST)*. No decelerations are seen.

FETAL HYPOXIA DURING LABOR

The fetus in utero is entirely dependent on the mother for its supply of oxygen, which it obtains from the maternal blood in the placental sinuses. Circulation of the blood through the sinuses is regulated by the mother's arterial blood pressure and by the activity of the uterine muscle. Maternal blood is injected into the sinuses in spurts from the open ends of spiral arterioles that are scattered, with corresponding venous channels, in the uterine wall beneath the placenta. Some of the blood is forced laterally into the marginal lakes, from which it is returned to the general circulation. Most of it, however, gravitates downward through the branching villi and leaves the intervillous space by way of the venous openings at the base.

The pressure within the intervillous space is about the same as or slightly higher than the amniotic fluid pressure, being about 5 to 10 mm Hg when the uterus is at rest and 55 mm Hg or more at the peak of a contraction. The intervillous pressure rises during a contraction because the veins are kinked and compressed by the uterine muscle fibers before the caliber of the more resistant arterioles is affected. Thus blood continues to flow into the spaces for some time after its means of egress are closed.

Under normal circumstances, during a uterine contraction the pressure within the intervillous space is lower than the capillary pressure in the placental villi, which is maintained by changes in fetal blood pressure. This prevents the villi from collapsing and impeding the flow of blood through the fetal vessels and permits the exchange of materials back and forth between the fetal and the maternal circulations even during a contraction.

The fetal oxygen supply can be reduced by any of the following:

1. *Reduction in blood flow through the maternal vessels.* The caliber of the arteries may be reduced by spasm in women with hypertensive complications of pregnancy, thus limiting blood flow. It is estimated that arterial blood flow can be reduced by as much as 50% in women with hypertensive disease.

   The flow of blood will also be impaired whenever the maternal systolic blood pressure is lower than the amniotic fluid pressure. Fetal hypoxia is likely to develop when maternal blood pressure levels fall below 60 mm Hg.

2. *Reduction in blood flow through the uterine sinuses.* Blood flow through the intervillous space will be reduced if the veins or arterioles are compressed over long periods of time by forceful, rapidly recurring or prolonged tetanic uterine contractions. A reduction in maternal blood pressure will have the same result.

3. *Reduction of the oxygen content of maternal blood.* The available circulating maternal hemoglobin can be reduced by profound chronic anemia or hemorrhage, thereby reducing the total oxygen capacity.

4. *Alterations in fetal circulation.* The circulation of blood through the vessels of the infant's body and placenta is maintained by the fetal heart. Anything that alters normal cardiac function will impair the circulation, as will compression of the umbilical cord. Placental infarction or separation will decrease the total area available for oxygen transfer from the maternal blood; if a considerable portion of placenta is involved, the infant cannot survive.

Although a minority of predelivery intrauterine deaths occur during labor, that short time segment, usually less than 24 hours, makes it the most important portion of pregnancy for continuous observation of the fetus for evidence of stress associated with uterine activity.

Accurate assessment of fetal well-being during labor depends on an understanding of the physiology of the fetal heart rate tracing, so that proper interpretation can be made. Periodic changes in fetal heart rate during labor have been classified according to their relationship to uterine contractions. In *early decelerations* the onset of the decrease in rate begins with the onset of the contraction, and normal rate resumes as the uterus relaxes; in *variable decelerations* there is no constant relationship of the deceleration to contractions; and *late decelerations* begin after the contraction starts, and recovery is prolonged (Fig. 32-4). These periodic changes provide the physician with information concerning the types of stress to which the fetus is being subjected and the physiologic mechanisms involved.

Early decelerations are reflex, are related to pressure on the fetal head, and are mediated by the vagus. They are not associated with a poor outcome. *Variable decelerations* are caused by cord compression. They are reflex changes characterized by a sudden drop in the fetal heart rate and a rapid return to normal. Whether this will

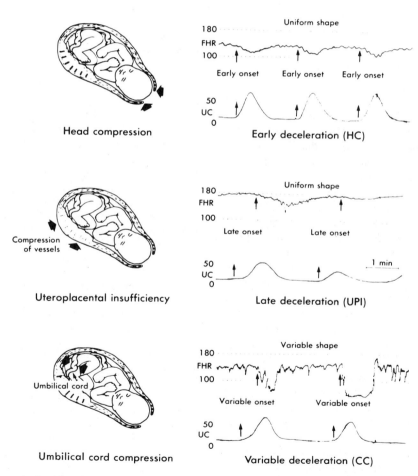

Fig. 32-4 Changes in fetal heart rate patterns related to various causes. (From Hon EH: An atlas of fetal heart rate patterns, New Haven, Conn, 1968, Harty Press, Inc.)

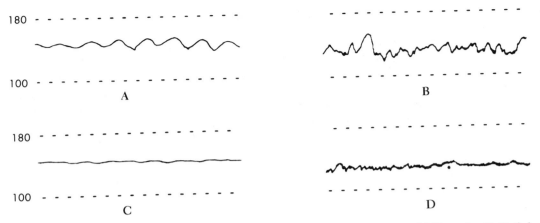

Fig. 32-5 Variability differences observed with fetal scalp electrode. **A,** Long-term variability only. **B,** Both long- and short-term variability. **C,** Neither long- nor short-term variability. **D,** Short-term variability only. (From Zanani B, Paul RH, Huey JR: Am J Obstet Gynecol 136:43, 1980.)

cause a problem for the fetus depends on the length of time the circulation is disturbed and the reserve of the fetus. *Late decelerations* are a sign of uteroplacental insufficiency.

The periodic changes in heart rate give the physician an understanding of the mechanisms of the stress to the fetus, but the most important point in the evaluation of the health of the intrauterine passenger is the presence or absence of significant *fetal distress*. This can be ascertained by the *beat-to-beat variability of the fetal heart rate* (Fig. 32-5). Good beat-to-beat variability indicates good fetal reserve. Poor beat-to-beat variability indicates either "distress" and little reserve or changes caused by exogenous medications such as meperidine given to the mother during labor. To differentiate these two conditions, *fetal scalp blood sampling* can be performed. Because fetal scalp Po_2 is technically difficult to measure and fluctuates rapidly, we generally use pH, Pco_2, and base excess to assess the fetal acid-base status. A low pH is evidence of anaerobic tissue metabolism. The normal pH of fetal scalp blood is above 7.25; values between 7.25 and 7.20 suggest that hypoxia may be developing. Hypoxia can be diag-

nosed if the pH is less than 7.20 in the absence of maternal acidosis.

Because timing of uterine activity is important in the assessment of periodic changes and beat-to-beat variability accurately reflects fetal health, it is important for the physician to understand the limitations of instrumentation in current labor monitoring technology. Judgments concerning the well-being of the fetus during labor should be made on the basis of the most complete data base. The *external tocodynamometer* provides incomplete information about uterine activity. This system usually assesses the frequency of uterine activity accurately but provides no information about resting uterine tone or the force of individual contractions. The accuracy of the tocodynamometer recording depends to a great extent on the ability of the patients to lie still and the frequency with which the labor floor staff will adjust the equipment. If there are problems in timing fetal heart rate accelerations, or when oxytocin is being administered, an *internal pressure catheter* to measure the force of uterine contractions and a *fetal scalp electrode* to record fetal heart rate should be introduced and connected to a transducer.

The major advantage of a fetal scalp electrode is that it provides an accurate fetal electrocardiographic signal. The R wave from this signal is used to count the

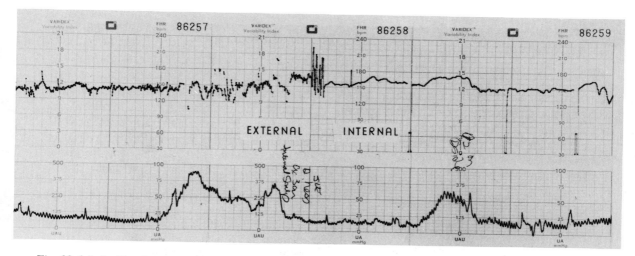

Fig. 32-6 Left side of upper portion of tracing shows good beat-to-beat variability with external monitor system. Immediately after internal electrode was applied, a much flatter fetal heart rate with decreased variability occurred.

heart rate, and the beat-to-beat variability is recorded on the monitor strip. None of the external systems can provide as accurate information about variability. The triggering signal from Doppler external monitoring is less clean; the recorded result shows more variability than is seen with the internal system. Poor beat-to-beat variability on the external system means poor variability, but good variability on the external system may be recorded as poor by an internal electrode (Fig. 32-6).

The health of every fetus should be accurately evaluated during almost every labor. Although one study indicated that frequent evaluation by nurse midwives could give equivalent newborn survival when compared with electronic monitoring, the vast majority of reports have shown a decrease in newborn morbidity and mortality with complete use of electronic monitoring. All patients admitted to the labor-delivery unit, except those who are about to deliver, should have an external monitor applied. If decelerations are observed, an internal electrode should be applied to the fetal scalp to determine the nature of the decelerations and the amount of beat-to-beat variability. If variable decelerations occur, a vaginal examination should be performed to check for

cord prolapse. If the cord cannot be felt, the patient should be positioned first on one side and then the other to determine if a change in maternal position will change the location of the cord and diminish cord compression during labor. So long as the variable decelerations do not get more severe and beat-to-beat variability persists, the labor can be allowed to continue. If late decelerations are seen, the patient should be positioned on her left side and given oxygen. If the late decelerations are mild and normal beat-to-beat variability is preserved, the labor can be allowed to continue. If variability is decreased, fetal scalp sampling is indicated. Labor may be allowed to continue if the pH is normal, but periodic scalp sampling will be necessary. If the fetus is acidotic, further labor is contraindicated, and cesarean section for fetal distress should be performed. If the capacity for fetal scalp sampling is not available, a cesarean section for fetal distress should be done if there are persistent late decelerations or severe variable decelerations, accompanied by loss of beat-to-beat variability.

Prolapsed umbilical cord. If a loop of the umbilical cord has prolapsed past the presenting part, it will be compressed against the pelvic wall with every uterine contraction. Each time this occurs, the blood flow through the umbilical vessels ceases, cardiac output is decreased, and the fetal blood pressure falls. The resultant hypoxia is indicated by a fall in the fetal heart rate and a variable deceleration pattern. Although prolapsed cord has no effect on the mother or the course of labor, the infant may die before delivery unless the obstruction to the fetal circulation is relieved.

The incidence of prolapse is about 0.5%; it occurs less frequently when the presenting part fits the pelvis snugly, as it does with normal vertex or frank breech positions, than with certain abnormalities. The principal etiologic factors are those that prevent the presenting part from occluding the pelvic inlet. These include (1) complete and footling breech positions; (2) transverse lies, particularly those in which the back lies superiorly; (3) low-lying placenta with marginal insertion of the cord; (4) a long cord; (5) hydramnios; (6) premature rupture of the membranes; and (7) upward displacement of the presenting part during examinations or operations for delivery. The cord can only prolapse after the membranes rupture.

Cord pressure can be suspected whenever the heart rate during a contraction decreases more than 20 beats/min. The diagnosis can usually be made by vaginal examination. If the membranes have not yet ruptured, the cord may be felt in the intact forebag below the presenting part. This is called a *forelying cord* and is somewhat less serious than a complete prolapse. The forewaters provide a cushion that may impede descent of the infant and thereby reduce the pressure on the umbilical vessels. With *complete prolapse* the cord falls through the cervix and descends into the vagina or even through the introitus. It can be seen or felt without difficulty.

An *occult prolapse* is one in which a loop of cord lies alongside the presenting part. The altered heart rate with each contraction is obvious, but the cord is so high that it may be impossible to feel it. Additional information can sometimes be obtained by manipulating the presenting part in

the inlet. It is pushed against each lateral pelvic wall, the pubis anteriorly and the sacrum posteriorly, while the heart rate is counted. A significant decrease in rate when the head is pushed against a specific area of the bony pelvis suggests that it may be compressing a loop of cord.

Treatment of prolapsed cord is unsatisfactory, and infant mortality is high because the cord often is extruded early in labor before the patient has even entered the hospital. By the time the diagnosis is made, the infant has already died.

If a forelying cord is diagnosed during early labor, cesarean section is almost always indicated. Labor may be allowed to continue if cervical dilation is almost complete, the presenting part is low in the pelvis, and the baby can be delivered promptly and easily when the membranes rupture. The patient should be transported to the delivery room, and the physician should scrub and be prepared to intervene at once if the cord prolapses.

When an actual prolapse is diagnosed during the first stage of labor, cesarean section should be performed if the fetus is alive and is likely to survive. While preparations for the operation are being made, the mother should be placed in the Trendelenburg position and given oxygen while the attendant holds the presenting part out of the pelvis with a sterile gloved hand in the vagina to present interruption of the fetal circulation. If the heart tones are absent, any form of operative interference is unwarranted.

If the cord prolapses during the second stage, it usually is possible to complete delivery by forceps or breech extraction.

Cord entanglement. If a long cord is looped several times around the neck, body, or extremities of the infant, it may be compressed as the loops are drawn tight during descent. The fetal heart rate decreases during each contraction, but no evidence of prolapse can be detected.

The patient suspected of having this condition is evaluated as are others exhibiting signs of hypoxia. Cesarean section should be performed if the variable deceleration pattern, which is characteristic of cord compression, increases and if beat-to-beat variability is lost. If variability and pH remain normal, the labor may be allowed to continue, even though the decelerations recur. One should be prepared to deliver the infant at any time if its condition deteriorates.

Head pressure. Occasionally, a marked depression in fetal heart rate will be detected late in the second stage when the head is distending the perineum. The decision concerning the need for prompt delivery can be made on the basis of beat-to-beat variability. If present, the labor can be allowed to continue.

CARE OF THE NEWBORN INFANT

Most infants make the change from intrauterine to extrauterine existence without difficulty, but some need the help of the physician and all should be observed closely during the immediate postnatal period. The normal infant cries and begins to breathe well within 1 minute of its birth without artificial stimulation. Mucus and blood should be aspirated from the mouth and nasopharynx after the head is born or soon after completion of the delivery. To minimize evaporative heat loss and subsequent cold stress, the infant should be dried and placed under a radiant heat source.

A standardized method for the assessment of the newborn was proposed by Apgar. It evaluates

the condition of the infant at 1 and 5 minutes after birth on the basis of five objective signs. Each is scored as 0, 1, or 2 (Table 32-1). The highest possible score is 10; most normal infants score between 7 and 10. The lower scores indicate increasing degrees of severity of asphyxia and depression. Infants who are moderately affected usually have scores between 4 and 7. The muscle tone is somewhat reduced, and the infant is cyanotic; the heart beats at a rate of 100 beats/min or more. They respond to stimulation and can be resuscitated without difficulty.

Those with scores below 4 are severely depressed and must be treated promptly if they are to survive intact.

Asphyxia neonatorum

Asphyxia is the result of intrauterine hypoxia suffered by the fetus, most commonly during labor or delivery or both. Any interference with the supply of oxygenated blood to the fetus may be a reason for asphyxia. The most frequent causes are maternal hypotension, placental abnormalities, abruptio placentae, and cord complications. Among the factors making up the Apgar scores, the heart rate is the most sensitive indicator of the infant's oxygenation. A sustained rate of over 100 beats/min is the goal of any resuscitative effort.

Apnea

Infants may fail to breath initially. In addition to intrauterine hypoxia, this may be caused by narcosis from drugs administered to the mother, especially anesthetic agents. Birth injuries or malformations such as pneumothorax and diaphragmatic hernia may also cause immediate respiratory difficulties.

Resuscitation

The important steps in resuscitating asphyxiated infants are the establishment of an airway, the delivery of oxygen, and the establishment of ventilation. Thus initial aspiration of the nasopharynx and, if necessary, the trachea is followed by artificial ventilation. Although the most

TABLE 32-1 Signs for determining condition of newborn infant

Sign	0	1	2
Heart rate	Absent	Below 100	Over 100
Respiratory effort	Absent	Slow, irregular	Good, crying
Response to catheter in nostril	None	Grimace	Cough or sneeze
Muscle tone	Limp	Some flexion of extremities	Active motion
Color	Blue, pale	Body pink, extremities blue	Completely pink

efficient means of artificial ventilation for new-born infants is the bag-to-endotracheal tube method, bag-to-mask ventilation is often useful while preparations for intubation progress rapidly. Artificial ventilation should not be used until the airway has been cleared. This is particularly important if the respiratory passages contain thick meconium; it will be forced into the lungs where it causes an intense reaction.

Aspiration of particulate meconium causes a chemical pneumonitis that, in turn, is the leading cause of death in full-term infants. Treatment of meconium aspiration is prevention that must be carried out in the delivery room. When thick meconium is present, the infant's mouth and nose should be suctioned as the head is delivered and before delivery of the thorax. After delivery, endotracheal intubation is performed, and the trachea suctioned. Ideally this should be performed before the first breath.

The infant should be positioned with a slightly dorsiflexed head. A laryngoscope with a newborn-sized blade is introduced at the right angle of the mouth, displacing the tongue to the left side. When the epiglottis is seen, the tip of the blade will be located between the tongue and the epiglottis and must be lifted forward. This will make the vocal cords visible. Any foreign material encountered should be suctioned before an endotracheal tube is inserted. The internal diameter of the tube should be 3.5 mm for term infants and 3.0 mm for premature infants.

A self-inflating bag is connected to the tube and compressed at a rate of 30 to 40 times a minute. Continued bradycardia and failure to initiate spontaneous breathing will necessitate further procedures such as cardiac massage and administration of sodium bicarbonate through the umbilical vein.

All resuscitative maneuvers should be performed gently; there is no place for rough and potentially traumatic procedures such as holding the baby upside down and slapping it.

Stimulant drugs are not indicated in the resuscitation of the newborn. If the infant's depression is caused by administration of morphine or other narcotics to the mother, naloxone (Narcan), 0.01 mg/kg, should be injected into the umbilical vein.

Ligation of the cord

The blood in the fetal circulation is distributed between vessels in the infant's body and those in the placenta. At the end of the second trimester about half of the total blood is in the placenta; as the baby grows larger, relatively more is contained within the infant itself. Blood volume of the newborn is only 250 to 300 ml. Consequently, blood loss from the umbilical cord must be avoided. The ultimate amount of blood retained in the infant will depend on the relative position of the placenta, blood pressure, cord obstructions, and the timing of the cord clamping.

The cord should be ligated with a tie or clamp placed about 2 cm from the skin edge. Subsequently, an antiseptic preparation such as triple dye should be applied to curtail colonization by pathogens, especially staphylococci.

The *absence of one umbilical artery* is associated with congenital malformations of the infant, which usually are severe and obvious. Infants with single umbilical arteries who are normal on examination need no further investigation, but the fact should be recorded because one should be alert for the increased chance of urinary tract anomalies.

The cord mummifies and drops off on about the fifth day of life, leaving a small area at the umbilicus that heals rapidly. Occasionally, the stump of the cord becomes infected and serves as a source of sepsis.

Treatment of the eyes

Credé in 1884 suggested that silver nitrate solution be instilled in the eyes of the newborn infant as an aid in preventing gonorrheal ophthalmia. This has eliminated one of the major causes of acquired blindness. A drop of 1% silver nitrate solution is instilled into each conjunctival sac. Because of an increasing carriage rate of chlamydia in pregnant women and the ineffectiveness of silver nitrate in preventing chlamydial eye infection in the newborn, most centers now use 0.5% erythromycin for eye prophylaxis.

SUGGESTED READING

Apgar V: Drugs in pregnancy, JAMA 190:840, 1964.

Ascari WQ, Allen AE, Baker WJ, and Pollack W: Rh$_0$ (D) immune globulin (human): Evaluation in women at risk of Rh immunization, JAMA 205:1, 1968.

Bowman JM and Manning FA: Intrauterine fetal transfusion: Winnipeg 1982, Obstet Gynecol 61:203, 1983.

Carson BS, Losey RW, Bowes WA Jr, and Simmons MA: Combined obstetric and pediatric approach to prevent meconium aspiration syndrome, Am J Obstet Gynecol 126:712, 1976.

Druzin ML, Gratacós J, Keegan KA, and Paul RH: Antepartum fetal heart rate testing. VII. The significance of fetal bradycardia, Am J Obstet Gynecol 139:194, 1981.

Evertson LR, Gauthier RJ, Schifrin BS, and Paul RH: Antepartum fetal heart rate testing, I. Evolution of the non-stress test, Am J Obstet Gynecol 133:29, 1974.

Feingold M, Fine RN, and Ingall D: Intravenous pyelography in infants with single umbilical artery, N Engl J Med 270:1178, 1964.

Freeman RK: The use of the oxytocin challenge test for antepartum clinical evaluation of uteroplacental respiratory function, Am J Obstet Gynecol 121:481, 1975.

Haverkamp AD, Orleans M, Langendoerfer S, McFee J, Murphy J, and Thompson HE: A controlled trial of the differential effects of intrapartum fetal monitoring, Am J Obstet Gynecol 134:399, 1979.

Herbst AL, Kurman RJ, Scully RE, and Postkanzer DC: Clear-cell adenocarcinoma of the genital tract in young females, N Engl J Med 287:1259, 1972.

Liley AW: Liquor amnii analysis in the management of pregnancy complicated by rhesus sensitization, Am J Obstet Gynecol 82:1359, 1961.

MacDonald D, Grant A, Sheridan-Pereira MS, Boyalan P, and Chalmers I: The Dublin randomized controlled trial of fetal heart rate monitoring, Am J Obstet Gynecol 152:524, 1985.

Manning FA, Morrison I, Lange IR, Harman CR, and Chamberlain PF: Fetal assessment based on fetal biophysical profile scoring: experience in 12,620 referred high-risk pregnancies, Am J Obstet Gynecol 151:343, 1985.

Morrow RF and Ritchie K: Doppler ultrasound velocimetry and its role in obstetrics, Clin Perinatol 16:771, 1989.

Neutra RR: Effect of fetal monitoring on neonatal death rates, N Engl J Med 299:324, 1978.

Reece EA, Copel JA, Scioscia AL, Grannum PA, DeGennaro N, and Hobbins: Diagnostic fetal umbilical blood sampling in the management of isoimmunization, Am J Obstet Gynecol 159:1057, 1988.

Schifrin BS and Dame L: Fetal heart rate patterns: prediction of Apgar score, JAMA 219:1332, 1972.

Thacker SB and Berkelman RL: Assessing the diagnostic accuracy and efficacy of selected antepartum surveillance techniques, Obstet Gynecol Surv 41:121, 1986.

Weinstein L: Irregular antibodies causing hemolytic disease of the newborn, Obstet Gynecol Surv 31:581, 1976.

Zanani B, Paul RH, and Huey JR: Intrapartum fetal heart rate: correlation with scalp pH in the preterm fetus, Am J Obstet Gynecol 136:43, 1980.

33

J. Robert Willson

Dystocia and prolonged labor

Objectives

RATIONALE: Deviations from the pattern of normal labor may be related to dysfunction of the uterine muscle, because of abnormal fetal size or abnormal positions. Prompt recognition and appropriate management reduce maternal and fetal complications.

The student should be able to:
  A. List the types of abnormal labor.
  B. Explain methods for evaluating fetopelvic disproportion.
  C. Describe complications resulting from abnormal labor.
  D. Demonstrate knowledge of the principles of managing dysfunctional labor, including the indications and contraindications for oxytocin stimulation.
  E. Describe diagnosis and principles of management of abnormal fetal positions.

The maximal duration of normal labor has been set arbitrarily at 24 hours; labor that extends beyond this period is termed *prolonged*. Some classify multiparous labors of more than 18 hours' duration as prolonged. Long or difficult labors, to which the term *dystocia* is applied, can be caused by ineffective uterine contractions, by abnormalities in the size or position of the fetus, and by alterations in the structure of the birth canal.

DYSTOCIA FROM UTERINE DYSFUNCTION

At the onset of normal labor, the uterine contractions often occur irregularly and last only a few seconds. Within 2 to 3 hours, however, they assume a more regular pattern and increase in frequency and intensity. The effect of normal uterine contractions is progressive cervical dilation and expulsion of the infant.

Uterine dysfunction can be suspected if the contractions of early labor do not assume a normal pattern within a few hours. Although the contractions of dysfunctional labor may cause almost as much discomfort as those of normal labor, they are far less effective in dilating the cervix.

The gradient of force exerted by the uterine contractions during normal labor is from the fundus to the cervix, and, as labor advances, the upper segment progressively becomes shorter and its walls thicker as the individual muscle fibers retract. The rising inferior border of the upper segment exerts traction on the lower segment and the effaced cervix, which are pulled upward around the presenting part as the latter is pushed through the gradually enlarging opening. This orderly sequence of events does not occur with uterine dysfunction.

As a result of incoordinate activity, the muscle fibers of the upper segment fail to retract, development of the lower segment is incomplete, the cervix remains thick and dilates slowly, or dilation may cease. The cervix often hangs down ahead of the presenting part instead of being applied tightly against it as in normal labor, and the cervix may become progressively thicker and more edematous. Under these circumstances, failure of the cervix to dilate in the usual manner is a result of incoordinate and ineffective uterine action rather than of local abnormality in the cervical tissues.

Abnormal progress in the latent or the active phase can be recognized promptly when cervical dilation is plotted on a normal labor curve.

Latent phase abnormality. Normal, well-coordinated uterine activity is essential for completing effacement of the cervix and subsequently for dilating it. The contractions of early dysfunctional labor are uncoordinated and do not accomplish this effectively. As a consequence, the time required to complete effacement and to enter the active phase is usually longer than during normal labor. This is called *prolonged latent phase* (Fig. 33-1).

The abnormal latent phases will be very short or very long. The major concern is in evaluating the patient who exhibits a possible prolongation of the latent phase. The obstetrician must make one or more of the following clinical decisions: whether the patient is in labor, whether she requires sedation, whether amniotomy should be performed, and whether she should be given oxytocin. There is no absolute amount of time that can be identified as normal for the latent phase; this can vary from service to service (see Fig. 29-14). *A latent phase of more than 10 to 12 hours in primigravidas and more than 6 to 8 hours in multiparas is considered prolonged.*

Active phase dysfunction. There are three possible *active phase patterns:* (1) *normal,* with cervical dilation progressing at the anticipated rate; (2) prolonged, with the cervix dilating steadily but at a rate less than normal *(prolonged active phase);* or (3) one in which the early active phase may appear to be normal or may be progressing slowly, but progress ceases before cervical dila-

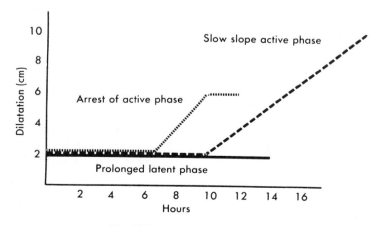

Fig. 33-1 Abnormal labor curves.

tion is complete *(active phase arrest)* (Fig. 33-1).

Because the cervix should dilate progressively during the active phase, abnormalities of this part of labor can be recognized early. A *prolonged active phase* can be diagnosed whenever cervical dilation progresses at a rate less than 0.7 cm/hr in primigravidas and less than 1.1 cm/hr in multiparas. An *active phase arrest* can be diagnosed if cervical dilation in the active phase does not change during a 2-hour period. By studying the slope of the active phase curve, the physician does not have to wait until the normal mean duration is exceeded to diagnose abnormal labor (Fig. 33-1).

Etiologic factors. Uterine dysfunction is almost always encountered in *primigravidas* and is unusual during subsequent labors. This fact eliminates structural abnormalities of the uterus or faulty nerve supply as etiologic factors. It is frequently stated that a prolonged latent phase can be caused by the administration of *analgesic drugs* too early in labor, but this is doubtful. Women who are given drugs during the normal latent phase continue to progress at a regular rate, and the quality of the contractions during early normal labor often improves after the patient is relaxed by medication. Analgesics certainly can increase an abnormality already present, but they probably do not cause it. *Overdistension of the uterus* by hydramnios or multiple pregnancy may decrease the efficiency of the uterine contractions, thus delaying progress. A prolonged *active phase,* during which the cervix dilates progressively but at a rate slower than anticipated, almost always occurs in primigravidas, and no specific cause can be found.

Active phase arrest, in which cervical dilation ceases during a 2-hour period, is an ominous sign because it is a pattern that is encountered with cephalopelvic disproportion in primigravidas. Active phase arrest is less likely to occur with cephalopelvic disproportion in multiparas (Fig. 33-2).

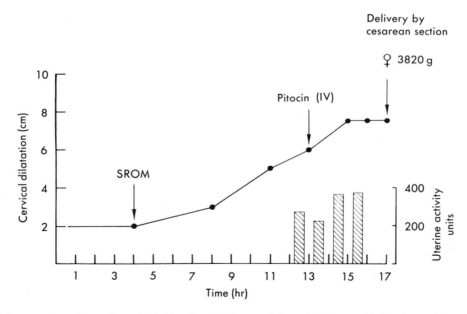

Fig. 33-2 Arrest active phase of cervical dilatation in 28-year-old gravida 3, para II. Uterine activity is noted in lower right portion of graph. In spite of improvement in uterine activity with intravenous administration of oxytocin (Pitocin), cervical dilatation stopped at 7 cm, and cesarean section was performed. *SROM,* Spontaneous rupture of membrane.

Effect of uterine dysfunction. Prolongation of labor and the consequent multiple vaginal examinations increase the risk of *endomyometritis,* particularly if a cesarean section is required.

The defective uterine contractions usually continue into the third stage, thereby increasing the incidence of *postpartum hemorrhage.* This is far more serious if labor has been so long that the mother is exhausted and dehydrated and the intravascular space is contracted. Blood loss may also be increased by injury from *operative delivery,* which is necessary more often than with normal labor.

Management of uterine dysfunction. Abnormal labor can usually be suspected within 6 to 8 hours after the labor begins because the contractions remain irregular and short and produce little change in the cervix or the station of the presenting part. The physician should not wait until a prolonged latent or an abnormal active phase can be diagnosed on the basis of elapsed time before starting the study and treatment.

Certain principles are essential to the proper management of any prolonged labor regardless of the cause. These include evaluation, protection against infection, sedation, and hydration.

EVALUATION. A sterile vaginal examination should be performed as soon as abnormal labor is suspected. Unanticipated abnormalities in fetal position or cephalopelvic disproportion may be diagnosed, and the consistency and dilation of the cervix can be determined.

PROTECTION AGAINST INFECTION. Vaginal examinations should be limited because bacteria are carried directly through the cervix on the fingers. Prophylactic antibiotics should not be necessary. There can be no need to treat infection if it is prevented by early recognition and proper management of abnormal labor.

SEDATION. Analgesic drugs administered as during normal labor may decrease both the force and the frequency of uterine contractions, but this is usually a short-term response. A phenothiazine preparation such as promethazine (Phenergan), 50 mg, will relax the patient and ease her tension without altering the contraction mechanism. If normal uterine activity can be achieved with oxytocics, any of the methods used to control pain during normal labor are applicable.

HYDRATION. Patients with prolonged labor should be kept well hydrated. From 2 to 3 L of fluid are necessary every 24 hours. Because absorption from the stomach is reduced during labor, the fluid should be given intravenously.

PROLONGED LATENT PHASE. The frequency with which the diagnosis of latent phase prolongation is made is in part determined by the obstetrician's decision as to when labor began. To use labor graphs effectively, one must make an arbitrary decision when the patient is admitted that labor began at the time she first felt painful uterine contractions. Some of these women will actually be in false labor and will be discharged, but initial decisions concerning the onset of labor permit early recognition of latent phase abnormalities. A latent phase that extends beyond normal on a labor graph should not be ignored.

An attempt should be made to correct the abnormality as soon as it becomes evident that contractions have not assumed a normal pattern, that there is no appreciable change in the cervix, and that labor is not progressing at a normal rate (Fig. 33-3). At the end of the sixth or eighth hour of latent phase labor a *sterile vaginal examination* is performed to determine fetal position and station and the condition of the cervix.

Amniotomy performed at the time of the vaginal examination may be followed by improved contractions and conversion to a normal pattern. Because amniotomy commits one to completing delivery within a reasonable time, the physician must be as certain as possi-

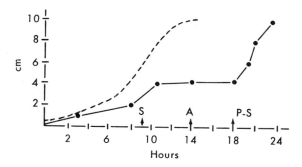

Fig. 33-3 Labor graph of primigravida with prolonged latent phase of labor. Sedative *(S)* was given at 9 hours, and amniotomy *(A)* performed at fourteenth hour. Latent phase persisted until oxytocin (Pitocin, *P*) was given. Position was right occipitoposterior; infant weight 2405 g.

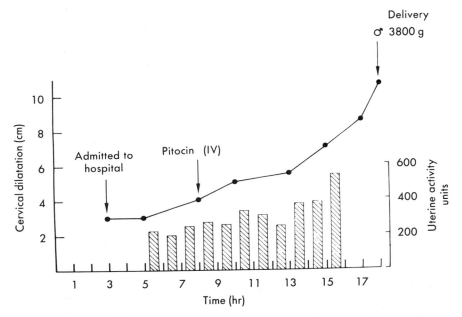

Fig. 33-4 Prolonged active phase in 20-year-old gravida 1, para 0. Progress of cervical dilation was slow and steady in spite of intravenous administration of oxytocin (Pitocin).

ble that the problem is a prolonged latent phase and not false labor before rupturing the membranes. One must also plan each step of the treatment in advance and be prepared to perform cesarean section while it is still safe if an effective contraction pattern cannot be established.

If normal progress has not been established within an hour after amniotomy, the uterus should be stimulated with *oxytocin*. The method by which this solution is administered is described in the discussion on induction of labor (Chapter 29). The dosage necessary to stimulate normal contractions is usually small, and at the beginning no more than 0.5 to 1 mU/min of oxytocin should be delivered. If this is not enough to induce a normal contraction pattern, the dosage can be increased gradually at 1 mU/min increments every 20 to 30 minutes. If the uterus does not respond to a dosage of 10 to 15 mU/min, a further increase is not likely to be effective. Intrauterine pressure and fetal heart recordings should be made during oxytocin infusion.

Almost all patients will enter the active phase with amniotomy and oxytocin stimulation, and in some the labor will progress normally without continued stimula-

tion, but many will develop active phase arrest if the oxytocin is stopped.

A *prolonged active phase* usually cannot be altered significantly by amniotomy or oxytocin. If cervical dilation is progressing at a regular but reduced rate and if there is no concern over the adequacy of the pelvis, no active treatment is necessary. Oxytocin should be used if uterine contractions occur irregularly and if the recorded contractions are of low amplitude (Fig. 33-4).

ACTIVE PHASE ARREST (Fig. 33-5). Arrest during the active phase of labor is cause for concern, because it may be an indication of fetopelvic disproportion in primigravidas. If the contractions are irregular and progressive cervical dilation ceases, vaginal examination is imperative. Treatment will depend on the degree of disproportion.

Amniotomy, if the membranes are still intact, and *oxytocin stimulation* are both indicated if there is no disproportion or only a minor degree, which can probably be overcome with normal contractions. Amniotomy should be performed even though the presenting part is still high, particularly if the vertex is well applied to

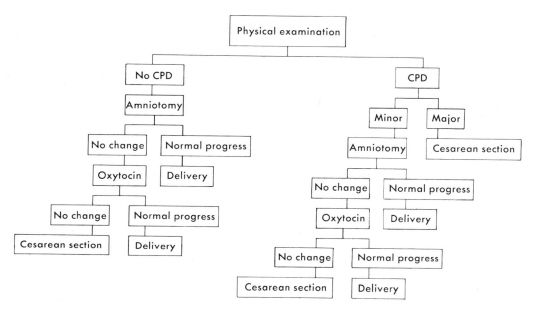

Fig. 33-5 Management of active phase arrest of cervical dilatation. *CPD,* Cephalopelvic disproportion.

the cervix. It may be all that is needed to correct the abnormality and to eliminate the need for oxytocin and cesarean section. The possibility of cord prolapse is slight and is outweighed by potential risks of active phase arrest. Oxytocin should be started if the contractions do not improve within an hour after amniotomy. Oxytocin must be continued throughout the rest of the labor; if it is stopped, the abnormal contraction pattern will usually recur.

Cesarean section may become necessary if oxytocin-stimulated contractions fail to overcome what is considered to be minor disproportion or if normal progress in labor cannot be established. A decision can almost always be made during the first 4 to 6 hours of stimulation; although delivery may not occur within this time, the physician can determine whether it can logically be anticipated.

DELIVERY. The decision as to when a patient should be delivered is made on the basis of observed progress and an estimate of how long the total labor will be. If a *prolonged latent phase* is terminated and active phase abnormality does not develop, one can anticipate nor-

mal delivery. If the prolonged latent phase is not terminated by amniotomy and oxytocin, there is no choice but cesarean section.

In general, there is no need to interfere in *prolonged active phase* if measured uterine activity is normal and cervical dilation and descent continue at a resonable rate. Cesarean section may be justified if uterine activity is inadequate and continues after the administration of oxytocin and arrest occurs. Vaginal delivery usually occurs when *active phase arrest* can be corrected by oxytocin, and there is no disproportion.

Whether a patient can be delivered vaginally will be determined by the size of the pelvis; the position, station, and size of the infant; and the amount of difficulty anticipated. There is a natural tendency to terminate abnormal labor as soon as possible. This is reflected in the fact that "poor progress in labor" is one of the leading indications for cesarean section in the United States. Because the pelvis generally is normal, as is the mechanism of labor under the influence of oxytocin, there is little need for difficult midforceps delivery. If intervention is necessary, an atraumatic delivery should be the goal. A cesarean section is preferable to a difficult midforceps delivery.

Cesarean section should not be considered a last resort measure in the treatment of dysfunction labor. With this attitude, perinatal morbidity and mortality can only increase. Cesarean section should be performed when (1) uterine dysfunction cannot be corrected by amniotomy and oxytocin stimulation, (2) delivery becomes necessary because of fetal distress before the cervix is dilated, or (3) during the second stage unless easy forceps delivery is possible. Nevertheless, cesarean section should not be used indiscriminately because abnormal labor usually occurs only in primigravidas and a uterine scar may complicate subsequent deliveries that are likely to be normal.

The incidence of hemorrhage following delivery is increased because the abnormal contractions continue during the third stage and because injury occurs more frequently than with normal delivery.

DYSTOCIA OF FETAL ORIGIN

Dystocia of fetal origin may be the result of excessive size, abnormal development, or unusual positions in the birth canal.

Excessive development

The usual infant at term weighs slightly more than 3200 g (7 pounds) and is about 50 cm (19.5 inches) long. About 10% weight at least 4000 g (9 pounds), but in no more than 1 or 2% is the birth weight over 4500 g (10 pounds).

The *birth weight often increases progressively in each pregnancy,* so the third or fourth infant may weigh much more than the first. Because of this the physician cannot assume that a multiparous woman will deliver without difficulty simply because she has before. The present infant may be too large to pass through the pelvis, although the measurements indicate that it is normal. Approximately 10% of primary cesarean sections in multiparas are performed because of disproportion. *Babies whose parents are large generally weigh more than those born to smaller individuals.* Fortunately, large women usually have large pelves that will permit the delivery of oversized infants without difficulty. *Maternal diabetes* is such an important factor that a glucose tolerance test should be performed in any woman who has been delivered of an infant weighing more than 4000 g. Fetal weight can be correlated with *maternal weight gain.* Women who gain more than 13.5 kg (30 pounds) during pregnancy are likely to have large babies. *Postmature babies* may be larger than those delivered before 42 weeks.

The normal-sized pelvis should be adequate for the delivery of infants weighing 4000 to 4500 g if the uterine contractions are forceful enough. If the baby is too large, however, disproportion similar to that encountered with normal infants and contracted pelvis can occur; as a consequence, the infant may be injured during difficult extraction.

The physician must be on the lookout for large babies, particularly in women in whom there is a reason for their development. The size cannot always be determined accurately by palpation. *Sonographic measurements of the biparietal diameter and body circumference* are helpful in determining fetal size.

During labor the findings are similar to those in disproportion from contracted pelvis, except that the latter more often occurs in primigravidas. The head may fail to enter the pelvis, or descent may be slow despite what appear to be normal uterine contractions.

It is important to recognize fetopelvic disproportion early in the course of labor. The uterus may rupture in multiparas with insurmountable disproportion because strong, forceful contractions continue despite the lack of descent. The primigravid uterus is more likely to respond by active phase arrest.

If disproportion is not too great, the head may descend and deliver, but the broad shoulders are not able to pass the inlet *(shoulder dystocia)* (Fig. 33-6). When this occurs, the chin will be pulled back tightly against the perineum as soon as the head is delivered through the introitus. Unless the infant is extracted promptly, it will die because its chest is compressed, preventing respiratory efforts, and the circulation through the cord is reduced.

The posterior shoulder usually has descended into the true pelvis below the promontory of the sacrum, but the bisacromial diameter is so long that the anterior shoulder, which lies above the pubis, cannot enter the pelvis. Under such circumstances forceful downward traction on the infant's head not only is ineffectual but may well stretch and injure the brachial plexus or even fracture the cervical spine. The physician should first attempt to push the anterior shoulder into the pelvis by direct pressure on it through the abdominal wall. If this cannot be accomplished, another maneuver must be tried at once. The hand is inserted into the vagina until the first and second fingers can be hooked in the poste-

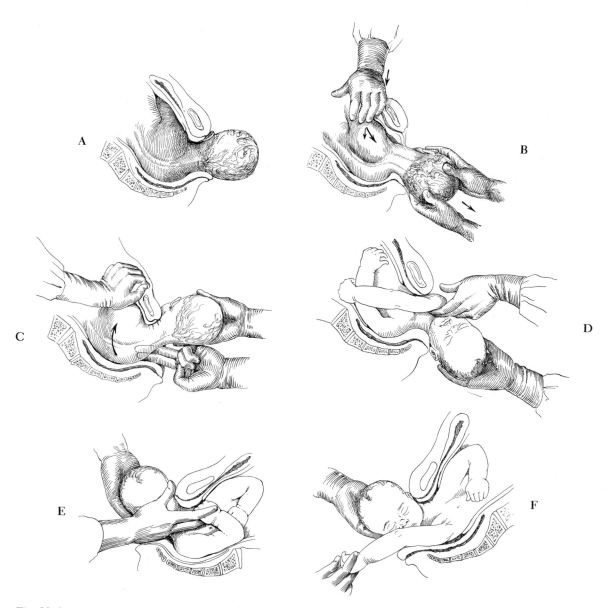

Fig. 33-6 Shoulder dystocia. **A,** Anterior shoulder cannot enter inlet. **B,** Attempt to push shoulder beneath pubis. **C** and **D,** Rotation of shoulders. **E** and **F,** Extraction of posterior arm.

rior axilla. The posterior shoulder is rotated anteriorly and pulled downward simultaneously with a corkscrew motion. If this maneuver is successful, the anterior shoulder is rotated into the true pelvis below the sacral promontory while the posterior shoulder is delivered from underneath the symphysis anteriorly. From this point, delivery can be completed with little difficulty (Fig. 33-6, *A* to *D*).

If the shoulders are wedged into the inlet so tightly that they cannot be rotated, the hand is passed over the posterior shoulder and along the chest until the baby's hand can be seized and pulled downward over the chest and through the introitus. This releases the posterior shoulder and will permit its anterior rotation and delivery (Fig. 33-6, *E* and *F*).

All of these maneuvers to achieve vaginal delivery can result in soft tissue injury to the fetus. One new approach is to push the head back into the vagina and do an immediate cesarean section. The results seem to be good.

Developmental abnormalities

Developmental anomalies seldom cause dystocia, but in rare instances they may. This is particularly true of deformities such as hydrocephalus, enlargement of the body or abdomen, or conjoined twins.

With *hydrocephalus,* labor is delayed because the head is too large to enter the inlet. The diagnosis can be suspected if a large mass is felt over the inlet. On vaginal palpation the presenting part is above the pelvic inlet; the sutures, if they can be reached, are wide; and the fontanels are huge. Ultrasonographic examination will provide confirmatory evidence. With breech position, hydrocephalus is sometimes not diagnosed until it is impossible to extract the aftercoming head.

If a decision is made for vaginal delivery, the head must usually be decompressed by draining fluid off through a needle or trocar. If the predelivery sonogram shows a significant amount of cerebral tissue, cesarean section may be considered.

The fetal body may be enlarged by *tumors of the liver, abnormal development of the kidneys, urinary retention* from obstruction in the lower urinary tract, or other anomalies. In the past these abnormalities did not become apparent until after the head had been delivered

and the body did not follow. More widespread use of antepartum ultrasonography has increased the frequency of early diagnosis. Their management is determined by the cause of the obstruction and whether it can be relieved by manipulation or operation through the maternal vagina.

DYSTOCIA FROM ABNORMALITIES IN POSITION AND PRESENTATION

Abnormalities in position and presentation frequently cause dystocia. If they are recognized promptly and are corrected, the results for both the mother and infant should be reasonably good.

Transverse lie

With transverse lie, the long axis of the infant lies at right angles to the longitudinal axis of the mother; its head lies in one flank, and its buttocks in the other. One of the shoulders lies over the inlet, the presenting part being the scapula or the achromial process. If the infant's back is directed toward the maternal spine, the presenting part will lie in the right or left posterior quadrant of the pelvis (right or left *scapuloposterior position*). If the back is directed anteriorly, the presenting part will lie in the right or left anterior quadrant (right or left *scapuloanterior position*) (Fig. 33-7). In an *oblique lie* the long axis of the fetus lies obliquely across the abdomen, with the head or the buttocks directed toward one or the other maternal iliac fossa.

Transverse lie occurs more often in multiparas than in primigravidas, but it complicates only about 0.25% to 0.5% of all pregnancies. If the placenta is implanted in the fundus or over the cervix, the infant may be forced to assume a transverse or an oblique position because the length of the uterine cavity is reduced. *In about one third of all transverse lies, the placenta occupies the lower segment.* Transverse lie is more common in *bicornuate or arcuate uteri* than in those that have developed normally. It may occur because of *hydramnios,* which permits the fetus considerable freedom of motion.

Diagnosis. Transverse lie can be suspected if the abdomen looks wider than it does long. If the uterus is relaxed, the head can be felt on one side, and the breech on the other; there is no presenting part in the inlet. It may be possible to palpate the shoulder through the vagina, but if the membranes are intact, the presenting part is often so high that it cannot be reached. During labor, the membranes can be felt bulging

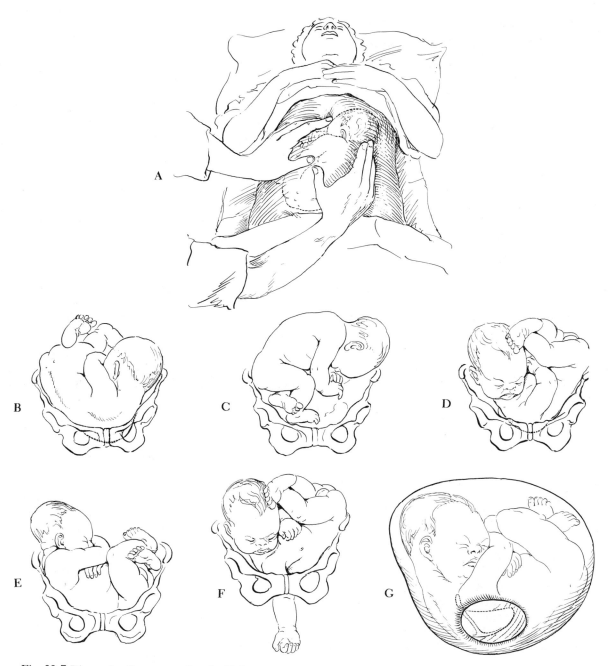

Fig. 33-7 Diagnosis of transverse lie. **A,** Oblique lie. **B,** Left scapuloanterior. **C,** Ventral surface of infant directed toward pelvic inlet and back toward fundus. **D,** Right scapuloposterior. **E,** Ventral surface of infant directed toward fundus and backlying over pelvic inlet. **F,** Right scapuloposterior with prolapsed arm. **G,** Transverse lie with back down.

through the partially dilated cervix with each contraction. Between contractions the scapula, the clavicle, the axilla, and the rib cage can be palpated. Sonographic examination will confirm the position of the fetus as well as that of the placenta.

Vaginal or rectal examinations should not be performed in the physician's office on patients suspected of having transverse lies. If placenta previa is present, profuse bleeding can be precipitated.

Course of labor. Spontaneous delivery of a living normal-sized infant should not be anticipated with shoulder presentation.

Prognosis. If the abnormality is recognized early and treated properly, the *maternal mortality and morbidity* should not be increased.

Perinatal deaths are caused by anoxia from prolapsed cord, which occurs more often than with normal presentation; by infection; or by injury from prolonged labor or attempts at delivery. The perinatal mortality is as high as 30% to 50% with vaginal delivery, but most babies who are reasonably mature and in good condition should survive if delivered by cesarean section.

Management. If transverse or oblique lie is recognized during late pregnancy, *external version* to a breech or a vertex position should be attempted. If this is impossible, a sonographic examination for placental site should be obtained, and other possible causes of the abnormal lies sought. Many transverse presentations correct themselves spontaneously before labor begins.

External version can also be attempted during early labor if placenta previa has been eliminated. If the position cannot be corrected, cesarean section offers the best prognosis for the infant in either primigravidas or multiparas.

Occipitoposterior position

In about a fourth of all vertex deliveries the occiput points toward one of the posterior quadrants during early labor. Almost all infants rotate to an anterior position spontaneously or deliver in the posterior position without difficulty, but, in a few patients, particularly those with abnormal pelves, the labor is prolonged and difficult.

One of the most important reasons for the occipitoposterior position (Fig. 33-8) is the shape of the bony pelvic inlet. If the transverse diameter of the inlet is

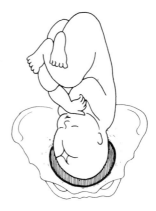

Fig. 33-8 Left occipitoposterior position.

narrowed and if the anteroposterior diameter is lengthened, as in an anthropoid pelvis, the head must descend with its long axis in an anteroposterior diameter. The occiput may be directed posteriorly or toward the pubis. If the anterior segment of the superior strait is narrow and of the android type, the head is also likely to descend in an oblique posterior position. The forehead fits the anterior segment of the inlet better than does the wider occipital area. In contrast, the infant's head is more likely to enter the gynecoid or the platypelloid pelvis in a transverse diameter, with its long axis in the longest axis of the inlet because it fits better; however, it can be in a posterior position if the pelvis is large.

Anterior rotation can be anticipated if the head is in an oblique occipitoposterior position and flexes as it descends, if the uterine contractions are effective, and if the pelvic size and shape and the levator muscles are normal. In primigravidas the second stage may be slightly longer than usual, but in multiparas the head often descends to the pelvic floor in the posterior position and rotates and delivers with one or two contractions.

Failure to rotate may be the result of inadequate uterine contractions that do not provide enough force to push the baby downward or of relaxation and separation of the levator muscles, eliminating the inclined plane up which the occiput is forced, or it may be because the transverse diameter of the bony pelvis is so narrow that the head cannot turn within the birth canal.

The occiput also may fail to rotate anteriorly because

the head is slightly deflexed, making some anterior portion rather than the occiput the presenting part. This area will naturally rotate anteriorly, thereby directing the occiput to the hollow of the sacrum, where it stays. This can occur when complete head flexion is not necessary because the head is small and the pelvis large.

If the head descends to the pelvic floor with the occiput in an oblique posterior position, the patient should be given an opportunity to rotate it herself. No interference is necessary as long as rotation is progressing, even though it is slow and the conditions of the mother and the baby are good. Conversely, delivery is indicated if the maternal or the fetal condition should change or if no progress in descent or rotation is made during a period of an hour.

If the head descends in a direct occipitoposterior position, anterior rotation is not likely to occur because the presenting part lies over the sacrum in the trough formed by the two levator muscles rather than on the inclined plane. In many instances, particularly in multiparas with roomy pelves and relaxed soft tissues and in those with anthropoid pelves, spontaneous or low forceps delivery with the occiput in a posterior position is not only possible but is preferable to operative rotation. The longer diameters of the head may increase perineal injury slightly, but damage from rotation if the pelvis is abnormal may be even greater. Cesarean section is indicated for an occipitoposterior position if descent ceases while the head is too high for safe forceps extraction.

Face position

When the head is completely deflexed, face position can be diagnosed (Fig. 33-9). The chin (mentum) is the presenting part, and relatively large diameters are presenting. Face positions occur in about 0.25% of all deliveries.

Complete deflexion may be primary, or it develops during descent of the head through the inlet; something holds the occiput up, thereby encouraging the anterior portion of the head to descend first. Deflexion increases as the head descends. Face positions may develop in women with *inlet contraction;* the bitemporal diameter is narrower than the biparietal and fits better in the inlet. The situation with a *large baby* is comparable. The *pendulous uterus in a multiparous woman* allows the infant to fall forward or to one side, thereby favoring abnormal positions. Flexion of the head may be prevented by *abnormalities of the neck or thorax* or by *loops of cord around the neck.* Almost all *anencephalic infants* present by the face.

Diagnosis. The fetal spine is extended, and the head is deflexed, with the occiput in contact with the back. On *abdominal examination* the smooth curve of the spine, which is characteristic of flexed attitudes, cannot be felt, but the extremities may be unusually prominent. The cephalic prominence can be felt on the side opposite the small parts. It often is difficult to make a diagnosis by abdominal palpation.

On *vaginal examination* the face may feel like a breech, but if the cervix is partly dilated, the supraorbital ridges, nose, eyes, and mouth can be palpated (Fig. 33-10). The deflexion can be confirmed by sonographic examination.

Course of labor. The mechanism of labor for the face position is similar to that in the vertex position, but the chin rather than the occipital portion of the head is the presenting part. As the head descends, extension increases until the head is completely deflexed, with the occiput in contact with the infant's back. The chin is rotated because it is forced downward against the levator sling and the bony side walls of the lower pelvis; as labor continues it gradually rotates anteriorly until it lies beneath the pubic arch, with the occipital portion of the head directed toward the sacrum. The submandibular area stems beneath the pubis, while the occiput is forced upward over the perineum until it is free of the vagina. The head therefore is delivered by flexion. The delivery of the shoulders and body is like that in occiput positions.

If anterior rotation of the chin fails to occur, *persistent mentoposterior position* can be diagnosed (Fig. 33-11). It is almost impossible for a normal-sized infant to deliver in a mentoposterior position because the chin, which lies in the hollow of the sacrum, can only be forced over the perineum by further extension of the head; this is impossible because it already is completely deflexed.

Delay from mentoposterior position often occurs when the presenting part is relatively high in the pelvis. If the head descends with the chin pointed directly posteriorly, rotation is not likely to occur. If it is directed obliquely posteriorly, rotation can be anticipated, especially in multiparas, but it usually does not occur until the presenting part begins to bulge the perineum.

It is important to remember that when the face is presenting, the biparietal diameter does not pass the

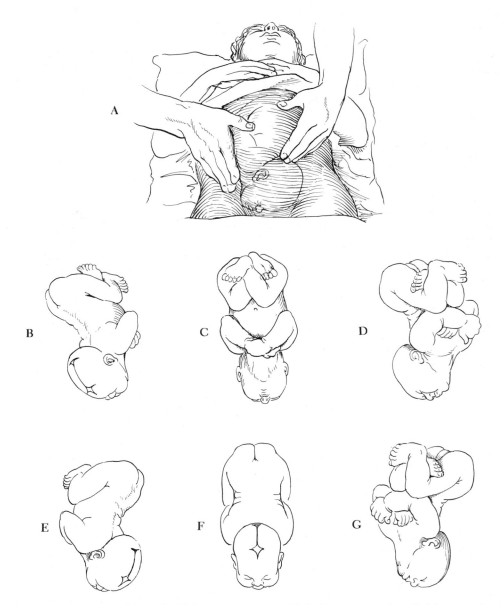

Fig. 33-9 Diagnosis of face positions. **A,** Right mentotransverse. **B,** Left mentoposterior. **C,** Mentoanterior. **D,** Left mentoanterior. **E,** Right mentoposterior. **F,** Mentoposterior. **G,** Right mentoanterior.

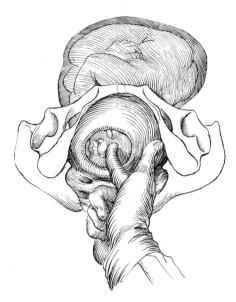

Fig. 33-10 Vaginal palpation of right mentotransverse.

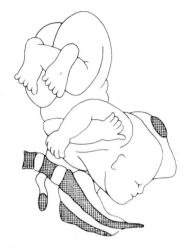

Fig. 33-11 Persistent mentoposterior position.

pelvic inlet until the chin reaches the pelvic floor; consequently, engagement occurs late in labor.

Management. The management of the face position depends on pelvic size, stage of labor, efficiency of the contractions, and parity. If an abnormal attitude is suspected by abdominal or rectal palpation, the patient should be examined vaginally. If there is no obvious disproportion, and particularly if the chin is in an anterior or a transverse position, labor may be allowed to continue. If the chin is directed posteriorly and the head is wedged into the upper pelvis, the outlook for normal delivery is unfavorable. In many instances, particularly in multiparas, face positions are not diagnosed until the patient is delivering.

Cesarean section is indicated when progress ceases with the presenting part high in the pelvis or when mentoposterior positions cannot be corrected. It is more often necessary in primigravidas than in multiparas, many of whom deliver rapidly and spontaneously despite the abnormal position.

Brow position

Deflexed attitudes in which the brow is the presenting part occur about once in every 500 to 1000 deliveries and result from any of the factors that tend to prevent flexion and increase extension. Such causes are a large pelvis or a small infant, contracted pelvis, and abnormalities in the shape of the head.

Spontaneous delivery in the brow position will not always occur even if the pelvis is of normal size because the presenting diameter of the fetal head (occipitomental, 13.5 cm) is too large to come through the inlet without extensive molding (Fig. 33-12). However, the brow is frequently a transient position, and enough alteration in position may occur as labor progresses to permit pelvic delivery.

Diagnosis. The diagnosis of brow position is made by palpating the anterior fontanel in the middle of the cervical opening with the supraorbital ridges at one side (Fig. 33-13). Ordinarily, the presenting part is well above the spines. On abdominal examination the deflexion may be suspected by the straight fetal spine with a cephalic prominence palpable on each side (Fig. 33-14).

Management. The management depends on the stage of labor, size of the infant, and the shape and size of the pelvis. Vaginal delivery can be anticipated if the infant is small and if the presenting part is below the

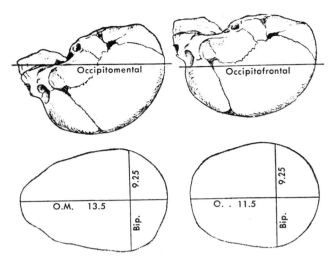

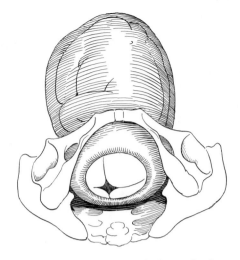

Fig. 33-12 With brow position, longest anteroposterior diameter of head (occipitomental) must pass through pelvis. (From Beck AC: Obstetrical practice, Baltimore, 1955, The Williams & Wilkins Co.)

Fig. 33-13 Brow position vaginal examination.

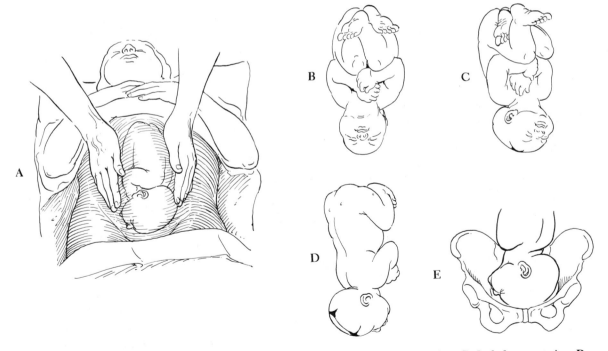

Fig. 33-14 Diagnosis of brow positions. **A,** Right frontotransverse. **B,** Frontoanterior. **C,** Left frontoanterior. **D,** Left frontoposterior. **E,** Right frontotransverse.

spines at the time the abnormal position is recognized. Often the presenting part is unengaged and cannot be depressed into the pelvis. In this event, delivery without altering the position is not to be expected. Flexion of the head to an occiput position or extension to a face position might solve the problem, but neither of these is easy if the head is molded. Cesarean section frequently is the preferred method for delivery, particularly in the primigravida, when progress ceases with incomplete cervical dilation or if the pelvis is contracted.

Compound presentation

Compound presentation can be diagnosed whenever one or more of an infant's extremities prolapse alongside the presenting head or breech. This occurs once in 700 to 1000 deliveries of viable infants. In most instances an upper rather than a lower extremity is involved. Compound presentation occurs most often if the pelvic inlet is contracted or if the infant is premature and so small that it does not occlude the birth canal. It is encountered more often in multiparas than in primigravidas.

Labor usually progresses normally. Occasionally, however, the prolapsed extremity may be responsible for abnormal rotation of the presenting part, or, if large

enough, it may even delay descent. Prolapsed cord occurs frequently with compound presentation, particularly if an extremity is prolapsed through the cervix.

No treatment for compound presentation is necessary unless labor is delayed. A hand lying beside the infant's head, for example, will usually not prolapse completely because the increasing pressure against it as the head descends will hold it up. If an entire arm or leg has descended through the cervix, it may be necessary to disengage the head and replace the extremity within the uterine cavity. Neither cesarean section nor version and extraction is often warranted.

SUGGESTED READING

Gopelrud J and Eastman NJ: Compound presentation: survey of 65 cases, Obstet Gynecol 1:59, 1953.

Phillips RD and Freeman M: The management of the persistent occiput posterior position, Obstet Gynecol 43:171, 1974.

Sack RA: The large infant, Am J Obstet Gynecol 104:195, 1969.

Seitchik J and Castillo M: Oxytocin augmentation of dysfunctional labor, Am J Obstet Gynecol 144:899, 1982.

Van Dorsten JP: Safe and effective external cephalic version with tocolysis, Contemp Ob/Gyn 19:44, 1982.

34

J. Robert Willson

Pelvimetry; dystocia from contracted pelvis

Objectives

RATIONALE: Dystocia related to fetopelvic disproportion may occur because the fetus is too large to pass through a bony pelvis with normal diameters or because the pelvis is so small that vaginal delivery of the baby is either impeded or prevented.

The student should be able to:

A. Describe the normal bony pelvis including the inlet, the midpelvis, and the outlet.

B. Name the four normal pelvic growth types and indicate how they differ from each other.

C. State the important measurements of the inlet, the midpelvis and the outlet in a normal gynecoid pelvis.

D. Describe how alterations in pelvic size and shape may influence the course of normal labor.

A clinical estimation of pelvic size is usually made at the initial prenatal visit because it is convenient to measure the pelvis at that time. Some physicians prefer to obtain the internal measurements later when the tissues are more supple and relaxed and when the patient is less tense. It makes little difference when the pelvis is measured as long as it is done before labor begins.

Most abnormal pelves can be at least suspected by clinical examination, but x-ray film study is necessary to obtain precise measurements and to determine pelvic shape accurately. Weighing the benefits derived from x-ray film pelvimetry

against the risks to the mother and the fetus, it is indicated only under unusual circumstances.

NORMAL PELVIS

For obstetric purposes the pelvis is divided into the *false pelvis* and the *true pelvis,* or *pelvic cavity,* at the level of the sacral promontory; the linea terminalis is on each side; and the upper border of the pubis anteriorly. The false pelvis serves no important obstetric purpose except to support the enlarging uterus and to direct the presenting part downward. The true pelvis—which is bounded by the sacrum posteriorly; the pelvic bones, mus-

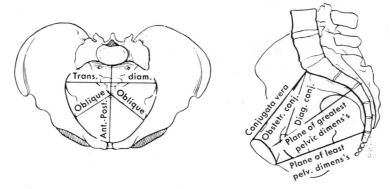

Fig. 34-1 Planes of pelvic inlet. (From Moloy HC: Evaluation of the pelvis in obstetrics, Philadelphia, 1951, WB Saunders Co.)

cles, and ligaments laterally; and the posterior surfaces of the rami of the pubis and the ischii anteriorly—is far more significant. Alteration in the size and shape of the pelvis may interfere with the mechanism of labor or even prevent normal delivery.

Pelvic inlet (Fig. 34-1). The pelvic inlet, or superior strait, the entrance to the true pelvis, is bounded by the promontory and alae of the sacrum, the lineae terminalis laterally, and the superior surface of the pubic bones anteriorly. It is oval in shape and its *angle of inclination,* the angle the plane of the inlet makes with the horizon with the patient standing, is about 55 degrees.

The *conjugata vera,* or *true conjugate,* extends from the midpoint of the sacral promontory to the superior surface of the symphysis and measures 10.5 to 11.5 cm. The *obstetric conjugate* extends from the promontory to the closest point on the convex posterior surface of the symphysis, which is about 0.5 to 1 cm below the upper margin. This measures about 0.5 cm less than the true conjugate. The *diagonal conjugate* extends from the promontory to the lower border of the symphysis and measures about 12.5 cm. This is the only anteroposterior measurement that can be obtained clinically (Fig. 34-1).

The *transverse diameter* of the inlet represents the greatest distance between the linea terminalis and usually forms a right angle with the true conjugate approximately 5 cm anterior to the promontory. It measures about 13.5 cm. The *oblique diameters* extend from each sacroiliac synchondrosis to the opposite iliopectineal eminence and measure about 12.5 cm. The right oblique diameter originates at the right sacroiliac synchondrosis and the left oblique diameter on the left side posteriorly (Fig. 34-1).

Pelvic cavity. The *plane of greatest pelvic dimensions,* the roomiest portion of the pelvic cavity, lies above the ischial spines at the level of a line that extends from the junction of the second and third sacral vertebrae to the middle of the posterior surface of the pubis. This measures about 12.75 cm (Fig. 34-2). The transverse diameter between the two iliac bones just above the superior surface of each acetabulum measures about 12.5 cm.

The *plane of least pelvic dimensions,* or the *midplane,* extends from the lower border of the pubis anteriorly to the lower sacrum at the level of the ischial spines and measures about 11.5 to 12 cm (Fig. 34-2). The transverse *bispinous diameter* is the smallest in the normal pelvic cavity, measuring about 10.5 cm.

Pelvic outlet. The pelvic outlet, or inferior

strait, is even less a "plane" than is the inlet. Actually, it is made up of two triangles sharing a common base at a line joining the two ischial tuberosities. The apex of the anterior triangle is the lower border of the symphysis, and the sides are the descending pubic rami and the ascending ischial rami. The apex of the posterior triangle is the tip of the sacrum, and the sides are the pelvic ligaments. The *bituberous* diameter measures 8 to 11 cm; and the *anteroposterior diameter,* or the distance between the lower border of the symphysis and the tip of the sacrum, is 11.5 cm (Fig. 34-2).

Many variations in the normal pelvis are produced by heredity and by variations in hormone stimulation, pressure, and disease during child-

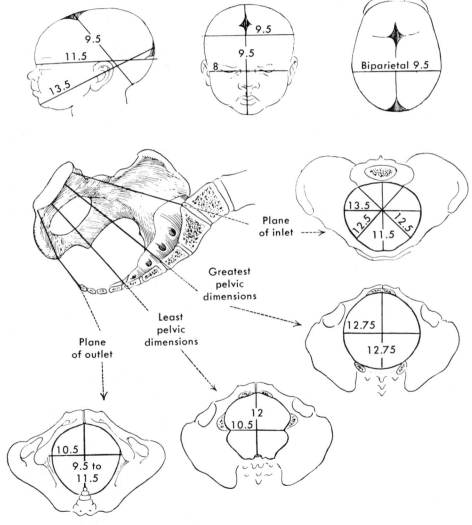

Fig. 34-2 Diameters in centimeters of various planes of pelvis and of fetal head that must pass through it.

hood. Most pelves are adequate for childbearing, but in some the deviation may be sufficient to disturb the mechanism of labor.

Classification. Caldwell and Moloy have suggested a classification of normal pelves on the basis of the configuration of the inlet and the corresponding changes in the midpelvis and lower pelvis as demonstrated by x-ray film examination. This provides an accurate method for visualizing pelvic contour and for predicting the mechanism of labor and its outcome.

The pelvic inlet is divided into a *posterior segment,* behind the line representing the widest transverse diameter, and an *anterior segment* in front of it (Fig. 34-1). The information necessary to classify the inlet includes the length of the transverse diameter and the anteroposterior length of each segment.

The sacrosciatic notch can be visualized by a lateral film: a wide notch means that the sacrum is displaced posteriorly or that the curve is deep, thus increasing the anteroposterior diameter at the midpelvis. A narrow notch indicates a reduced anteroposterior diameter because the sacrum lies farther forward than usual.

Evaluation of the midpelvis and outlet includes measurement of the bispinous diameter and observation of the shape of the spinous processes and the length, width, and curve of the sacrum. The subpubic angle is estimated, and the contour of the arch is noted. The degree of convergence or divergence of the lateral walls (splay) is also of importance; with considerable convergence toward the outlet, delay may be anticipated.

Female pelves are grouped into four pure types—*gynecoid, android, anthropoid,* and *platypelloid*—on the basis of morphology as determined by stereoscopic x-ray film study (Fig 34-3).

GYNECOID PELVIS. Gynecoid pelvis occurs in 40% to 45% of women. The inlet of the typical female pelvis is rounded or slightly oval with both anterior and posterior segments rounded and spacious. The sacrum is well curved and of average length, and the sacrosciatic notch is of medium width. The subpubic angle is wide, and the sides of the arch are curved. The bispinous and bituberous diameters are wide, and the side walls are straight.

ANDROID PELVIS. Android pelvis, which occurs in 25% to 35% of white women and 10% to 15% of black women, is a masculine type of pelvis with a wedge-shaped inlet. The posterior segment is wide and relatively flat, and the anterior segment is narrow with a narrow retropubic angle. The sacrum is straight and inclined forward, and the sacrosciatic notch is narrow. The subpubic angle is narrow, and the bones of the arch are straight. The side walls converge, reducing the bispinous and bituberous diameters. This is the typical *funnel pelvis.*

ANTHROPOID PELVIS. Anthropoid pelvis occurs in 20% to 30% of white women and 40% to 45% of black women. The transverse diameter of the inlet is reduced, making it a long narrow oval with an increase in the lengths of both the anterior and posterior segments. The sacrosciatic notch is wide and shallow, and the sacrum has an average curvature but is long and narrow. The subpubic arch is narrowed. The side walls of the pelvis are straight, but both the bispinous and the bituberous diameters are shortened.

PLATYPELLOID PELVIS. Platypelloid (flat) pelvis occurs in 2% to 5% of white women and only occasionally in black women. The transverse diameter of the inlet is lengthened, and the anteroposterior diameter is reduced. Both segments are rounded but flat, and the retropubic angle is rounded. The sacrum is normal, but the sacrosciatic notch is narrowed. The subpubic angle is wide. The side walls are straight, but the bispinous and bituberous diameters are increased.

MIXED TYPES. Pelves in which the anterior and posterior segments are of different types are frequently encountered. They are named by mentioning first the shape of the posterior segment and then that of the anterior segment.

ESTIMATION OF PELVIC CAPACITY
Clinical pelvimetry

Clinical measurements are less accurate than those obtained by x-ray film examination, but they are adequate for almost all patients. Internal measurements can be made at any period of normal pregnancy and, if carefully performed, will

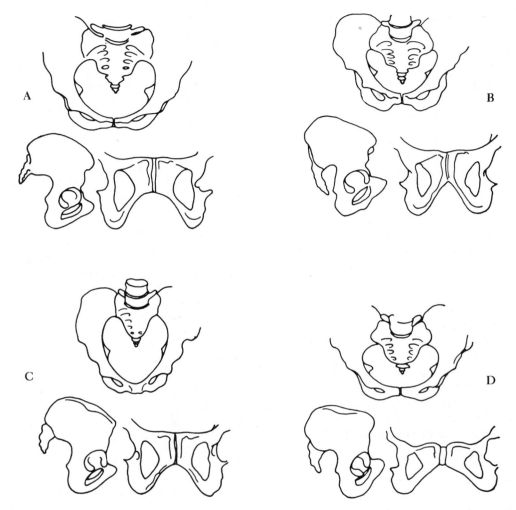

Fig. 34-3 Female pelvis showing normal growth types. **A,** Gynecoid. **B,** Android. **C,** Anthropoid. **D,** Platypelloid.

provide a considerable amount of information concerning the pelvis.

Pelvic inlet. The only diameter of the inlet that can be measured with even reasonable accuracy is the *diagonal conjugate* (Fig. 34-4). From this measurement the length of the conjugata vera can then be estimated.

With the patient in lithotomy position, legs abducted, and the buttocks slightly over the edge of the table, the examiner's index and second fingers are inserted through the introitus until the sacrum is reached. When the tip of the second finger touches the promontory or can be inserted no farther, the entire hand is pivoted forward until the radial surface of the index finger or its metacarpal presses against the apex of the pubic arch. The index finger of the opposite hand marks the point on the examining hand that touches the inferior border of the pubis, and the fingers are withdrawn from the vagina. The depth of insertion can be determined by measuring the distance between the tip

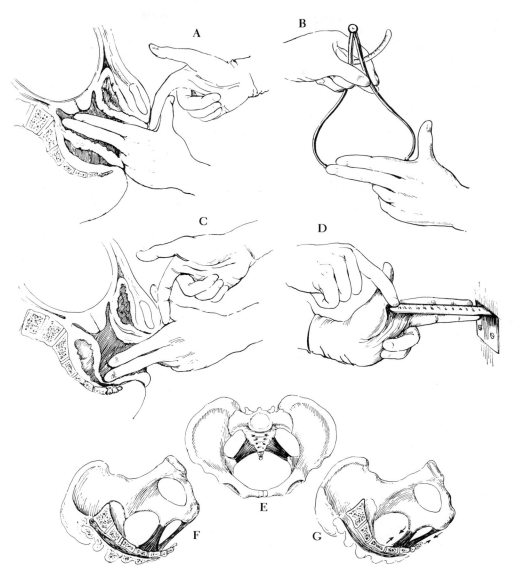

Fig. 34-4 Manual measurement of pelvic inlet and midpelvis. **A,** Estimation of diagonal conjugate diameter. **B** and **D,** Methods for measuring anteroposterior diameters. **C,** Estimation of anteroposterior diameter of outlet. **E** to **G,** Differences in length of sacrospinous and sacrotuberous ligaments estimated by sweeping examining finger along them.

of the second finger and the point at which the symphysis was contacted. If the promontory is touched, this represents the length of the diagonal conjugate (DC). If the promontory is not reached, the measurement should be recorded as the distance the fingers were inserted plus (DC = 10 cm plus), which will indicate that the greatest distance is greater than that noted.

The *conjugata vera* is estimated by subtracting 1.5 to 2 cm from the DC. If the pubic depth is short, 1.5 cm is subtracted; and if long, 2 cm. Physicians cannot even estimate the true conjugate if they fail to touch the promontory, but if the fingers can be inserted at least 11.5 cm, the anteroposterior diameter probably is normal.

The *transverse diameter* cannot be measured, but the width of the inlet can be estimated by attempting to palpate the linea terminalis. If the entire lateral border of the inlet can be touched on each side, the transverse diameter probably is shortened.

Midpelvis. The *bispinous diameter* cannot be measured clinically, but an impression as to the adequacy of the midpelvis can be obtained. The normal ischial spine projects only slightly into the cavity. If the spines are long, sharp, and heavy, the physician should suspect that the midpelvis is small. This is more likely to

be true if the subpubic arch is narrow and if there is considerable resistance as the fingers are swept from one side of the pelvis to the other (Fig. 34-5).

If the sacral curvature is flattened, or if the sacrum is rotated farther anteriorly than usual, the anteroposterior diameter at the midpelvis and the outlet will be reduced. This is associated with shortening of the sacrospinous ligaments, which ordinarily are about 4 cm long. Posterior rotation of the sacrum increases both the anteroposterior diameter and the length of the sacrospinous ligaments (Fig. 34-4). The sacrum, the ischial spines, and the ligaments can be felt most accurately by rectal palpation.

Pelvic outlet. The *angle of the pubic arch* can be estimated by laying a thumb or forefinger along the inner aspect of each ramus with their tips meeting at the symphysis (Fig. 34-6). The normal subpubic angle is at least 85 degrees. The angle probably is reduced if it is impossible to separate the index and second fingers placed side by side beneath the symphysis. The curvature of the pubic rami should also be studied.

The length of the *bituberous diameter* (Fig. 34-7) alone does not determine the adequacy of the outlet because the distance between the tuberosities varies with the depth of the pelvis and the subpubic angle. If the

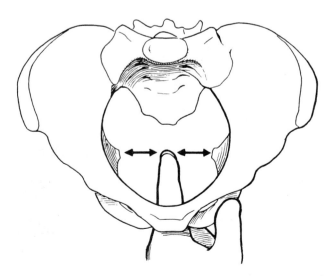

Fig. 34-5 Estimation of bispinous diameter. (From Moloy HC: Evaluation of the pelvis in obstetrics, Philadelphia, 1951, WB Saunders Co.)

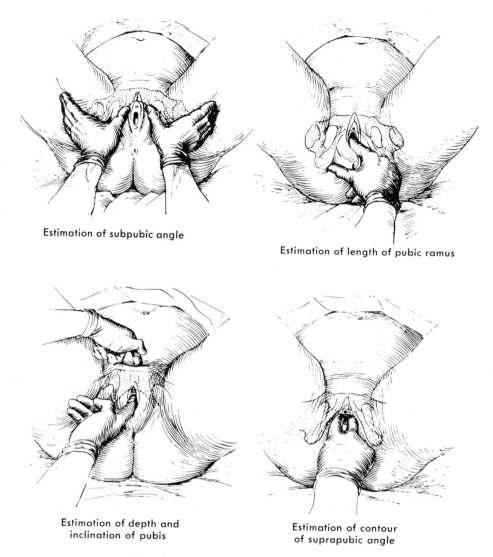

Estimation of subpubic angle

Estimation of length of pubic ramus

Estimation of depth and
inclination of pubis

Estimation of contour
of suprapubic angle

Fig. 34-6 Manual measurement of pelvic outlet.

true pelvis is deep, the bituberous diameter may be of normal length even though the subpubic angle is considerably below normal (Fig. 34-8).

The bituberous diameter can be measured with a suitable pelvimeter, but the measurement is not particularly accurate. The amount of fat overlying the bone varies, and it may be difficult to determine exactly where the most widely separated points on the tuberosities are located. The measurement will be short if taken too far anteriorly. The physician can also estimate the adequacy of the outlet by attempting to insert a clenched fist between the tuberosities. If the average-sized male fist can be placed between the tuberosities, the outlet should be of ample size.

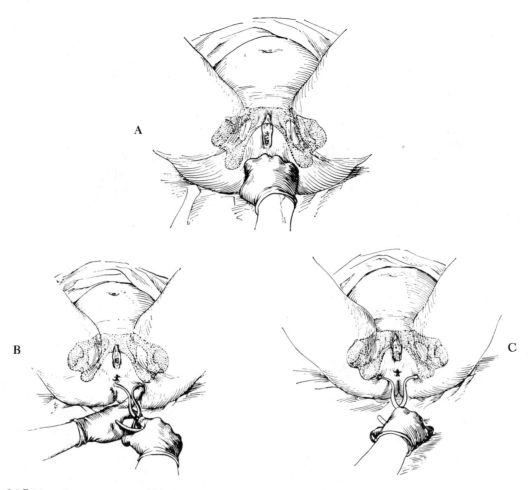

Fig. 34-7 Manual measurement of bituberous diameter. **A,** Bituberous diameter is probably normal if average-sized clenched fist can be inserted between tuberosities. **B** and **C,** Measurement with DeLee pelvimeter taken between inner surfaces of tuberosities as far posteriorly as possible.

The *anteroposterior diameter* of the outlet is obtained in much the same manner as the diagonal conjugate. The fingers are inserted until the sacrococcygeal junction can be palpated, and the distance between the fingertip and the point at which the index finger contacted the lower border of the symphysis is measured.

Although each of these measurements is described individually and the pelvis is divided into the three main areas, variations rarely affect only one portion.

For example, if the sacrum is straight and the bispinous diameter is reduced, the side walls usually converge, and the subpubic angle and the bituberous diameter are reduced.

CONTRACTED PELVIS

Any pelvis that is reduced in size or distorted enough to interfere with normal labor can be considered as contracted.

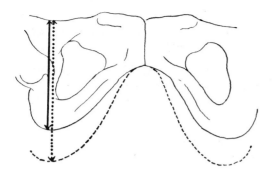

Fig. 34-8 Variations in width of bituberous diameter with differences in length of pubic rami. With deep pelvis, bituberous diameter may be normal even though angle is narrow. (From Caldwell WE and Moloy HC: Am J Obstet Gynecol 26:479, 1933.)

Classification. The classification of Caldwell and Moloy includes the normal growth types, as well as abnormalities caused by disease, injury, or congenital defects.

1. *Normal growth types:* Gynecoid, android, anthropoid, and platypelloid
2. *Abnormal growth types:* Infantile and dwarf
3. *Types caused by disease of the pelvic bones and joints:* Rachitic, congenital, inflammatory, atypical, and traumatic
4. *Types secondary to abnormalities of the spinal column:* Kyphotic, scoliotic, kyphoscoliotic, and spondylolisthetic
5. *Types secondary to abnormalities of the lower extremities:* Femoral luxation, atrophy, or loss of extremity

Other common terms used to describe abnormal pelves are *generally contracted,* which is equivalent to a gynecoid type; *funnel* or *masculine,* which is equivalent to the android type; and *simple flat,* which is equivalent to the platypelloid type. The configuration of each is like that of its normal parent growth type, but the measurements are reduced.

Effect on pregnancy. There usually is no change during pregnancy except in patients with pronounced contractions of the pelvic inlet. Because of the reduced measurements, the fetus is more likely to be carried high, and lightening is less likely to occur.

Effect on labor and delivery. Because lightening may not occur in women with inlet contraction, the head is likely to be unengaged or even above the pelvic brim when labor begins. Abnormal positions and presentations occur more frequently in women with contracted pelves; deflexed attitudes of the head, shoulder presentations, and compound presentations are encountered two to three times as often. The labor is likely to be prolonged and more difficult, and the incidence of cesarean delivery is increased.

Mechanism of labor. Significant alterations in the size or shape of the bony pelvis naturally affect the course of labor, but, because the shapes of many contracted pelves are like those of the normal growth types, the mechanism is often similar to that which occurs normally.

GYNECOID PELVIS. The mechanism in the small gynecoid pelvis is like that in the normal pelvis except that the head must flex at a higher level and mold more to descend through the inlet. Because all the diameters are reduced, resistance to descent is encountered at all levels of the birth canal.

PLATYPELLOID PELVIS. The main alteration in shape and size in the platypelloid pelvis involves the anteroposterior diameter of the inlet; consequently, delay occurs during the first and the early second stages of labor. The head must engage in the transverse diameter; therefore, descent will be impeded if the anteroposterior measurement of the inlet is less than the biparietal diameter of the fetal skull (9.5 cm). The mechanism by which the head enters the small inlet is an exaggeration of the normal. With each contraction, the parietal bones are forced against the sacrum posteriorly and the pubis anteriorly, gradually causing their edges to approximate each other at the sagittal suture while the two parietal plates are elevated in relation to the frontal and occipital bones. This is called *molding* and serves to decrease the biparietal diameter. While the head is being molded, the anterior parietal bone is forced downward behind the pubis where it remains fixed, acting as a fulcrum on which lateral flexion takes place as the uterine contractions force the posterior parietal eminence past the promontory. As this occurs, the sagittal suture gradually approaches the anterior segment of the inlet. As soon as the biparietal diameter has passed the inlet, the head descends through the pelvis in the transverse diameter, usually not rotating until it reaches the pelvic floor.

If the parietal bosses ride above the promontory posteriorly and the pubis anteriorly with the sagittal suture near the center of the pelvis (synclitism), another mechanism may occur. Because the head cannot descend, it extends slightly with each contraction until the relatively short bitemporal diameter is forced into the inlet. This is one of the mechanisms by which deflexed attitudes are produced.

The primary effect of inlet contraction is on engagement, but it may also interfere with normal termination of labor. If much molding, elongation of the head, and caput formation occur, the lowest portion of the head can descend well down into the pelvis before the biparietal diameter passes through the inlet. The anteroposterior pelvic diameters are so short, and the head fits the inlet so tightly that it can neither rotate to an anterior position nor follow the curve of the sacrum anteriorly, so it remains wedged in the transverse position; consequently, descent ceases even though the capacity of the lower pelvis is ample. This is called *transverse arrest* of the head. *Deep* transverse arrest occurs with the lowest portion of the head below station 2, and *high* transverse arrest with the head near the spines.

ANDROID PELVIS. In the android pelvis the anterior segment of the inlet is wedge shaped, and the posterior segment is flattened; consequently, the head often descends in an oblique occipitoposterior position. In this position the relatively narrow frontal portion of the head fits better into the forepelvis than does the broad occipital area. The occiput usually descends to a point just below the ischial spines, but progress may cease at this level if convergence of the bony side walls is pronounced and if forward displacement of the sacrum considerably reduces the posterior sagittal diameter at the midpelvis. If the head can descend farther, the narrow lower pelvis may prevent anterior rotation of the occiput.

ANTHROPOID PELVIS. In the anthropoid pelvis occipitoposterior positions are common; in fact, it may be impossible for the head to enter the pelvic inlet except in an occipitoposterior or occipitoanterior position. Because the transverse diameter is reduced along the entire length of the pelvis, the head usually descends and delivers without rotating. Occasionally, the head fails to enter the inlet, either because of extreme transverse narrowing or because it lies in a transverse or oblique

position rather than an occipitoanterior or occipitoposterior position, which is more favorable in transversely contracted pelves.

Management of labor. For purposes of treatment, abnormal pelves can be divided into those in which the primary contraction is at the inlet and those in which the primary contraction involves the midpelvis and outlet.

Abnormal labor can be anticipated in women with reduced pelvic measurements or those in whom dystocia has occurred during previous labors. An unusual fetal position or a floating head at term should suggest the possibility of inlet disproportion, even though the measurements are normal.

A *sterile vaginal examination* with the patient in lithotomy position should be performed during early labor in any woman whose pelvic measurements are reduced or in whom there is any suggestion of disproportion. The biparietal diameter of the fetal head can be measured accurately by *sonography,* but this examination is of little help when disproportion is suspected.

INLET CONTRACTION. Inlet contraction can be diagnosed if the conjugata vera is 10 cm or less in length or if the diagonal conjugate measures 11.5 cm or less. The outcome of labor is in part dependent on the length of the true conjugate, but other important factors are pelvic configuration, size and position of the infant, and the effectiveness of the uterine contractions. Although it may not always be possible to prognosticate the eventual outcome, inlet contractions are usually relatively easy to manage as compared with the abnormalities involving the lower pelvis.

A reasonably accurate evaluation of whether the head will pass the inlet can be obtained at vaginal examination. Disproportion can be diagnosed if it is impossible to insert the first two fingers between the head in the inlet and the posterior surface of the pubis or if the head is overriding the pubis and cannot be forced into the inlet by downward pressure on the uterine fundus or on the suprapubic portion of the head. If the head can be pushed down to station minus 1 or 0, the size of the inlet probably is adequate. However, the inability to impress the head into the pelvis does not prove that there is significant disproportion. Reevaluation of cervical dilation and descent after a period of electronically monitored active labor should provide the answer for the route of delivery.

An elective cesarean section may be indicated in

women at least 38 weeks pregnant when labor begins if the conjugata vera is 8.5 cm or less with vertex presentation. This is particularly true if the head is floating and does not descend with adequate uterine contractions. Any abnormality in pelvic shape and size justifies cesarean section for breech presentations.

Trial labor. Because most women with mild inlet contractions and some of those with more pronounced deformities will deliver vaginally if the uterine contractions are forceful enough, almost all should be allowed to undergo a trial labor. If the uterine contractions are of normal quality and recur every 3 to 5 minutes, the physician can ordinarily decide within 8 to 10 hours whether vaginal delivery is possible. If the inlet contraction can be overcome, the cervix will dilate, and the head will descend through the superior strait. If this occurs, labor can be permitted to continue with the expectation that it will terminate normally even though it may take longer than usual.

The physician must make certain that descent and engagement actually are occurring. In some instances the lower portion of the head descends into the pelvis, giving the appearance of steady progress in labor. In reality the apparent descent is a result of extreme molding and elongation of the skull and edema of the scalp (caput succedaneum) while the biparietal diameter remains stationary above the plane of the inlet. If there is any question concerning descent, a lateral x-ray film or sonographic study should be done. If descent does not occur, cesarean section can be performed safely after an adequate trial labor.

The membranes usually rupture spontaneously during the course of labor, but, if they do not, they should be ruptured artificially. Intact membranes will sometimes prevent the head from descending, even though the pelvic capacity is perfectly adequate for delivery. The head often descends and delivers after amniotomy. There is some danger of the cord prolapsing if the amniotic sac is perforated while the presenting part is high. If this should occur, it is immediately obvious, and the infant can be delivered alive by cesarean section.

Unfortunately, a good trial labor is not always possible. Many women with contracted pelves also have abnormal labors with irregular, ineffective uterine contractions. Others will begin what appears to be a normal labor, cervical dilation progressing to 6 to 7 cm after which the contractions become irregular and ineffective—an *active phase arrest.* This is a common

response to cephalopelvic disproportion in primigravidas. Oxytocin stimulation is justified if the physician determines that the disproportion is minor. If it seems obvious that vaginal delivery will not occur, even with forceful uterine contractions, cesarean section should be performed. If the disproportion is insurmountable, the uterus can rupture.

Sedatives may be administered if the labor is normal. If the labor is abnormal, an intrauterine pressure catheter should be used, and the uterine activity improved with intravenous Pitocin. The patient should be kept comfortable with sedation and/or an epidural anesthetic. Orificial examinations should be kept at a minimum to reduce the chance of infection; descent can be followed by palpating the anterior shoulder and measuring its distance above the pubis.

MIDPELVIC AND OUTLET CONTRACTION. There is no reliable method for evaluating the adequacy of the lower pelvis, and a trial labor is much less satisfactory than with inlet contractions. Sterile vaginal examination should be performed early in the course of labor; if the head has already reached the level of the spines and can be depressed farther, it probably will continue to descend and will deliver unless the outlet is too small. On the other hand, if the head is high, in a posterior position, and cannot be depressed past the long spines and the anteriorly projecting sacrum, the outlook is less favorable. Cesarean section is always preferable to a traumatic forceps extraction.

If the head descends beyond station plus 2, vaginal delivery usually is possible. If the attempt at delivery is unsuccessful or if it appears that extraction will be traumatic, cesarean section should be performed.

Complications. Infant mortality and morbidity should not increase if the fetus is monitored electronically during labor and if a traumatic vaginal delivery is avoided. Injury to the brachial plexus may occur during attempts to overcome shoulder dystocia.

SUGGESTED READING

Caldwell WE and Moloy HC: Anatomical variations in the female pelvis and their effect on labor with a suggested classification, Am J Obstet Gynecol 26:479, 1933.

Caldwell WE and Swenson PC: The use of the roentgen ray in obstetrics. II. The mechanism of labor, Am J Roentgenol 41:719, 1939.

Javert CT and Steele KB: The transverse position and the mechanism of labor, Int Abstr Surg 75:507, 1942.

Kaltreider DF: Pelvic shape and its relation to midplane prognosis, Am J Obstet Gynecol 63:116, 1952.

Moloy HC: Pelvic model manikins to show pelvic shape and to demonstrate labor mechanisms, Am J Obstet Gynecol 48:149, 1944.

Steer CM: Evaluation of the pelvis in obstetrics, Philadelphia, 1959, WB Saunders Co.

Tancer ML and Vandenberg W: Disproportion in the multipara, Obstet Gynecol 14:753, 1959.

35

Russell K. Laros, Jr.

Multifetal pregnancy

Objectives

RATIONALE: An understanding of the physiology of multifetation enables the student to comprehend the abnormalities that may occur during the antepartum and intrapartum periods.

The student should be able to:
A. Describe the process of multifetation.

B. List antepartum complications frequently seen in multiple pregnancies.
C. Demonstrate knowledge of antepartum and intrapartum management of multiple pregnancies.

Pregnancies in which more than one fetus is produced are associated with more complications than are single births.

Types. Twins are either *dizygotic* (double-ovum, or fraternal) or *monozygotic* (single-ovum, or identical). In *dizygotic twins,* two separate ova produced during the same period of ovulation are fertilized by two spermatozoa. The twins need not be of the same sex, and often they do not resemble each other any more than singly born siblings. There are two separate placentas with no communication between the two circulatory systems, although the placentas may be so completely fused that they look like a single structure. The infants are separated from each other by two layers of amnion and two of chorion (Fig. 35-1). About two thirds of all twin pregnancies are dizygotic.

Monozygotic twins occur in about a third of all twin pregnancies. Because both infants develop from a single fertilized ovum, they are always of the same sex and are either almost identical in appearance or are mirror images. In 25% to 30% of monozygotic twins, the two daughter cells separate within 3 to 4 days after fertilization; as a consequence, each twin has its own complete placenta and membranes (Fig. 35-2). Occasionally, the separation into two distinct embryos occurs 7 to 13 days after fertilization but after the amniotic cavity has formed. In this type, *monoamniotic twins,* there is a single placenta, and both infants develop in a common amniotic cavity. The *monochorionic-diamniotic placenta characteristic of 70% to 75% of monozygotic twin pregnancies* develops when separation occurs between these two

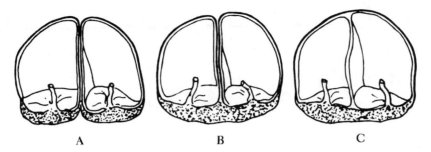

Fig. 35-1 Placenta and membranes in twin pregnancy. **A,** Dizygotic twins with two complete placentas and membranes. **B,** Dizygotic twins with double membranes and fused placenta. **C,** Monozygotic twins with double amniotic cavities enclosed within one chorion.

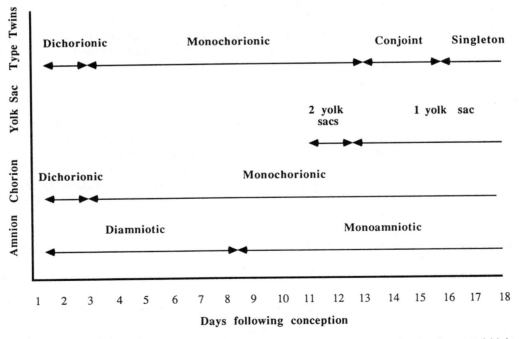

Fig. 35-2 Schematic representation of the events in monozygotic twinning based on the developmental biology of the involved tissues and when separation occurs. Thus separation during the first 3 days produces diamniotic, dichorionic twins; days 3 to 8, diamniotic, monochorionic twins; days 8 to 12, monoamniotic, monochorionic twins; days 12 to 15, conjoint twins. (From Benirschke K and Kim CK: N Engl J Med 288:1276, 1973.)

extremes. If separation occurs on days 13 through 15, conjoint twins will result; thereafter, only a singleton pregnancy is possible. The circulations of the two fetuses communicate with each other through the blood vessels in the shared placenta, and each fetus is enclosed in its own amniotic sac, but both sacs are surrounded by a single chorionic membrane. Thus, in contrast to dizygotic twins, monochorionic-diamniotic fetuses are separated from each other by only two layers of amnion.

Conjoined twins are formed when separation is incomplete. The degree of the deformity is determined by which area of the fetus failed to separate.

More than two fetuses develop by the same mechanisms as do twins, but there are more opportunities for variation in each pregnancy. For example, two of triplets may be monozygotic and the third from a second ovum, all may be fraternal if three ova were fertilized, or all may arise from one ovum. The same possibilities hold true for any number of fetuses.

Superfecundation is a term indicating that two ova produced at the same ovulation were fertilized after two separate acts of coitus. The pregnancies, of course, are always dizygotic. Superfecundation can be suspected if individuals of two or more races are involved; each offspring will have the characteristics of its father superimposed on those of the mother. It can be proved by HLA testing of the children and the putative fathers. The HLA haplotypes are so varied that it is unlikely that they are often duplicated by chance. Thus superfecundation can be substantiated if the haplotypes of each of two suspected fathers match those of each of two twins.

INCIDENCE

The incidence of twins in the United States is currently about 1:80. Factors influencing the frequency of multiple gestations include maternal race, parity and age, heredity, and iatrogenic etiologic factors. In a study of 21 million births, the natural occurrence of multifetal pregnancies was found to be approximately as follows: twins 1:85; triplets, 1:7,630; quadruplets, 1:671,000; and quintuplets, 1:41,600,000. In recent years these frequencies have been altered by both the use of various regimens for ovulation induction and by older average maternal age.

Racial differences in the rate of multiple gestation are striking with a ratio of 1:74 in black women and 1:92 in whites. Comparable figures for triplets are 1:5,631 and 1:9,828. The highest rate is 1:19 in rural Nigeria, whereas the lowest is 1:125 for Asians. This variation in frequency is seen only in dizygotic twinning with the frequency of monozygosity (1:250) apparently unaffected by race, heredity, or other factors.

The influence of *heredity* is predominantly through the mother. The father has little influence on twinning. Women who themselves are dizygotic twins produce twins at a rate of 17.1/1000 deliveries, whereas the rate for wives of husbands who are dizygotic twins is only 7.9/1000 deliveries. Female siblings of dizygotic twins behave like female twins in this regard, but the male siblings behave like male twins.

The differences in dizygotic twinning probably are related to *differences in gonadotropin production*. The number of ovulations that can be stimulated in experimental animals is determined by the dosage of gonadotropin administered. It is well known that multiple ovulations can occur in women treated with clomiphene and human FSH. The hereditary factor in twinning may be that gonadotropin production is higher in women who produce dizygotic twins than in those who produce only singletons.

Both *maternal age and parity* influence the rate of multiple pregnancy. In a Swedish study, twins were delivered by 1.27% of women having their first pregnancy as compared with 2.67% of women who were gravida 4 or higher. A similar study in Canada confirmed the effect of age and parity but also showed a seasonal variation in dizygotic twinning with the highest rate associated with October conceptions.

Infertility therapy has had a profound effect on

the frequency of multiple gestations and also has provided new data on the frequency of the spontaneous loss of one or more members of a multiple gestation. Clomiphene therapy, in vitro fertilization, human postmenopausal gonadotropin yield multiple gestation rate of 1:8, 1:5, and 1:3, respectively.

All of the these frequencies relate to delivery rather than conception. Although the increased use of ultrasound has suggested a loss rate as high as 78%, this figure is undoubtedly too high; a more realistic figure based on prospective evaluation of a large number of viable pregnancies suggests a frequency of 21%.

Sex ratios. The proportion of male to female fetuses in multifetal pregnancy is less than in single births. The discrepancy is exaggerated as the number of fetuses increases: 50.85% of twin fetuses are male as compared with only 46.48% of quadruplets.

FETAL DEVELOPMENT

Each twin at birth is usually smaller than a single infant of the same gestational age, but the combined weights of the babies are likely to be much more. More than 50% of individual twins weigh less than 2500 g.

Intrauterine growth retardation (IUGR) is more common in multiple pregnancies and can be either concordant (fetuses affected equally) or discordant (disparity between the fetuses). Serial ultrasound is essential to early diagnosis and should be performed at about 28 and 34 weeks of gestation. The causes for concordant IUGR are the same as for singletons (see Chapter 32). Discordant IUGR is a difference in weight of ≥25% ([weight of larger − weight of smaller] ÷ weight of larger). It is important to calculate weight and not rely on biparietal measurements alone. When discordant IUGR is present, the perinatal mortality is increased 2.5-fold and is of greatest concern in monochorionic twins where twin-twin transfusion may be present. Careful placental evaluation shows vascular anastamoses in the majority of monochorionic twins. Most commonly these are artery-to-artery but venous-to-venous and arterial-to-venous anastomoses are also observed. These anastomoses are of practical significance at the time of delivery, as the second twin may exsanguinate if a vasa previa of the first twin ruptures or if the cord of the first twin is not clamped.

Large anastomoses can lead to significant shifts of blood between fetuses that produce the classical *transfusion syndrome*—the small (donor) twin is anemic and has a pale placenta and oligohydramnios, whereas the larger (recipient) is plethoric and has a large placenta and hydramnios. When one dies, a sudden shift of fluid may lead to the death of the other. Rare cases of disseminated intravascular coagulation have been described after the death of one twin. The mechanism postulated is that thromboplastins from the dead twin are slowly infused into the survivor. When the transfusion syndrome is present, the perinatal mortality rate has been reported to be as high as 70%.

In some instances one of the twins fails to develop and is deformed. One may die early and become compressed while the other grows normally. This is called *fetus papyraceus* (Fig. 35-3).

Malformations occur twice as often in twins as in singletons. Anomalies are usually discordant, even in monozygotic twins. Cleft lip and palate show a 40% concordance in monozygotic twins and 6% in dizygotic twins. The rate of concordance from Down's syndrome is similarly 84.6% and 2.5%.

The *stuck twin* occurs with diamniotic-monochorionic twins where one resides in a sac with markedly diminished fluid and appears stuck to the uterine wall. Often the membrane between sacs is very difficult to see; however, the other twin is really in a large, hydramniotic sac. The position of the stuck twin does not change with alterations in the mother's position. This is really a variant of the transfusion syndrome appearing in the second trimester and is associated with very high perinatal mortality.

In the past, multiple gestations have been thought to be a cause of hydramnios. Although recent series substantiate the increased incidence of hydramnios in twin gestations, virtually every case of hydramnios was associated with a fetal anomaly.

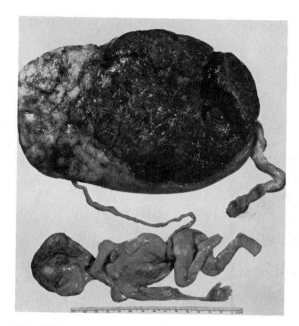

Fig. 35-3 Fetus papyraceus. Infarcted nonfunctioning placenta to which degenerated is attached can be seen at left. Other infant was normal.

CLINICAL COURSE

Nausea and vomiting may be more severe and persistent than in single-fetus pregnancies. Women with multifetal pregnancies are more uncomfortable because of the large uterus, and discomfort increases with each additional fetus. *Varicosities, backache, pelvic pressure, hemorrhoids, edema,* and *difficulty in breathing* occur frequently.

Pregnancy-induced hypertension occurs in approximately 23% of multiple pregnancies and occurs at an earlier gestational age than in singleton pregnancies. Diagnosis and treatment are discussed in Chapter 26. *Renal function* can be reduced significantly if the uterus is large enough to compress the ureters; renal function returns to normal after delivery. *Anemia* can be prevented by administration of supplemental iron (60 to 80 mg/day) and folic acid (1 mg/day). Increased folate meets needs created by the increased DNA synthesis required for growth of the multiple gestation and the additional iron facilitates the red

cell mass and plasma volume expansion that occurs.

Premature labor occurs in more than 50% of twin and 75% of triplet pregnancies and is the major cause of the increased perinatal mortality observed in multiple pregnancies. The role of bed rest after 26 weeks of pregnancy remains controversial. Although several studies show a reduction in prematurity and perinatal mortality, others show either no benefit or an increase in prematurity when women with twin pregnancies were placed at bed rest in the hospital during the third trimester. The prophylactic use of beta-mimetic agents, progesterone, and cerclage have been shown to be of no benefit.

The *duration of labor* usually is normal. *Uterine dysfunction* may occur if the uterus is greatly overdistended. For the same reason *postpartum blood loss is often excessive.* Cephalopelvic disproportion is seldom encountered because each baby is relatively small.

The *position* of the infants is variable. Both heads may present, or one presentation may be a vertex and the other a breech. Occasionally, both present as breeches, or one may lie longitudinally and the other transversely. Abnormal position, particularly of the second twin, occurs more often than in single pregnancies (Fig. 35-4).

Monoamniotic twins present a special problem because of the risk of cord entanglement. The overall perinatal mortality is 50%, with mortality most commonly occurring in the last 6 to 8 weeks of gestation. The diagnosis should be suspected when a membrane separating the two sacs cannot be defined after careful sonographic evaluation. Sonographic demonstration of a confluence of umbilical cords is diagnostic. If a conglomeration cannot be seen, the diagnosis should be confirmed by amniography at 34 weeks. It is accomplished by injecting 20 ml of a water-soluble contrast medium such as Hypaque-M 75%. At the same time a specimen of amniotic fluid should be analyzed for demonstration of fetal lung maturity. If the diagnosis is confirmed and the lungs are mature, delivery is indicated. If the lungs are not mature, beta-methasone is administered, and delivery is carried out 48 hours later.

DIAGNOSIS

The diagnosis should be suspected if the uterus seems larger than it should for the calculated period of

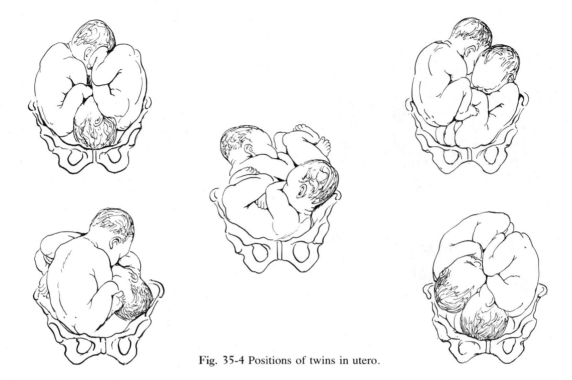

Fig. 35-4 Positions of twins in utero.

gestation, in the presence of an excessive amount of fluid, or if a profusion of small parts or more than one head or more than two fetal poles can be felt (Fig. 35-5). Unfortunately, multifetal pregnancy is often overlooked and, in as many as 12% of cases, is not diagnosed until late in pregnancy or after the first baby has been delivered.

The circumference of the abdomen at the umbilicus usually measures less than 100 cm in normal women at term; with multifetal pregnancy, it is usually larger. If two separate sets of fetal heart sounds that are widely separated and of different rates when counted simultaneously are heard, the diagnosis is certain.

Multifetal pregnancy can be diagnosed by *sonography* before the twelfth week if more than one gestational sac can be demonstrated and when the fetal skulls can be outlined. An ultrasound examination should be ordered whenever twin pregnancy is suspected and whenever pregnancy occurs after ovulation induction. It is preferable to x-ray film examination for confirming a clinical impression of multifetal preg-

nancy. Unless the entire abdomen is scanned, however, the additional fetus(es) may be missed. This will permit the physician to anticipate problems that may arise during labor or delivery.

Concentrations of *chorionic gonadotropin, alpha-fetoprotein,* and *placental lactogen (chorionic somatomammotropin)* in maternal plasma are higher with twins than with a single fetus. These tests are not diagnostic of multifetal pregnancy.

All the evidences of twin pregnancy are exaggerated when three or more infants develop. An exact count can be made only by x-ray film examination or sonography.

MANAGEMENT

Most women with multifetal pregnancy will be more comfortable with a maternity garment to support the large abdomen. Cervical effacement occurs earlier than with a single pregnancy, and, because labor usually begins before term, women with multifetal pregnancies should not travel during the last trimester.

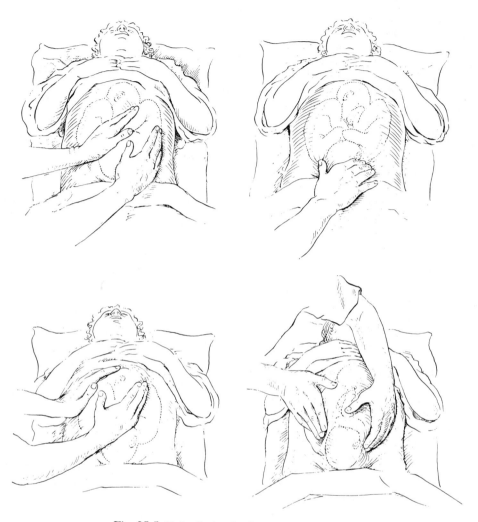

Fig. 35-5 Abdominal palpation of twin pregnancy.

Labor and delivery. Compatible blood should be available to use if bleeding following delivery is excessive, and an intravenous infusion should be started through an 18-gauge needle when labor is well established. Twin pregnancy has little effect on the length of labor in either primigravidas or multiparas, but dysfunctional labor occurs more often than with single pregnancies. Artificial rupture of the presenting sac to reduce distension will generally improve labor.

If labor begins weeks before term, sedation must be used with caution; when the pregnancy has progressed to 37 weeks or more, analgesic drugs ought not to harm the infants. However, *regional nerve block* is usually preferable.

The labor and delivery should be managed by an obstetrician who is experienced in the delivery of twins and who is capable of performing the operative maneuvers required for the delivery of both fetuses. If such a person is not available, most patients with twins should be transferred to a perinatal center for delivery, unless the fetuses are so immature that they have little chance of surviving. If there is no facility in the area, *cesarean section* is more appropriate than vaginal delivery if the fetuses are mature enough to survive.

Cesarean section should also be used more often for the delivery of premature twins, whenever breech or transverse presentations are diagnosed in one or both fetuses, when the second infant is considerably larger than the first, and for other complications such as premature rupture of the membranes when labor cannot be induced, dysfunctional labor that does not improve after amniotomy and the cautious administration of oxytocin, fetal distress during labor, prolapsed cord, and placenta previa or abruptio placentae or when delivery is necessary because of medical complications.

Vaginal delivery is appropriate when labor starts so early that the fetuses have little chance of surviving. It also may be selected for the delivery of mature infants when both are in vertex positions, if there are no contraindications to vaginal delivery, and if an experienced obstetrician, a capable anesthesiologist or anesthetist, and two attendants who are able to resuscitate depressed infants can be present at delivery.

Because the second twin may ultimately present as a breech, a decision as to the capacity of the maternal pelvis for delivery of a breech should be made before labor begins or during its early stages. Thus CT pelvimetry should be performed after 37 weeks of gestation and, if the inlet anterior-posterior and transverse diameters are greater than or equal to 11 and 12 cm, respectively, and the transverse of the midpelvis is at least 10 cm, the patient is a candidate for vaginal breech delivery. CT pelvimetry is preferred to standard radiologic techniques because of the precision of the measurements and a 95% reduction in the radiation to which the fetus is exposed.

The first child may be allowed to deliver spontaneously, or a low forceps delivery can be performed. The cord should be cut between two hemostats to prevent exsanguination of the second of monozygotic twins.

The position or even the lie of the second twin may change as the first baby leaves the uterus; consequently, the presenting part of the second infant should be identified soon after the first is delivered so that plans can be made for its delivery. This can be accomplished either by palpation or by ultrasound examination. As a general rule the membranes should be rup-

tured artificially, after which the vertex or breech usually descends into the upper pelvis. One must make sure that the cord did not prolapse after amniotomy. Uterine contractions usually recur when the membranes are ruptured; if they do, spontaneous delivery can be anticipated. If they do not, dilute oxytocin can be administered, or, depending on the conditions, a forceps extraction or breech extraction can be performed by an experienced obstetrician. As an alternative, cesarean section may be indicated for those who have had little experience in operative vaginal delivery or in cases where pelvic measurements do not meet the criteria for vaginal delivery of the breech. The fetal heart must be monitored constantly until the infant is delivered. The baby should be delivered immediately if bleeding suggesting placental separation occurs or for abnormal fetal heart rate patterns.

A prolonged wait after the delivery of the first fetus subjects the second to an undue hazard. The placenta may separate as the uterine muscle contracts, and cord prolapse is favored by the fact that the second presenting part is usually high or because the infant lies transversely. The results are best when the second twin is delivered within 10 to 15 minutes of the first.

If the second infant is lying transversely after the first delivers, a decision must be made promptly as to how it can be delivered with the least chance of injury. If the back is directed toward the fundus of the uterus, an experienced obstetrician can usually deliver it by bringing the legs through the cervix and extracting it as a breech *(version and extraction)*. The major problems are those encountered in any breech extraction. If the back lies over the cervix with the extremities in the fundus, version is difficult to perform, and the fetus is likely to be injured. Under these conditions cesarean delivery usually is preferred. Cesarean section may also be performed if the position of the second twin changes from vertex to breech or transverse during the delivery of the first infant and the operator has had little experience in delivering babies in these positions.

In cases in which the second twin presenting as a breech but the pelvis is inadequate or in which the operator is inexperienced in breech delivery, an alternative to cesarean section is to attempt external version after the first twin is delivered. In many instances either a transverse lie or breech can be converted to a vertex presentation. However, the version must be carried out promptly after delivery of the first twin to take advantage of the 3 to 5 minutes of profound uterine relaxation that usually occurs.

Regional anesthesia is preferable to inhalation anesthesia for vaginal twin delivery because pregnancy often terminates prematurely and because the distended uterus tends to contract poorly. Pudendal block alone or supplemented by nitrous oxide–oxygen during the delivery may be adequate. Intrauterine manipulation for delivery of the second twin usually cannot be performed with pudendal block or conduction anesthesia alone; hence deep inhalation anesthesia is necessary.

Occasionally, the placenta of the first infant will deliver while the second twin is still in the uterus, but more often both placentas are extruded simultaneously after both babies have been born. If the placenta cannot be expressed by the usual maneuvers, it must be removed manually. The placenta may separate partially after the first child is born. When this occurs, the second infant must be delivered or it will die of anoxia.

Most triplet and quadruplet pregnancies should be terminated by cesarean section in a perinatal center.

Complications. *Prolapsed cord* occurs more often than in single pregnancies and is more likely to complicate the delivery of the second infant than the first.

Collision between two fetal poles attempting to enter the inlet simultaneously may delay descent. Cesarean section usually is preferable to trying to manipulate the fetuses into more favorable positions. If the first infant presents as a breech and the second as a vertex, *the heads may lock at the inlet* after the body of the presenting twin has been delivered.

Locking occurs most commonly with premature twins whose heads are both small enough to allow simultaneous entry into the pelvis. In a large series of twin pregnancies, the incidence of locking was 1:813 overall; it was 1:88 when the presentations were breech-vertex. Overall the mortality was 50%, with an 80% mortality rate associated with the first twin. The problem can be prevented by early cesarean section in cases of premature twins in the breech-vertex presentation.

Prognosis. The perinatal mortality, 10 to 15%, is considerably higher than that for single births. The principal causes of death are the complications of prematurity, infection, prolapsed cord, anoxia during delivery of the aftercoming head,

and injury. The mortality for monozygotic twins is two to three times that for dizygotic.

Many of the complications can be prevented if the labor and delivery are managed by an experienced obstetrician in a perinatal center. This is particularly true if vaginal delivery is planned. The mortality for the second twin is higher than that for the first because it may assume an abnormal position, making vaginal delivery difficult; and because it may be larger than the first baby, the size may impede its delivery. The number of deaths can be reduced if the second infant is delivered promptly by forceps or breech extraction or by version and extraction, if the obstetrician has been trained to perform these operations, or by cesarean section if that seems to be more appropriate.

The maternal risk is somewhat increased because of the relatively high incidence of postpartum hemorrhage. Postpartum hemorrhage from uterine atony is more common after delivery of a multiple gestation. Because of this, venous access with a large-bore cannula is mandatory. If significant atony occurs, it should be treated promptly with oxytocin by rapid intravenous infusion in a dose of 50 to 100 mU/min. If this is unsuccessful, 0.2 mg of methylergonovine should be given intravenously. An effective alternative is 250 to 500 μg IM of prostaglandin $F_{2\alpha}$-15 methyl.

SUGGESTED READING

Acker D, Lieberman M, Holbrook RH, James O, Phillippe M, and Edlin KC: Delivery of the second twin, Obstet Gynecol 59:710, 1982.

Barrett JM, Staggs SM, Van Hooydonk JE, Growdon JH, Killam AP, and Boehm FH: The effect of type of delivery upon neonatal outcome in premature twins, Am J Obstet Gynecol 143:360, 1982.

Benirschke K and Kim CK: Multiple pregnancy, N Engl J Med 288:1276, 1973.

Cherouny PH, Hoskins IA, Johnson TRB, and Niebyl JR: Multiple pregnancy with late death of one fetus, Obstet Gynecol 74:318, 1989.

Chervenak FA, Johnson RE, Berkowitz RL, and Hobbins JC: Intrapartum version of the second twin, Obstet Gynecol 62:160, 1983.

Chervaenak FA, Johnson RE, Berkowitz RL, Grannum P, and Hobbins JC: Is routine cesarean section necessary for vertex-breech and vertex-transverse twin gestations? Am J Obstet Gynecol 148:1, 1984.

Cohen M, Kohl SG, and Rosenthal AH: Fetal interlocking complicating twin gestation, Am J Obstet Gynecol 91:407, 1965.

Crane JP, Tomich PG, and Kopta M: Ultrasonic growth patterns in normal and discordant twins, Obstet Gynecol 55:678, 1980.

Elwood JM: Maternal and environmental factors affecting twin births in Canadian cities, Br J Obstet Gynaecol 85:351, 1978.

Erkkola R, Ala-Mello S, Piiroinen O, Kero P, and Sillanpaa M: Growth discordancy in twin pregnancies: a risk factor not detected by measurement of biparietal diameter, Obstet Gynecol 66:203, 1985.

Farooqui JH, Grossman JH, and Shannon RA: A review of twin pregnancy and perinatal mortality, Obstet Gynecol Surv 28:144, 1973.

Gilstrap LC, Hauth JC, Hankin GDV, and Beck A: Twins: prophylactic hospitalization and ward rest at early gestational age, Obstet Gynecol 69:578, 1987.

Gummerus M and Halonen O: Prophylactic long-term oral tocolysis of multiple pregnancies, Br J Obstet Gynaecol 94:249, 1987.

Hanna JH and Hill JM: Single intrauterine fetal demise in multiple gestation, Obstet Gynecol 63:126, 1984.

Hashimoto B, Callen PW, Filly RA, and Laros, RK: Ultrasound evaluation of polyhydramnios and twin pregnancy, Am J Obstet Gynecol 154:1069, 1986.

Itzkowicz D: A survey of 59 triplet pregnancies, Br J Obstet Gynaecol 86:23, 1979.

Jeffries RL, Bowes WA, and DeLaney JJ: Role of bedrest in twin gestation, Obstet Gynecol 43:822, 1983.

Kovacs BW, Kirschbaum TH, and Paul R: Twin gestation: I. Antenatal care and complications, Obstet Gynecol 74:313, 1989.

Landy HJ, Weiner S, Corson SL, Batzer FR, and Bolognese RJ: The 'vanishing twin': ultrasonographic assessment of fetal disappearance in the first trimester, Am J Obstet Gynecol 155:14, 1986.

Laros RK and Dattel BJ: Management of twin pregnancy: the vaginal route is still safe, Am J Obstet Gynecol 158:1330, 1988.

McCarthy BJ, Sachs BP, Layde PM, Burton A, Terry JS, and Rochat R: The epidemiology of neonatal death in twins, Am J Obstet Gynecol 141:252, 1981.

O'Connor MC, Arias E, Royston JP, and Dalrymple IJ: The merits of special antenatal care for twin pregnancies, Br J Obstet Gynaecol 88:222, 1981.

O'Connor MC, Murphy H, and Dalrymple IJ: Double blind trial of ritodrine and placebo in twin pregnancies, Br J Obstet Gynaecol 86:706, 1979.

Olofsson P and Rydhstrom H: Twin delivery: how should the second twin be delivered? Am J Obstet Gynecol 153:479, 1985.

Rabinovici J, Barkai G, Reichman B, Serr DM, and Mashlach S: Randomized management of the second nonvertex twin: vaginal delivery or cesarean section, Am J Obstet Gynecol 156:52, 1987.

Sakala EP: Obstetric management of conjoint twins, Obstet Gynecol 67:21s, 1986.

Saunders MC, Dick JS, Brown IM, McPherson K, and Chalmers I: The effects of hospital admission for bed rest on the duration of twin pregnancy: a randomized trial, Lancet 2:793, 1985.

Szymonowicz W, Preston H, and Yu VY: The surviving monozygotic twin, Arch Dis Child 61:454, 1986.

Yarkoni S, Reece EA, Holford T, O'Connor TZ, and Hobbins JC: Estimated fetal weights in the evaluation of growth in twin gestations: a prospective longitudinal study, Obstet Gynecol 69:636, 1987.

36

Russell K. Laros, Jr.

Breech delivery

Objectives

RATIONALE: Although breech presentation occurs in only 3% to 5% of deliveries, an understanding of the cause, diagnosis, and method of delivery is important.

The student should be able to:

A. List etiologic factors in breech presentation.

B. Explain the techniques of diagnosis.

C. Discuss the role of external version.

D. Demonstrate knowledge of the principles of breech delivery.

Breech positions, which occur in about 3% to 5% of all singleton deliveries, are longitudinal lies in which the buttocks alone or the buttocks and some portion of one or both lower extremities descend through the birth canal first. The sacrum is the guiding point; therefore the possible positions in the maternal pelvis are sacroanterior (SA), left and right sacroanterior (LSA-RSA), left and right sacrotransverse (LST-RST), left and right sacroposterior (LSP-RSP), and direct sacroposterior (SP) (Fig. 36-1).

VARIETIES OF FETAL ATTITUDE
(Fig. 36-2)

In the *frank breech*, which is present in about two thirds of all breech deliveries of babies weighing more than 2500 g, the infant's hips are flexed on the abdomen, and the knees are extended so that the feet lie in front of the face or the head. In a *complete breech*, the attitude is one of complete flexion; both the hips and knees are flexed, and the feet present with the buttocks. With the less common *incomplete breech* attitudes, one foot *(single footling)* or both feet *(double footling)* descend through the cervix ahead of the buttocks because the hips and knees are partially extended. In the other type of incomplete breech, one or both *knees present* because of partial or complete extension of the hips, whereas the knees remain flexed.

ETIOLOGIC FACTORS

Premature labor and delivery are the most common cause of breech delivery. Before week 32 of

463

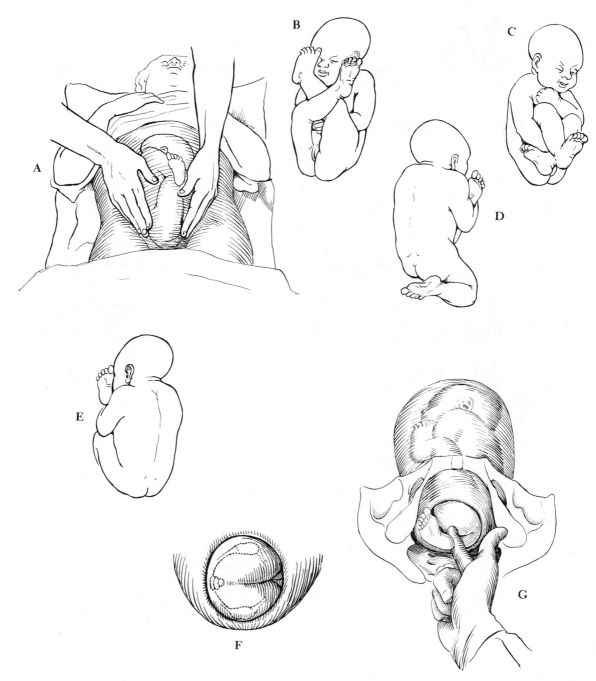

Fig. 36-1 Breech positions. **A,** Right sacrotransverse. **B,** Left sacroposterior. **C,** Right sacroposterior. **D,** Right sacroanterior. **E,** Left sacroanterior. **F,** Right sacrotransverse. **G,** Vaginal palpation of left sacrotransverse.

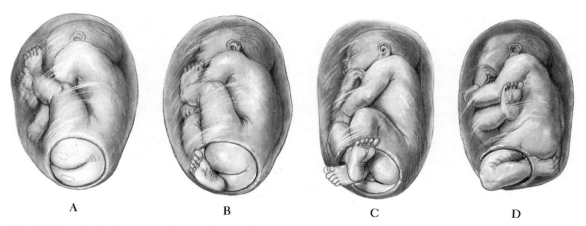

Fig. 36-2 Fetal attitudes in breech positions. **A,** Frank breech. **B,** Incomplete breech. **C,** Complete breech. **D,** Knee presentation.

gestation, the fetus can move freely within the uterus because the volume of amniotic fluid is relatively greater than it will be later in pregnancy. Breech presentation is found in approximately 41% of fetuses with birth weights of 500 to 999 g, 15% weighing 1500 to 1999 g, 5% weighing 2500 to 2999 g, and 2% weighing 3000 g or more.

The capacity of the fundal area of the uterus is decreased when the placenta is implanted in one of the cornua. With cornual implantation the head may fit better in the fundus than will the larger mass of buttocks, feet, and legs. Cornual placental implantations are present in 73% of women with breech presentations at or near term but in only 5% of those with cephalic presentations. When breech positions recur in successive pregnancies, congenital uterine anomalies such as bicornuate uterus may be a cause. Other factors include multiparity, hydramnios, multifetal pregnancy, fetal anomalies, and low implantation of the placenta. Because the incidence of congenital anomalies is threefold higher in the term breech, careful ultrasound evaluation is an important part of management.

Fetal motion plays an important part in decreas-ing the rate of occurrence of breech positions as pregnancy advances. When the knees are extended, the ability of the fetus to make crawling motions is eliminated, and conversion does not occur. Extension of the knees may account for the high percentage of frank breech positions in late pregnancy, most of those with flexed knees having converted to vertex. A small dead fetus, however, can be changed from breech to vertex position by uterine activity.

PROGNOSIS

Breech presentations should not influence *maternal mortality*, but *morbidity* is likely to be increased. Cervical and vaginal lacerations and even uterine rupture may occur during vaginal delivery, particularly when breech extraction is performed. These, of course, increase blood loss and predispose to infection. *Hemorrhage* may also be caused by uterine atony from deep anesthesia required for breech extraction. Complications, particularly infection and those related to blood loss, are increased severalfold after *cesarean delivery*.

The gross uncorrected *perinatal mortality* may be as high as 20% to 30%, but for the normal fetus this should be reducible to a rate comparable to that for vertex presentation at a comparable gestational age. The most important causes of perinatal mortality are associated with vaginal delivery and include the following:

1. *Anoxia* resulting from delay in delivery of the aftercoming head and from prolapsed cord, which occurs about ten times more often than in vertex positions.
2. *Injuries,* the most serious of which are those that cause intracranial hemorrhage, fractures of the spine associated with spinal cord injury, and rupture of the liver, spleen, and adrenals
3. *Complications of prematurity*
4. *Developmental anomalies,* which are present two to three times more often than with vertex presentations

DIAGNOSIS

The diagnosis of breech position can usually be made by abdominal examination alone (Fig. 36-1), but it may be necessary to perform other studies to confirm the impression obtained by palpation.

Abdominal examination. The firm, round, ballottable head can be felt in the fundus of the uterus and the irregular, softer breech over the pelvic inlet. A cephalic prominence cannot be palpated above the pubis. The fetal heart is usually best heard on the side of the abdomen toward which the back is directed and at or above the level of the umbilicus.

Vaginal examination. If the cervix is partly dilated, the physician can feel the triangular sacrum and coccyx with an ischial tuberosity on either side (Fig. 36-1). One or both feet can be palpated in the incomplete or complete breech attitudes. If the membranes are ruptured, fresh meconium may be present on the examining finger.

The most frequent error is mistaking the breech for a face or a shoulder. If the face is presenting, the bony orbits can be outlined, the sucking action of the mouth can be recognized, and there is no fresh meconium. With a shoulder presentation, the scapula and ribs can be identified.

Ultrasound. Ultrasound is as accurate as is x-ray film for determining the exact position of the feet and legs and for identifying fetal anomalies. If the presentation is in doubt as term approaches, an ultrasonographic study is certainly in order.

MECHANISM OF LABOR (Fig. 36-3)

The cervix dilates at the usual rate in both primigravidas and multiparas if the uterine contractions are normal, but the presenting part may remain at or just above the level of the ischial spines until cervical dilation is complete, after which it descends. The fact that the breech remains high during the first stage does not indicate fetopelvic disproportion, as does failure of the presenting vertex to descend. The diameters of the breech are less than those of the head; consequently, size alone is usually not a factor in the presenting part's remaining high.

The presenting part usually enters the inlet with its widest diameter, the bitrochanteric, in the transverse or in one of the oblique diameters of the pelvis. It descends in this diameter until the anterior hip meets the resistance of the muscular pelvic floor and the bony pelvis. As descent continues, the increasing pressure of the anterior hip against the levator sling causes the hip to rotate 45 degrees anteriorly to a position beneath the pubic arch; the opposite hip is now directed toward the maternal sacrum, and the infant's spine is directed toward the lateral pelvic wall. With further descent, the anterior hip becomes visible in the introitus, at which time it impinges beneath the symphysis and remains relatively stationary while the posterior hip is forced upward and anteriorly over the perineum as the infant's spine bends laterally. After the posterior hip clears the perineum, it falls backward, permitting the expulsion of the anterior hip from the vagina.

With a few more contractions, the shoulders enter the inlet in the same oblique diameter that was occupied by the bitrochanteric diameter or in the transverse. They too descend until the anterior shoulder strikes the levator sling and rotates 45 degrees or more to a position beneath the pubic arch with the axilla visible; the posterior shoulder now lies in the hollow of the sacrum. The continuing uterine contractions force the posterior shoulder anteriorly over the perineum until it and the arm are delivered, after which it falls backward, permitting the anterior shoulder and arm to emerge from beneath the symphysis.

The head is usually incompletely flexed and enters

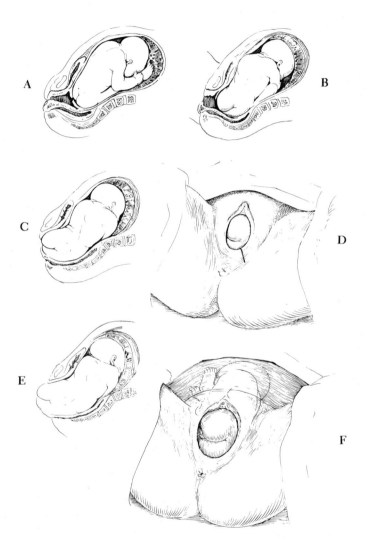

Fig. 36-3 Mechanism of breech labor. **A,** Breech enters inlet in oblique diameter. **B,** Rotation to sacrum left. **C** and **D,** Anterior hip appears in introitus. **E** and **F,** Both hips distending introitus.

the inlet with its long axis in either the transverse or in an oblique diameter, with the occiput directed obliquely anteriorly. The head descends, and the occiput is rotated anteriorly until the neck impinges beneath the pubis, after which the head becomes progressively more flexed as it descends; as a result the chin, nose, forehead, vertex, and occiput are forced over the perineum.

Variations. The previous description applies to most breech deliveries in women with normal pelves. Variations can be expected if the pelvis is small or with frank or incomplete varieties.

MANAGEMENT

Breech positions cannot be regarded lightly because, even though the deliveries are managed by experts, the perinatal mortality is greater than when the vertex presents. All breech deliveries should take place in a hospital. Family physicians and house staff should ask for consultation as soon as the position is recognized.

During pregnancy. If the breech can be converted to a vertex by *external version* (Fig. 36-4), the danger to the infant and likelihood of cesarean section will be reduced. This maneuver should be attempted after the thirty-fifth week, when most spontaneous versions will already have occurred, but it may also be possible to change the position at a later stage of pregnancy or even during early labor.

Several publications document the feasibility and value of external version at term. Although the reported success rate varies from 50% to 97%, most large series suggest that version succeeds in 75% to 80% of cases. Factors that appear to decrease the success rate include increased gestational age at the time of the procedure, primigravidity, frank breech, anterior placenta, and maternal obesity. Contraindications to attempting external version are placenta previa, a uterine anomaly, undiagnosed vaginal bleeding, oligohydramnios, a nonreactive nonstress test, and intrauterine growth retardation. Relative contraindications include a prior cesarean section, advanced cervical dilation, and a nuchal cord.

Complications are rare and relate to fetal distress, premature rupture of the membranes, and premature labor. Transient bradycardia is seen in 30% to 40% of cases, and prolonged bradycardia requiring immediate cesarean section occurs in <1% of cases. Fetal-maternal hemorrhage has been reported in 6% to 15% of cases, and Rh immune globulin should be given to all Rh-negative women in whom version is attempted.

External version should be done in or near the labor delivery suite. First, an ultrasound examination is done to confirm the fetal position, to locate the placenta, and to look for a nuchal cord. After a reactive fetal heart rate has been documented, an intravenous infusion of 5% dextrose in normal saline is started, and terbutaline or ritodrine is administered to achieve uterine relaxation. Terbutaline can be given either as a bolus of 0.125 mg or an infusion of 5 µg/min; ritodrine is given by infusion at 100 µg/min. The patient is then placed in the moderate Trendelenburg position, and a lubricant or talcum powder is applied to the mother's abdomen. One hand manipulates the head toward the pelvis while the other attempts to mobilize the buttocks in the lower segment and push the breech toward the fundus of the uterus. The head is rotated in the direction that provides the shortest course to the pelvis. The fetal heart must be checked frequently during attempted version because cord entanglement or pressure or anything else interfering with fetal oxygen supply will be reflected in an alteration of cardiac rhythm. If the manipulations produce pain, the physician should desist.

The fetus will usually remain in the vertex position, but some will revert. This is likely to occur when the reason for the breech position is still present.

During labor. The principal responsibility of the obstetrician during late pregnancy and early in labor is to decide whether to deliver the patient vaginally or by cesarean section. The decision is made on the basis of parity, duration of pregnancy, estimated fetal size, pelvic capacity, condition of the cervix, quality of the uterine contractions, station, fetal attitude, and reaction of the patient to her pregnancy and delivery. One of the most important factors in the decision is the experience of the physician who will conduct the delivery.

That cesarean section is not always necessary can be documented by a number of recent reports describing carefully selected patients who have been allowed to

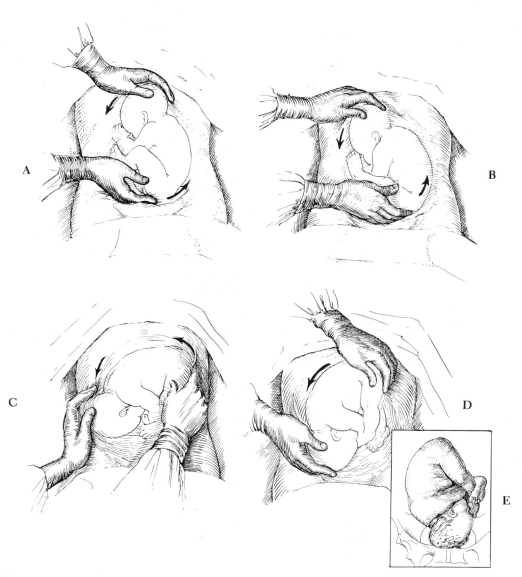

Fig. 36-4 External cephalic version. **A,** Buttocks are dislodged, and head is flexed. **B,** Buttocks are pushed upward and head downward until infant lies in transverse position. **C** and **D,** Version is completed by further manipulation. **E,** Position of fetus after completed version.

deliver vaginally. These studies show no perinatal morbidity or mortality attributable to the route of delivery. However, the protocols have fairly stringent criteria that must be met if labor and vaginal delivery are to be allowed.

An important factor in choosing between vaginal delivery and cesarean section is the experience of the obstetrician. Those who have trained since cesarean section has been used more liberally have had little opportunity to learn the techniques for breech delivery. The possibility of disabling or lethal fetal injury is substantially increased when vaginal delivery is attempted by inexperienced operators.

Vaginal delivery should be considered only if one anticipates a normal labor and delivery. Abdominal and vaginal examinations should be performed soon after labor begins to estimate fetal weight and to determine the amount of cervical effacement and dilation, the status of the membranes, and the pelvic capacity. An ultrasound study to confirm fetal attitude and size is helpful in making the decision.

The fetus should weigh between 2500 and 3800 g. Vaginal delivery for premature breeches weighing less than 1500 g is associated with a higher perinatal morbidity and mortality. Complications include difficulty in delivering the aftercoming head (which is larger than the thorax until week 32 of gestation) through an incompletely dilated cervix as well as the fragility of the very premature infant. At present insufficient data are available to allow a definitive conclusion as to the best route of delivery for infants weighing between 1500 and 2500 g. Oversized babies are likely to be injured by the manipulation necessary for vaginal delivery. Although determining fetal size accurately is difficult, a combination of clinical examination and ultrasound provides the best available information on which to base a management decision.

The pelvis should be of normal size and shape. A trial of labor when the pelvis is thought to be small or misshapen is not appropriate when the breech is presenting. The body can descend through a pelvis too small to permit the passage of an unmolded aftercoming head. If the head is forcibly extracted, the baby will be injured. If it is allowed to mold and deliver gradually, the infant will die of anoxia.

We obtain CT pelvimetry either before or soon after the onset of labor. This technique provides precise pelvic measurements with radiation dose of only 60 mrad. Our criteria for allowing a trial of labor are pelvic inlet measurements of 12 cm in the transverse and 11 cm in anterior-posterior diameter and a midpelvic transverse measurement of 10 cm. In the past many obstetricians have felt that multiparity—and thus delivery through a "proven pelvis"—confers an element of safety in electing to do a vaginal breech delivery. Data in the literature refute this assumption and indicate that parity has no influence on outcome. Furthermore, the pelvic delivery of a fetus as a vertex does not guarantee that breech delivery will be safe, and thus CT pelvimetry is indicated regardless of a woman's parity.

The most favorable fetal attitude is the frank breech with a well-flexed head. The cord is less likely to prolapse if the cervical opening is plugged by the buttocks alone than it is with the footling varieties. The latter provide many chinks through which a loop of cord can slip. The fetal cervical spine and spinal cord is likely to be damaged during vaginal delivery if the head is extended.

Labor should be progressing at a normal rate by the time the patient enters the hospital. Oxytocin induction of labor is allowed but not stimulation of an abnormal labor.

An obstetrician experienced in breech delivery is essential to a favorable outcome. Cesarean delivery is almost always preferred when the fetus is mature enough to survive if the responsible physician has not had considerable experience with breech delivery.

The membranes should not be ruptured artificially in normal labors because this may permit the cord to prolapse past the irregular presenting part, which occludes the cervix less completely than does the firm, round head.

The fetal heart tones should be recorded constantly by an electronic monitor, as occult or complete prolapse of the cord occurs so frequently. The *passage of meconium* is of no significance during breech labors, but an attempt must be made to determine a cause for abnormal fetal heart tones whenever they are detected.

Delivery. The physician must be certain that the cervix is completely dilated before attempting breech delivery. The buttocks, the body, and even the shoulders can descend through a cervix that is not sufficiently dilated to permit passage of the head. This is particularly true with premature infants whose heads are larger than their shoulders. With a frank breech, the presenting part is smaller than the combined buttocks, feet, and legs of an infant in the complete breech attitude and will pass through a cervical opening much smaller than that required for the complete variety.

SPONTANEOUS DELIVERY. With spontaneous delivery the entire delivery is completed without manipulation by the attendant. This most often occurs with small, premature infants and in multiparas with large pelves and rapid labors.

PARTIAL BREECH EXTRACTION. Partial breech extraction, also known as *assisted breech delivery,* consists of spontaneous, controlled expulsion as far as the umbilicus, after which the shoulders and the head are extracted by the physician. When the breech begins to distend the introitus and about 8 to 10 cm of the presenting part is visible during a contraction, an episiotomy is performed if necessary. If this is done at the proper time, the next few contractions force the buttocks and the abdomen through the introitus, after which the rest of the body is extracted.

Downward traction is applied to the pelvic girdle with the thumbs placed parallel to each other over the sacrum or along the femurs, and the index fingers encircling the iliac crest (Fig. 36-5). Pressure and traction should be on bones rather than soft tissues, particularly the abdomen, to reduce the possibility of injury. Several studies have described a number of soft-tissue injuries, including adrenal hemorrhage, attributable to trauma inflicted during breech delivery.

The body is gradually pulled downward, keeping the back directed anteriorly until the anterior axilla comes into view and the scapula emerges from beneath the pubic arch. Two fingers are introduced beneath the arch to a position along the humerus, and the arm is wiped down over the infant's chest and delivered (Fig. 36-6). The body is then lifted upward, and the posterior arm is delivered in the same manner (Fig. 36-7).

The head can usually be delivered by manual manipulation alone with the Celsus-Wigand-Martin maneuver (Fig. 36-8), by which it can be brought through the inlet in the transverse or oblique diameter and then ro-

tated to the anteroposterior diameter of the lower pelvis and delivered over the perineum by flexion. The head can also be delivered by forceps after it has descended to the pelvic floor and has rotated to an anteroposterior position. This is comparable to low forceps extraction of a presenting head. Forceps should never be used to try to bring the head through the pelvic inlet or through an incompletely dilated cervix.

If the pelvis is small, if the cervix is incompletely dilated, or if the fetus is extracted too rapidly, the arms may be swept upward beside the head *(extended arms).* From there they can be rotated to a position behind the fetal neck *(nuchal arms)* as the body is turned. This complication can usually be prevented by slow deliberate extraction of the body. Both can be corrected by freeing the arms and manipulating them downward across the fetal chest.

At this stage of the delivery the umbilical cord is compressed against the bony pelvis, and the blood flow is cut off. The fetus will become anoxic if it cannot begin to breathe. It is not necessary to deliver the entire head at this time; only the mouth must be exposed. More problems are caused by undue haste and forceful attempts at extraction than by deliberate performance of the required maneuvers.

COMPLETE BREECH EXTRACTION. In complete breech extraction the entire infant is extracted from the birth canal. This is one of the most difficult and potentially traumatic of all the obstetric operations and, even when performed by experts, results in unacceptably high perinatal morbidity and mortality. Cesarean section is preferable in almost every instance.

CESAREAN SECTION. The decision to proceed with vaginal delivery of a breech warrants careful judgment and skillful management of labor and delivery. Although the weight of evidence available indicates that vaginal delivery can be accomplished safely, long-term follow-up studies are not yet available. We believe that the patient must be an active participant in the decision-making process and give a fully informed consent.

Following are the indications for cesarean section for breech presentation:

1. *An estimated fetal weight between 750 and 2500 g*
2. *Suspected fetopelvic disproportion.* The time when the fetus is most likely to be in-

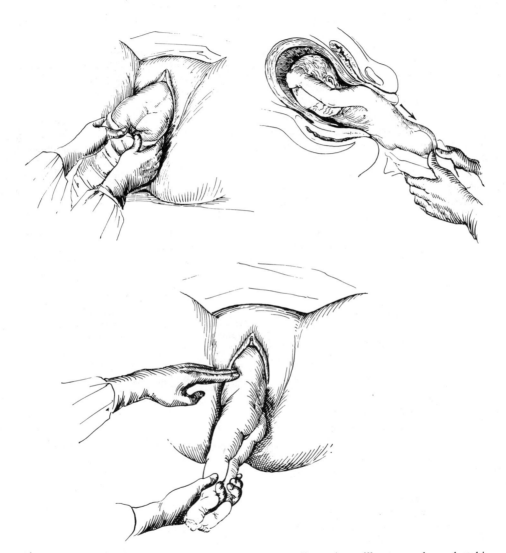

Fig. 36-5 Partial breech extraction. Traction is downward until anterior axilla appears beneath pubic arch.

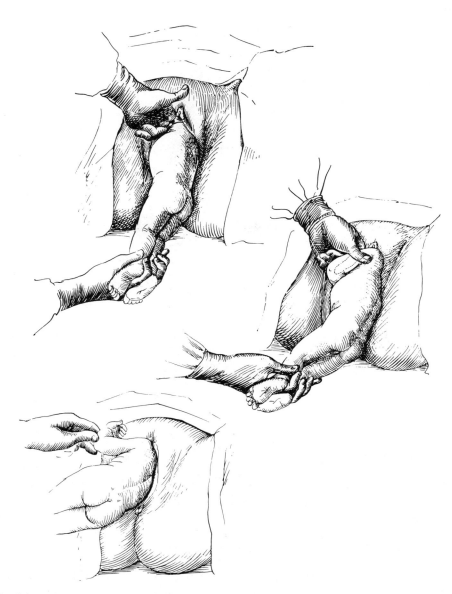

Fig. 36-6 Partial breech extraction. Anterior arm is wiped across chest by pressure with index and second fingers.

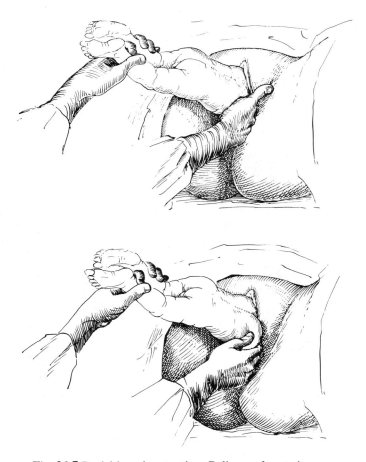

Fig. 36-7 Partial breech extraction. Delivery of posterior arm.

jured is during the delivery of the aftercoming head. Anoxia may lead to death or long-term disability if the head cannot be delivered relatively promptly. Conversely, forceful attempts to extract the head through a small pelvis may cause intracranial hemorrhage or injury to the spinal cord and nerve roots or to abdominal viscera.

3. *Hyperextension of the fetal head.* The manipulations necessary for vaginal delivery are associated with a high frequency of long-term neurologic disability.

4. *Abnormal labor.* The presence of an active phase abnormality of the first stage of labor

or a protracted descent in the second stage is associated with fetopelvic disproportion and an increased frequency of fetal injury.

5. *The absence of an obstetrician experienced in vaginal breech delivery.* Both the decision to allow a trial of labor and the techniques of vaginal delivery require skill and experience.

Cesarean section does not guarantee an atraumatic delivery. The same maneuvers used for vaginal delivery of the breech are required at the time of cesarean section. Ample abdominal and uterine incisions are essential. A low-segment, transverse incision can be used if the lower uter-

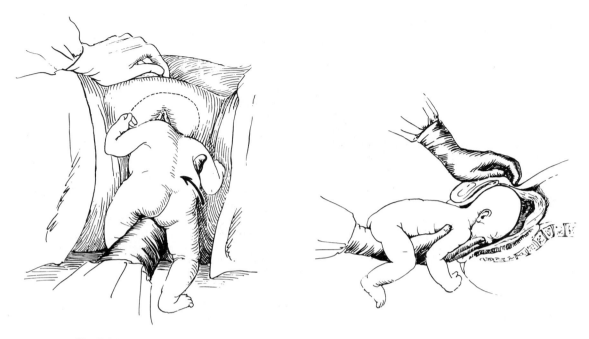

Fig. 36-8 Partial breech extraction. Delivery of head by Celsus-Wigand-Martin maneuver.

ine segment is well developed; otherwise, the uterine incision should be vertical.

SUGGESTED READING

Benson W, Boyce DC, and Vaughn DL: Breech delivery in the primigravida, Obstet Gynecol 40:417, 1972.

Bowes WA, Taylor ES, O'Brien M, and Bowes C: Breech delivery: evaluation of the method of delivery on perinatal results and maternal morbidity, Am J Obstet Gynecol 135:915, 1979.

Brenner WE: Breech presentation, Clin Obstet Gynecol 21:511, 1978.

Caterini H, Langer A, Sama J, Devanesan M, and Pelosi MA: Fetal risk in hyperextension of the fetal head in breech presentation, Am J Obstet Gynecol 123:631, 1975.

Collea JV, Chein C, and Quilligan EJ: The randomized management of term frank breech presentation: a study of 208 cases, Am J Obstet Gynecol 137:235, 1980.

Crawford JS: An appraisal of lumbar epidural blockade in patients with a singleton fetus presenting by the breech, J Obstet Gynaecol Br Commonw 81:867, 1974.

Faber-Nijholt R, Juisjes HJ, Touwen BCL, and Fidler VJ: Neurologic follow-up of 281 children born in breech presentation, Br Med J 286:9, 1983.

Fall O and Nilsson BA: External cephalic version in breech presentation under tocolysis, Obstet Gynecol 53:712, 1979.

Ferguson JE II and Dyson DC: Intrapartum external cephalic version, Am J Obstet Gynecol 152:297, 1985.

Fianu S and Vaclavinkova V: The site of placental attachment as a factor in the aetiology of breech presentation, Acta Obstet Gynecol Scand 57:371, 1978.

Flanagan TA, Mulchahey KM, Korenbrot CC, Green JR, and Laros RK Jr: Management of term breech presentation, Am J Obstet Gynecol 156:1492, 1987.

Friedman EL: Labor, clinical evaluation and management, New York, 1978, Appleton-Century-Croft.

Gimovsky ML, Wallace RL, Schifrin BS, and Paul RH: Randomized management of the nonfrank breech presentation at term: a preliminary report, Am J Obstet Gynecol 146:34, 1983.

Goldenberg RL and Nelson KG: The premature breech, Am J Obstet Gynecol 127:240, 1977.

Green JE, McLean F, and Smith LP: Has an increased cesarean section rate for term breech delivery reduced the incidence of birth asphyxia, trauma, and death? Am J Obstet Gynecol 141:643, 1982.

Hofmeyr GJ: Effect of external cephalic version in late pregnancy on breech presentation and cesarean section rate, Br J Obstet Gynaecol 90:392, 1983.

Ingemarsson I, Westgren M, and Svenningsen NW: Long-term follow-up of preterm infants in breech presentation delivered by cesarean section, Lancet 2:172, 1978.

Kitchen W, Ford GW, Doyle LW, Richards AL, Lissenden JV, Pepperell RJ, and Duke JE: Cesarean section or vaginal delivery at 24 to 28 weeks' gestation: comparison of survival and neonatal and two-year morbidity, Obstet Gynecol 66:149, 1985.

Phelan JP, Stine LE, Mueller E, McCart D, and Yehs: Observations of fetal heart rate characteristics related to external cephalic version and tocolysis, Am J Obstet Gynecol 149:658, 1984.

Ranney B: The gentle art of external cephalic version, Am. J. Obstet. Gynecol. 116:239, 1973.

Rovinsky JJ, Miller JA, and Kaplan S: Management of breech presentation at term, Am J Obstet Gynecol 115:497, 1973.

Sachs BP, McCarthy BJ, Rubin G, Burton A, Terry J, and Tyler CW Jr: Cesarean section: risks and benefits for mother and fetus, JAMA 250:2157, 1983.

Stine LE, Phelan JP, Wallace R, Eglinton GS, van Dorsten P, and Schifrin BS: Update on external cephalic version performed at term, Obstet Gynecol 65:642, 1985.

Tatum RK: Vaginal breech delivery of selected infants weighing more than 2000 grams, Am J Obstet Gynecol 152:145, 1985.

Todd WD and Steer AB: Term breech: review of 1006 term breech deliveries, Obstet Gynecol 22:583, 1963.

Van Dorsten P, Schifrin B, and Wallace RL: External cephalic version under tocolysis: prospective randomized study, Am J Obstet Gynecol 141:422, 1981.

Watson WJ and Benson WL: Vaginal delivery for the selected frank breech infant at term, Obstet Gynecol 64:638, 1984.

Westgren M, Grindsell H, Ingemarsson I, and Svenningsen NW: Hyperextension of the fetal head in breech presentation: a study with long-term follow-up, Br J Obstet Gynaecol 88:104, 1981.

37

Russell K. Laros, Jr.

Forceps and vacuum delivery

Objectives

RATIONALE: An understanding of the indications for and proper use of forceps and vacuum is essential to the practice of safe obstetrics.

The student should be able to:

A. Name the indications for the use of forceps and vacuum.
B. Describe the technique of application of forceps and the vacuum extractor.

Obstetric forceps and vacuum extractors are instruments designed to *extract* the infant from the birth canal or to *rotate* its head within the vagina. They are never used to compress the head or to aid in dilating the cervix and are applied only to the head of the infant and never to any other part of its body.

More than 600 types of forceps and four types of vacuum extractors have been designed. Many of the forceps are for a specific purpose such as extraction of the aftercoming head in breech delivery or for rotation of the head from certain abnormal positions. All forceps are alike in that they consist of two blades that articulate at the point where the shafts cross and lead into the handles. The blades have a *cephalic curve,* which conforms to the contours of the infant's head, and

most forceps have a *pelvic curve,* which approximates the curve of the pelvic canal. The blades may be fenestrated or solid. The left blade is the one that is inserted into the left half of the pelvis, the handle being held in the operator's left hand. This blade articulates with the right one by means of a flanged lock on the shafts of the instrument (Fig. 37-1).

Three types of vacuum extractors are currently available in the United States: the classical Malmström instrument, the Bird modification, and Silastic modifications. The Bird modification replaces the traction chain with a nylon cord; the Silastic devices have a different, more trumpetlike shape. Metal cups are available with 40-, 50-, and 60-mm opening diameters, and the Silastic device has a 65-mm opening.

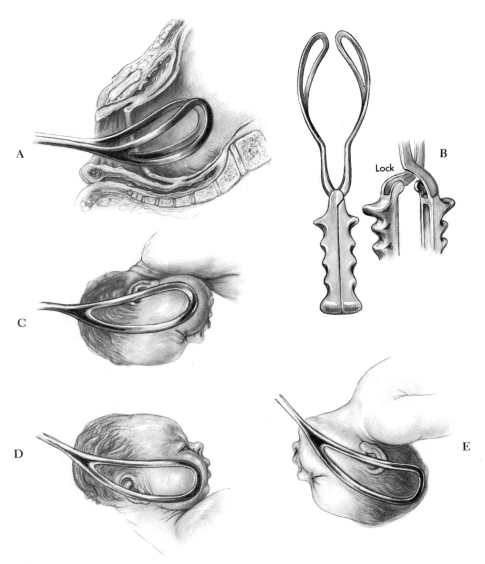

Fig. 37-1 Obstetric forceps. **A,** Forceps in transverse position with pelvic curve corresponding to curve of birth canal. **B,** Cephalic curve of blades and lock. **C** to **E,** Cephalic application. **C,** Occipitoanterior (ideal application). **D,** Occipitoposterior. **E,** Application to aftercoming head in breech presentation.

TYPES OF FORCEPS AND VACUUM APPLICATIONS

Forceps and vacuum operations are classified according to the station and position of the presenting part at the time the instrument is applied. The American College of Obstetricians and Gynecologists has recently enunciated a revised definition of operative pelvic deliveries (Fig. 37-2).

Outlet forceps or vacuum application. An *outlet* application indicates that the scalp is visible at the introitus, the fetal skull is on the pelvic floor, the sagittal suture is in the anterior-posterior or in the left or right anterior or posterior oblique diameter, and rotation does not exceed 45 degrees. After a patient has been anesthetized for delivery, particularly with spinal or epidural anesthesia, which eliminates perineal sensation and the urge to bear down, the head may retract slightly in the birth canal. This application would still be classified as outlet if the criteria had been met before the anesthetic had been administered.

Low forceps or vacuum application. If the station of the fetal head meets the criteria for an outlet application but rotation exceeds 45 degrees,

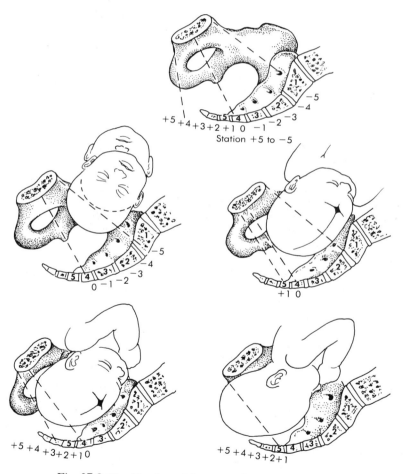

Fig. 37-2 Classification of forceps and vacuum deliveries.

the application is defined as *low*. Alternatively, the application is low if the station is between plus 2 and the pelvic floor and the rotation is 45 degrees or less.

Midforceps or vacuum application. A *midpelvic* application indicates that the head is engaged, but the leading part of the skull is above plus 2 station. Any degree of rotation is acceptable.

High forceps or vacuum application. A *high* application exists when the head lies between the plane of the pelvic inlet and the level of the ischial spines. There is virtually no indication for the use of high forceps or vacuum in modern obstetrics.

Merely naming the type of application is not sufficient because some midpelvic and low applications are extremely easy and others are difficult. Much more information is provided by an exact description of the station and position of the head and the difficulties encountered during the application and delivery of the infant in the hospital record.

The *position* of the forceps in the pelvis is determined by the pelvic diameter that passes at a right angle through the center of the fenestra. If each blade is applied to the lateral pelvic wall with its pelvic curve directed anteriorly, the forceps are in the transverse diameter of the pelvis. If the blades are then rotated 45 degrees, they lie in an oblique diameter. If they are rotated another 45 degrees, the pelvic curve is directed toward the lateral pelvic wall with one blade overlying the sacrum and the other beneath the pubic arch; they are now in the anteroposterior diameter.

The blades are said to be in the *cephalic* or *ideal application* if they have been applied to the head in the occipitomental diameter and equidistant from the sagittal suture (Fig. 37-1). If the blades are applied to the sides of the pelvis with the front of the forceps directed anteriorly without regard to the position of the fetal head, they are in *pelvic application*.

INDICATIONS FOR OPERATIVE VAGINAL DELIVERY

The use of forceps or vacuum is indicated whenever terminating the second stage of labor is in the best interest of either the mother or the fetus and when an operative vaginal delivery is the easiest and safest method of delivering the baby.

The principal reason for operative vaginal delivery is *cessation of progress during the second stage of labor*. This can be expressed either as an arrest of descent in station or an overall prolongation of the second stage. The length of the second stage is influenced by both the mother's parity and the use of regional anesthesia. The second stage is prolonged (exceeding the 95th percentile) if the following limits are exceeded:

Primipara with regional anesthesia: >3 hours
Primipara with no regional anesthesia: >2 hours
Multipara with regional anesthesia: >2 hours
Multipara without regional anesthesia: >1 hour.

Fetal distress is also an indication for prompt delivery. Either forceps or vacuum can be used; however, forceps usually allow a more rapid delivery.

Several maternal disorders dictate *avoidance of pushing* and the attendant Valsalva maneuver. Examples include certain types of maternal heart disease, unoperated Berry aneurysms and arteriovenous malformations, and poorly controlled myasthenia gravis.

REQUIREMENTS

Although a true indication for forceps delivery may be present, such an operation may be dangerous both to mother and baby unless the following requirements or conditions are met.

The operator must be familiar with the normal mechanism of labor and trained in the application and use of forceps and vacuum. The physician who has not had special training in operative obstetrics should usually not perform forceps or vacuum extractions. Consultation should be sought for all such problems.

The cervix must be completely dilated. No one can forcibly extract an infant through an undilated cervix without producing a laceration that may extend into the lower uterine segment.

There can be no marked disproportion between the size of the baby and the size of the pelvis.

The head must be engaged. The lower the head

in the pelvis, the safer and easier will be the delivery. The physician must ascertain by pelvic and, if there is a question, by radiologic examination that the head actually is engaged before attempting operative vaginal delivery from a midpelvic location. If a huge caput has formed or if the head is molded and greatly elongated, its most dependent part may be deep in the vagina while the biparietal diameter is still above the plane of the inlet.

Forceps extraction from a high station, particularly in primigravidas, often results in deep soft-tissue lacerations as the head is drawn through the unprepared vagina. This is substantially less of a problem if vacuum extraction is used.

The vertex or the face must be presenting in a position that will permit delivery, and the head must be large enough to be grasped by the blades.

Anesthetic must be adequate for the procedure. Pudendal block is satisfactory for most low and outlet deliveries but inadequate for more difficult procedures, particularly when the head must be rotated. Spinal, epidural, caudal, or inhalation anesthesia will provide the muscle relaxation and pain relief required for these deliveries.

The membranes must be ruptured.

Contraindications. The use of forceps and vacuum is contraindicated in certain *abnormal positions* such as impacted mentoposterior and brow, which cannot usually be corrected and delivered safely through the vagina, or for breech delivery, except to extract the aftercoming head. Operative vaginal delivery also is contraindicated when progress is delayed by *significant cephalopelvic disproportion, before the presenting part has descended well below the level of the ischial spines,* and *when the cervix is incompletely dilated.* Cesarean delivery is almost always preferred under these circumstances.

SELECTION OF PATIENTS

The best results from operative vaginal delivery are obtained when the operations are performed by expert obstetricians, but technique is not the only factor that influences the outcome. The operator must know when to interfere and when to allow labor to continue. Patient observation or oxytocin stimulation often permits spontaneous delivery or at least makes a potentially difficult operation easy if the head descends deeper into the pelvis. A reduction in unindicated and traumatic forceps extractions will improve both fetal and maternal outcomes.

Outlet and low extraction. Forceps extraction, when properly executed, does not add to the risk for the mother or the infant. This operation may be performed electively, or it may become necessary if the patient is unable to use her secondary powers to aid in the expulsion of the infant or if the uterine contractions become ineffectual late in the second stage. Under such circumstances, forceps delivery may be preferable to oxytocin stimulation.

Technique

The patient, in lithotomy position and properly anesthetized, is examined to determine the exact position of the fetal head. The left blade of the forceps is introduced between the head and the guiding fingers of the physician's right hand until it lies in proper cephalic and pelvic application (Fig. 37-3, *A*). The right blade is then introduced into the right side of the pelvis (Fig. 37-3, *B*). The forceps are locked after any necessary adjustments in their position have been made. If the forceps cannot be locked easily, the physician should suspect that the blades are not properly applied.

After a final examination to ascertain that the application is correct, the head is extracted (Fig. 37-3, *C* and *D*). Traction at first is directed toward the floor to pull the head through the proper axis of the birth canal. As soon as the occiput appears beneath the pubic arch, the handles of the forceps are elevated each time traction is applied. This tends to extend the head as it descends, a duplication of the sequence of events during normal labor. The forceps are removed in the reverse order of their application, the right one first and then the left (Fig. 37-3, *E* and *F*).

The vacuum should never be applied to a face, brow, or breech presentation. The largest possible cup should be applied, taking great care that no cervix or vagina is caught between the head and the cup. Low vacuum is

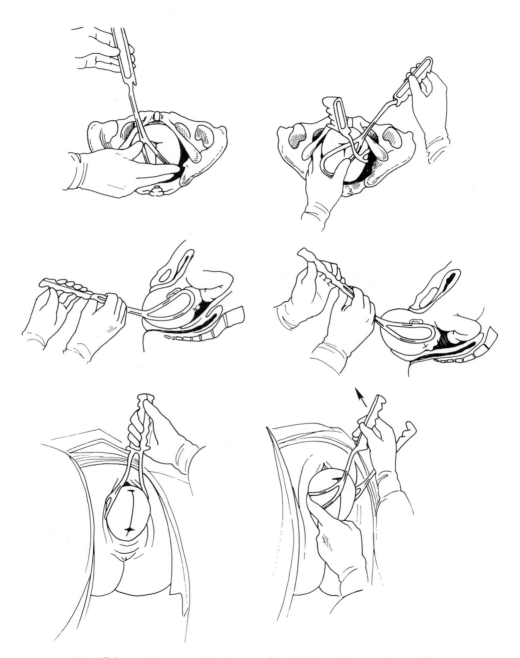

Fig. 37-3 Low forceps application to a fetus in the occiput anterior position.

applied, and the application rechecked to be certain that the cup is free of all maternal tissue. The vacuum is then rapidly increased to 600 mm Hg. If fetal distress is not present, waiting 5 to 10 minutes to allow a chignon to form and fill the cup is advantageous. Axis traction is then applied (Fig. 37-4, *A*), and rotation is allowed to occur spontaneously. *Never rotate the head by turning the cup*. Traction should be applied at the time of uterine contractions and as a supplement to maternal pushing. Delivery should usually be accomplished with three to five pulls (Fig. 37-4, *B* to *D*). If the vacuum seal is broken, the cup pops off and should be reapplied carefully. The maximum number of pop offs should be limited to three and the total traction time to 30 minutes. If a fetal scalp electrode is in place, the cup can

be applied over the wire leads; however, if a pop off occurs, the electrode should be removed and an external monitor used. Prior performance of a fetal scalp blood sample is only a relative contraindication to the use of the vacuum extractor.

Midpelvic extraction. Midforceps and midvacuum extraction is generally contraindicated unless there is a clear-cut reason to terminate labor. The techniques of application and traction are as described previously. When midpelvic application is required, the head has usually not yet rotated to an anterior position. Although a transverse or posterior position does not contraindicate a midforceps delivery, it makes the application and subsequent extraction more difficult.

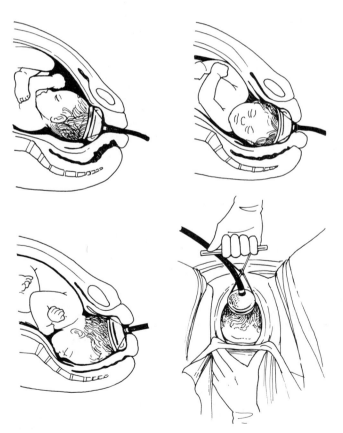

Fig. 37-4 Low vacuum application to a fetus in the occiput posterior position.

High pelvic extraction. High forceps and vacuum deliveries can rarely be justified. Cesarean section is almost always preferable when the need for delivery arises before the head is engaged.

Trial forceps or vacuum. All midpelvic vaginal deliveries should be approached as a trial, implying that a ready alternative exists. This can only occur if the facility to do an immediate cesarean section (an operating room team and an anesthesiologist) is available. If gentle traction does not lead to descent or if persistent fetal bradycardia develops, the forceps or vacuum should be removed and the patient delivered abdominally.

RESULTS

The morbidity and mortality for both the mother and infant should be minimized if operative vaginal delivery is properly performed. Several contemporary studies show that outlet and low forceps and vacuum, when properly used, do not increase morbidity. However, midpelvic delivery does carry a significant risk for fetal morbidity. Traumatic lesions for the infant include skull fracture, intracranial hemorrhage, cephalohematomas, seventh-nerve palsy, and soft-tissue lacerations. There is also a higher incidence of acidemia and low Apgar scores in infants delivered by midforceps or vacuum. The alternative to a midpelvic delivery is cesarean section, which poses increased risk of infection, blood loss, and a longer hospital stay for the mother. However, these maternal risks are usually far more acceptable than any permanent fetal injury.

SUGGESTED READING

Angell LK, Robb RM, and Berson FG: Visual prognosis in patients with ruptures in Descement's membrane due to forceps injuries, Arch Ophth 99:2137, 1981.

Baerthlein WC, Moodley S, and Stinson SK: Comparison of maternal and neonatal morbidity in midforceps deliveries and midpelvis vacuum extractions, Obstet Gynecol 67:594, 1986.

Blennow G, Svenningsen NW, Gustafson B, Sunden B, and Gronquist S: Neonatal and prospective follow-up study of infants delivered by vacuum extraction, Acta Obstet Gynecol Scand 56:189, 1977.

Bowes WA and Bowes C: Current role of the midforceps operation, Clin Obstet Gynecol 23:549, 1980.

Boyd ME, Usher RH, and others: Failed forceps, Obstet Gynecol 68:779, 1986.

Broekhuizen FF, Washington JM, Johnson F, and Hamilton PR: Vacuum extraction versus forceps delivery: indications and complications, Obstet Gynecol 69:338, 1987.

Dennen EH: Forceps deliveries, Philadelphia, 1955, FA Davis Co.

Dierker LJ, Rosen MG, Thompson K, Debanne S, and Linn P: The midforceps: maternal and neonatal outcomes, Am J Obstet Gynecol 152:176, 1985.

Douglass LH and Kaltreider DF: Trial forceps, Am J Obstet Gynecol 65:889, 1953.

Federle MP, Cohen HA, Rosenwein MF, Brant-Zanadzki MN, and Cann CE: Pelvimetry by digital radiography: low-dose examination, Radiology 143:733, 1982.

Friedman EA: Labor: clinical evaluation and management, 2d ed, New York, 1978, Appleton-Century-Croft.

Friedman EA, Sachtleben-Murray MR, Dahrouge D, and Neff RK: Long-term effects of labor and delivery on offspring: a matched-pair analysis, Am J Obstet Gynecol 150:941, 1984.

Gilstrap LC, Hauth JC, Schiano S, and others: Neonatal acidosis and method of delivery, Obstet Gynecol 63:681, 1984.

Halme J and Ekbladh L: The vacuum extractor for obstetric delivery, Clin Obstet Gynecol 25:167, 1982.

Healy DL and Laufe LE: Survey of obstetric forceps training in North America in 1981, Am J Obstet Gynecol 151:54, 1985.

Jouppila R, Jouppila P, and Hollmen A: Segmental epidural analgesia in labour: related to the progress of labour, fetal malposition and instrumental delivery, Acta Obstet Gynecol 58:135, 1979.

Kilpatrick SJ and Laros, RK: Characteristics of normal labor, Obstet Gynecol 74:85, 1989.

Maryniak GM and Frank JB: Clinical assessment of the Kobayashi vacuum extractor, Obstet Gynecol 64:431, 1984.

Plauche WC: Vacuum extraction, Obstet Gynecol 52:289, 1978.

Punnonen R, Aro P, Kuukankorpi A, and Pystynen P: Fetal and maternal effects of forceps and vacuum extraction, Br J Obstet Gynaecol 93:1132, 1986.

Richardson DA, Evans MI, and Cibils LA: Midforceps delivery: a critical review, Am J Obstet Gynecol 145:621, 1983.

Robertson PA, Zhao RL, and Laros RK: Neonatal and maternal outcome in low and midpelvic operative deliveries, Am J Obstet Gynecol 162:1436, 1990.

Shnider S and Levinson G: Anesthesia for obstetrics, Baltimore, 1986, Williams & Wilkins.

Traub AI, Morrow RJ, Ritchie, and others: A continuing use for Kielland's forceps? Br J Obstet Gynaecol 91:894, 1984.

Varner MW, Cruikshank DP, and Laube DW: X-ray pelvimetry in clinical obstetrics, Obstet Gynecol 56:296, 1980.

38

Russell K. Laros, Jr.

Cesarean section

Objectives

RATIONALE: Cesarean section plays an important role as a mode of delivery used by the contemporary obstetrician. It also has become the most common operation performed in the United States.

The student should be able to:
A. Name the indications for cesarean section.
B. List the different types of cesarean section.
C. Describe the postoperative complications most commonly seen.

Cesarean section is an operative procedure by which the infant is delivered through incisions in the abdominal and uterine walls. This term should not be applied to the removal of an extrauterine abdominal pregnancy.

INCIDENCE

According to the National Institutes of Health Task Force on Cesarean Childbirth (Rosen), the cesarean birthrate in the United States increased from 5.5% in 1970 (195,000 operations) to 15.2% in 1978 (510,000 operations) and is still rising. In fact, cesarean section is now the most frequent operation performed in the United States. In part the change has resulted from the increasing safety with which cesarean delivery can be performed: infection can be prevented or controlled, anesthetic techniques have been improved, and more labors that end in cesarean delivery are managed by trained obstetrician-gynecologists in sophisticated perinatal units. The improvements in neonatal care for the infant have permitted the extension of indications for the operation to include the delivery of infants of low birth weight and those who might be injured by prolonged labor or traumatic operative vaginal delivery.

The factors that have contributed most to the rising incidence of cesarean delivery are *dystocia* (30% increase), *repeat operations* (25% to 30% increase), *breech presentation* (10% to 15% increase), and *fetal distress* (10% to 15% increase).

It was hoped that increased use of a trial labor in subsequent pregnancies (or vaginal birth after cesarean section [VBAC]) would achieve a leveling off and even a decline in the rate of cesarean section. Although the frequency of VBAC has steadily increased, the rate of cesarean delivery has not yet begun to decline.

If obstetricians are to halt and reverse this trend, we must actively encourage trials of labor after previous sections, critically reexamine the indications for primary section, and change our environment to eliminate the practice of defensive medicine. Hopeful reports are beginning to appear. One Chicago hospital was able to decrease the rate of cesarean section from 17.5% to 11.5% over a 3-year span. It was accomplished by instituting the following policies: a formal second opinion was required for all cesarean sections; all patients previously delivered by cesarean section were counseled at their first prenatal visit that a trial of labor was anticipated; a rigorous protocol for the diagnosis and treatment of dystocia was utilized; the diagnosis of fetal distress based on fetal heart rate monitoring had to be corroborated by sampling fetal blood whenever feasible; vaginal delivery of fetus in the breech presentation was expected if specific selection criteria were met; and an ongoing peer review process was instituted to assure adherence to departmental protocols.

INDICATIONS

The major indications for cesarean delivery, which are discussed in detail in the chapters concerned with specific complications, are reviewed briefly here.

Mechanical dystocia. Fetopelvic disproportion can result from abnormalities in the bony pelvis, excessive fetal size, or adnexal or uterine tumors that block the birth canal. Most decisions for cesarean section because of disproportion between pelvic and fetal size are made during labor, when it becomes evident that the fetus cannot be delivered safely through the vagina. Ovarian tumors that are recognized and removed during early pregnancy obviously cannot interfere with labor, but myomas located low in the posterior uterine wall may because they cannot be removed during pregnancy.

Dysfunctional labor. An increasing number of cesarean operations are performed because of "failure to progress." Many of these are considered to be caused by fetopelvic disproportion, but in a substantial number the lack of progress is caused by dysfunctional labor. Cesarean delivery will certainly improve the outcome for the fetus if normal progress cannot be established by oxytocin stimulation.

Placenta previa. Almost all patients with complete placenta previa and most of those with incomplete varieties can be delivered more safely by cesarean section than through the vagina.

Abruptio placentae. Cesarean section may be performed to control profuse bleeding associated with complete placental separation when the conditions are not appropriate for induction of labor and vaginal delivery or for partial placental separation if one cannot anticipate early vaginal delivery and there is no indication that the fetus is seriously compromised.

Malposition of fetus. Cesarean section is indicated for most stable transverse lies, unless the baby already is dead or is so small that it is unlikely to survive; for abnormal vertex positions that cannot be corrected and delivered vaginally; and for some breech presentations.

Maternal medical conditions. If deterioration of a medical complication of pregnancy places either the mother or the fetus in jeopardy and induction fails, delivery by cesarean section is indicated. Severe preeclampsia, eclampsia, and diabetes are examples.

Previous cesarean section. A previous cesarean section in and of itself *is not* an indication for cesarean section. Ample data show the safety and effectiveness of a trial of labor after cesarean delivery.

Uterine and vaginal operations. Pregnancies that occur after reconstructive surgery of an anomalous uterus; deep, multiple myomectomy; or tubal reimplantation are usually best terminated by elective cesarean section. Prior repair of a rectovaginal or vesicovaginal fistula and the presence of an abdominally placed cerclage are also indications.

Fetal indications. Fetal indications for cesarean delivery include well-documented fetal distress, umbilical cord prolapse when the cervix is not fully dilated or operative vaginal delivery is contraindicated by the fetal position or station, the premature breech, and fetal anomalies or conditions for which passage through the birth canal would be harmful and increase fetal morbidity. Examples of this last group include hydrocephalus, osteogenesis imperfecta, active herpes simplex, multifetal gestations greater than twins, and isoimmune thrombocytopenia.

CHOICE OF OPERATION

Classic section. In classic cesarean section, the uterine incision is made through the upper contractile portion of the fundus above the dome of the bladder (Fig. 38-1). It is easy to perform but has certain disadvantages that make it undesirable. The incision in the thick, active upper segment bleeds more and may not heal as well as the low segment incision. It also cannot be peritonized; thus there is more chance for the development of adhesions and for infected uterine contents to seep into the peritoneal cavity, producing infection and ileus and distension. The risk of infection is high after this operation if the membranes have been ruptured or if the patient has been in labor. Rupture of the uterine scar in sub-

sequent pregnancies occurs more often after the classic than the lower segment operations.

Classic cesarean section may be preferable to the lower segment operations if the bladder is firmly adherent to the uterus, for transverse lie, when the fetal back is directed toward the pelvic inlet, for anterior wall placenta previa, and when it is necessary to empty the uterus rapidly.

Low segment section. In low segment cesarean section, the uterine incision is made in the thin lower segment after the vesicouterine peritoneum has been cut and the bladder separated and pushed downward from its attachment to the anterior uterine wall. One advantage is that the incision is behind the bladder and can be completely covered by peritoneum; thus the seepage from the uterus is reduced and postpartum peritoneal infection is less likely to occur than with the classic method. The low segment section can be used more safely after the membranes have been ruptured or labor has been in progress for some hours.

A transverse incision in the lower segment is preferable to a vertical one because it requires less mobilization of the bladder and because the incidence of rupture in subsequent pregnancies is lower. Its major disadvantages are that it can extend into the huge uterine veins and that the manipulations necessary to deliver a fetus presenting as a frank breech or transversely are more

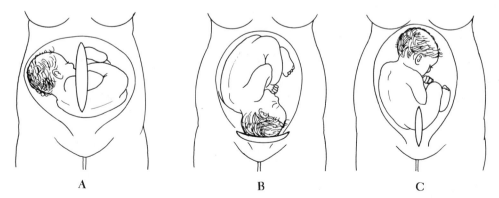

Fig. 38-1 Cesarean section showing position of uterine incision. **A,** Classic incision. **B,** Low segment transverse incision. **C,** Low segment longitudinal incision.

difficult through a transverse opening. A vertical incision can extend downward through the cervix or upward into the upper segment of the uterus and is more likely to separate during subsequent labors. Involvement of the contractile portion of the uterus, by deliberate incision or by traumatic extension, explains the increased possibility of rupture during a later pregnancy.

Extraperitoneal section. In extraperitoneal cesarean section, the uterine incision is made in the lower segment behind the bladder after the peritoneum has been dissected off the dome of the bladder without entering the peritoneal cavity. The bladder is then pushed downward to expose the uterine wall. The extraperitoneal section is more difficult to perform, requiring a skilled operator, and bladder and ureteral injuries are more common than with the other operations. It does not solve the problem when infection has extended through the uterine wall, and it is not necessary in the potentially infected patient; therefore its value is limited.

Cesarean hysterectomy. Cesarean section followed by removal of the uterus is indicated if there is a definite reason for hysterectomy, for example, multiple fibroid tumors or uterine rupture. Its value in the infected patient is greatest if the uterine wall is deeply and heavily infected and contains multiple small abscesses that may produce a constant source of infected emboli.

Cesarean hysterectomy should not usually be considered as an alternative to cesarean section and tubal sterilization. The morbidity and potential mortality associated with hysterectomy is far greater than with tubal ligation.

ANESTHESIA

There should be no increase in maternal or fetal mortality from the anesthetic. The same factors that influence the administration of medication and anesthetic in vaginal delivery hold true with cesarean section. The fetus is narcotized or anesthetized by all the medication given the mother. Conduction anesthesia, except when contraindicated, is usually preferable to inhalation technics.

Conduction anesthesia provides excellent pain relief with limited effects on the fetus, unless the blood pressure falls to a level too low to maintain uterine perfusion. *Inhalation anesthesia* is preferable for patients who are bleeding and when rapid delivery is essential. The effects of the inhaled agent on the fetus can be minimized if the abdomen is prepared and draped and the surgical team is ready to start the operation as soon as an adequate anesthetic level has been reached. If the infant is delivered within 6 or 8 minutes, it will be little affected by the anesthetic.

An important cause of maternal morbidity and mortality is aspiration of vomitus as anesthesia is being induced or as the patient is reacting after inhalation techniques. The effects of aspiration can be reduced by giving the mother 30 ml of an antacid solution preoperatively.

TRIAL OF LABOR AFTER CESAREAN SECTION

Trials of labor should be carried out in most women previously delivered by cesarean section. Studies from both the United States and abroad report success rates between 38.6% and 97.1%, with an average of 74%. A prior classical section is an exception because the risk of uterine rupture is about 10%; the rupture is usually catastrophic, resulting in significant blood loss for the mother and death for the fetus. In contrast, patients with prior uterine incisions that are known to be completely within the lower segment should be encouraged to attempt a trial of labor. Furthermore, a woman with two or more previous cesarean deliveries should not be discouraged from a trial of labor.

When a lower uterine segment scar separates during a subsequent labor, the separation is usually minor or may be a totally asymptomatic dehiscence. Separation is heralded by vaginal bleeding, uterine pain, and fetal distress. Because pain is such a nonspecific sign, maternal bleeding and fetal distress ought to be considered the primary signs of rupture.

Numerous reports in the literature show that the risk of scar separation is less than 1% and that the risk of perinatal mortality is no greater for fetuses delivered by a trial of labor than for those delivered by elective, repeat cesarean section.

In the past, many authors have cautioned against the use of oxytocin during a trial of labor after cesarean section. However, recent reports show a clear trend toward the cautious use of oxytocin in physiologic doses. In fact, the success rate appears to be related to the willingness to use oxytocin, especially in women whose prior cesarean delivery was performed because of the indication of dystocia.

The requirements for allowing a trial of labor are minimal and include the availability of a physician who is capable of performing a cesarean delivery, an operating room, and an anesthesiologist. These requirements are really no different from those for dealing with acute fetal distress during labor.

Elective repeat cesarean section. This procedure should be reserved for patients who have a significant cause such as severe, documented pelvic contracture or breech presentation with pelvic measurements that fail to meet the minimum required for vaginal breech delivery. When an elective cesarean section is performed before the onset of labor, maturity of the fetal lung must first be assured. Fetal maturity can be assumed if at least two of the clinical criteria and one of the laboratory criteria as follows are met:

Clinical criteria—39 weeks since the onset of the last normal menstrual period in woman with regular cycles, fetal heart tones documented before 20 weeks by nonelectronic fetoscope, and congruous uterine size and gestational age by pelvic examination performed before week 16 of gestation.

Laboratory determinants—26 weeks since the taking of a positive serum pregnancy test, or an ultrasonic examination performed before 20 weeks of gestation that confirms gestational age.

STERILIZATION

The fact that a woman must be delivered by cesarean section does not necessarily limit her reproductive career, but repeated abdominal operations are more dangerous than an equal number of vaginal deliveries. A tubal ligation may be performed in conjunction with cesarean section if the patient requests it, but there is no reason to insist on the operation simply because of previous cesarean deliveries.

COMPLICATIONS

The mortality associated with cesarean section even under the most favorable conditions is five to seven times greater than for normal delivery. The deaths are not all direct results of the operation itself; many are caused by the complication that made the cesarean delivery necessary. However, cesarean section is a very safe operation. In fact, the Boston Women's Hospital reported more than 10,000 consecutive cesarean sections without a maternal death. The more important issue is the increased maternal morbidity and length of hospital stay associated with cesarean delivery.

Infection. Infection, one of the most common of the complications of cesarean section, occurs more often after emergency operations performed during labor than after planned elective procedures. The number of serious infections can be reduced significantly by early decision to deliver patients in abnormal labor, by meticulous surgical technique, and by the judicious use of prophylactic antibiotics (see Chapter 40).

Bleeding. Cesarean section is not a blood-conserving procedure; the blood loss averages at least 1 L, and many patients lose much more. Red blood cell transfusion should be required in only 3% to 4% of patients delivered by cesarean section. The only circumstance in which autologous blood donation is indicated in anticipation of a cesarean section is that of placenta previa. Only in this clinical setting is adequate time available for donation coupled with the probability of blood loss sufficient to require transfusion.

Anesthetic. Unless the anesthetic is carefully controlled, it may contribute substantially to the mortality. Many of the deaths associated with aspiration of gastric contents can be prevented if the mother is given 30 ml of an antacid solution orally just before the anesthetic is administered.

This neutralizes gastric acid and reduces lung damage if she aspirates vomitus.

Perinatal mortality. Cesarean delivery does not guarantee infant survival; in fact, the perinatal mortality associated with the operation is higher than that for delivery in general. Many deaths occur because of the complications that make delivery necessary.

Although cesarean section can now be used more liberally for small babies who are delivered in hospitals that provide excellent perinatal intensive care, there is a limit beyond which it offers no advantage. Several reports have documented that cesarean section does not improve the outcomes for very small babies unless they are in other than a cephalic presentation.

Not everyone agrees that the increased incidence of cesarean section is necessary to maintain low perinatal mortality rates. A report from Ireland, noted a decrease in perinatal mortality in 76,547 births from 42.1 in 1970 to 16.8 in 1980 at the National Maternity Hospital, Dublin. During this same period the cesarean section rate increased from 4.2% to only 4.8%. They accomplished this by being more aggressive in their management of dysfunctional labor, by encouraging vaginal breech delivery, and by reducing the number of repeat cesarean sections.

The figures in most reports relate only to mortality. One of the advantages of the increasing rate of cesarean section is decreased perinatal morbidity and mortality for breech presentation, transverse lie, cephalopelvic disproportion, placenta previa, and other complications. In the past, many babies were damaged during the vaginal management of these complications. Such babies are now much more likely to be born without injury.

SUGGESTED READING

Barrett JM, Boehm FH, and Vaughan WK: The effect of type of delivery on neonatal outcome in singleton infants of birth weight of 1000 g or less, JAMA 250:625, 1983.

Chestnut DH, Eden RD, Gall SA, and Parker RT: Postpartum hysterectomy: a review of cesarean and postpartum hysterectomy, Obstet Gynecol 65:365, 1985.

Flamm BL, Lim OW, Jones C, Fallon D, Newmann LA, and Mantis JK: Vaginal birth after cesarean section: results of a multicenter study, Am J Obstet Gynecol 158:1079, 1988.

Gibbs CE: Planned vaginal delivery following cesarean section, Clin Obstet Gynecol 23:507, 1980.

Kitchen W, Ford GW, Doyle LW, Richards AL, Lissenden JV, Pepperell RJ, and Duke JE: Cesarean section or vaginal delivery at 24 to 28 weeks' gestation: comparison of survival and neonatal and two-year morbidity, Obstet Gynecol 66:149, 1985.

Lowe JA, Klassen DF, and Loup RJ: Cesarean sections in U.S. PAS hospitals, PAS Reporter 14:1, 1976.

Meier PR and Porreco RP: Trial of labor following cesarean section: a two-year experience, Am J Obstet Gynecol 144:671, 1982.

Myers SA and Gleicher N: A successful program to lower cesarean section rates, N Engl J Med 319:1511, 1988.

Nielsen TF: Cesarean section: a controversial feature of modern obstetric practice, Gynecol Obstet Invest 21:57, 1986.

O'Driscoll K and Foley M: Correlation of decrease in perinatal mortality and increase in cesarean section rates, Obstet Gynecol 61:1, 1983.

Olshan AF, Shy KK, Luthy DA, Hickok D, Weiss NS, and Daling JR: Cesarean birth and neonatal mortality in very-low-birth-weight infants, Am J Obstet Gynecol 64:267, 1984.

Paul RH, Phelan JP, and Yeh S: Trial of labor in the patient with a prior cesarean birth, Am J Obstet Gynecol 151:297, 1985.

Phelan JP, Ahn MO, Diaz F, Brar HS, and Rodriguez MH: Twice a section, always a section, Obstet Gynecol 73:161, 1989.

Phelan JP and Clark SL, editors: Cesarean section, New York, 1988, Elsevier.

Rosen MG: NIH consensus development statement on cesarean childbirth, Obstet Gynecol 57:537, 1981.

Sachs BP, McCarthy BJ, Rubin G, Burton A, Terry J, and Tyler CW Jr: Cesarean section: risks and benefits for mother and fetus, JAMA 250:2157, 1983.

Saldana LR, Schulman H, and Reuss L: Management of pregnancy after cesarean section, Am J Obstet Gynecol 135:555, 1979.

39

J. Robert Willson

Immediate and remote effects of childbirth injury; uterine retrodisplacement

Objectives

RATIONALE: Relaxation of the pelvic supporting structures is a common cause of symptoms in women. The student should be familiar with the anatomy of normal pelvic support and of the types of defects, the symptoms, and the principles of management of each.

The student should be able to:

A. Demonstrate knowledge of the etiology of pelvic relaxation.

B. Describe anatomic alterations, symptoms, and physical findings for each type of relaxation.

C. List the types of urinary incontinence and explain the diagnostic measures by which each type of incontinence can be diagnosed.

D. Discuss the principles of management of urinary incontinence.

Some damage to the soft-tissue structures of the birth canal and adjacent organs occurs during every delivery. It usually is more pronounced in primigravidas, whose relatively firm tissues offer more resistance to the descent of the baby than do those of multiparas. In some women the soft tissues are so readily distensible that they stretch without tearing to permit expulsion of the infant. Thus the supports remain intact even after several pregnancies. In contrast, extensive damage may occur in others, even though every effort is made to preserve the structures; these women may also develop varicose veins and diastasis recti, suggesting that they may have a generalized supporting-tissue deficiency that is basically responsible for the failure to heal properly.

The cervix, vagina, and perineum should be inspected after each hospital delivery, and obvious injuries should be repaired immediately unless there is a good reason for delay. Approximation of the injured tissues permits them to heal faster and limits the extent of the residual damage.

The primary support of the uterus and the upper vagina is offered by the *cardinal ligaments* (Mackenrodt's ligaments), which are connective tissue condensations that extend laterally and posteriorly from the endopelvic fascia surrounding the cervix and upper vagina to fuse with the fas-

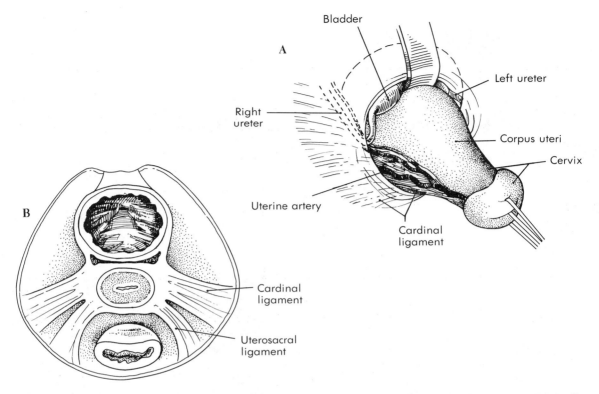

Fig. 39-1 Cardinal ligaments. **A,** Relationships of cardinal ligament as seen during vaginal hysterectomy. **B,** Cardinal and uterosacral ligaments and paracervical fascia at level just above internal cervical os.

cia overlying the obturator and levator muscles. The round ligaments and the broad ligaments have relatively little supporting function (Fig. 39-1).

The muscles making up each levator ani sweep downward from their attachments along the iliopectineal line and form the pelvic diaphragm, the superior surface of which is covered by a strong layer of endopelvic fascia (Fig. 39-2). The pubococcygeus portion of the levator surrounds the rectum and is intimately connected to the lateral walls of the urethra and vagina. The levator bundles are held together between the rectum and the vagina by the fascia, which, with the tissues in the lower portion of the rectovaginal septum, make up the perineal body (Fig. 39-3, *B*). The bladder and the rectum are supported by the mus-

cle in the wall of each of the organs and the extensions of the endopelvic fascia in the rectovaginal and vesicovaginal septa.

PERINEAL LACERATIONS

Perineal lacerations are divided into four types, depending on their depth. In a *first-degree laceration,* the tear extends through the skin and the superficial structures above the muscles. In a *second-degree laceration,* the tear extends through the muscles of the perineal body but does not involve the sphincter ani. A *third-degree laceration* severs the sphincter, and with a *fourth-degree laceration* the anterior rectal wall is also torn. Perineal injuries usually occur as the structures at the vaginal outlet are overdistended during delivery of the head.

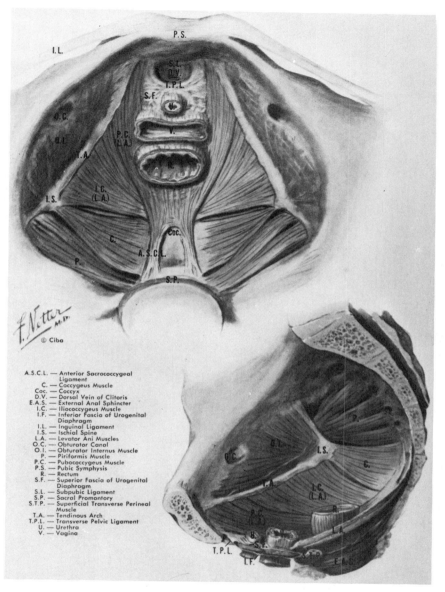

A.S.C.L. — Anterior Sacrococcygeal
　　　　　Ligament
　C. — Coccygeus Muscle
Coc. — Coccyx
D.V. — Dorsal Vein of Clitoris
E.A.S. — External Anal Sphincter
I.C. — Iliococcygeus Muscle
I.F. — Inferior Fascia of Urogenital
　　　　　Diaphragm
I.L. — Inguinal Ligament
I.S. — Ischial Spine
L.A. — Levator Ani Muscles
O.C. — Obturator Canal
O.I. — Obturator Internus Muscle
P. — Piriformis Muscle
P.C. — Pubococcygeus Muscle
P.S. — Pubic Symphysis
R. — Rectum
S.F. — Superior Fascia of Urogenital
　　　　　Diaphragm
S.L. — Subpubic Ligament
S.P. — Sacral Promontory
S.T.P. — Superficial Transverse Perineal
　　　　　Muscle
T.A. — Tendinous Arch
T.P.L. — Transverse Pelvic Ligament
U. — Urethra
V. — Vagina

Fig. 39-2 Muscles within pelvic cavity. (© Copyright 1954, 1965, CIBA Pharmaceutical Company. Division of CIBA-GEIGY Corporation. Reprinted with permission from The CIBA Collection of Medical Illustrations illustrated by Frank H. Netter, MD. All rights reserved.)

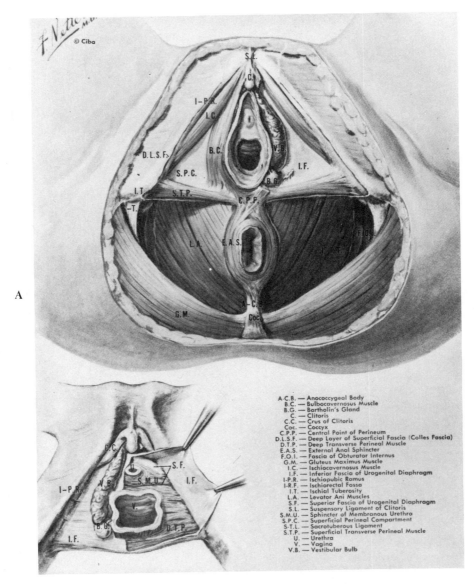

A.C.B. — Anococcygeal Body
B.C. — Bulbocavernosus Muscle
B.G. — Bartholin's Gland
C. — Clitoris
C.C. — Crus of Clitoris
Coc. — Coccyx
C.P.P. — Central Point of Perineum
D.L.S.F. — Deep Layer of Superficial Fascia (Colles Fascia)
D.T.P. — Deep Transverse Perineal Muscle
E.A.S. — External Anal Sphincter
F.O.I. — Fascia of Obturator Internus
G.M. — Gluteus Maximus Muscle
I.C. — Ischiocavernosus Muscle
I.F. — Inferior Fascia of Urogenital Diaphragm
I.P.R. — Ischiopubic Ramus
I-R.F. — Ischiorectal Fossa
I.T. — Ischial Tuberosity
L.A. — Levator Ani Muscles
S.F. — Superior Fascia of Urogenital Diaphragm
S.L. — Suspensory Ligament of Clitoris
S.M.U. — Sphincter of Membranous Urethra
S.P.C. — Superficial Perineal Compartment
S.T.L. — Sacrotuberous Ligament
S.T.P. — Superficial Transverse Perineal Muscle
U. — Urethra
V. — Vagina
V.B. — Vestibular Bulb

Fig. 39-3 A, Levator and superficial muscles from below. (© Copyright 1954, 1965, CIBA Pharmaceutical Company, Division of CIBA-GEIGY Corporation. Reprinted with permission of The CIBA Collection of Medical Illustrations illustrated by Frank H. Netter, MD. All rights reserved.)

At least the lower vagina is involved whenever the perineum is injured. The vaginal portion of the tear often extends up one or both lateral sulci rather than up the midline; the depth depends on the extent of the perineal injury. The levator fascia is injured in all but the most superficial perineal lacerations (Fig. 39-4, *A*).

Treatment

Perineal lacerations should be repaired immediately with chromic no. 3-0 or 4-0 catgut or polyglycolic sutures. The most superficial ones can be closed with one layer of interrupted sutures, but two or more layers may be necessary for the more extensive injuries. It often is advantageous to use no. 4-0 sutures on an atraumatic needle to close the wounds near the clitoris because the small needle and suture will provoke less bleeding. It is particularly important to repair third- and fourth-degree lacerations so that the patient can retain fecal continence (Fig. 39-4).

Late results

Perineal injuries that do not involve the levator ani usually produce no permanent disability, even though they are not repaired. If the severed ends

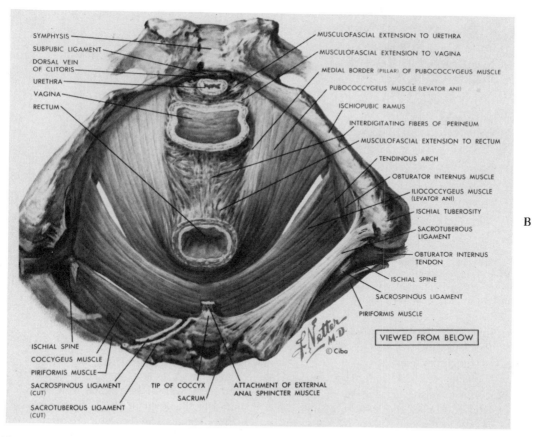

B

Fig. 39-3, cont'd B, Levator muscles from below; superficial muscles removed. (© Copyright 1954, 1965, CIBA Pharmaceutical Company, Division of CIBA-GIEGY Corporation. Reprinted with permission of The CIBA Collection of Medical Illustrations illustrated by Frank H. Netter, MD. All rights reserved.)

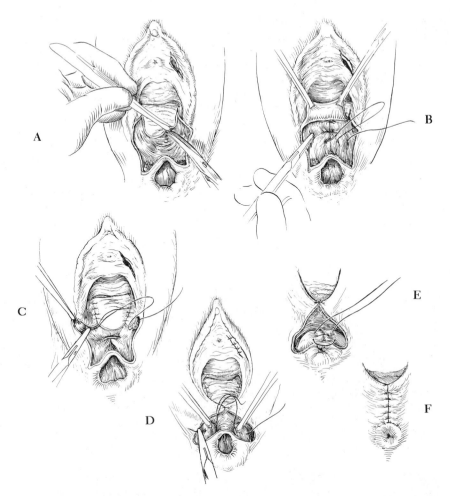

Fig. 39-4 Perineal lacerations. **A,** Bilateral sulcus tears, periurethral tear, and separation of anal sphincter. **B,** Exposure and approximation of levator structures. **C,** Approximation of torn bulbocavernosus muscle. **D and E,** Approximation of ends of anal sphincter. **F,** Complete repair.

of the superficial perineal muscles, particularly the bulbocavernosus, are not approximated, the vaginal introitus may gape.

If a sphincter tear is overlooked, the patient will probably be incontinent of feces unless the puborectalis portion of the levator ani muscle is strong enough to compensate for the torn sphincter. Because the levators and the sphincter are both involved in the injury, this usually does not occur.

VAGINAL LACERATIONS

Perineal injuries usually extend up the vaginal sulci and, if deep enough, will separate the levator ani from its attachments to the lateral vaginal and rectal walls. The vaginal wall may also be injured at the level of the ischial spines or in the vault. The tears in the vault are often circular and may be the result of forceps rotation, particularly if there is some degree of cephalopelvic disproportion.

INJURIES TO THE LEVATOR SLING

Perineal and vaginal lacerations may be relatively superficial, leaving the important deep supporting structures intact, or they may extend more deeply and interrupt the integrity of the levator sling and the endopelvic fascia. The extent of the visible laceration is usually obvious, but extensive damage to the deep supporting structures can occur even though there is no visible injury involving the skin or the vaginal wall.

As the presenting part descends through the birth canal and distends the lower vagina, the levator bundles are separated, and the levator fascia is stretched. If the fascial layer is unusually resilient, it can stretch enough to permit the birth of the baby and then return to normal, but more often it tears, permitting the levator muscles to separate and retract laterally.

The accompanying perineal and vaginal lacerations disrupt the fascial layer in the rectovaginal septum, destroying the support of the rectum anteriorly. The levator pillars may also be detached from the lateral walls of the rectum, further reducing its support. The lacerations usually are irregular, and the involved tissue is often badly bruised.

Serious lacerations can occur because labor terminates so forcibly and rapidly that the structures are torn apart rather than stretched slowly or because of disproportion between the size of the infant and that of the pelvis. Another common cause is a narrow pubic arch. As the head is delivering, it cannot fit snugly beneath the symphysis but is forced backward toward the posterior pelvis, putting undue strain on the soft tissues as it passes through the introitus.

Treatment

Immediate approximation of the torn levator structures and of the vaginal and perineal injuries will permit the tissues to heal and will reduce subsequent deformity. However, there may be a rather considerable amount of permanent relaxation of the repaired structures because they usually have been rather seriously injured by the extreme distension that preceded their final bursting.

Prevention

Even though the physician makes every possible effort to eliminate traumatic deliveries, the supporting structures will be injured unless special precautions are taken. *The most important measure for preventing serious posterior wall injury is episiotomy, or incision of the perineum and the underlying supporting structures.* Episiotomy should be performed on almost every primigravida and on most multiparas with intact pelvic supports.

If episiotomy is to offer maximum protection, the perineum must be incised before the tissues have already been stretched and injured by the advancing presenting part. The incision, which must be long enough to cut all the tissues holding the levator bundles together in the midline, is made when the perineum is flattened and bulging and when the vaginal opening is dilated about 6 cm during a contraction. A mediolateral or a median episiotomy (Figs. 39-5 to 39-7) will produce equally good results if the incision is made properly and at the right time and if it is carefully repaired.

Regional or general anesthesia is essential for the performance of an adequate episiotomy because it must be made before the tissues have been injured. The practice of making a small incision without anesthesia in the overstretched and blanched perineum offers no protection to the deep fascia and muscle; they already have been stretched to their maximum and have retracted so that only the superficial structures are cut.

The entire episiotomy is repaired meticulously with chromic no. 3-0 or 4-0 catgut or polyglycolic sutures, which produce relatively little local reaction. The repair should not be started until the placenta has been delivered and the uterus is well contracted. It is difficult to explore the uterus after the wound is closed unless the sutures are removed.

Late results

If injuries are left unrepaired, permanent defects in support may result. Occasionally, however, the same lesions develop in women whose

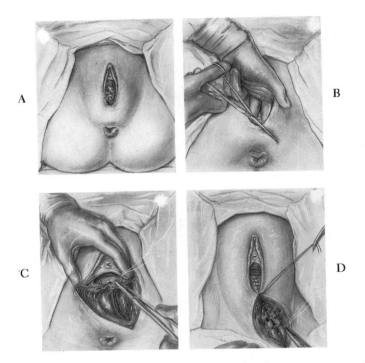

Fig. 39-5 Left mediolateral episiotomy. **A,** Incision is made before perineal structures are damaged. **B,** Incision from midline toward ischial tuberosity. **C,** Repair of vaginal wall. Sutures must include muscle layer, as well as epithelium. **D,** Approximation of levator bundles.

injuries have been carefully repaired, in those in whom an attempt has been made to prevent lacerations, and even in those who have never been pregnant.

Rectocele (Fig. 39-8). Unrepaired posterior lacerations disrupt the fascial support of the rectal wall, permit the levator bundles to retract laterally, and destroy the perineal body, thereby eliminating the normal support of the lower vagina. One of the functions of the perineal body is to deflect stool posteriorly toward the anal canal, through which it is evacuated. Loss of the midline support in the lower vagina and introitus permits the rectum and the posterior vaginal wall to sag anteriorly. Each time a woman with such a defect strains in an attempt to evacuate her rectum, the fecal mass is forced downward against the rela-

tively thin rectovaginal wall, stretching it a little more. The rectum gradually protrudes more and more into the vagina until eventually a large pouch may be visible through the relaxed introitus. This lesion, which is called a *rectocele,* is the most common late result of childbirth injury. Most rectoceles are small and produce few symptoms, but some are huge and bulge outside the vaginal canal whenever the patient stands up.

SYMPTOMS. The symptoms produced by a rectocele are related to the loss of muscular and fascial support and the consequent disturbance of bowel function. If the lesion is large, most women will experience "bearing down" and a sensation of lack of support when on their feet. They feel as though all the pelvic organs are going to fall out

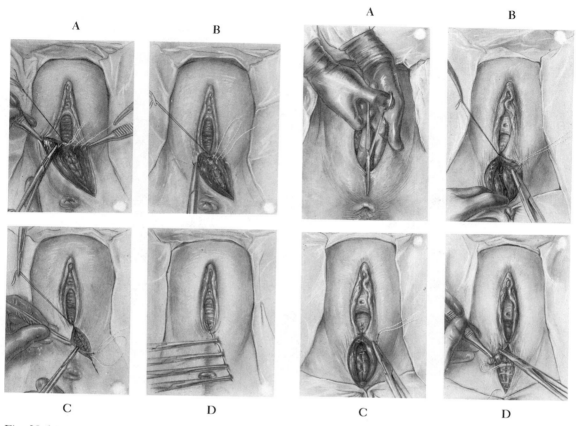

Fig. 39-6 Left mediolateral episiotomy, continued. **A,** Repair of bulbocavernosus muscle. **B,** Reconstruction of urogenital diaphragm. **C** and **D,** Skin closure.

Fig. 39-7 Median episiotomy. **A,** Incision to anal sphincter. **B,** Approximation of levator bundles. Vaginal incision has already been closed. **C,** Reconstruction of urogenital diaphragm. **D,** Skin closure.

through the introitus. They may also complain of the protrusion of a mass. Those with large rectoceles find it difficult to evacuate the rectum because the fecal material is pushed into the rectal pouch instead of being deflected toward the anal opening by the structures of the perineal body and the levator support of the lower rectum, which have been destroyed (Fig. 39-8). If questioned, these women usually state that they must hold the mass up with the fingers in the vagina to permit evacuation of fecal material. The fingers substitute for the intact vaginal wall and perineal body

and divert the fecal mass downward into the anal canal rather than toward the vagina. The symptoms disappear when these women lie down.

DIAGNOSIS. The diagnosis is made by observing the mass protruding from the vagina and identifying it as a rectocele by performing rectal and vaginal examinations. The relaxed posterior vaginal wall can be inverted through the introitus by the rectal finger.

TREATMENT. Symptom-producing rectoceles can be corrected only by an operative procedure by which the

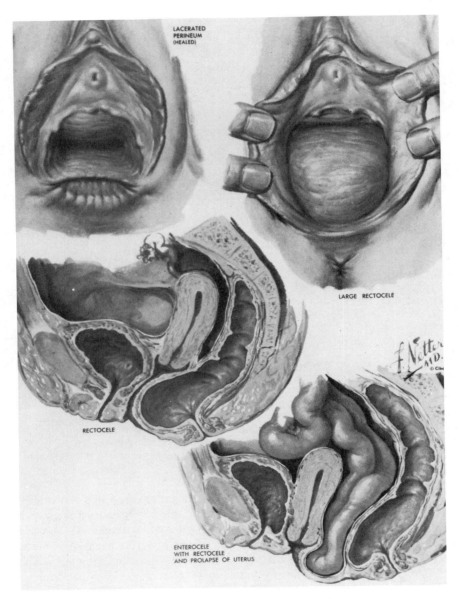

Fig. 39-8 Chronic posterior wall injuries. (© Copyright 1954, 1965, CIBA Pharmaceutical Company, Division of CIBA-GEIGY Corporation. Reprinted with permission from The CIBA Collection of Medical Illustrations illustrated by Frank H. Netter, MD. All rights reserved.)

separated levator muscles and their fascia and the structures of the perineal body are approximated in the midline between the anterior rectal and the posterior vaginal walls, thereby restoring the continuity of the supports. This procedure is performed with a vaginal approach and is called *perineorrhaphy* if the repair involves only the structures of the perineal body and lower rectum, *posterior colpoplasty* if the repair is more extensive, or more simply *posterior vaginal repair.*

Enterocele (Fig. 39-8). Enterocele, also called *posterior vaginal hernia* or *cul-de-sac hernia,* consists of herniation of the peritoneum of the posterior cul-de-sac downward between the uterosacral ligaments into the rectovaginal septum. The cul-de-sac in women who develop this defect probably is deeper than usual, and when its support is disrupted by childbirth injury, the weight of the intestine and omentum when the patient is on her feet gradually enlarges the sac and forces it downward between the rectum and the vagina. This lesion occurs frequently in association with prolapse of the uterus and after vaginal hysterectomy, particularly when it is performed as part of the treatment of vaginal relaxation.

SYMPTOMS. Enterocele produces few symptoms except pressure and a bearing-down sensation, which may be caused primarily by the relaxation of the other structures. Large enteroceles may protrude through the introitus.

DIAGNOSIS. On superficial inspection, an enterocele may resemble a rectocele, and in fact both lesions often are present in the same patient. Unless it is recognized and repaired, the first indication of its presence may be a persistent posterior wall bulge after rectocele repair or a herniation of the vaginal vault after vaginal hysterectomy.

TREATMENT. The hernia is usually treated by vaginal operation because rectocele and uterine prolapse are almost always present. An abdominal operation that accomplishes the same thing can also be performed but is not usually necessary.

INJURIES TO THE ANTERIOR VAGINAL WALL

In nulliparous women the bladder is supported by the integrity of the vesical and vaginal walls and by an extension of the endopelvic fascia between the inferior vesical wall and the anterior vaginal wall. During labor the bladder, which is attached to the anterior surface of the uterus, is pulled up out of the pelvis as the lower uterine segment elongates. As a consequence, only the urethra, the vesical neck, and a portion of the bladder floor are vulnerable to injury.

As the presenting part descends and dilates the vagina, the structures in the vesicovaginal septum are stretched or even torn in multiple areas beneath the vaginal epithelium. If the infant is unusually large, the delivery precipitous, or the bony pelvis small, more damage occurs than from the usual delivery. If there is some degree of disproportion, there may be so little room between the head and the bony walls of the pelvis that the soft-tissue structures are pushed down ahead of the presenting part while the bladder is pulled upward each time the uterus contracts. The combination of counterforces may damage the supporting structures of the upper uretha, the vesical neck, and the bladder itself. The same effect is produced if the soft tissues are relatively rigid and do not dilate properly as labor progresses.

Treatment

The vaginal epithelium covering the anterior wall is seldom torn during delivery; consequently, there is little obvious soft-tissue damage and nothing can be repaired at the time of delivery. Tears in the lateral or posterior vagina and those in the vault do not affect the bladder.

Prevention

Injuries to the anterior wall can be minimized by a few simple procedures. The performance of episiotomy will eliminate the resistance offered by the muscle and fascia posteriorly and will permit the head to descend through the posterior portion of the outlet, thereby decreasing pressure on the urethra and vesical neck. Low forceps extraction combined with episiotomy, if the delivery of the head is delayed, will also reduce anterior soft-tissue trauma, but difficult forceps operations may increase it.

Late results

Relaxation of bladder and urethral supports can develop as a result of pregnancy even though there was no obvious soft-tissue damage at the time of delivery.

Cystocele (Fig. 39-9). A cystocele, the protrusion of the bladder downward into the vaginal canal, develops because the supporting structures in the vesicovaginal septum have lost their integrity. As with rectocele, anterior wall relaxation is not present immediately after delivery but develops over time and often after the patient has had several babies. The weakened anterior vaginal wall descends because of the force of gravity and the weight of the abdominal organs when the patient is on her feet. Repeated stresses, for example, increases in intraabdominal pressure from lifting, straining, and coughing and the weight of accumulated urine in the bladder, gradually stretch the vesicovaginal septum until the bladder bulges into the vagina. With time a cystocele enlarges until it may protrude through the introitus.

The urethra may also be involved in anterior wall relaxation because it, too, can be injured during the expulsion of the baby. *Urethrocele* rarely develops unless the bladder also is injured. The combined lesion is a *cystourethrocele* (Fig. 39-9).

SYMPTOMS. Small cystoceles, and even some huge ones, produce few symptoms. Some women complain only of bearing-down sensations in the pelvis and the protrusion of a mass through the introitus when they are on their feet. The pressure and the mass disappear when they lie down. Urinary control is maintained unless urethral and vesical neck function is disturbed. In fact, many women with large cystoceles find it difficult to initiate voiding unless they push the sagging bladder upward with their fingers. The bladder usually empties itself reasonably well, and in most instances there is little residual urine.

DIAGNOSIS. The diagnosis of cystocele is made by identifying the vaginal bulge as involving the anterior wall. Unless there is an associated urethral injury, the urethra and bladder neck may be well supported behind the pubis even when the patient strains and the cystocele is pushed downward. The size of the pouch and the degree of protrusion can often be better appreciated by examining the patient while she stands upright.

TREATMENT. The bulge of the cystocele is obliterated by plicating the bladder wall with interrupted sutures after the cystocele has been exposed by deflecting the vaginal mucosa off it. This can be accomplished only by a vaginal approach because the involved area cannot be reached through an abdominal incision. The fact that a cystocele is present does not mean that treatment is necessary; only those that produce symptoms should be operated on.

Urinary incontinence. Many women experience uncontrollable leakage of urine, which in most instances is the result of an injury sustained during childbirth. However, other causes must also be considered. Five major categories of conditions can disturb urinary control:

1. *Stress urinary (anatomic) incontinence.* The loss of urine occurs with sudden increases in intraabdominal pressure such as that generated by sneezing or from sudden jarring movements. The loss is caused by structural injuries to the urethra and bladder neck.
2. *Detrusor dyssynergia.* The incontinence results from involuntary detrusor activity, which is triggered by a variety of stimuli.
3. *Urge incontinence.* Urge incontinence is characterized by the inability to keep from urinating when the urge to void occurs suddenly. Urge incontinence usually is caused by intrinsic disorders of the bladder and urethra, the most common being urethritis and urethral stricture, trigonitis, and cystitis.
4. *Neuropathies.* Neurologic disorders such as multiple sclerosis, diabetic neuritis, and diseases of or injuries to the spinal cord disturb the nerve control of bladder function. Such disorders usually cause overflow or uninhibited detrusor incontinence.
5. *Congenital and acquired urinary tract abnormalities.* Urinary tract abnormalities in-

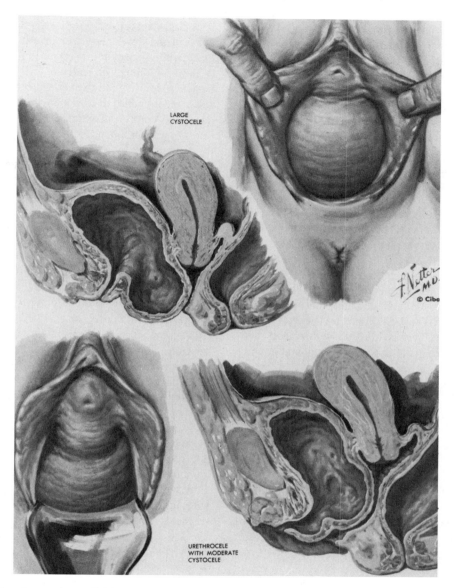

Fig. 39-9 Chronic anterior wall injuries. (© Copyright 1954, 1965, CIBA Pharmaceutical Company, Division of CIBA-GEIGY Corporation. Reprinted with permission from The CIBA Collection of Medical Illustrations illustrated by Frank H. Netter, MD. All rights reserved.)

clude congenital defects such as ectopic ureter, abnormal muscular development of the vesical neck, neurologic disorders, and acquired lesions such as urinary fistulas (p. 512) and destruction of all or part of the urethra. The incontinence is usually constant and unrelated to voiding, to activity, or to position.

Continence of urine is dependent on normal urethrovesical support, normal anatomic configuration, innervation and function of the structures involved in voiding, and normal urethrovesical pressure relationships. In women who are continent, the intraurethral pressure is always greater than the intravesical pressure except during voiding. When intravesical pressure is in the normal range, the differential is maintained principally by the primary urethral sphincter, an extension of the smooth muscle layers of the bladder wall that makes up the proximal 3 cm of the urethra. The tension provided by the voluntary muscle, fascia, and blood vessels that surround the urethra adds to the effect of the sphincter. Muscles in the lower urethra have little to do with urinary control; the entire distal third can be amputated without disturbing function.

When intravesical pressure is increased, for example, with coughing or straining, additional urethral pressure is supplied by voluntary contraction of the pubococcygeus muscle, which compresses the upper urethra and pulls it upward behind the pubis. The upper urethra and the urethrovesical junction lie within the abdominal cavity above the levator plate; hence increases in intraabdominal pressure are transmitted equally to the bladder and to the proximal urethra. Therefore changes in intraabdominal pressure do not affect the urethrovesical pressure relationships (Fig. 39-10, *A*).

Voiding is initiated by relaxation of the voluntary muscles and the urethral sphincter and by contraction of the detrusor muscles. As a consequence, the urethral lumen is widened and shortened as its relaxed proximal wall is drawn up and funneled by the contracting longitudinal muscle fibers in the bladder wall. The short, relaxed urethra offers little resistance to the flow of urine from the contracting bladder.

STRESS URINARY INCONTINENCE. Stress incontinence is the involuntary loss of urine precipitated by coughing, sneezing, laughing, or lifting and by walking, running, or sudden jarring changes in position. Many multiparous women have slight stress incontinence during menstruation but maintain good control at other times. If the dysfunction is more pronounced, incontinence is present throughout the month. In the most severe cases the patient loses urine with the slightest provocation and must wear protective pads constantly.

Some women develop mild incontinence after the birth of their first babies; in others it does not appear until they have had several. Many women first become incontinent after the menopause, and in most the symptoms become more annoying as the effects of estrogen deprivation on the tissues and blood vessels in the bladder neck, the urethra, and the surrounding structures increase.

Stress incontinence, also called *anatomic incontinence,* usually results from changes in the structure and function of the urethra and the urethrovesical junction caused by injury during childbirth. The extent of the dysfunction is determined by how much the tissues were disrupted during delivery and how completely they recovered. The basic problem is that the mechanism for increasing intraurethral pressure is disturbed, and it cannot respond rapidly and completely enough to compensate for sudden rises in intravesical pressure such as those that occur with coughing or sneezing. When intraabdominal pressure and, simultaneously, intravesical pressure is increased suddenly, urine spurts from the incompetent urethra. The principal anatomic defects associated with stress incontinence are *changes in the posterior urethrovesical angle* and *changes in the relationship of the urethra to the pubis (urethral axis).* The net result is that support of the vesical neck and the proximal urethra is altered and function is disturbed.

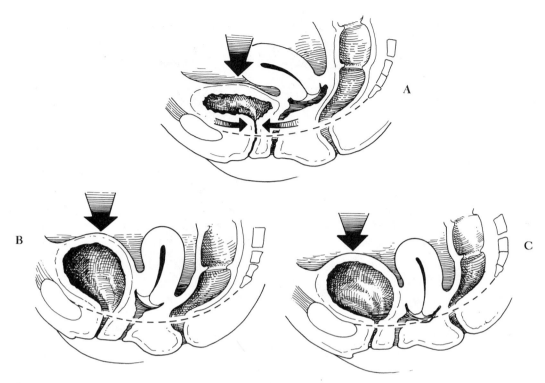

Fig. 39-10 Changes in urethrovesical angle and angle of inclination of urethra to perpendicular in normal women and with stress urinary incontinence. **A,** Vesical neck and proximal urethra above levator plate *(dotted line)*. Stress of increased intraabdominal pressure on bladder and proximal urethra *(arrows)*. **B** and **C,** Descent of proximal urethra and descent and funneling of vesical neck. Full force of increased intraabdominal pressure *(arrows)* and intravesical pressure against incompetent vesical neck and urethra.

In the normal bladder the posterior wall of the urethra and the flat base of the bladder form a 90- to 100-degree angle with each other. In women with stress incontinence the angle is lost, and the bladder neck is funneled and lies at the most dependent portion of the bladder (Fig. 39-11). Because these changes are like those that occur in continent women when micturition is initiated, patients with stress urinary incontinence are always in the preliminary voiding phase. Any increase in the intravesical pressure forces urine through the urethra.

The urethral axis, the angle of inclination of the upper urethra to the perpendicular while in the upright po-

sition, is another important factor in urinary control. In normal women the angle is no more than 30 degrees. In incontinent women it is increased, often to more than 90 degrees, because the urethra is displaced backward and downward (Fig. 39-11). The degree to which the posterior urethrovesical angle is lost and the urethra is displaced is an indication of how much the urethral support was altered by the injuries sustained during delivery.

An additional factor that may affect urinary control when urethral support has been disrupted is related to the transmission of intraabdominal pressure changes to the structures. If the vesical neck is displaced down-

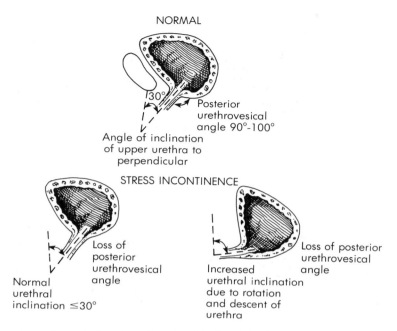

Fig. 39-11 Changes in urethrovesical angle and angle of inclination of urethra to perpendicular in normal women and those with stress urinary incontinence.

ward because the levator plate is weakened, it may lie outside the abdominal cavity. Increases in intraabdominal pressure are then transmitted to the bladder but not to the urethra. The difference between the elevated intravesical pressure and the unchanged intraurethral pressure is followed by a spurt of urine (Fig. 39-10, *B* and *C*).

Diagnosis. The diagnosis of stress incontinence is made on the basis of an accurate history, physical examination, and a variety of testing procedures. It is essential that stress incontinence be differentiated from other causes of incontinence because the treatment of each varies.

The typical patient with stress incontinence is multiparous, and many are already postmenopausal. The incontinence has gradually become more troublesome, and in some patients it may be so severe that they are wet much of the time. Characteristically, a small amount of urine spurts from the urethra immediately whenever the in-

traabdominal pressure is increased by laughing, sneezing, or coughing or when they walk, run, or even step off curbs. The loss of urine can usually be stopped by voluntary muscle contraction. It does not occur at night, it usually does not occur with simple changes in position, and there is no discomfort associated with voiding.

Relaxation of the structures that support the urethra and bladder neck can be demonstrated by asking the patient to bear down. The axis of the normally supported urethra in the lithotomy position is usually horizontal; if the supports are weakened, the bladder and the urethra will rotate backward and downward when intraabdominal pressure is increased.

The degree of change can be measured by the *Q-tip test* (Fig. 39-12). One inserts a lubricated cotton swab into the urethra to the level of the vesical neck and observes its change in relationship to the horizontal as the patient bears down.

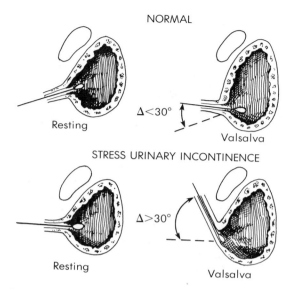

NORMAL

Resting

$\Delta < 30°$

Valsalva

STRESS URINARY INCONTINENCE

Resting

$\Delta > 30°$

Valsalva

Fig. 39-12 Q-tip test. With increased intraabdominal pressure the vesical neck descends and the handle of the Q-tip rotates more than 30 degrees with stress incontinence. Little movement occurs with normal support.

When the relaxed anterior vaginal wall and vesical neck descend as intraabdominal pressure is increased, the handle of the Q-tip rotates upward around the lower border of the pubis. If the structures are relaxed, the handle of the swab will rotate through an arc of at least 30 degrees. There is little motion if the vesical neck is well supported.

The integrity of the sphincter mechanism can be tested by having the patient cough vigorously or by having her hold her breath and bear down. Urine will spurt from the urethra if muscle control is defective. Of course, this test is uninformative when the bladder is empty. If the patient has voided shortly before examination, enough water should be instilled into the bladder to produce an urge to void. If she does not lose urine in the lithotomy position, the test should be repeated with the patient standing.

The *cystometrogram* in stress incontinence is normal, in contrast to that in detrusor dyssynergia, uninhibited neurogenic bladder, or irritable bladder. *Urethral closure pressure profiles* measure pressure at various levels of the urethra. The pressure, particularly in the upper urethra, is reduced in women with stress urinary incontinence. Defective bladder neck function can be seen by *urethroscopy,* and bladder lesions with *cystoscopy; urograms* usually are not necessary.

Treatment. In some women, particularly those with relatively little descent of the bladder and urethra, stress incontinence can be corrected by *systematic muscle exercise.* The patient is taught how to contract the pubococcygeus muscles that pull the bladder neck upward and angulate it to constrict the distal urethra. If the patient contracts the muscles 80 to 100 times a day and attempts to check the flow of urine suddenly while she is voiding, the pubococcygeus may become strong enough to prevent leakage. The exercise must be continued indefinitely. The administration of *estrogen* may improve urinary control in postmenopausal women with a good bit of local atrophic change but little obvious tissue relaxation. In addition to estrogen an alpha-receptor stimulating drug (phenylpropanolamine) may increase baseline urethral tone.

Another simple treatment, which often is effective, is to insert a *Smith-Hodge vaginal pessary.* The retropubic portion of the ring elevates the vesical neck, lengthens the urethra, and may improve urinary control. This may be used to indicate which patients will benefit from surgical repair.

Surgical treatment should be selected for patients with true stress incontinence that is not improved by muscle exercises and those who have large structural defects. Operation will make incontinence caused by neurogenic problems worse.

Most surgical procedures are directed toward restoring the integrity of the lost supports and particularly toward improving the function of the sphincter mechanism. If there is a large cystocele, this can usually be accomplished by a vaginal operation that obliterates the cystocele, elevates the bladder neck, reestablishes the urethrovesical angle, and narrows the urethral orifice. For some women, particularly those whose angles of inclination approach 90 degrees but with little additional anterior wall relaxation, an abdominal approach is preferred. In these operations, the urethra and vesical neck are pulled upward by sutures that attach the structures to the posterior surface of the pubis or to other pelvic fascias; this restores the urethrovesical angle and prevents the bladder neck from descending. More complicated procedures in which slings of rectus fascia or of plastic strips are used to support the bladder neck are seldom necessary.

DETRUSOR DYSSYNERGIA. Detrusor dyssynergia or unstable bladder is the responsible factor in incontinence in at least 10% of affected women. It can be suspected from the history and physical examination, but it can be diagnosed precisely only by urethrocystometry. The loss of urine occurs because of involuntary detrusor activity. The urine flow cannot be controlled voluntarily.

Diagnosis. Detrusor dyssynergia must be differentiated from both urge and stress incontinence, with which it shares some symptoms. The treatment for each varies.

The only symptom of mild detrusor dyssynergia may be frequency and urgency of micturition with occasional urge incontinence. The patient is unable to hold her urine long enough to get to the toilet after she first feels the urge to void. Incontinence is more troublesome in advanced cases.

In contrast to those with stress incontinence in whom a small amount of urine is lost simultaneously with an increase in intraabdominal pressure, the flow of urine in women with detrusor dyssynergia may start 10 to 20 seconds *after* the stress and continues for 5 to 10 seconds. A large amount of urine is lost, and the stream cannot be stopped voluntarily. Incontinence may be triggered by running, walking, or a change in position, but it does not characteristically follow coughing and sneezing. Some women lose urine when they hear water running. Incontinence caused by detrusor dyssynergia usually does not occur during the night, but the patient may lose urine as soon as she arises from bed in the morning.

Bladder and urethral support usually is normal, and the patient generally cannot demonstrate incontinence by coughing and straining, even though the bladder is full. Neurologic examination is normal. Abnormal detrusor activity can be detected by measuring the urethral and bladder pressures simultaneously or, if instrumentation for this procedure is not available, by cystometry alone.

The volume of urine that stimulates detrusor activity measures the functional capacity of the bladder. Normal women experience a strong urge to void when the bladder contains 400 to 500 ml of urine. Voiding is voluntary and can be prevented. In contrast, in the patient with an unstable bladder, detrusor activity is usually stimulated at a lower volume of urine, and voiding cannot be inhibited. Uninhibited contractions can often be induced during the test if the patient changes position, walks in place, or bounces up and down on her heels.

Treatment. The treatment of detrusor dyssynergia is medical; the incontinence is usually made worse by surgical procedures. The patient should be reassured that there are no structural or neurologic abnormalities, and she should be urged to try to gradually prolong the intervals between voiding. *Anticholinergic drugs,* which decrease excessive spontaneous bladder activity and uninhibited contractions, will usually relieve, or at least lessen, the symptoms.

OTHER CAUSES OF INCONTINENCE. Other than stress incontinence and detrusor dyssynergia, the major cause of incontinence in adult women is *urge incontinence* associated with urethral and bladder disorders. These include chronic urethrocystitis, the urethral syndrome, which may be caused by *Chlamydia* infection, urethral strictures, and other intrinsic bladder disorders. Urge incontinence must be differentiated from detrusor dyssynergia. Dysuria is not often a symptom of unstable bladder, but it often is present in women with urge incontinence because of the local disorder. The diagnosis is made by urethroscopy, cystoscopy, and urine culture. The incontinence can usually be corrected by treating the local condition appropriately.

Other causes of incontinence can be diagnosed by urologic and neurologic examinations.

INJURIES TO THE UTERUS
Cervical lacerations

The cervix is usually torn during delivery, but most lacerations are shallow and bleed little; consequently, they rarely constitute a major cause of postpartum hemorrhage and need no repair. More extensive lacerations that extend upward and particularly those that involve the lower segment may produce serious bleeding. These are most often caused by precipitous delivery or by ill-advised attempts to "dilate" the cervix artificially or to extract the infant before dilation is complete.

The cervix should be exposed and inspected after each hospital delivery. If a laceration other than a shallow nick is found, the defect should be closed with interrupted chromic no. 3-0 catgut sutures.

Rupture of the uterus

Rupture of the uterus is the most serious of the childbirth injuries, but fortunately it occurs only once in 1500 to 2000 deliveries. The uterus may rupture during pregnancy, but usually the wall gives way during labor.

Etiologic factors. During pregnancy the most frequent cause of rupture of the upper segment is *separation of a scar* from a previous classical cesarean section. Rupture of the normal uterus except by direct trauma seldom occurs. The ruptures that occur during labor also may involve a scar, but an intact uterus also can rupture. Injuries to the lower segment are frequently the result of *obstructed labor* from cephalopelvic disproportion or malposition. The presenting part cannot descend through the pelvis, and the continuing contraction and retraction of the muscle fibers in the upper segment stretch and thin the lower segment to a point at which separation occurs. Uterine rupture occurs more often in multiparas than in primigravidas. In the latter the response to fetopelvic disproportion is usually active phase arrest. The multiparous uterus continues to contract until it ruptures.

Other traumatic causes are the *administration of oxytocin* in doses that are too large or to a patient in whom stimulation is contraindicated (for example, obstructed labor, abnormal positions) and *operative deliveries* such as version and breech extraction. The uterus almost never ruptures during dysfunctional labor because the ineffective contractions do not stretch and thin the lower segment to a point at which the muscle fibers separate.

A *complete rupture* is one that extends through the entire uterine wall into the peritoneal cavity if the injury involves the upper segment, or into the broad ligament if the tear is in the lower segment; with an *incomplete rupture* the visceral peritoneum remains intact. There may be some external bleeding, but the major hemorrhage is often concealed within the broad ligament or the abdominal cavity unless the cervix as well as the uterine wall is involved.

Diagnosis. Rupture should be suspected when a woman in labor experiences sudden sharp, agonizing pain, uterine contractions cease, and clinical evidence of bleeding develops rapidly. If the baby has been extruded into the peritoneal cavity, it may be possible to palpate it outside the uterus, and the presenting part can no longer be felt through the cervix.

Rupture of a low segment cesarean section scar occurs infrequently and may produce no symptoms (Chapter 38).

Treatment. The possibility that the uterus may rupture during abnormal labor should always be considered, and necessary precautions should be taken to prevent its occurrence. *Elective repeat cesarean section* in those whose scars are most likely to separate will reduce the incidence of ruptures in these patients (Chapter 38). Recognition of the cause and proper management of *prolonged labor,* adequate *anesthesia* for operative deliveries, and the judicious use of *oxytocic drugs* will also serve as preventive measures.

Expectant management of a ruptured uterus is almost never warranted. Prompt transfusion with blood and laparotomy are usually indicated; it is necessary to perform hysterectomy unless the laceration is small, in which event it may be possible to repair it and leave the uterus intact.

Prognosis. The *perinatal mortality* is almost 100% if the fetus is extruded from the uterus into the peritoneal cavity. If labor is well advanced and the presenting part is deep in the pelvis at the time of the rupture, the infant may remain within the birth canal, and prompt delivery can save its life. The *maternal mortality* is primarily from hemorrhage and can be kept at a minimum by prompt and adequate treatment, but it may be as high as 20% to 50%.

INJURIES INVOLVING UTERINE SUPPORT

The major support for the uterus and the upper vagina is provided by the thickenings of the endopelvic fascia known as the cardinal or Mackenrodt's ligaments. They extend from about the level of the internal os and upper vagina laterally to blend with the fascia covering the obturator internus muscle (Fig. 39-1). The uterosacral ligaments are attached to the cervix posteriorly and below the level of the internal os. They pull the cervix upward and backward, thus rotating the fundus anteriorly.

Tearing of the cardinal ligaments during labor and delivery is rare, but they can be unduly stretched if descent is delayed by cephalopelvic disproportion, because of prolonged bearing-down efforts before the cervix is dilated, or if attempts are made to complete delivery forcibly before the cervix is fully dilated.

Late results

The axis of the uterus ordinarily forms an acute angle with the axis of the vagina, which in itself tends to prevent prolapse. Descent of the uterus can occur only when supporting structures such as the uterosacral ligaments and the cardinal ligaments relax, thereby altering the relationship of the uterus to the vaginal axis. This relaxation permits the cervix to sag downward into the vagina while the body of the uterus rotates posteriorly until its long axis lies in the axis of the vagina. If vaginal wall support also is compromised, the pressure of the abdominal organs on the uterus will gradually force it downward through the vaginal tube. The latter is inverted, carrying the bladder and rectum with it as the uterus descends toward the introitus.

Descensus, or *prolapse,* of the uterus may occur in infants, nulliparous women, and multiparas (Fig. 39-13). Defects in innervation and in the ba-

sic integrity of the supporting structures account for descensus in the first two groups and childbirth trauma for the third.

The uterus seldom descends immediately after delivery, but the defect develops gradually. The enlarging cystocele and rectocele that almost always accompany prolapse pull down on the uterus and cervix. As the cystocele enlarges and the cervix elongates, the ligaments become weaker until they can no longer hold the uterus in place. The more advanced stages of uterine prolapse are most often encountered in women past the menopause. Atrophy of the tissues eliminates whatever support was left.

A *first-degree prolapse* is one in which the cervix lies between the level of the ischial spines and the vaginal introitus. In *second-degree prolapse,* the cervix protudes through the introitus, while the corpus remains within the vagina. In *third-degree,* or *complete, prolapse* both the cervix and the body of the uterus have passed through the introitus, and the entire vaginal canal is inverted.

Symptoms. The symptoms of prolapse are primarily those related to the weight of the descending organs and their protrusion through the introitus. If the prolapsed cervix becomes ulcerated, it may bleed.

Diagnosis. The diagnosis is made by pelvic examination. The prolapse may reduce itself spontaneously when the patient lies down. Consequently, to determine the extent of the lesion it often is necessary to have the patient strain and push the cervix down, to exert traction on it with a tenaculum, and to examine her in an upright position. Prolapse must be differentiated from simple hypertrophy and elongation of the cervix that do not involve loss of uterine support.

Treatment. In general, the treatment of prolapse is operative, but, in certain poor-risk patients or those who are very old, a pessary may be inserted to hold the uterus in place. The physician should be certain that the patient actually is a poor operative risk before advising pessary support. Advanced age alone does not necessarily contraindicate surgical treatment (Fig. 39-14).

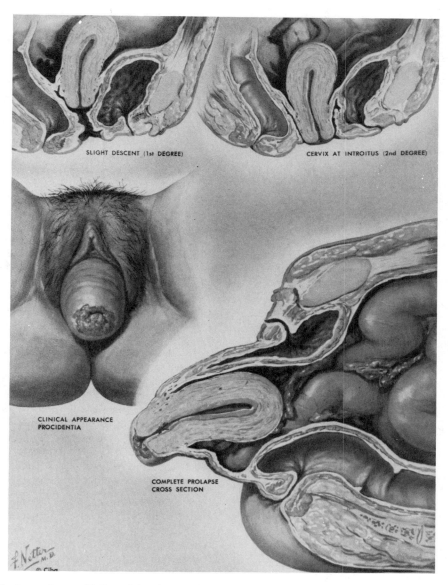

SLIGHT DESCENT (1st DEGREE)

CERVIX AT INTROITUS (2nd DEGREE)

CLINICAL APPEARANCE
PROCIDENTIA

COMPLETE PROLAPSE
CROSS SECTION

Fig. 39-13 Uterine prolapse. (© Copyright 1954, 1965, CIBA Pharmaceutical Company, Division of CIBA-GEIGY Corporation. Reprinted with permission from The CIBA Collection of Medical Illustrations illustrated by Frank H. Netter, MD. All rights reserved.)

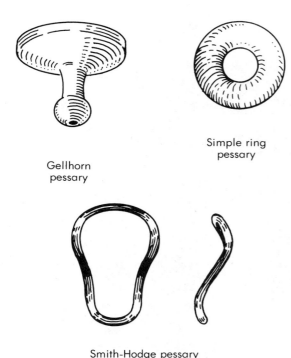

Gellhorn
pessary

Simple ring
pessary

Smith-Hodge pessary

Fig. 39-14 Types of pessaries used to support prolapsed uterus (Gellhorn and ring) and retrodisplaced uterus (Smith-Hodge).

Operative correction of prolapse rarely requires an abdominal operation. The faulty supporting structures can only be approached vaginally; hence procedures such as abdominal suspension of the uterus often fail because they do not correct the fundamental pathologic change. An effective operation usually includes vaginal hysterectomy; repair of the cystocele, rectocele, and enterocele; and shortening of the cardinal ligaments that are used to support the vaginal vault.

GENITAL FISTULAS

Fistulous openings between the bladder and the genital tract (vesicovaginal, vesicocervical, or vesicouterine), between the ureter and the vagina (ureterovaginal), and between the rectum and the vagina (rectovaginal) are caused by radiation, operative trauma, or injuries during labor and delivery.

Urinary tract fistulas

The most common urinary tract fistula is that which forms in the anterior vaginal wall, a *vesicovaginal fistula*. In past years almost all such fistulas were caused by necrosis of the vesicovaginal septum from pressure during delayed labor, but today the majority follow hysterectomy.

As a result of the abnormal opening, the patient is partially or completely incontinent of urine, and the constant flow of urine from the vagina excoriates the vulva and thighs. If the defect is large, all the urine will be passed through the vagina, but if it is small, the patient may void normally even though some of the urine seeps through the fistulous opening.

The diagnosis of vesicovaginal fistula is confirmed by demonstrating the opening between the bladder and the vagina and cystoscopic examination. If a small pack is placed in the vagina and methylene blue is instilled into the bladder, the dye will seep through the opening and discolor the pack.

Ureterovaginal fistulas usually develop because of devascularization or direct injury during radical operations for uterine cancer. The defect in the ureter develops near the ureterovesical junction, and the seepage of urine is usually first observed during the third week after the operation.

Indigo carmine, when injected intravenously, will be excreted in the urine, and, if there is a ureterovaginal fistula, some of the dye will enter the vagina and stain a pack. Because this will also occur with a vesicovaginal fistula, one more test is necessary to differentiate the two lesions: methylene blue instilled into the bladder will enter the vagina through a vesicovaginal fistula, but this will not occur if the defect is in the ureter. These tests combined with cystoscopy and pyelography should localize any urinary tract fistula accurately.

Treatment. Most vesicovaginal fistulas can be closed satisfactorily by an experienced gynecologist through a vaginal approach. The treatment of a ureterovaginal fistula is determined by its location. The injured ureter can either be implanted into the bladder (ureteroneocystostomy) or the severed ends can be anastomosed.

Rectovaginal fistulas

Rectovaginal fistulas are caused by infection in an episiotomy, a suture placed through the rectal wall during repair, or an unrecognized rectal injury incurred during delivery or vaginal repair.

They may also be caused by extension of cervical cancer or from radiation necrosis after its treatment. Most of the traumatic lesions are found near the vaginal opening, whereas those caused by radium and cancer are higher. All result in fecal incontinence and passage of fecal material from the vagina. These lesions can be differentiated from incontinence caused by complete perineal laceration by the fact that with a fistula the sphincter ani is intact.

Treatment. Rectovaginal fistulas can almost always be corrected by a surgical procedure, but, because the operative field is infected, the repair may break down. Colostomy may be necessary before surgery for complicated rectovaginal fistulas.

SEPARATION OF THE SYMPHYSIS PUBIS

The *symphysis pubis* always separates to some extent during delivery, but, if the baby is forcibly extracted or unusually large, a serious injury can be produced.

When the patient attempts to move or stand on her feet after delivery, she experiences severe pain in the region of the symphysis and in the sacroiliac joints. The symphyseal area is tender, and the ends of the pubic bones are widely separated. The bone ends are unusually mobile and can be felt to shift several centimeters when the patient shifts her weight from one foot to the other. The bladder neck and the urethra may be injured, and as a result the urine may be bloody.

Treatment of separation of the symphysis consists of immobilization of the pelvic girdle by a tight binder or adhesive strapping until the pubis heals. The symptoms diminish rapidly.

HEMATOMA FORMATION

A hematoma may form in the rectovaginal septum, in the episiotomy (Fig. 39-15), or in the base of the broad ligament after delivery. A large amount of blood can accumulate in the loose subcutaneous tissue of the labium without any evi-

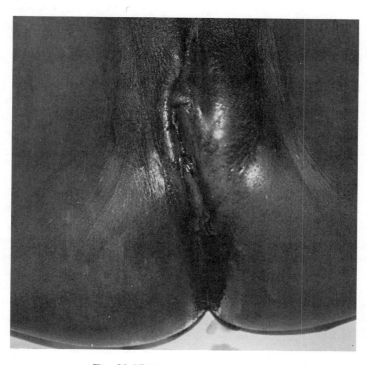

Fig. 39-15 Hematoma in episiotomy.

dence of external bleeding. The hematoma can also extend upward retroperitoneally, sometimes as high as the diaphragm. Evidence of shock may be one of the first signs of blood loss.

An enlarging hematoma causes pelvic pain and rectal pressure soon after delivery. Unfortunately, this is frequently attributed to the episiotomy and is treated symptomatically without examination. Inspection of the perineum generally reveals it to be distended and ecchymotic, and, when rectal examination is performed, it is easy to feel the tender mass.

A hematoma in the episiotomy, unless it is small and stable, must be evacuated. If the bleeding vessel can be demonstrated, it should be ligated. Occasionally, it is necessary to pack the cavity to check diffuse oozing, but the bleeding can almost always be controlled by resuturing the episiotomy. Small hematomas in the vaginal wall generally need no treatment.

RETRODISPLACEMENT OF THE UTERUS

The term *retrodisplacement* includes several situations in which the body of the uterus is displaced from its usual location overlying the bladder and occupies a position in the posterior pelvis. With *retroflexion* the fundus lies posteriorly, while the cervix retains its usual position in the vagina; the uterus is flexed in the region of the isthmus, the axis of the body forming an angle with the cervix. In *retroversion* the fundus rotates posteriorly and the cervix anteriorly around an axis at the level of the internal os. *Retrocession* indicates that the entire uterus has sagged backward into the posterior pelvis.

Retrodisplacement, which can be detected in 20% to 30% of all women, is caused by an alteration in the supporting structures of the pelvis. The uterus rotates in an anterioposterior plane around an axis situated approximately at the level of the internal os. Therefore anterior traction on the corpus or posterior and upward traction on the cervix will tend to rotate the uterus into an anterior position, with the fundus overlying the pubis and the cervix pointing toward the rectum, the long axis of the uterus forming an acute angle with the axis of the vagina. The anterior position

of the uterus is maintained by a number of forces: the *uterosacral ligaments* pull the cervix backward and upward, and the *round ligaments* help return the fundus to an anterior position if for some reason it is rotated posteriorly.

When a woman assumes an erect posture, the *intraabdominal pressure* and the loops of *intestine* pressing on the posterior surface of the uterus force the fundus toward the pubis, thereby rotating the cervix backward and upward until it lies above the level of the corpus. With the patient lying on her back, the fundus is directed toward the ceiling and may fall anteriorly or posteriorly; thus its position may vary from one examination to the next. If the bladder is distended, the fundus will be pushed posteriorly.

In some women the uterus is congenitally displaced and can be found lying posteriorly throughout their entire lives. In others, retrodisplacement develops after childbirth when the supporting structures are injured.

Symptoms. A retrodisplaced uterus may produce symptoms, but, when groups of women with retrodisplacements are compared with those whose uteri are in an anterior position, the same symptoms occur in about the same ratio in each group.

If the body of the retrodisplaced uterus is enlarged, boggy, heavy, and tender, it may cause pelvic pressure, low backache, and dyspareunia; it may even interfere with evacuation of the rectum. The uterus can be bound down in the posterior pelvis by the adhesions of endometriosis or those of the residua of pelvic infection, in which event symptoms are more often caused by the disease process itself than by the position of the uterus. A normal-sized, freely movable, retrodisplaced uterus rarely produces symptoms.

Diagnosis. The diagnosis of retrodisplacement is made by bimanual examination and by rectovaginal palpation. Either the axis of the cervix lies parallel with the axis of the vagina, or the tip of the cervix may point anteriorly toward the bladder. The body of the uterus can be felt lying in the posterior cul-de-sac by palpating behind the cervix through the posterior fornix (Fig. 39-16).

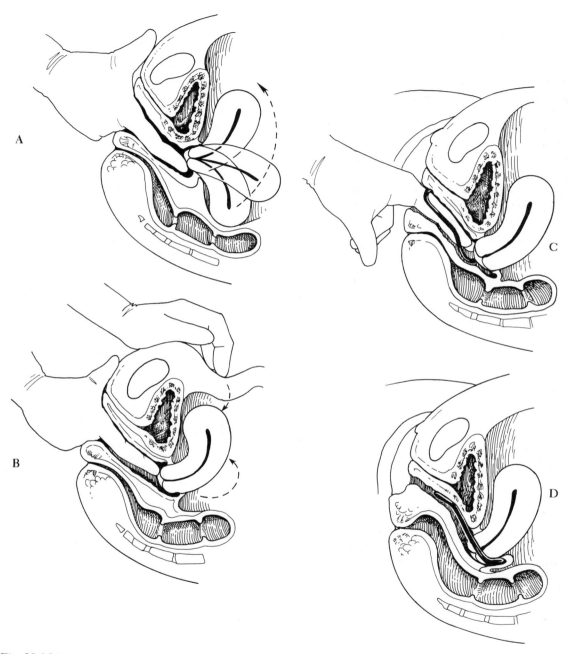

Fig. 39-16 Diagnosis and pessary support of retrodisplaced uterus. **A,** The fundus of the uterus can be felt in the posterior cul-de-sac. **B,** Uterus returned to anterior position by combined vaginal and abdominal manipulation. **C,** Pessary insertion. **D,** Pessary in place with superior bar elevating the posterior fornix, inferior bar beneath symphysis pubis, and lateral bars resting on levator muscles.

It sometimes is difficult to differentiate a retro-displaced uterus from one in normal position with a fibroid arising from the posterior wall and occupying the cul-de-sac or from an ovarian tumor prolapsed behind the uterus. If a sound is inserted into the uterine cavity, the physician can usually tell which way the fundus points.

Treatment. There is no need to suggest treatment for a retrodisplacement unless the patient has symptoms such as pelvic pain, dysmenorrhea, pressure, or infertility that could possibly be related to the position of the uterus. If the symptom is relieved after the uterus has been replaced and held in an anterior position by a proper pessary and recurs when it is permitted to fall posteriorly, the physician can suspect a relationship between the position of the uterus and the symptom. If, on the other hand, the symptom is still present after the retrodisplacement has been corrected, no such relationship can be assumed.

The initial therapeutic step in studying a patient with a retrodisplaced uterus and a pelvic symptom is actually diagnostic. The uterus is elevated by combined vaginal and abdominal manipulation, and a suitable pessary is inserted into the vagina to maintain the anterior position. The pessary is left in place for 2 to 3 months.

If the symptoms are not eliminated by elevating the uterus, they obviously are not caused by its posterior position. If they are relieved while the pessary is in place and recur when the uterus falls backward after it is removed, it can be assumed that the symptoms are caused by the retrodisplacement, and surgical correction can be considered. Operation to correct retrodisplaced but otherwise normal uteri should rarely be necessary. In many instances the uterus falls back without the support of the pessary, but the symptoms do not recur. In such patients no further treatment is necessary. Long-continued pessary treatment is generally unwarranted.

Uteri that are fixed in the cul-de-sac by endometriosis or chronic tuboovarian infection are not suitable for pessary treatment because the uterus usually is so firmly bound down that it cannot be moved without an operation.

SUGGESTED READING

Bhatia NN, Bergman A, and Gunning JE: Urodynamic effects of a vaginal pessary in women with stress urinary incontinence, Am J Obstet Gynecol 147:876, 1983.

Bhatia NN and Ostergard DR: Urodynamics in women with stress urinary incontinence, Obstet Gynecol 60:552, 1982.

Byrne DJ, Stewart PA, and Gray BK: The role of urodynamics in female urinary stress incontinence, Br J Urol 59:288, 1987.

DeLancey, JOL: Structural aspects of urethrovesical function in the female, Neurourol Urodyn 7:509, 1988.

Fantyl JA: Urinary incontinence due to detrusor instability, Clin Obstet Gynecol 27:474, 1984.

Gainey HL: Postpartum observation of tissue damage, Am J Obstet Gynecol 70:800, 1955.

Golan A, Sandbank O, and Rubin A: Rupture of the pregnant uterus, Obstet Gynecol 56:549, 1980.

Green TH Jr: Urinary stress incontinence: differential diagnosis, pathophysiology, and management, Am J Obstet Gynecol 122:368, 1975.

Hajj SN: Female urinary incontinence: a dynamic evaluation, J Reprod Med 23:33, 1979.

Kegel A: Progressive resistance exercise in functional restoration of perineal muscles, Am J Obstet Gynecol 56:238, 1948.

Langmade CF and Oliver JA Jr: Simplifying the management of stress incontinence, Am J Obstet Gynecol 149:24, 1984.

Mengert WF: Mechanics of uterine support and position, Am J Obstet Gynecol 31:755, 1936.

Ostergard DR and McCarthy TA: Diagnostic procedures in female urology, Am J Obstet Gynecol 137:401, 1980.

Plauche WC, von Almen W, and Muller R: Catastrophic uterine rupture, Obstet Gynecol 64:792, 1984.

Ranney B: Enterocele, vaginal prolapse, pelvic hernia: recognition and treatment, Am J Obstet Gynecol 140:53, 1981.

van Geelen JM, Lemmens WAJG, Esokes TKAB, and Martin CB Jr: The urethral pressure profiles in pregnancy and after delivery in healthy nulliparous women, Am J Obstet Gynecol 144:636, 1982.

40

William J. Ledger

Obstetric and gynecologic infections

Objectives

RATIONALE: Although there has been a surge in our understanding of the microbiology of pelvic infection and the introduction of a plethora of new antibacterial agents, pelvic infections still occur in the 1990s.

The student should be able to:
  A. Describe a multibacterial pelvic infection.

  B. List the organisms that often cause a mild inapparent infection in the mother with the capability of seriously damaging the newborn.
  C. Describe an antibiotic strategy for the treatment of soft tissue pelvic infection.

The range of response of women to infection is wide. Although serious problems are much less common now, physicians cannot ignore the potential problems of infection. Sepsis from gram-negative aerobes and coagulase-positive *Staphylococcus* can be life-threatening in the 1990s, and pelvic abscesses from gram-negative anaerobic bacteria, which often require operative intervention for a cure, still occur. In contrast to these obvious clinical problems, infections can have a subtle clinical presentation. Many women with salpingitis, which results in blocked tubes, have minimal symptoms without fever, and serious newborn infections can occur with no maternal symptomatology. These varying patient pre-

sentations require physician awareness of the potential of serious outcomes, plus knowledge of diagnostic and therapeutic interventions.

INFECTIONS DURING PREGNANCY THAT CAN AFFECT THE FETUS

Pregnant women are as susceptible to infection as other women. In most instances, infections neither affect the infant nor alter the course of the pregnancy. However, there are exceptions.

Maternal infections with a potential for unfavorable fetal outcome have many common clinical characteristics, even though they are caused by a wide variety of pathogens ranging from viruses to protozoa. In most cases, the maternal in-

---

TORCH SYNDROME

T	Toxoplasmosis
O	Other organisms
R	Rubella
C	Cytomegalovirus
H	Herpes

---

fection is inapparent or mild; however, the impact on the fetus can be severe. To help categorize these infections, the acronym the *TORCH* syndrome cateorizes the different infections based upon the first letter of the offending organisms (see the box above). As the number of other offending organisms has grown with continued medical observation, the list has become quite long. In spite of these obvious shortcomings, this classification does provide a framework for discussion.

Toxoplasmosis

Toxoplasmosis, an important infection, is poorly understood by most obstetricians. It is important because, although uncommon, it is a more frequent infection of the newborn than syphilis, and it responds to treatment with therapeutic agents. It is poorly understood because 90% or more of patients are asymptomatic, and many obstetricians too often become confused by the serologic tests used to confirm the diagnosis.

The parasite *Toxoplasma gondii,* which causes toxoplasmosis, can be transmitted to humans from raw meat or cat feces, both of which can contain infective oocytes. The fetus can be infected as a result of parasitemia during the initial acute attack. *Fetal infection does not occur as a result of chronic maternal infection.*

The infant response to infection can be predicted by the timing of the infection. If exposed in the first trimester, a small number of babies will be infected, but those infected are more likely to have serious problems including encephalitis, microcephaly, hydrocephaly, chorioretini-

tis, convulsions, hepatosplenomegaly, jaundice, and mental retardation than the babies of women infected later. Infants infected in third trimester are more likely to be infected at birth and are less likely to have serious problems because the disease has not been present long enough to progress to the point of irreversible tissue damage. Detection of infection immediately after birth is important because chemotherapeutic agents that can stop the progression of the disease are available.

Physician may not detect infection in women with no clinical symptomatology because toxoplasmosis is usually diagnosed by the appearance of antibodies in the serum. A prepregnancy antibody titer is a helpful starting point because the presence of antibodies indicates a previous exposure to toxoplasmosis and means the patient need have no concern about toxoplasmosis during this or any subsequent pregnancy. Too often, unfortunately, antibodies are first detected at the time of the first antepartum visit. In these instances, the antibody test can be repeated and an IgM antibody test done as well, which, if positive, indicates an acute infection. The diagnosis of an acute infection during pregnancy is not the end of the evaluation unless it is detected in the first trimester and the patient wants the pregnancy to be terminated. Alternatively, fetal blood sampling in utero should be done to evaluate fetal blood for IgM and determine if this infant has been infected. Treatment with spiramycin can be initiated during pregnancy. This drug is not approved by the FDA at present and requires individual clearance before it can be given. Although this treatment does not prevent all newborn infections, it does cut down the frequency and severity of subsequent problems.

Other infections

Hepatitis B. Hepatitis B virus can cause serious problems for the newborn. The virus from an asymptomatic mother can be transmitted to the fetus across the placenta. If undetected, the newborn can become a carrier of the virus and later develop chronic hepatitis and in some cases a liver malignancy. The mother's carrier state can be discovered by blood testing during the pregnancy; if she is found to carry the virus, the newborn can be treated at birth with hepatitis B immunoglobulin. Simultaneously, hepatitis B vaccine should be given so that the newborn can manufacture his or her own antibodies and thus not become a carrier.

An influx of immigrants from the Far East and the Caribbean, both areas in which hepatitis B is an endemic disease, as well as the widespread use of intravenous drugs among the poor in the United States, has increased the incidence of hepatitis B. Although high-risk groups have been identified, the current recommendation is to screen all pregnant women for the hepatitis B antigen to detect those who are asymptomatic carriers of the hepatitis B virus.

Human immune deficiency virus. The human immune deficiency virus (HIV) has become a new problem for the newborn in the United States in the past decade, particularly among urban poor pregnant women who have been intravenous drug users or whose male sexual partners are intravenous drug users. The obstetrician caring for these asymptomatic women has two potential problems. The newborn can become infected transplacentally and succumb to one of the opportunistic infections in the nursery after birth, often before the mother becomes symptomatic. In addition, the secretions of infected mothers and babies, particularly blood, are potential sources of HIV infection to the medical attendants.

The medical care of patients infected with HIV has been a complex problem. In the United States to date, they have been concentrated in those hospitals that care for the urban poor. Attempts to screen the high-risk population selectively were as unsuccessful as they were for hepatitis B. Too many carriers were missed. The solution to this dilemma is the same as it was for hepatitis B. For an urban poor population with a known incidence of prior exposure and infection with HIV, universal screening is medically indicated. However, many unresolved aspects prevent implementation

of this policy. It has become more of a political than a medical issue, because of justified concerns about confidentiality of test results and knowledge that false-positive results would be devastating for individuals from a population that has a low incidence of disease. These concerns to date have taken priority over needs for medical information about the carrier state.

This situation was probably partially justified when no medical intervention was available for those women who were HIV antibody positive. However, several new additions to the equation add weight to the argument for more HIV screening. For those who are HIV positive, AZT (zidovudine), has the potential to prolong survival. Close observation, testing, and treatment for *Pneumocystis carinii* pneumonia, tuberculosis, and syphilis are indicated in this population. In addition, these women can be given the option to terminate the pregnancy, with the knowledge that close to 50% of such newborns will be infected with the virus and are likely to die subsequently of complications of HIV infection. Nevertheless, to date the clinical experience has been that most pregnant women who know they are HIV positive do not elect termination, and many have repeated pregnancies. For the medical team, awareness of the HIV status of the mother should result in more careful techniques during pregnancy and at the time of delivery to prevent any contamination of the medical team with maternal and newborn blood and secretions.

Group B beta hemolytic streptococcus. The Group B beta hemolytic streptococcus can be the cause of severe infection in the newborn, resulting in significant mortality and among the survivors central nervous system morbidity. The fetus most at risk is the premature newborn following vaginal delivery from a mother with heavy vaginal colonization of the group B streptococcus and absent maternal serum antibodies. Prevention of this problem remains difficult. Many women who are infected deliver infants who are free of infection. The ratio in some series is 100:1. Using systemic antibiotics during pregnancy to eliminate colonization is usually ineffective. All high-risk mothers—those with premature labor and those with premature rupture of membranes—should be cultured for the presence of this organism. Treatment of the mother in labor with antibiotics such as penicillin (or erythromycin for the penicillin-allergic mother) is associated with an improved infant survival rate. The development of rapid techniques to detect the group B beta hemolytic streptococcus will be an important addition to more selective therapy.

Syphilis. The spirochete *Treponema pallidum* can cross the placenta and infect the fetus. The fetal manifestations are protean, with bone and soft-tissue lesions the most frequently seen. In nearly every case, the mother is asymptomatic; thus the physician must depend on serologic testing for syphilis to confirm the diagnosis. The universal screening tests for syphilis are reagin tests. They have the advantage of being simple to do, with reproducible results and titers, and they can be used as a measure of the patient's response to treatment. They have the major disadvantage of being nonspecific, so that a positive test does not always indicate infection by *Treponema pallidum*. In a pregnant patient with a positive reagin test, a specific antibody test for *Treponema pallidum* should be done. The fluorescent treponemal antibody-absorption test (FTA-ABS) can be performed to confirm the diagnosis. If the tests are positive, treatment is indicated for the mother and the fetus. Because *Treponema pallidum* is quite susceptible to penicillin and replicates slowly (approximately every 24 hours), a long-acting penicillin that does not achieve high levels in maternal or newborn sera is the treatment of choice. If the physician can confirm that the infection was acquired within the past year, a single shot of 2.4 million units of benzathine penicillin suffices. If the infection was acquired more than a year before or at an unknown time, this first dose should be followed by two subsequent doses at weekly intervals. Erythromycin has not proven effective because of the low levels achieved in the fetus. Therefore, the penicillin-allergic mother should be desensitized and given penicillin. The incidence of syphilis in the United States has risen markedly in the past few years, and obstetricians should be more aware of it as a diagnostic possibility, particularly in an urban poor population.

Tuberculosis. *Mycobacterium tuberculosis* can infect the placenta and then be disseminated to the newborn. The primary site of infection is nearly always the lungs. It is an important clinical entity, the incidence of which is increasing in the United States, particularly among the urban poor. This disease is frequently found in women who are HIV antibody positive.

Over the years, a diagnostic formulation has evolved that may not be appropriate for a high-risk population. In order to reduce radiation exposure, pregnant women are skin tested and, if positive, receive chest x-rays to see if any active lung lesions could be detected. This skin test screening may be inappropriate for a high-risk population in which some women with disseminated disease are skin test negative. In these groups, a routine chest x-ray screening examination is a better course of action.

Fortunately, chemotherapeutic agents are available for treatment. Two drugs are used in combination because they are more effective and resistance occurs much more slowly. Ethambutol is often used with isoniazid (INH). Supplemental pyridoxine should be used with INH, to prevent any deficiency from developing.

Varicella (chickenpox). Varicella can be a life-threatening infection in an adult, and transplacental infection can occur. It can cause skin scarring in the fetus, as well as limb defects and low birth weight if acquired early in pregnancy. If active maternal disease is detected just before delivery, the newborn can be given specific varicella zoster immune globulin (VZIG). Although most adults have had chickenpox, many are not aware of their past history with the organism. In these cases, a prenatal varicella antibody titer is helpful, for it eliminates maternal concerns if an exposure to a child with chickenpox occurs sometime later during pregnancy.

Rubella (German measles)

Gregg reported a high incidence of congenital defects in the eyes of infants whose mothers had contracted rubella during early pregnancy. Swan later calculated that 74.4% of infants would develop a congenital malformation if the maternal infection occurred during the first 4 months of pregnancy.

Cooper and Krugman, studying 344 infants with congenital rubella diagnosed during the first 18 months of life, found 73 to be normal and 271 abnormal. Defects diagnosed included congenital heart disease (142), hearing loss (140), cataract or glaucoma (107), psychomotor retardation (109, of which 65 were severe or moderate), and neonatal purpura (58). Thirty-five infants died. Other manifestations of congenital rubella found in 58 infants with neonatal purpura included hepatomegaly (72%), splenomegaly (69%), congenital heart disease (67%), eye lesions (45%), adenopathy (22%), bone lesions (22%), hepatitis (19%), anemia (17%), and genitourinary defects (7%). Progressive sclerosing panencephalitis has been reported to occur during the second decade of life as a late complication of congenital rubella.

Many infants who survive have prolonged active viral infections. Rubella virus has been cultured from infected infants well past the second year of life. An infant who sheds virus obviously can serve as a source of infection for others. Susceptible nurses and physicians who are or might become pregnant should not care for infants with congenital rubella unless they have antibodies to the disease. This testing should be a condition for employment in hospitals. Those without antibodies can be immunized. This precaution is necessary not only for their own protection but also to protect susceptible pregnant women who will have contact with them during the antepartum period.

Other effects of rubella during early pregnancy are spontaneous abortion, premature delivery, and intrauterine fetal death.

Therapeutic abortion is justifiable whenever unquestioned rubella is contracted during the first 20 weeks after the onset of the last menstrual period, unless the parents are willing to accept the risk of the infant's being affected.

Termination should also be considered for women who acquire infections late in the second trimester. Hardy and coworkers found only 7 normal children among a group of 22 whose mothers had had rubella between the thirteenth and thirty-first weeks. Two others died. Only 4 of 11 infants of women who had rubella after the twentieth week were normal. Of the 7 abnormal infants four had psychomotor disturbances (3 were retarded), 2 others had congenital anomalies, 5 had small heads, and all 9 infants who were examined shed virus.

Before abortion is approved, it must be ascertained that the patient actually had rubella. An exact clinical diagnosis, particularly in retrospect, is difficult because the course of rubella is much like that of several other viral infections. A precise diagnosis can be made on the basis of antibody studies. Hemagglutination-inhibition (HI) antibodies are not present in susceptible persons, but they can be detected within 48 hours after the appearance of the rash and reach a peak within 2 weeks.

The HI titers can be used to differentiate rubella from other nonteratogenic virus infections only by demonstrating a rise in titer after the acute infection. It is essential therefore that the titer be determined within 2 or 3 days after the appearance of the rash and again about 2 weeks later. A significant increase in titer on the second test indicates that the infection actually was rubella.

A high HI titer on a single test 1 to 2 weeks after a presumed rubella infection is of no diagnostic significance; there is no way to determine from such a single examination whether the elevated titer occurred in response to an infection years or days before the study.

A test for complement-fixing antibodies can provide an answer. These antibodies appear a few days after the onset of the rash and reach peak levels 3 to 5 weeks later. If both HI and complement-fixing antibodies are elevated, the infection was a recent one. An elevated HI titer without complement-fixing antibodies suggests a remote infection that will not affect the embryo. Rubella-specific IgM antibody response can be demonstrated shortly after the rash appears. Because the response rises and falls fairly rapidly, the absence of response several weeks after exposure or illness does not eliminate rubella.

A rubella antibody study should be performed at the first prenatal visit. If the titer is 1:8 or more, the woman is immune. If it is less than 1:8, she is susceptible, and the appearance of antibodies after an acute illness will be diagnostic of rubella.

Approximately 10% of women of childbearing age in this country are susceptible to rubella. If unprotected women are discovered and vaccinated before they become pregnant, the chances of their developing clinical rubella are minimal. Although rises in HI and complement-fixing antibody responses occur in as many as 80% of vaccinated persons during rubella epidemics, the clinical evidence is that the fetuses of the vaccinated women are protected.

Rubella antibody testing should be a part of every premarital and prepregnancy examination if it has not already been done. Those who are susceptible can then be immunized. The possibility of pregnancy must be eliminated before a woman is vaccinated.

Rubella vaccinelike virus has been recovered from fetal tissues after vaccination during pregnancy, but there is no danger of congenital abnormality with the vaccination. Preblud and colleagues determined the outcome of the pregnancies of 633 women who were vaccinated between 4 weeks before and 16 weeks after the estimated date of conception. The immune status of two thirds of the women was not known, 27.6% were susceptible, and 5.7% were immune when they were vaccinated. Of the total, 24 aborted spontaneously, abortion was induced in 197, and the outcome was unknown in 48. None of the 364 newborn infants, including the 112 whose mothers were known to be susceptible to infection when they were vaccinated, had congenital anomalies.

Patients should be advised not to become pregnant for three months after vaccination. If they do, abortion can be offered because the virus is live even though there is no risk of congenital defect. One of the best times to immunize a woman whose susceptibility has been discovered during pregnancy is while she is still in the hospital after delivery.

Cytomegalovirus

Cytomegalovirus disease is the most common of all congenital infections. About 10 of 1000 newborn infants excrete cytomegalovirus, and characteristic immediate or remote changes caused by infection with the virus can be recognized in at least one of 1000. The most serious effects include microcephaly, hydrocephaly, cerebral calcification, deafness, chorioretinitis, hepatosplenomegaly and jaundice, thrombocytopenia, hemolytic anemia, and convulsions. Some of those in whom the initial infection was mild and unrecognized have impaired intelligence and hearing defects.

The precise mechanism by which the fetus or newborn infant is infected is not known. At least 60% of the general population have acquired antibodies to the virus by the age of 35 to 40. The virus can be transmitted across the placenta to the fetus as a result of a new maternal infection or much less commonly by a new infection in a patient with previous antibodies. The virus is present in the cervical secretions of at least 5% of all women during pregnancy, and the recovery rate increases as pregnancy advances; hence the infant may become infected during delivery. The virus can be recovered from breast milk, urine, tears, and saliva; thus infection can also occur during the neonatal period.

Griffiths, Campbell-Benzie, and Heath found cytomegalovirus complement-fixing antibodies in 57% of 5575 women at the first prenatal examination. Repeat studies in 1608 who had been seronegative at the first test indicated that 14 (0.87%) had experienced a primary infection during pregnancy. Although 14 infants appeared normal at birth, one child subsequently developed a hearing defect, and another was microcephalic. The presence of maternal antibody is not totally protective for the fetus, but the most serious newborn outcome occurs in those women who have a primary infection during pregnancy. There is a significant acquisition of cytomegalovirus by mothers with infants in day care centers. Susceptible pregnant women should be aware of this danger.

Because acute cytomegalovirus infection in adults may cause only minor symptoms, there is no good way to anticipate the birth of an affected fetus. It may be worthwhile to evaluate pregnant women for the presence of antibodies to cytomegalovirus in the first trimester and repeat the testing in the third trimester in susceptible women. No effective treatment is available for either the mother or an infected newborn, although much research has been done to develop a vaccine.

Chlamydial infections. These infections are caused by an obligatory intracellular parasite, *Chlamydia trachomatis*. It has been isolated mainly from the lower genital tract of both males and females and is one of the most common sexually transmitted diseases. Chlamydial cervicitis, like gonorrhea, can be asymptomatic; in fact, the two are often found concomitantly in the cervix. Acute and chronic chlamydial infections in the female involve the cervix and fallopian tubes. In the male, nongonococcal urethritis and epididymitis are usual effects. Maternal chlamydial cervicitis poses a risk to the neonate or newborn infant. *Inclusion conjunctivitis* of the newborn, an acute mucopurulent infection, is now several times more often the cause of ophthalmia than is gonorrhea. *Neonatal pneumonia* caused by *C. trachomatis* does not occur as frequently, and symptoms tend to develop insidiously after discharge from the hospital. Infections usually respond to treatment with tetracycline or erythromycin.

Laboratory diagnosis is difficult, but new techniques hold promise. Rapid evaluation using a monoclonal antibody technique provides an accurate diagnosis in most cases and has replaced cell culture techniques in most hospitals.

Herpes (Herpes simplex)

Herpes simplex can be a serious problem for the newborn, but the mode of spread is different from most of the other members of the TORCH family. Transplacental infection is rare; instead, the fetus is infected by exposure to the virus in the birth canal.

The prevention of newborn infection by herpes simplex is still in a state of flux because so little is known about mechanisms of transmission. Much information has been obtained. Clearly women whose first genital herpes infection occurred just before delivery are more likely to deliver infected newborns than are those who have previously had genital herpes and who have serum antibodies. If a woman has active genital herpes lesions at term and when membranes have been ruptured for less than 4 hours, cesarean section decreases the risk of newborn infection. What is not known is the exact method of transmission. The majority of newborn infections occur in women with no genital herpes lesions, many of whom have no history of genital herpes. Some studies have indicated that asymptomatic women can shed herpes virus at delivery and that many more mothers shed virus than deliver babies who become infected. The characteristics of women at risk for delivering infected newborns is not known.

The newborn infection can be serious with severe central nervous system damage. Physicians should be alert to the presence of any genital tract lesion of a patient in labor. If the physician is suspicious of herpes, a cesarean section should be done. The pediatrician should be alerted to isolate the baby and to consider the use of antiviral agents.

Listeria monocytogenes. A non-spore-forming, gram-positive aerobic rod, *Listeria monocytogenes* can cross the placenta and infect the fetus in utero. In a recent epidemic of maternal infections in Los Angeles, the source of the infection was contamination of commercial cheese with this organism. In this epidemic, the maternal infections were associated with high maternal fevers, general malaise, and subsequent intrauterine fetal deaths. In contrast to this epidemic, sporadic cases have been seen in New York City in which the suspected but not proven source of infection was imported cheeses. These women were not acutely ill but instead had flulike symptoms and no localizing signs. The diagnosis is best made by a positive blood culture on these women; cervical cultures can show no growth of this organism even when the fetus is infected. Fortunately, this organism is susceptible to penicillin. Alternatively, sulfamethoxazole-trimethoprim can be given to penicillin-allergic patients. These antibiotics cross the placenta and effectively treat the fetus as well as the mother. This is a rare but treatable cause of perinatal morbidity and mortality.

Lyme disease. A new concern for obstetricians, Lyme disease has protean manifestations, with a skin rash, occasionally fever, joint pain, and late-developing central nervous system symptomatology. It is caused by the spirochete *Borrelia burgdorferi* and is usually transmitted by the bite of an infected ixodes tick. In pregnant women, the spirochete can cross the placenta to infect the fetus. This infection has been associated with congenital cardiac malformations and encephalitis.

This disease is a difficult problem of detection. The maternal symptoms are often vague, and diagnosis is dependent upon antibody testing, which has not been standardized. To date, clinicians are most aware of this infection in those sections of the country, particularly the East Coast, where the disease is endemic. In these areas, knowing the maternal antibody state before pregnancy occurs is helpful in the interpretation of antibody testing. In endemic areas, the discovery of a typical skin lesion, erythema migrans, which begins as a red macule or papule that expands to form a large annular erythema with a bright red outer border and partial central cleaving, should arouse suspicion. Some women have no skin lesions but are found to have rising antibody titer with joint symptoms. This is an indication for antibiotic treatment. Fortunately, penicillin is effective, and erythromycin can be given to the penicillin-allergic pregnant patient. Although uncommon thus far, it is an increasing cause of newborn infection in the United States.

Parvovirus (fifth disease). This infection, caused by human *Parvovirus* B19, can result in a serious problem for the fetus. The infection can be mild or inapparent in the mother. The virus can cross the placenta and cause disseminated disease often presenting as nonimmune hydrops fetalis in the newborn. It should be suspected when an ultrasound evaluation of hydramnios reveals fetal ascites that cannot be explained on the basis of maternal-fetal blood incompatibilities. Fetal blood can be obtained by cordocentesis to confirm the in utero diagnosis. Prompt delivery with exchange transfusion can help the baby.

IMMUNIZATION DURING PREGNANCY

The decision of whether a pregnant woman should be immunized is influenced by several factors: susceptibility to the disease, the possibility of exposure, the effect on mother and fetus if the disease is contracted, and the risk of the fetus from immunization.

Although information about the effects of acute infectious diseases on the course of pregnancy and the fetus is incomplete, clearly many of the risks involved can be eliminated by preventive immunization. An important part of premarital and prepregnancy examinations, therefore, is learning which infectious diseases the patient has had, testing for susceptibility to diseases known to be teratogenic, and vaccinating susceptible women before they conceive.

Pregnant women with chronic cardiac, pulmonary, or metabolic diseases should be considered candidates for immunization against influenza and pneumococcal pneumonia; as a general rule, however, immunization is best avoided during pregnancy. Immunoglobulins, toxoids, and vaccines made from inactivated organisms are usually safe for pregnant women, but, except in emergencies, those made from live organisms should be avoided because they may infect the fetus.

SOFT-TISSUE PELVIC INFECTIONS

The most important of the many developments that have changed our concepts of infections of the female reproductive organs are (1) a better understanding of the bacteria involved; (2) a new classification of pelvic infection that differentiates low-risk from high-risk patients; and (3) a proliferation of new antibiotics, particularly cephalosporins, penicillins, imipenem, aztreonam, and quinolones, with broader spectrums of antibacterial activity.

In the past, every effort was made to identify a single "pathogenic" bacterial species, (for example, *Neisseria gonorrhoeae*) to account for a specific infection. An antibiotic effective against that organism could then be prescribed. For the most part, only aerobic cultures were examined; hence anaerobic bacteria were not identified. As a consequence, cultures of pus from pelvic abscesses, which almost always contain anaerobes, were usually reported to be "sterile." This concept is too simplified; infections of the female pelvic organs are usually multibacterial, and often three or more organisms can be isolated from the infected tissues. In addition, the importance of anaerobic bacteria, which can be recovered in about 70% of pelvic infections, is now appreciated. Few pelvic abscesses actually are "sterile." Anaerobes can be recovered in almost every instance, and a specific organism, *Bacteroides fragilis,* is isolated frequently. Anaerobic bacteria can also be cultured from the blood in 25% or more of women with pelvic infections and an associated bacteremia.

Organisms other than anaerobic bacreria are important in the microbiology of pelvic infections. *Gram-negative aerobes* have been associated with serious infections, particularly in patients with septic shock. The gram-positive aerobe *group B beta hemolytic streptococcus* has been implicated in both maternal and newborn infections. *Mycoplasma* species appear to be significant in some infections. Of greater clinical significance is *Chlamydia trachomatis,* which is assuming an important role in the genesis of pelvic infections.

Pitfalls abound in the evaluation and treatment of women with pelvic infection. Definitive recommendations concerning proper treatment are not yet available because some of the end points of therapy have not been studied. For example, whether the results of hospital treatment of salpingo-oophoritis are better than those obtained by outpatient therapy is not known. There is insufficient information to suggest that any one antibiotic regimen is superior to another. Of special significance is that we know little of one of the most important end points of therapy: the number of women whose tubes will function normally after antibiotic treatment is completed. A judgment about the patient's immediate response is usually easy to make: she becomes asymptomatic, or she does not. If she fails to respond to the initial treatment, she may require different antibiotics, heparin for the treatment of septic pelvic thrombophlebitis, or some form of operative intervention to effect a cure.

The microbiologic identification of the bacteria at the site of infection before treatment is started, and proof that the bacteria have been eliminated by the antibiotic regimen that results in clinical cure is information that is often impossible to obtain. The only access routes to the site of infection through which material for culture can be obtained are the vagina and the cervix. Both contain abundant aerobic and anaerobic bacterial flora that usually cannot be conclusively identified as either normal or pathogenic. The organisms listed in Table 40-1 have been recovered from pelvic sites of infection and can also be recovered from the lower genital tract of asymptomatic women.

Because of the difficulties of clinical evaluation in multibacterial pelvic infections, considerable effort has been exerted to develop an animal model applicable to human infections. The work of Weinstein and associates has had a profound impact on the antibacterial treatment of pelvic infections. In their experimental model, a gelatin capsule filled with rat feces is placed in the peritoneal cavity of rats. As the capsule dissolves, a biphasic response occurs to the heavy bacterial insult of the organisms in the rat feces. Peritonitis develops during the early onset phase. At this stage gram-negative *aerobic bacteria* can be isolated from the blood of the affected animals. Approximately 40% of the animals die as a result of the peritonitis. The survivors look fairly well for 2 to 3 days but then become sick as a result of the development of intraabdominal abscesses in which *anaerobic bacteria* predominate. Thus, the

TABLE 40-1 Organisms found in pelvic infections that can also be recovered from the lower genital tract of asymptomatic women

Gram-positive bacteria	Gram-negative bacteria
Aerobes	
Group B beta-hemolytic streptococcus	*E. coli*
Enterococcus	*Klebsiella* species
Coagulase-positive staphylococcus	
Anaerobes	
Peptostreptococcus species	*Veillonella* species
Clostridium perfringens	*Bacteroides* bivius
	B. disiens
	B. fragilis
	B. melaninogenicus
	Fusobacterium species

response to a massive bacterial insult of mixed bacteria is biphasic: an early onset phase with sepsis and death in which gram-negative aerobic bacteria are involved, and a late onset phase in which abscesses form and anaerobic bacteria predominate. This model is appealing because the end points of the bacterial insult and the treatment are so clear. The presence of intraabdominal abscesses can be easily identified, and death is a specific end point.

After having demonstrated a predictable response to multibacterial insult, the investigators attempted to modify the course of the infections by administering antibiotics. They discovered that if the animals are pretreated with an aminoglycoside (gentamicin) before the bacterial insult, the early onset phase of the infection can be almost completely eliminated, but those that survive develop intraabdominal abscesses. With clindamycin, which is effective against anaerobic bacteria but not gram-negative aerobes, the early onset phase of infection is not influenced, but the survivors form few abscesses. Finally, if a combination of clindamycin and gentamicin is given, both phases of the infection can be almost completely eliminated.

Two questions must be answered before the results of animal experiments can be applied clinically: is the experimental infection similar to those that occur in humans, and can the regimen used in the animal model be applied to the treatment of mixed bacterial pelvic infections in women?

Many parallels exist between the model infections in animals and those that develop in humans. Early onset infections are often seen in obstetric practice. The cause of infection is obvious because of the temporal relationship between the event initiating the infection (for example, a delivery) and the onset of symptoms. In addition, gram-negative aerobes, usually *E. coli,* can often be isolated from the bloodstream during the early stage of the infection. However, other aspects of human experience are less like those in the animal model. Gram-positive aerobes such as the group

B betahemolytic streptococcus and anaerobic bacteria, both gram-positive and gram-negative, are often recovered from the bloodstream of patients who have a bacteremia associated with the early phase of a pelvic infection. Another major difference from the animal model is that death from sepsis is now an uncommon event in humans.

The late onset problems, however, are similar in human and experimental infections. In each, the abscesses develop relatively late after the initiating cause, and anaerobes are most often involved. Late infections may be difficult to recognize because of the long interval between the initiating procedure, the pelvic operation, and the development of the clinical signs of infection.

The next question involves the reproducibility of the therapeutic results in the animal model as compared with human experience. The effectiveness of systemic antibiotics in experimental infections depends upon the administration of the antibiotics before or at the time of the multibacterial insult. One of the realities of clinical experience is that infections are already established when the physician first has an opportunity to recognize and treat them. All patients have symptoms before treatment begins. In addition, some patients have had an infection for several days before they seek care. There are important differences in the results of treating well-established infections as compared with those in which treatment can be started early in the clinical course of the disease. I evaluated a total of 501 patients who were treated for varying degrees of soft-tissue pelvic infections to delineate this particular point. The patients were classified retrospectively as having had early infections if symptoms had been present for fewer than 5 days and if an indurated pelvic mass could not be felt when treatment was started. Patients with well-established infections had one of two clinical findings: symptoms for 5 days or more or an indurated pelvic mass that was considered to be a pelvic abscess.

The results were striking. A significantly higher number of successful responses to the initial treatment occurred in women who were seen early in the clinical course of infection; more of the patients who were treated for a well-established infection required some form of operative intervention to effect a cure. This clinical classification is important for prognosticating the outcome of the treatment of soft-tissue pelvic infections. The prognosis for unsuccessful antibiotic therapy and the need for operative intervention are greater when treatment has not begun until the infection is well established.

An additional aspect of antibiotic therapy is the tremendous proliferation of new agents. There are now second- and third-generation cephalosporins and new penicillins that have a broader spectrum of activity against the anaerobic bacteria that are most often responsible for obstetric and gynecologic infections. The great appeal of all of these agents is their low toxicity. In addition, imipenem has a broad spectrum of antibacterial activities. Some new antibiotics have appeal because of specific antibacterial actions. Aztreonam has great activity against gram-negative aerobes, whereas the quinolones seem effective against gram-negative aerobes and chlamydia.

There is justifiable concern regarding renal and eighth cranial nerve toxicity when aminoglycosides are prescribed and about the toxicity associated with the use of clindamycin and chloramphenicol.

CATEGORIES OF INFECTION

The two broad categories of infection are those that are community acquired, that is, the patient already has the infection when she is admitted to the hospital, and those that are hospital acquired, or nosocomial. Nosocomial infections include those that can be associated with the more resistant microorganisms.

Community-acquired infections

Infected abortion. A striking change has occurred in the medical problems related to infected abortion. The number of such infections has decreased, in part because of increased use of effective contraceptives and, probably of more signifi-

cance, because of the ready availability of legal pregnancy termination services. Not only has there been an overall decrease in the number of patients with infected abortions but also the infections that occur are far less serious than were those encountered in the past. Patients with infected abortions have a much better prognosis for cure than do women with other types of community-acquired infection.

CLINICAL EVALUATION. The evaluation of each patient with an infected abortion includes assessment by physician examination, accurate recording of the vital signs, and appropriate laboratory tests. *Hypotension* or an *oral temperature above 39° C* places the patient in a high-risk category because of the possibility of septic shock. *Generalized peritonitis,* an indication of extensive extrauterine involvement, also places the patient at higher risk. Uterine size is assessed, and the cervix is inspected for the presence of products of conception. Placental tissue can be removed from the cervical canal with ring forceps without causing significant discomfort. Perhaps the most important aspect of the pelvic examination is a careful assessment of the extent of the infection. More prolonged medical treatment is required when the infection has extended beyond the confines of the uterus than when it is localized.

Laboratory studies include a *complete blood count with a differential.* Anemia and/or leukopenia identifies patients at higher risk. A low white blood cell count may be an early manifestation of septic shock. A number of *microbiologic samples* should be obtained before antibiotic therapy is started. The most important of these is a *blood culture,* which, when positive, identifies the most significant organisms involved with the infection. Anaerobic bacteria can often be identified in the bloodstream if appropriate culture techniques are used. This information will be particularly helpful if the patient fails to respond to the antibiotics that are administered first.

There is little justification for relying on the results of anaerobic cultures obtained from the endocervical canal because of the high frequency of surface anaerobic bacterial contamination. However, aerobic cultures should be obtained from the cervix to ensure that serious pathogens are not present. The recovery of an aerobe such as the group A beta hemolytic streptococcus has great significance; these bacteria require strict isolation techniques for the patient.

X-ray film examination or other imaging evaluations of the abdomen can be helpful. Free air beneath the diaphragm suggests that the uterus was perforated during an abortion attempt. Radiolucent foreign bodies that have been pushed through the wall of the uterus into the peritoneal cavity can also be seen. Either of these indicates the need for an exploratory operation to estimate the extent of the infection and to remove the foreign body.

TREATMENT. The treatment of a patient with an infected abortion should be directed toward correcting the pathologic changes: infection that begins in the necrotic trophoblastic tissue within the uterine cavity and that can extend into or through the uterine wall.

Bacteria are introduced into the uterus during the manipulations necessary to disrupt the pregnancy. The risk is slight if the abortion is performed early in the pregnancy with sterile technique by a skilled physician. The most serious infections follow abortion done by nonprofessional persons without concern for antisepsis. Such infections are infrequently seen in the United States since the liberalization of laws regulating termination of unwanted pregnancy.

The point of entry for bacteria is through the placental site or through vaginal or uterine injuries. The bacteria advance by way of the veins (phlebitis) or the lymphatics (lymphangitis). The most common extrauterine infection is *parametrial cellulitis*, which may progress to *abscess* formation. Pelvic and even generalized *peritonitis* also occurs with the most serious infections.

The use of *antibiotics* that usually are appropriate for the responsible organisms, primarily gramnegative aerobes and anaerobes, should be combined with curettage to remove the infected products of conception. Chow, Marshall, and Guze have shown that removal of the residual infected placental tissue is probably a more important factor in recovery than is antibiotic therapy. Although there is debate over the timing of curettage and concern about seeding the bloodstream with bacteria, it is usually safe whenever therapeutic levels of antibiotics have been achieved.

In most women with infected abortions, one of the *second-generation cephalosporins* such as cefoxitin should be the first drug administered. If there is evidence of septic shock, a combination of clindamycin and gentamicin (alternatively, metronidazole, penicillin, and gentamicin) is also appropriate; they provide better coverage against *B. fragilis*. Either cefoxitin alone or the combinations with clindamycin or metronidazole provide good coverage for the important gramnegative aerobes and the anaerobes so frequently involved in extrauterine infection associated with abortion.

Patients who are critically ill require more extensive therapy. Many such patients were more than 12 weeks pregnant when termination was attempted; the tissues are more likely injured during second-trimester abortions. These serious infections may occur in many ways. The infection can be caused by *C. perfringens*, with widespread dissemination of its virulent exotoxins. This diagnosis should be considered in any patient with an infected abortion who has renal failure and evidence of intravascular hemolysis. It can be confirmed by x-ray film examination of the pelvis; the enlarged uterus has an onionskin appearance because of gas formation in its wall. Additional supporting evidence is the presence of gram-positive bacilli with swollen ends in the endocervical smear. In addition to antibiotic therapy, hysterectomy can be required to remove the nidus of infection. This aggressive American approach is not universally agreed upon; British physicians do hysterectomies less frequently, and the majority of women they treat are cured. This may be a result of differences in the interpretation of microbiologic results.

Clostridium perfringens can be recovered from the lower genital tract of normal, asymptomatic women; hence isolation of this organism in a culture from a patient with an infected abortion is not an indication for laparotomy unless serious infection is demonstrated. Fortunately for the practitioner today, these infections are rare, in contrast to the more frequent problems with "gas gangrene" of the uterus when elective termination of pregnancy was not permitted.

Patients other than those with uterine infections may require operative intervention. Women with extensive uterine damage or infected pelvic hematomas may remain septic despite the use of appropriate antibiotics. In these patients, laparotomy to drain or remove an abscess or pelvic organs will effect a cure.

PELVIC ABSCESS. In some patients, fever, pelvic pain, and signs of peritonitis persist in spite of antibiotic therapy and evacuation of the uterus. This situation suggests advancing parametritis and pelvic cellulitis, which may eventually end with pelvic abscess formation. Pelvic examination and sonogram should be performed in such patients in an attempt to detect the first evidence of an abscess. Many abscesses point into the vagina and can be drained by posterior colpotomy. In many cases imaging techniques and directed needle aspiration can be employed.

RUPTURED UTERUS. Laparoscopy and laparotomy should be performed if uterine perforation is diagnosed by x-ray film examination or is thought to be a possibility because of intraperitoneal bleeding or obvious local injury or if the uterus is perforated during surgical evacuation of the necrotic, infected contents. This concern applies to any lateral perforations of the uterus and if the perforation occurs and a suction instrument has been turned on while outside the uterus. With extensive lacerations it usually is necessary to remove the uterus. The bowel should be inspected because it can be damaged if the uterus is perforated.

THROMBOPHLEBITIS. Puerperal infection extends from its source in the uterine cavity through the wall and into the parametrium by progressive phlebitis and lymphangitis, as well as by direct tissue involvement. Thrombophlebitis eventually involves the veins on the lateral pelvic walls, the ovarian veins, and the vena cava. Septic emboli are transported to distant parts of the body where they set up secondary areas of infection from which the patient may eventually die, even through the pelvic lesion clears. When embolization continues even in the presence of adequate antibiotic and anticoagulant therapy, ovarian and vena caval ligation can be indicated. With better knowledge of anaerobic organism involvement in infection and early use of antibiotics effective against anaerobes, this entity is rarer now than it was in the 1960s.

SEPTIC SHOCK. Septic shock associated with an infected abortion is now an unusual clinical event. The successful treatment of the potentially lethal condition requires an understanding of the pathophysiologic changes and a marshaling of all available intensive care resources. Bacterial products, usually endotoxins from gram-negative aerobic bacteria, are disseminated from the site of infection, attach to macrophages, and release tumor necrosis factor with unfavorable effects on other vital organ systems throughout the body, including hypotension with reduced tissue perfusion, which becomes evident as urine output decreases or ceases completely. The hematocrit may be normal or elevated, even though blood loss has been excessive, because of the hypovolemia. The white blood cell count may be within the normal range even though it had been greatly elevated before signs of shock appeared.

The basic requirements for the successful treatment of septic shock include (1) the reduction of peripheral resistance, (2) the restoration of circulating blood volume, and (3) the treatment of infection. The response to the treatment program is monitored by determining the blood pressure, pulse rate, respiration rate, and urine output at 30-minute intervals and by measuring central venous pressure.

Serious therapeutic mistakes can be made in the care of these women if the physician focuses on symptoms while ignoring the underlying pathophysiologic conditions. A delay in performing a necessary operation while repeatedly administering fluid challenges to stimulate urine production, using vasopressors to restore blood pressure, or prescribing repeated steroid doses to combat the effects of endotoxic shock may cause the death of a patient who would have survived with proper care. *Septic shock in a patient with an infected abortion will be perpetuated as long as the nidus of infection exists. It requires curettage as the minimal operative procedure and hysterectomy if the infection is more extensive.*

Salpingo-oophoritis. The criteria for the diagnosis of salpingo-oophoritis have changed remarkably in the last decade. Until the late 1970s, physicians were required to adhere to strict criteria for making a diagnosis of acute salpingo-oophoritis to prevent the indiscriminate ordering of antibiotics when another form of treatment was indicated. A major concern was that inappropriate antibiotic therapy would delay operations for ectopic pregnancy. Following are the criteria formerly used for establishing a clinical diagnosis of salpingo-oophoritis:

1. Acute pelvic pain of a few days' duration
2. Temperature of 38° C (100.4° F) or higher
3. Tender adnexal swelling or mass
4. Increased erythrocyte sedimentation rate or elevated white blood cell count

Studies in which laparoscopy was performed on patients admitted with a clinical diagnosis of salpingitis have revealed the shortcomings of this approach. Nearly half of women with laparoscopic evidence of acute salpingitis are afebrile at the time of admission, unilateral salpingitis is an accepted clinical entity, and elevated white blood cell counts or an increased sedimentation rate do not differentiate salpingitis from other noninfectious types of pelvic disorders. These facts indicate that the physician should consider pelvic infection in any woman with acute pelvic pain.

A wide variety of bacterial species has been implicated in the pathogenesis of salpingo-oophoritis, but a continuing emphasis on *N. gonorrhoeae* has been maintained in the United States. Gonococci are often recovered from the endocervix of patients with salpingitis but less often from peritoneal fluid. The gonococcus was considered to be a bacterial trailblazer paving the way for subsequent colonization and infection of the endosalpinx with other bacteria. Studies by Sweet, Draper, and Hadley confirm the concept that salpingitis is a multibacterial infection and that the greatest variety of bacterial isolates can be recovered early in the course of the disease. Many gram-positive and gram-negative aerobes and anaerobes, in addition to *N. gonorrhoeae,* are involved in such multibacterial pelvic infections.

Many observations suggest that *Chlamydia species* play a significant role in pelvic infections. These organisms were isolated in six of 20 biopsies of the fimbriae of fallopian tubes obtained at the time of laparoscopy in women with acute salpingitis. Chlamydia also can be recovered from biopsies of pelvic adhesions in women with a past history of salpingitis. Women with blocked tubes from previous infection as the cause of their infertility have a higher than expected incidence of chlamydia antibodies in their blood. Confirmation of these findings will have an impact on future antibiotic strategies in women with salpingitis; chlamydia are relatively susceptible to tetracycline, erythromycin, and clindamycin, but they are usually resistant to the cephalosporins and the newer penicillins.

The role of other organisms is currently being evaluated. *Mycoplasma species* have been isolated occasionally from women with salpingo-oophoritis; its significance has not yet been established.

Community-acquired infections caused by these organisms are also classified as sexually transmitted diseases because they are disseminated almost entirely by heterosexual or homosexual contact. *Gonorrhea and chlamydial infections* are the most common of the sexually transmitted diseases. The highest rates of gonorrhea, in order of frequency, occur between the ages 20 and 24, 15 and 19, and 25 and 29. The bacteria grow in the cervical crypts and produce an acute cervicitis, which may eventually become chronic and relatively asymptomatic. In less than half of cases, the bacteria are carried upward through the uterus to the tubes. During the upward extension, which usually occurs during menstruation, a transient endometritis and then endosalpingitis develop. The tubal mucosa responds to the bacteria by producing a purulent exudate. The fimbriae become agglutinated in an attempt to prevent the infection from extending to the peritoneal cavity. The distended pus-filled tube is called a *pyosalpinx.* If *peritonitis* is associated with the disease, the bowel and omentum adhere to the involved tubes in an attempt to keep the infection confined in the pelvis. Both fallopian tubes usually are involved.

Variations from this clinical picture occur. Many patients obviously have had extensive endosalpingitis and even peritonitis because the tubes are closed, clubbed, and adherent, but they have no history of an acute infection. In others, particularly women who are using an intrauterine contraceptive device when they become infected, only one tube is involved.

DIAGNOSIS. Because of these variations, the clinical diagnosis of acute salpingo-oophoritis may be difficult to establish. It should be suspected in all sexually active women who complain of lower abdominal discomfort or pain. Westrom has found that all women with laparoscopy-confirmed salpingitis have white blood cells in their vaginal fluid. In addition, needle culdocentesis is a helpful diagnostic technique in afebrile patients. The presence of bacteria in fluid obtained from the posterior cul-de-sac suggests intraperitoneal infection and indicates antibiotic therapy. A Gram stain should be made, and the fluid sent for aerobic and anaerobic culture.

Two other examinations are important: the physician should try to determine whether inflammatory masses are present (an exact evaluation may be difficult because pronounced tenderness limits the accuracy of bimanual examination), and a sample of the cervical secretions should be sent for gonococcal culture and a Gram-stained specimen examined for gonococci.

TREATMENT

Antibiotic therapy. Although guidelines for the antibiotic treatment of salpingitis are not yet based on properly designed prospective clinical studies, some observations influence therapeutic strategies. The recovery of *N. gonorrhoeae* from the endocervical canal of patients with clinical evidence of salpingitis identifies a population with specific risk characteristics. These women usually respond rapidly to antibiotic therapy and subsequently have a lower rate of irreversible tubal damage. The sexual partners should also be treated before activity is resumed. In contrast to many stated beliefs, 20% to 40% of men from whom *N. gonorrhoeae* can be cultured are symptomatic and can reinfect successfully treated women.

The results of treatment are also influenced by the status of the infection when the patient is first seen. Those with early infections are far more

---

MANAGEMENT OF PID

Ambulatory treatment
Recommended regimen
Cefoxitin, 2 g IM *plus* **probenecid,** 1 g orally concurrently, *or* **ceftriaxone,** 250 mg IM, *or* equivalent **cephalosporin**

plus

Doxycycline, 100 mg orally 2 times a day for 10-14 days

or

Tetracycline, 500 mg orally 4 times a day for 10-14 days

Inpatient treatment
One of the following:
Recommended regimen A
Cefoxitin, 2 g IV every 6 hours, *or* **cefotetan,** IV 2 g every 12 hours

plus

Doxycycline, 100 mg every 12 hours orally or IV

The above regimen is given for at least 48 hours after the patient clinically improves.
After discharge from hospital, continuation of:
Doxycycline, 100 mg orally 2 times a day for a total of 10-14 days
Recommended regimen B
Clindamycin, IV 900 mg every 8 hours

plus

Gentamicin, loading dose IV or IM (2 mg/kg) *followed by* a maintenance dose (1.5 mg/kg) every 8 hours

---

likely to respond successfully to antibiotic treatment than are those in whom the processes are well established.

The clinical decisions concerning treatment of salpingo-oophoritis are made most logically on the basis of an overall view of the most effective antibiotic regimen. Following are the antimicrobial agents recommended by the Centers for Disease Control (see box above).

More intensive antibiotic therapy is indicated for patients with indurated pelvic masses. Clindamycin, 600 mg intravenously every 6 hours, and gentamicin, 3 to 5 mg/kg/day in divided doses at 8-hour intervals, should be given. Because of the variations in serum levels achieved in patients receiving gentamicin, peak and trough blood concentrations of the antibiotics should be measured after 24 hours of therapy. The results will guide necessary dosage adjustment. Ultrasonography may be helpful in differentiating a tuboovarian complex from a tuboovarian abscess and in identifying patients who may need an operation or aspiration of the abscess.

Surgical therapy. In recent years, the operative care of women with salpingo-oophoritis has been modified. There is general consensus on a number of therapeutic points. A ruptured tuboovarian abscess represents an operative emergency. Women can die unless the infected pelvic structures are removed, the peritoneal cavity is lavaged, appropriate antibiotics are administered, and shock is treated. This diagnosis should be considered in every woman with diffuse peritonitis and a tachycardia out of proportion to the temperature elevation. The suspected diagnosis can be confirmed by a culdocentesis in which a free flow of purulent material is obtained. A pelvic abscess bulging into the vagina through a distended posterior cul-de-sac can be treated with transvaginal drainage. Operative evacuation of pelvic abscesses usually results in a clinical cure, with no further operative care needed. Removing the pelvic organs is usually necessary if the infection persists after it has been drained or if infection recurs.

Other indications for surgery are more controversial. There is no standard definition of failure to respond to medical therapy. Although some gynecologists advocate laparotomy if there is no response after 48 hours of antibiotic therapy, most have been more conservative. The need for early operative intervention has decreased since more emphasis has been placed on the use of antibiotics such as clindamycin, metronidazole, or cefoxitin, which are effective against *B. fragilis* and other anaerobes, and not longer periods of antibiotic therapy before deciding that the medical treatment has failed. A decrease in temperature, pain, and pelvic tenderness after treatment has been started is an indication for continuing medical therapy.

Traditional teaching has stressed the bilaterality of pelvic infection and the need to remove both adnexa when an operation is necessary. However, unilateral tubal abscesses do occur. In such patients only the involved adnexum need be removed. Some women respond initially to antibiotic therapy but have recurrent bouts of pain. In the past, total abdominal hysterectomy and bilateral salpingo-oophorectomy were recommended to relieve the pain. This solution is still appropriate if repeated acute attacks have left the pelvic structures extensively damaged, but it is not always necessary. Lysis of adhesions to free the adherent tubes and ovaries, resection of structures that are most involved, and instillation of a high-molecular-weight dextran solution to help prevent reformation of adhesions may relieve the symptoms. The isolation of *Chlamydia* organisms from the adhesions is an indication for the use of a tetracycline.

Nosocomial infections

Postoperative infections. Any patient who has undergone a pelvic operation may develop a postoperative infection. These infections are categorized as those of the operative site, such as an infection in the abdominal incision or at the vault of the vagina after hysterectomy, and those that are separate from the surgical field, for example, a postoperative respiratory tract infection.

PREVENTION. An important responsibility of surgeons who perform pelvic operations is to make every effort to prevent postoperative infection, but a number of time-honored hospital and operating room rituals may actually increase the infection rate. The longer the preoperative stay, the greater the postoperative infection rate. Shaving the operative site the evening before the operation, the use of cautery rather than a sharp knife, and using plastic adhesive drapes instead of towels or wound drapes all increase the number of abdominal wound infections.

Swartz and Tanaree have shown that closed suction T-tube drainage of the space between the peritoneum and the vaginal cuff lowers the incidence of postoperative pelvic infections after hysterectomy. Several controllable procedures favorably influence the rate of postoperative urinary tract infection. Meticulous attention to maintaining a closed drainage system while an indwelling catheter is in place minimizes the occurrence of urinary tract infections. A correlation exists between the length of time a transurethral catheter is in place and postoperative urinary tract infection. Indwelling catheters should be removed as soon as the patient is able to void. The number of infections can be reduced even more by the use of suprapubic bladder drainage instead of a transurethral catheter. These facts should be considered during the preoperative planning for the care of women scheduled for elective operations.

Systemic *antibiotic prophylaxis* has been used increasingly to lower the incidence of postoperative site infection. This represents a remarkable change in philosophy; prophylaxis had been condemned by many leaders in the field of infectious disease. The change was made on the basis of a number of carefully controlled double-blind clinical studies that demonstrated the favorable impact of a short course of perioperative antibiotic prophylaxis on the postoperative infection rate. There is little disagreement that prophylactic antibiotics are effective in women undergoing vaginal hysterectomy. Although there has been less enthusiasm for prophylaxis with abdominal hysterectomy, most recent studies have shown that it does decrease postoperative infections after abdominal hysterectomies for benign disease and after radical operations for uterine cancer. The most commonly used antibiotics have been the cephalosporins, but penicillins have been equally effective. Although no carefully controlled studies have been done, antibiotic prophylaxis has also been used widely in women undergoing salpingolysis and elective tubal reconstruction. Since chlaymdiae can sometimes be recovered from the pelvic adhesions that appear to be old and inactive, tetracycline would probably be a better choice than a penicillin or cephalosporin in these women.

TREATMENT. In spite of preventive measures, postoperative infections still occur. Women with these infections should be studied systematically so that an appropriate treatment plan can be developed. A complete physical exaination should be performed on every postoperative patient who is febrile in an attempt to determine the site of infection. This is important because the antibacterial agents selected for the treatment of a multibacterial pelvic infection differ from those that will eradicate a urinary tract infection caused by a single species of bacteria. In addition, a postoperative infection associated with a collection of infected material such as a *vaginal cuff* or an *abdominal wound abscess* is more effectively treated by drainage than by systemic antibiotics. Unless purulent material can be aspirated directly from the site of infection, culture for anaerobic bacteria is of little help; bacteria that grow may represent surface contaminants. Blood cultures for aerobic and anaerobic bacteria should be obtained before treatment is started.

If the infection is manifested only by induration and tenderness without fluctuation, good clinical results can usually be achieved with second-generation cephalosporins such as cefamandole and cefoxitin. Some patients who have been discharged from the hospital after what seems to have been an uneventful recovery will require readmission because they have developed clinical evidence of a postoperative infection. These patients' conditions usually respond best to a combination of gentamicin and clindamycin. An operation to remove or drain an abscess or to remove the infected structure should be performed if the infection does not respond promptly to antibiotic therapy.

Abdominal wound infections are best treated by opening the entire wound. This ensures adequate drainage and permits the clinician to determine the integrity of the fascia. Systemic antibiotics are seldom needed unless there is spreading involvement of the wound edge. Rapidly spreading inflammation of the skin adjacent to the wound may herald the presence of a dangerous synergistic infection. If there is a possibility that this is occurring, wide debridement may be lifesaving.

Most nonoperative site infections in the postoperative period involve the urinary tract. These problems usually are easily managed. Uncomplicated urinary tract infections usually respond promptly to sulfonamides or nitrofurantoins, which have limited antibacterial activity outside the urinary tract. However, any postoperative patient who develops acute pyelonephritis should be investigated for the possibility of ureteral injury related to the pelvic operation.

Postpartum (puerperal) infections. In the tradition of Semmelweiss, obstetricians have maintained a consistent focus on maternal postpartum infections. In the past, statistics concerning obstetric infection rates were based on temperature recording. "Infectious morbidity" was defined as an oral temperature of 38° C (100.4° F) or more on any 2 of the first 10 postpartum days, excluding the first 24 hours. This standard is now much less useful than it was in the past. In the era of diagnostic-related groups, no women remain in the hospital for 10 days after normal delivery; some are discharged within a few hours, and most have left by the third day. As a consequence, the first abnormal temperature elevation may occur after the patient has gone home. The day on

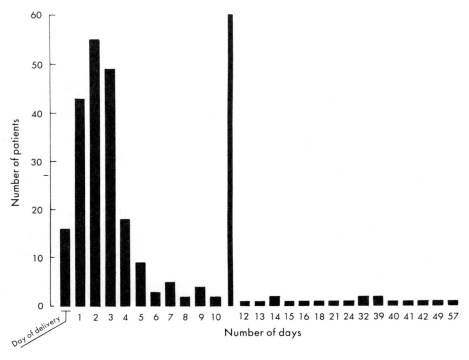

Fig. 40-1 Graph depicting first day of temperature elevation in postpartum patients with clinical diagnosis of bacterial infection. (From Ledger WJ, Reite AM, and Headington JT: Obstet Gynecol 37:769, 1971.)

which the temperature first rose in a series of women who developed puerperal infection is shown in Fig. 40-1. Unless the infection is serious, these patients are treated without readmission, thus they are not included in hospital statistics as having developed postpartum infections. Another source of inaccuracy in compiling statistics on the basis of temperature morbidity is that systemic antibiotics are often prescribed for postpartum patients soon after the first temperature elevation and are continued for long periods. Many women receiving this treatment will not have postpartum infections that satisfy the definition based on temperature; hence reported infection rates do not reflect the reality of what is happening on a service. The postpartum infection rate should include the total number of patients who received systemic antibiotics, as well as those who met the temperature definition of infection.

PREVENTION. The prevention of postpartum infection requires a knowledge of the factors that increase risk. Women with a consistently high infection rate include those whose delivery is by cesarean section, particularly those who have been in labor and those from the lower socioeconomic populations. One might suspect that factors such as prolonged labor, prolonged rupture of membranes, frequent internal examination during labor, or the use of invasive monitoring techniques would increase the risk of infection, but they do not do so consistently.

Cesarean section, particularly in patients who have been in labor, is followed by a high postpartum infection rate. The experience with prophylaxis with vaginal and abdominal hysterectomy suggests that systemic preventive antibiotics might be of value because the operative field is usually contaminated by the bacteria present in the amniotic cavity. Prospective, double-blind studies of antibiotic prophylaxis for cesarean section indicate that the infection rate is lower in patients who have been given systemic antibiotics. There is concern about timing of antibiotic administration. Ideally for the mother, the antibiotics should be given before the operation is started, but this strategy results in a therapeutic level of antibiotics in the fetus, as well as in the mother. To prevent this problem, the first dose of the prophylactic is administered intravenously in the operating room as soon as the umbilical cord has been clamped. This approach is effective but not the risk of cardiovascular collapse has been reported in patients after the intravenous injection of cephalothin in the operating room. The mechanism of action of this adverse effect is not known.

TREATMENT. In spite of these preventive techniques, postpartum infections still occur. Since effective treatment regimens must be established on the basis of the changes produced by the infection, an understanding of the pathophysiology of puerperal infections is essential to their treatment.

Puerperal infection is for all practical purposes a wound infection. The point of entry for the bacteria from the uterine cavity is the placental site. From there they extend through the uterine wall by way of the veins (phlebitis), the lymphatics (lymphangitis), or direct extension through the muscle.

Endomyometritis, the most common type of puerperal infection, involves the endometrium and the superficial muscle layer of the uterine wall. Bacteria can be cultured from the uterine cavity in most women during prolonged or difficult labor and soon after normal delivery. Adherent bits of placenta in the area of the placental site, the shaggy decidua, and blood clots in the uterus serve as excellent media for the growth of bacteria, and as a consequence almost every recently delivered woman has a mild but inconsequential endometritis.

The clinically important infections are more obvious. With these infections, generally the temperature is slightly elevated from the day of delivery on, but by the third day, it may be as high as 38.3° to 39° C (101° to 102° F). The patient has

few symptoms other than malaise and perhaps slight abdominal tenderness. The lochia is often purulent, and malodorous.

The clinical course of infections caused by group A or group B beta hemolytic streptococcus is different from that of endomyometritis caused by other bacteria. The temperature rises abruptly to 39° to 40° C (102° to 104° F), frequently during the first 12 hours after delivery, and the patient looks and feels acutely ill. There may be little or no discharge from the uterus, and that present usually is not purulent.

Absence of the lochia is more often an evidence of *lochial block* than of beta hemolytic streptococcal infection. This is produced by an obstruction to drainage of the uterine cavity by a sheet of retained membrane, a blood clot, or an abnormal position of the uterus. With this condition, the temperature rises abruptly, often after slight daily temperature rises.

The uterus in women with endomyometritis is usually boggy, larger, and less well contracted than it should be. It is tender, but the parametrial areas can be palpated without producing any great amount of discomfort. Unless the symptoms are caused by lochial block, there usually is a purulent discharge coming from the cervix.

In the more serious cases of endomyometritis, the entire thickness of the uterine wall is involved and may even be the site of multiple small abscesses. This type of infection usually follows the early use of antibiotics ineffective against gram-negative anaerobes. All the symptoms and the findings that characterize endomyometritis are exaggerated, and there usually is parametrial tenderness.

Further extension of the organisms along the blood vessels and lymphatics produces cellulitis within the peritoneal folds of one or occasionally both broad ligaments *(parametritis)*. The signs are similar to those with endomyometritis but are much more severe. The temperature may reach 39.5° to 40° C (103° to 104° F). The pulse is elevated, and the white blood cell count may be 30,000 or more. The uterus is boggy and tender, limited in mobility, and sometimes pushed to one side by tender induration filling half of the pelvis; the other side may be relatively normal.

An *abscess* may develop in the center of the area of cellulitis. As it enlarges, it may eventually dissect downward to point in the posterior cul-de-sac, or it may extend upward until it can be felt above the inguinal ligament. In either event, as an abscess develops, the evidence of pelvic infection becomes more pronounced.

Peritonitis almost always accompanies parametritis and pelvic cellulitis. It varies in severity from relatively mild involvement of the peritoneal covering of the broad ligaments to widespread generalized infection.

Because *phlebitis* in the pelvic and the ovarian veins occurs as part of every serious puerperal infection, bacteremia is common. An unexpected result of a study of bacteremia from Texas indicated that those patients with an endomyometritis and a bacteremia were no more seriously ill than those without a bacteremia—that is, they responded well to the use of appropriate antibiotics.

A general physical and pelvic examination should be performed before treatment is begun. Evaluation of the pelvis provides information concerning the extent of the involvement of the pelvic structures and facilitates the removal of membranes or placental tissue visible in the endocervical canal. In patients with lochial block the discharge of uterine secretions is reestablished and the temperature returns to normal after the obstructing issue is removed with ring forceps.

Aerobic cultures from the lochia should be obtained in all febrile women suspected of having postpartum endomyometritis. There should be particular concern if the group A beta hemolytic streptococcus is found because it places the mother at risk as well as its being contagious. Attempts have been made to obtain anaerobic cultures uncontaminated by normal vaginal and cervical flora by using double-lumen aspirators to sample the endometrial cavity, transabdominal transfundal aspiration, and needle culdocentesis to obtain peritoneal fluid. None of these ensures that contamination has been eliminated. It is difficult to interpret standard blood studies in postpartum women. Normal women have a leukocytosis with a shift to the left.

There are rational guidelines for treating women with postpartum endomyometritis. Infections that develop after vaginal delivery are much less complicated than that following cesarean section. This is particularly true on services with a high cesarean section rate because of a reduced rate of operative vaginal deliveries such as midforceps and breech extraction. Because of this, a single antibiotic agent such as cefoxitin is often appropriate. Chlamydia may be a factor in late postpartum endomyometritis following vaginal delivery; that is, the patient has been discharged and, in a week to 10 days, is seen with an elevated temperature and a tender uterus. For such infections one of the newer tetracyclines such as doxycycline is a logical choice.

Endomyometritis that follows cesarean section is more serious than that which develops after vaginal delivery. Traditionally, these patients have been treated with a combination of penicillin and an aminoglycoside, but in the past two decades, studies have demonstrated the superiority of using clindamycin and either gentamicin or ampicillin as initial therapy. Better results have also been achieved with the newer cephalosporins and the newer penicillins. An abdominal wound infection should be suspected when patients fail to respond to systemic antibiotic therapy.

Many febrile postpartum patients will have urinary tract infections. This diagnosis can be suspected in a patient with no other clinical findings, the presence of bacteria on microscopic examination of an unspun catheterized urine sample, and a significant bacterial colony count. Women with these infections are best treated with nitrofurantoins whose activity is limited to the urinary tract. Any antibiotic given to the mother will appear in her breast milk.

THROMBOPHLEBITIS

Prenatal thrombophlebitis. Deep vein thrombophlebitis does not often occur during pregnancy. Anticoagulant therapy is indicated, but treatment is complicated by the pregnancy. Warfarin (Coumadin) crosses the placenta and may cause fetal death and hemorrhage in newborn infants. Heparin is preferable because it does not cross the placenta. In most instances the patient can learn to administer it. For serious infections, heparin should be continued throughout the entire pregnancy. It is discontinued when labor begins and restarted a few hours after delivery.

Puerperal thrombophlebitis. Although thrombophlebitis is an integral part of all puerperal infections, it is generally confined to the blood vessels in the uterine wall and is of little consequence. If the process extends laterally and involves the ovarian veins and the large vessels along the lateral pelvic wall, the prognosis becomes worse. Pelvic thrombophlebitis often is first suspected during the latter part of the first postpartum week, although in most instances the temperature has never been normal after delivery. The early use of antibiotics effective against gram-negative anaerobic bacteria had made this a much less frequent clinical entity than in the past.

Ovarian vein thrombosis is a distinct entity that should be suspected in any woman who develops unilateral lower abdominal pain, tenderness, and fever during the first few days after delivery. The pain is deep and constant and may radiate to the groin, the flank, or the costovertebral angle. Gastrointestinal symptoms usually are minimal, but ileus may be present. The abdomen is tender but soft, and a tender elongated mass can generally be felt on deep palpation. This differentiates it from pyelonephritis and the more common postpartum infections. Laparotomy often is necessary to confirm the diagnosis and to eliminate other lesions such as appendicitis.

The most serious involvement of the veins of the extremities is that of the *femoral vein,* which produces the process known as "milk leg." It usually appears at the end of the second week or later, and the patient experiences edema and pain in the affected leg and chills and fever. It seems likely that most postpartum involvements of the leg veins represent retrograde extensions from a pelvic thrombophlebitis.

DIAGNOSIS. The diagnosis of pelvic thrombophlebitis is difficult because involvement of the pelvic veins is difficult to discern. The physician should suspect the diagnosis in any postpartum patient with persistent unexplained fever, particularly if it is associated with a uterine infection and increasing pelvic pain and tenderness.

Heparin may be helpful in establishing the diagnosis. Puerperal pelvic thrombophlebitis can be diagnosed with reasonable accuracy when fever, which persists despite adequate antibiotic therapy, resolves within 48 hours after an appropriate dosage of heparin is added to the regimen.

TREATMENT. The treatment of postpartum thrombophlebitis is like that for nonpregnant women. Antibiotics will already have been prescribed for most women suspected of having puerperal thrombophlebitis; in fact, failure to respond to antibiotics is an important diagnostic feature of the condition. Because *Bacteroides* species and other anaerobes are recognized as the organisms often responsible for thrombophlebitis, drugs to which they are susceptible should be added to the therapeutic regimen. Anticoagulation with heparin instituted early is essential in controlling the infection and in preventing serious vascular sequelae.

MASTITIS

Postpartum mastitis usually begins at least 2 weeks after delivery and is most common in women who are nursing or have attempted to nurse their infants. The bacteria are usually introduced through the nipples, and the incidence is not influenced by elaborate breast care. Infection is far more common in white than in black patients.

The patient may have pain in one quadrant of the breast, followed by fever, chills, and enlargement of the affected gland. The systemic reaction to a small area of infection may be pronounced. The breast is erythematous, indurated, and tender; if the process is far enough advanced, fluctuation may be detected.

Treatment consists first of prevention, by prohibiting nursing by women whose nipples are inverted and abnormal, those in whom cracks and fissures do not heal promptly, those who have bleeding from the nipples, and those whose nipples are injured by the baby.

Curative treatment must be started early to be effective. Nursing is immediately stopped, the breast is immobilized with a tight binder, and ice is applied. Many breast infections are caused by penicillin-resistant staphylococci; consequently, an antibiotic preparation such as oxacillin is generally more appropriate than penicillin. A Gram stain and culture of milk expressed during the examination may help determine appropriate treatment.

Such treatment usually aborts or cures the infection, but if the temperature remains elevated and fluctuation appears, incision and drainage become necessary. Extensive destruction of breast tissue may result from unrecognized abscess formation.

PELVIC TUBERCULOSIS

Tuberculosis of the pelvic organs usually is caused by tuberculous infection in some other part of the body, but frequently the primary source is quiescent at the time the pelvic involvement is discovered. The infection reaches the tube by hematogenous transmission or, less often, from an infection involving the peritoneum. It spreads downward along the tubal mucosa to the endometrium and then to the cervix and vagina. Because the extension is from above downward, the structures in the lower genital tract are not often involved. It is possible, however, that lesions on the external genitals, vagina, and cervix can come from an extrinsic source such as tuberculosis epididymitis.

Tuberculous pelvic infection is encountered less frequently in the United States than in other parts of the world, where it is said to account for about 5% of all cases of salpingitis. Tuberculosis is found in from 5% to 10% of all women studied for infertility in Israel, Scotland, and some other countries, but much less often here. This picture may change. Refugees from the Caribbean and Southeast Asia have a high incidence of tuberculosis. In urban centers, an increase in the number of infertile women with unexpected pelvic tuberculosis has been seen.

The most characteristic lesions involve the tubes and the endometrium. There may be many small tubercles over the peritoneal surface, and the tube may be enlarged, thickened, and adherent. The lumen often contains cheesy, necrotic material, but, in contrast to the findings in other types of salpingo-oophoritis, the fimbriated end is open. Tubercles may be seen in any of the layers of the tubal wall. The ovarian involvement is usually superficial.

Endometrial tuberculosis is almost always a result of infection in the tubes and can usually be diagnosed microscopically without difficulty, particularly when the biopsy is obtained in the secretory phase of the cycle.

DIAGNOSIS. The symptoms are variable and are determined by the structures involved. Extensive tubal tuberculosis with distortion and fixation generally causes dysmenorrhea and dyspareunia and may interfere with descent of the ovum. If the endometrium is involved, the menstrual cycle often is altered, but there is no characteristic change. The flow is increased and irregular at least as often as it is decreased. Most of the patients are infertile. Lesions of the vagina and cervix may resemble cancer and can be differentiated from it only by biopsy.

The diagnosis should be suspected in any woman without a history of an acute pelvic infection who has pelvic pain and enlarged adherent adnexa, particularly in virgins. In such a patient, endometrial biopsy or curettage may demonstrate the lesion. If the endometrium is involved, the tubes are almost certain to be infected also; because the transmission is from above downward, however, tuberculous salpingitis can be present even though the endometrium is normal. Failure to demonstrate tubercles in the endometrium therefore does not eliminate the diagnosis. The lesion at this stage can sometimes be detected by culture of uterine discharge or from material obtained from aspiration of the endometrial cavity.

TREATMENT. Active and prolonged antibiotic treatment is indicated. Operation is less important now because the infection can usually be eradicated by the medications alone.

SUGGESTED READING

Adler SP: Cytomegalovirus and child day care, N Engl J Med 321:1290, 1989.

Anand A and others: Human Parvovirus infection in pregnancy and hydrops fetalis, N Engl J Med 316:183, 1987.

Bartlett JG and others: Therapeutic efficacy of 29 antimicrobial regimens in experimental intra-abdominal sepsis, Rev Infect Dis 3:535, 1981.

Berkeley AS and others: Imipenem/cilastatin in the treatment of obstetric and gynecologic infections, Am J Med 78:79, 1985.

Blanco JD, Gibbs RS, and Castaneda YS: Bacteremia in obstetrics: clinical course, Obstet Gynecol 58:621, 1981.

Brunham RC and others: Chlamydia trachomatis infection in women with ectopic pregnancy, Obstet Gynecol 67:722, 1986.

Burke DS and others: Measurement of the false positive rate in a screening program for human immunodeficiency virus infections, 319:961, 1988.

Centers for Disease Control: Current trends, tuberculosis—United States, 1983, MMWR 33:28, 1984.

Centers for Disease Control: Guidelines for the prevention and control of congenital syphilis, MMWR 37:S1, 1988.

Centers for Disease Control: Rubella and congenital rubella syndrome—United States, 1985-1988, MMWR 38:173, 1989.

Centers for Disease Control: 1989 Sexually transmitted disease treatment guidelines, MMWR 38:S8, 1989.

Chow AW, Marshall JR, and Guze LB: A double blind comparison of clindamycin with penicillin plus chloramphenicol in treatment of septic abortion, J Infect Dis 135:535, 1977.

Cohen MB and others: Septic pelvic thrombophlebitis: an update, Obstet Gynecol 62:83, 1983.

Cooper LZ and Krugman S: Clinical manifestations of postnatal and congenital rubella, Arch Ophthalmol 77:434, 1967.

Cooper LZ and others: Neonatal thrombocythopenic purpura and other manifestations of rubella contracted in utero, Am J Dis Child 110:416, 1965.

Curran JW and others: Female gonorrhea: its relation to abnormal bleeding, urinary tract symptoms, and cervicitis, Obstet Gynecol 45:195, 1975.

Daffos F and others: Prenatal management of 746 pregnancies at risk for congenital toxoplasmosis, N Engl J Med 318:271, 1987.

Dodson MG, Faro S, and Gentry LO: Treatment of acute pelvic inflammatory disease with aztreonam, a new monocyclic B-lactam antibiotic, and clindamycin, Obstet Gynecol 67:657, 1986.

Eschenbach DA: Acute pelvic inflammatory disease, Urol Clin North Am 11:65, 1984.

Eschenbach DA and others: Polymicrobial etiology of acute pelvic inflammatory disease, N Engl J Med 295:165, 1975.

Faro S: Group B beta hemolytic streptococcus—puerperal infections, Am J Obstet Gynecol 139:686, 1981.

Good JT Jr and others: Tuberculosis in association with pregnancy, Am J Obstet Gynecol 140:492, 1981.

Gregg NM: Further observations on congenital defects in infants following maternal rubella, Trans Ophthalmol Soc Aust 4:119, 1946.

Griffiths PD, Campbell-Benzie A, and Heath RB: A prospective study of primary cytomegalovirus infection in pregnant women, Br J Obstet Gynaecol 87:308, 1980.

Grossman JH III, Wallen WC, and Sever JL: Management of genital herpes simplex virus infection during pregnancy, Obstet Gynecol 58:1, 1981.

Hanshaw JB and others: School failure and deafness after "silent" congenital cytomegalovirus infection, N Engl J Med 295:468, 1976.

Hardy JB and others: Adverse fetal outcome following maternal rubella after the first trimester of pregnancy, JAMA 207:2414, 1969.

Hawkins DF and others: Management of septic chemical abortion with renal failure: use of a conservative regimen, N Engl J Med 282:722, 1975.

Henry-Suchet J, Catalan F, Loffredo PF, and others: Microbiology of specimens obtained by laparoscopy from controls and from patients with pelvic inflammatory disease or infertility with tubal obstruction: Chlamydia trachomatis and Ureaplasma urealyticum, Am J Obstet Gynecol 138:1022, 1980.

Horstmann DM and others: Rubella, reinfection of vaccinated and naturally immune persons exposed in an epidemic, N Engl J Med 283:771, 1970.

Immunization Practices Advisory Committee: Prevention of prenatal transmission of hepatitus B virus: prenatal screening of all pregnant women for hepatitus B surface antigen, MMWR 37:341, 1988.

Katz SL and Wilfert CM: Human immunodeficiency virus. Infection of newborns, N Engl J Med 320:1687, 1989.

Ledger WJ: Anaerobic infections, Am J Obstet Gynecol 123:111, 1975.

Ledger WJ: Selection of antimicrobial agents for treatment of infections of the female genital tract, Rev Infect Dis 5:98, 1983.

Ledger WJ, Gee C, and Lewis WP: Guidelines for antibiotic prophylaxis in gynecology, Am J Obstet Gynecol 121:1038, 1975.

Ledger WJ and Headington JT: Group A beta hemolytic streptococcus: an important cause of serious infections in obstetrics and gynecology, Obstet Gynecol 39:474, 1972.

Ledger WJ, Norman M, Gee C, and Lewis W: Bacteremia on an obstetric-gynecologic service, Am J Obstet Gynecol 121:205, 1975.

Ledger WJ and Peterson EP: The use of heparin in the management of pelvic thrombophlebitis, Surg Obstet Gynecol 131:1115, 1970.

Linnan MJ and others: Epidemic listeriosis associated with Mexican-style cheese, N Engl J Med 319:823, 1988.

Mann JM and others: Assessing risks of rubella infection during pregnancy: a standardized approach, JAMA 245:1647, 1981.

Mardh PA, Ripa T, Svensson L, and Westrom L: Chlamydia trachomatis infection in patients with acute salpingitis, N Engl J Med 296:1377, 1977.

Minkoff H and Mead P: An obstetric approach to the prevention of early onset Group B beta hemolytic streptococcal sepsis, Am J Obstet Gynecol 154:973, 1986.

New York City Department of Health: Congenital syphilis: its prevention and control, 8:1, 1989.

Paryani SG and Arvin AM: Intrauterine infection with varicella-zoster virus after maternal varicella, N Engl J Med 314:1542, 1986.

Preblud SR and others: Fetal risk associated with rubella vaccine, JAMA 246:1413, 1981.

Prober CG and others: Use of routine viral cultures at delivery to identify neonatals exposed to herpes simplex virus, N Engl J Med 318:887, 1988.

Reynolds DW and others: Maternal cytomegalovirus excretion and perinatal infection, N Engl J Med 289:1, 1973.

Rhame FS and Maki DG: The case for wider testing for HIV infection, N Engl J Med 320:1248, 1989.

Rotheram EB and Schick SF: Nonclostridial anaerobic bacteria in septic abortion, Am J Med 46:80, 1969.

Schachter J: Chlamydial infections (part I), N Engl J Med 298:428, 1978.

Schachter J: Chlamydial infections (part II), N Engl J Med 298:490, 1978.

Snydman DR: Hepatitis in pregnancy, N Engl J Med 313:1398, 1985.

Spruill FG, Minette LJ, and Stumer WC: Two surgical deaths associated with cephalothin, JAMA 229:440, 1974.

Stagno S et al: Congenital cytomegalovirus infection, N Engl J Med 306:945, 1982.

Steere AC: Lyme disease, N Engl J Med 321:586, 1989.

Swan C: Rubella in pregnancy, an etiologic factor in congenital malformations, stillbirths, miscarriages, and abortions, J Obstet Gynecol Br Commonw 56:591, 1949.

Swartz WH and Tanaree P: Suction drainage as an alternative to prophylactic antibiotics for hysterectomy, Obstet Gynecol 45:305, 1975.

Sweet RL, Draper DL, and Hadley WK: Etiology of acute salpingitis: influence of episode number and duration of symptoms, Obstet Gynecol 58:62, 1981.

Sweet RL and Ledger WJ: Puerperal infectious morbidity, Am J Obstet Gynecol 117:1093, 1973.

Weiss R and Thier SO: HIV testing is the answer—what's the question, N Engl J Med 319:1010, 1988.

Westrom L: Incidence, prevalence and trends of acute pelvic inflammatory disease and its consequences in industrialized counties, Am J Obstet Gynecol 138:880, 1980.

Woernle CH and others: Human parvovirus B19 Infection during pregnancy, J Infect Dis 156:17, 1987.

41

J. Robert Willson

The puerperium

Objectives

RATIONALE: During the puerperium the physiologic changes that occurred during pregnancy must be reversed and injuries to the reproductive tissues must heal. To provide appropriate care, physicians should be familiar with the physiologic process and the emotional needs during this phase of reproduction.

The student should be able to:

A. Demonstrate a knowledge of the normal physiologic changes during the postpartum period, including involution of the uterus, return of ovarian function and menstruation, lactation, alterations in general endocrine function, and regression of changes in nonreproductive organs.

B. Describe care after normal pregnancy and delivery.

C. Explain counseling of the patient, including contraception.

The puerperium is the period from 6 to 8 weeks after delivery during which the physical and physiologic changes produced by pregnancy regress.

NORMAL CHANGES

Uterus. The uterus, which at term weighs about 1000 g, returns to its nonpregnant weight of 60 to 80 g by a process known as *involution*. The uterus weighs about 500 g at the end of the first week and about 300 to 350 g at the end of the second week after delivery.

During involution the excess protein in the uterine muscle cells is broken down by autolysis and excreted in the urine, or it is used, at least partially, if the patient is lactating. The number of muscle cells does not change during involution, but rather the size of each individual cell decreases by about 90%.

After the lower segment has regained its tone during the first few hours after delivery, the superior surface of the fundus can be felt below the umbilicus. The size of the uterus decreases rapidly, so that at the tenth to twelfth day it is at the level of the upper border of the pubis, and by the sixth week it usually has returned to normal size.

The more superficial layers of the decidua become necrotic and slough, but the bases of the glands that dip into the muscularis remain intact and active. The new endometrium, which eventually will line the entire cavity, regenerates from the remaining glandular epithelium.

The placental site is reduced to about half its predelivery size as the uterus contracts after expelling the placenta. It becomes progressively smaller, measuring only about 3 by 4 cm at the end of the second week. Immediate control of bleeding from the open choriodecidual sinuses is obtained by compression and kinking of the blood vessels leading to them. This is followed by clot formation in the open vessels. The remaining decidual and trophoblastic tissue at the placental site, the thrombosed choriodecidual sinuses and blood vessels, and a superficial layer of myometrium beneath the placental site are infiltrated with leukocytes, and tissue necrosis begins by the second day. Eventually the crust, composed of decidua, thrombosed vessels, endometrial glands, and myometrium, separates from the normal uterine wall beneath. This permits healing without significant scarring.

Regeneration of the endometrium from the remaining glandular tissue begins on the third day and progresses rapidly. The entire uterine cavity, except for the placental site, is covered by endometrium by the end of the third week. The placental site is reepithelized within another 2 to 3 weeks by endometrium growing in from the edges and from the glands beneath the remaining crust.

The discharge from the uterus, which is made up of blood from the vessels of the placental site and debris from decidual necrosis, is called *lochia*. The discharge of pure blood from the open vessels soon changes to the *lochia rubra*, which is made up of necrotic decidua and blood. It gradually becomes less red as the vessels thrombose, but bloody discharge often persists for 4 to 5 weeks. The *serosanguineous lochia*, which is tan in color, contains less blood and soon changes to the white or yellow *lochia alba*. Bloody discharge may persist if placental fragments remain in the uterus or if for some reason involution does not proceed at its usual rate.

The endometrial cavity is sterile from 6 to 24 hours after normal delivery but then becomes contaminated from the upward migration of vaginal bacteria. Bacterial growth in the shaggy necrotic decidua contributes to the discharge.

Cervix. Immediately after delivery the cervix is relaxed and flabby, but it regains its tone fairly rapidly. Within a few days the canal reforms as both the internal and the external os contract; by the end of 10 to 14 days, the canal is well formed and narrow.

Vagina. The vagina never returns completely to the pregravid state, and sometimes there may even be some relaxation after primary cesarean section. The tags of tissue that represent the hymenal ring are called *carunculae myrtiformes*. The vaginal epithelium looks thin and smooth like that of postmenopausal women until the ovaries again begin to function and produce estrogen.

Urinary tract. The bladder may be edematous and hyperemic, and there may even be areas of submucosal hemorrhage from the trauma of delivery. The hydronephrosis and hydroureter regress rapidly if the urinary tract is normal and within 2 to 3 weeks may have disappeared completely. Diagnostic urography should be delayed for at least 6 weeks to make certain that the gestational changes have regressed.

A marked diuresis begins within the first 12 hours after delivery in normal women; this is the mechanism by which the excess tissue fluid is eliminated. Naturally, the diuresis is more pronounced in women who have been edematous than in those with normal fluid retention.

Breasts. During pregnancy the glandular and ductal tissues of the breasts are stimulated by rising concentrations of estrogen, progesterone, human placental lactogen (hPL), prolactin, cortisol, and insulin. The concentrations of these hormones decrease promptly after delivery, and the time required for them to return to prepregnancy levels is determined in part by whether the mother nurses her infant. The complicated interactions of the various hormones and breast tissue are not clear, but prolactin appears to be essential for lactation. Prolactin concentrations rise abruptly, but temporarily, as a result of the stimulus of sucking. Although prolactin stimulation is essential for initiation of milk production, there is no direct relationship between the level of prolactin secretion and maintenance of an adequate milk supply. Women without anterior pituitary function do not lactate.

Colostrum, a thin, yellow, alkaline fluid, is secreted by the glandular tissue of the breasts during late pregnancy and the first few days after delivery. Colostrum contains more protein but less fat and sugar than does milk. The concentration of globulin is greater than that of albumin.

On the third or fourth day after delivery, the breasts become *engorged* and are distended, firm, tender, and warm, and milk can be expressed from the nipples. Engorgement may involve axillary breast tissue or even that in other accessory nipples along the milk line (Fig. 41-1). The breast distension is primarily from engorgement of blood vessels and lymphatics rather than from an accumulation of milk.

There is no large supply of ready-made milk; much of it is produced in response to the stimulus of nursing. The activity of the suckling infant initiates a stimulus from the nipple that releases oxytocin from the posterior lobe of the pituitary gland. Oxytocin stimulates the myoepithelial cells surrounding the mammary glands to contract and force the milk into the ducts and from the nipples. This is called *milk ejection, or "letdown."* In some instances the sight of the baby or even the thought of nursing will initiate the reflex.

A normal pregnancy diet supplemented with an additional pint of milk each day will usually replace the materials secreted in breast milk.

Vital signs. There should be no great change in *body temperature* during the puerperium. A rise usually indicates infection. The *pulse rate* often is low. A rapid pulse should suggest the possibility of undue blood loss. *Blood pressure* should be altered only slightly in normal women.

Blood. The white blood cell count increases during labor and in the early puerperium. It may reach 20,000 to 30,000 if the labor has been prolonged. The rise is almost entirely the result of an

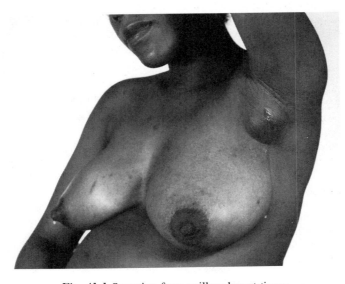

Fig. 41-1 Secretion from axillary breast tissue.

increase in granulocytes. The count usually returns to normal within a few days.

As the plasma volume diminishes during the puerperium, the hemoglobin reading and the red blood cell count rise. The patient who has had an adequate iron intake during pregnancy and who has not bled excessively at delivery should not be anemic.

Body weight. An immediate weight loss of 4.8 to 5.8 kg (10 to 12 pounds) occurs at delivery. During the first few days of the puerperium the weight will decrease by 1.9 to 2.4 kg (4 or 5 pounds) more as the excess tissue fluid is eliminated. If the patient has been edematous, the loss will be greater. A further decrease will occur as the uterus involutes and plasma volume contracts.

Endocrine status. The major sources of hormone production during pregnancy are the placenta and the adrenal, thyroid, and anterior pituitary glands. Hormone secretion changes considerably after delivery.

The hormones that are produced by the trophoblastic cells are of necessity all reduced after placental delivery. Only a small amount of *chorionic gonadotropin* can be detected in the urine after the first day. *Estrogen* production is largely a function of the fetoplacental unit and ceases with delivery. The concentrations of estrone and estradiol reach the nonpregnant range within a week, but the estriol concentration decreases more slowly, this hormone being present for 2 to 3 weeks. *Progesterone* can no longer be detected after the first week.

Adrenal function is increased during pregnancy and returns to normal rather rapidly after delivery. *Aldosterone* production decreases promptly after delivery, and the excretion of *corticoids, 17-ketosteroids,* and *11-oxycorticosteroids* usually returns to normal levels during the first week.

The changes in *thyroid function* are reversed by delivery and slowly return to the normal level.

Pituitary function, except for the production of *prolactin* and *oxytocin,* which are increased by suckling, appears to be unchanged by delivery. The production of anterior pituitary gonadotropic hormones is gradually resumed.

Ovarian function. Cyclic ovarian function is suspended after conception, but the ovaries continue to secrete estrogen and progesterone throughout the pregnancy. According to Acar, MacNaughton, and Coutts, the corpus luteum produces progesterone but little estrogen; the latter is secreted by other ovarian tissues. Estrogen and progesterone are also elaborated by trophoblastic tissues.

The anterior pituitary–inhibiting effects of estrogen and progesterone are removed when the placenta is delivered and FSH and LH secretions gradually rise, but the levels are lower than those during menstrual cycles. The time required for return of normal ovarian function is governed by the rapidity with which both hypothalamic-pituitary activity and ovarian response are restored. This is determined principally by whether the mother is nursing her infant.

The studies of Bonnar and colleagues explain why ovarian function is inhibited in nursing mothers. Even though FSH and LH levels are well above those during the early puerperium, the high levels of prolactin inhibit the ovarian response to gonadotropin stimulation. The studies of Konner and Worthman on !Kung hunter-gatherers, who have an interval of about 44 months between births, supports this concept. !Kung mothers nurse their infants briefly, but frequently, several times an hour, until the children are 3 or more years old. Konner and Worthman compared the concentrations of prolactin, estrogen, and progesterone in 16 nursing mothers with those in eight who were menstruating. Estrogen and progesterone concentrations in the lactating mothers were comparable to those found in women with hyperprolactinemic amenorrhea.

Most women who do not nurse their babies will have a period of bleeding within 4 to 6 weeks of the baby's birth, whereas those who are lactating are often, but not invariably, amenorrheic as long as they nurse. Sharman reported the return of menstrual function in 91% of nonlactating multiparas and in a third of lactating primiparas within 3 months after delivery. Multiparas more often started to menstruate earlier, even though lactating. The first period of bleeding may be heavier than a normal menstrual period and often is anovulatory. By the third or fourth period, bleeding and ovulation should have returned to normal.

Sharman, studying postdelivery endometrial regeneration by biopsy, first found secretory endometrium, presumably resulting from ovulation, on the forty-fourth postpartum day. Kava and co-workers obtained secretory endometrium from 15 women between the thirty-third and forty-seventh postpartum days and on the ninety-third day in another patient.

Ovulation can occur in women who are lactating, even though menstruation has not been reestablished. Perez and associates reported that ovulation occurred in 14.1% of women who were on a full nursing schedule and in 28.8% of those nursing partially. The earliest ovulation occurred on day 36, and the latest on day 422. These figures indicate the need for contraception in all recently delivered women.

CARE AFTER DELIVERY

The patient should be closely supervised for at least an hour after delivery. During this time her pulse and blood pressure should be checked every 15 minutes. The uterus should be palpated frequently to make certain that it remains well contracted, and the vulvar pad inspected for evidences of bleeding. The attendant should not have to manipulate and massage the uterus to prevent relaxation; if this is necessary, something is wrong.

The patient may be returned to her room at the end of an hour if the pulse is below 100, the blood pressure is stable, the uterus remains contracted, there is no unusual bleeding, and she is awake. She must be checked frequently in her room for several hours.

Puerperal care is directed toward returning the patient to normal as rapidly as possible. In general, the patients are not ill and need not be treated like those who have undergone major surgical procedures.

Ambulation. The normal woman may be out of bed and become completely ambulatory as rapidly as she is able. Those who have had spinal or epidural anesthesia for delivery should not be allowed up until both sensation and voluntary muscle control have returned.

Diet. A general diet may be ordered as soon as the patient wants it. The diet is similar to that during pregnancy, but mothers who are nursing their babies should have at least an additional pint of milk to replace the protein, calcium, and other ingredients secreted in breast milk.

Lactation. Breast milk is clean, inexpensive, and readily available, and mothers should be encouraged to nurse their babies. It is well known that nursing infants develop passive immunity against certain infectious diseases from maternal antibodies that cross the placenta and that are present in colostrum and milk.

Maternal IgG antibodies are transferred to the fetus across the placenta before birth. The predominant immunoglobulin in human milk is secretory IgA, which provides protection within the infant's gastrointestinal tract. IgA contains antibodies against certain bacteria, for example, *E. coli,* to which the infant is regularly exposed and against which it has little or no immunity. The intestine also protects the infant against certain IgG antibodies such as those in immunized Rh-negative women; the antibodies are not absorbed through the intestinal wall.

Many mothers notice painful contractions and an increase in vaginal discharge while the infant is at breast because nipple stimulation causes oxytocin release and uterine contraction.

The normal baby may be allowed to nurse before leaving the delivery room if the mother wishes. Babies and mothers, particularly primiparas, must be taught the techniques of nursing; consequently, the first attempts should be supervised by an experienced infant nurse. She can show the mother how to hold the infant and help it grasp the nipple.

Breast engorgement is temporary, the acute symptoms lasting only a day or two. The discomfort is mostly caused by lymphatic and venous engorgement rather than by distension with milk; pumping the breast may not be particularly helpful and may even increase the symptoms after relieving them temporarily. In most women the discomfort can be controlled with a tight, supporting binder, ice caps, and a simple analgesic.

Bromocriptine, 2.5 to 5 mg twice daily for 14 days, will usually prevent engorgement in women who choose not to nurse their infants. Some milk may be secreted while the patient is taking the drug, and engorgement may occur when she stops taking it.

The concentrations of drugs in milk are usually no greater than those in maternal serum. *Alcohol, heroin, cocaine,* and *methadone* are all excreted in breast milk and may have adverse effects on the infant. Low-dose oral contraceptives appear to have no ill effects on the baby.

A good practice to follow is similar to that during pregnancy: the only drugs to be prescribed are those that are necessary and known to be innocuous to the infant.

Bladder care. The renal excretion of urine is increased during the early puerperium, but the patient may have difficulty in voiding because of perineal pain or local edema from trauma. The bladder may be atonic and can become remarkably distended without producing discomfort. If the patient voids spontaneously after delivery, no particular care is necessary except to check for the adequacy of urinary output and to palpate the abdomen frequently to make certain the bladder is not distended.

The patient who has not voided during the first 6 hours after delivery should be encouraged to try. If she is unsuccessful, the administration of codeine and aspirin orally or of a belladonna and opium suppository by rectum to relieve perineal pain may relax muscle spasm and aid in voiding. If she still is unable to void, she should be catheterized. This may be repeated every 2 to 4 hours, or more often if she is uncomfortable or if the distended bladder can be felt above the pubis, until she can urinate voluntarily. An indwelling catheter can be left in place for 24 to 48 hours if it is necessary to empty the bladder more than two or three times.

Bowel. Many women are constipated during the puerperium. Normal bowel function can be established by the use of stool softeners, suppositories, or mild laxatives such as milk of magnesia. Enemas are not often necessary.

Perineal care. If the patient must remain in bed, the vulva should be cleansed by the nurse two or three times daily and after each bowel movement. When she becomes ambulatory, she can cleanse the vulva herself after voiding and bowel movements with soft tissues and soap and water; no antiseptics are necessary. The perineum should be wiped from its anterior aspect toward the anus; the paper is discarded at the end of each stroke.

Tenderness in the episiotomy is usually caused by edema from too much suture material or sutures that have been tied too tightly. The discomfort can be relieved by the use of a heat lamp for 20 to 30 minutes three times daily or by the administration of aspirin and codeine or the insertion of a belladonna and opium rectal suppository three or four times daily. Hot sitz baths can be taken as soon as the patient can get into the tub.

Afterpains. Multiparas often are troubled by painful uterine contractions during the first 48 hours after delivery. These usually are stronger while the baby is nursing. The pain can be relieved with aspirin and codeine or a prostaglandin synthesis inhibitor. Primiparas rarely experience afterpains.

Exercises. Exercises such as leg or body raising to strengthen the abdominal muscles can be started any time the patient can perform them comfortably.

The *pubococcygeus muscles* should be exercised systematically by contracting them slowly six to eight times in succession ten times daily. This will help prevent relaxation and urinary stress incontinence.

Blood count. The hematocrit should be determined before discharge. An iron preparation should be prescribed for all postpartum patients.

Bathing. Postpartum patients may shower whenever they are strong enough. Tub bathing may be resumed when the patient can get into and out of the tub comfortably.

Contraception. Most women will already have resumed intercourse before the first postpartum examination, and some of those who use no contraception will have conceived. Breast-feeding provides some protection against pregnancy because prolactin appears to reduce ovarian response to gonadotropins. However, the contraceptive effect of suckling cannot be relied on, particularly when the interval between nursings is increased to several hours. Ovulation may occur before the first period of uterine bleeding in both nursing and nonnursing mothers. Pregnancy spacing should be discussed with the patient before she leaves the hospital, and a suitable and reliable method of contraception should be prescribed.

Low-dose oral contraceptives can be started soon after delivery, even though the infant is being breastfed.

If oral contraceptives are contraindicated, condoms or foam or both should be suggested. Diaphragms cannot be fitted or intrauterine devices inserted safely until the reproductive organs have involuted completely. Intercourse can be resumed when the episiotomy is healed and coitus is comfortable.

CARE OF THE INFANT

Ideally, the baby should not be separated from its mother, but practically this is impossible. The most important time during which effective *bonding* is established seems to be the first hours of life; hence, whenever possible, the newborn infant should remain with its mother during this critical period. Skin stimulation, eye contact, and suckling appear to be important factors in establishing the relationship. The initial contact is expanded with rooming-in if it is available.

The infant may remain with the mother constantly, or the plan can be modified to include daytime care at the bedside, returning the baby to a central nursery or smaller peripheral nursery during the night. With the modified program, the baby is brought to the mother's bedside early each morning. During the day she assumes responsibility for its care under the supervision of the nurses, but before midnight the infant is returned to the nursery. The father should be encouraged to hold the baby and to change and feed it.

DISCHARGE FROM THE HOSPITAL

Most women who have had normal pregnancies and labors can be discharged by the third postpartum day; many will want to leave sooner.

Before the patient is discharged, the breasts, abdomen, perineum, and uterus should be inspected and palpated. The physician should be sure that she is voiding normally, that her blood pressure has stabilized, and that she is physically able to cope with her responsibilities at home. Each patient should be instructed specifically as to what she may and may not do after leaving the hospital. It is preferable that she limit her activity for a week or two after delivery, but this may be impossible if she has no help. Contraception should be discussed with her and a suitable method proposed.

The increasing interest in *alternative methods of providing obstetric care* has led to some significant changes in hospital stay. Hospital delivery with a brief period of hospitalization is an acceptable alternative to home delivery with all its potential dangers. Patients may be offered all the advantages of hospital delivery and be discharged in 6 to 12 hours if the delivery is normal and the immediate puerperium is uncomplicated.

SUBSEQUENT EXAMINATIONS

Normal patients return to the office for examination when the infant is 6 to 8 weeks old. Those with abnormalities must, of course, be seen earlier. At the first visit the patient is weighed; her blood pressure is recorded; and the breasts, abdomen, and pelvis are examined. A clean-voided urine specimen should be examined, a urine culture should be ordered if she has had a urinary tract infection, and a blood count should be obtained. This is also a good time to obtain material for a cervical cytologic examination.

If involution is complete, and if she appears normal physically, she should be instructed in some form of contraception if she wishes it and is not already using a birth control method and asked to return in 12 months. Any abnormalities present at this time should be corrected before the patient is discharged.

POSTPARTUM COMPLICATIONS

Bleeding. Abnormal bleeding can occur in any stage of the puerperium. Its management is discussed in Chapter 31.

Hemorrhoids. During labor and delivery, pressure from the presenting part impedes the flow of blood through the hemorrhoidal veins, and the resultant distension of the vessels may produce permanent injury to their walls. The hemorrhoids usually decrease in size rapidly and cause little discomfort, but some may produce severe pain, particularly if they thrombose.

The local application of witch hazel packs or ice reduces the distension and relieves discomfort. Belladonna and opium rectal suppositories provide relief for hemorrhoids that are more painful. The clot should be evacuated from those that thrombose. Hot sitz baths may also be ordered.

Backache. Backache occurs frequently in puerperal women and is most often caused by the unusual activity necessary for the care of the new baby. A suitable support, rest, and heat will usually control it.

Pubic separation. The symphysis may be unusually mobile, and there may be considerable separation of the pubic bones. This causes severe pain when the patient attempts to walk. The area is tender to palpation, and the defect can be palpated readily. The only treatment necessary is adhesive strapping or a tight supporting garment to immobilize the pelvic girdle and rest in bed. Recovery usually is rapid.

Subinvolution. Involution of the uterus may be delayed by endometritis, inadequate uterine drainage, retention of placental fragments, uterine fibroids, and other less obvious causes. It occurs most often in multiparas.

With delayed involution, bloody discharge is more profuse and lasts longer than usual. The uterus is large, soft, and boggy and may be retrodisplaced. Generally, it is freely movable, and there is no evidence of infection.

Normal involution can be aided by promoting adequate uterine drainage during the early puerperium. This is best accomplished by ambulation and upright posture. The course of involution is influenced only slightly by oxytocic drugs, and they ordinarily need not be prescribed during the puerperium.

If the uterus has not yet reached normal size and if bloody discharge is still present 6 weeks after delivery, *subinvolution* can be diagnosed. Unless the delay in involution is a result of retained placental fragments or a far more serious but unusual complication such as choriocarcinoma, hot vaginal douches taken twice daily for a week or two will usually hasten the return to normal.

Amenorrhea. Return of menstruation may be delayed after delivery because of minor and easily correctable dysfunctions of the endocrine organs. Other disorders such as anterior pituitary necrosis (Sheehan's syndrome) are more difficult to treat. The *galactorrhea-amenorrhea syndrome,* which is characterized by amenorrhea and persistent lactation, is discussed in Chapter 9.

Uterine retrodisplacement. During the early puerperium the large, heavy uterus will often fall posteriorly, particularly when the patient lies on her back. As involution progresses, the uterus will assume its normal prepregnancy position unless the pelvic supports have been extensively damaged.

Most retrodisplaced uteri produce no symptoms and need no treatment, but if the uterus is large, boggy, subinvoluted, and retrodisplaced at the first postpartum visit, it can be replaced and held forward with a pessary. This may aid drainage and promote involution. When involution is complete, the pessary should be re-

moved. If the uterus again assumes a retrodisplaced position and is producing symptoms, it can be managed as described in Chapter 39.

Cervicitis. The cervix is almost always injured during labor and delivery, and most multiparous women have some sort of cervical lesion, of which cervicitis is the most common.

An unepithelialized area is often observed around the external os of recently delivered women, particularly if involution is not yet complete. If such a lesion is found at the first postpartum office visit, it can be treated with hot cautery or freezing if the pelvic organs have already returned to their normal nonpregnancy state. If the uterus is still enlarged and boggy, the cervical lesion may well heal spontaneously as involution progresses. Such patients should be advised to return for examination in 4 to 6 weeks. If the lesion is still present, it can be treated at that time; if it has healed, no therapy is necessary.

SUGGESTED READING

Acar B, MacNaughton MC, and Coutts JRT: Ovarian function in women immediately post partum, Obstet Gynecol 57:468, 1981.

Anderson WR and Davis J: Placental site involution, Am J Obstet Gynecol 102:23, 1968.

Beer AE and Billingham RE: Immunology and the breast, Perinatology, p. 13, Jan-Feb. 1981.

Bonnar J, Franklin M, Nott PN, and others: Effect of breast-feeding on pituitary-ovarian function after childbirth, Br Med J 4:82, 1975.

Bunner DL, VanderLaan EP, and VanderLaan WP: Prolactin levels in nursing mothers, Am J Obstet Gyencol 131:250, 1978.

Delvoye P, Demaegd M, and Vwayitu-Nyampeta RC: Serum prolactin, gonadotropins, and estradiol in menstruating and amenorrheic mothers during two years' lactation, Am J Obstet Gynecol 130:635, 1978.

Howie PW, McNeilly AS, McArdle T, Smart L, and Houston M: The relationship between suckling-induced prolactin response and lactogenesis, J Clin Endocrinol Metab 50:670, 1980.

Kava HW, Klinger HP, Molnar JJ, and Romney SL: Resumption of ovulation post partum, Am J Obstet Gynecol 102:122, 1968.

Konner M and Worthman C: Nursing frequency, gonadal function, and birth spacing among !Kung hunter-gatherers, Science 207:788, 1980.

Little RE, and others: Maternal alcohol use during breastfeeding and infant mental and motor development at one year, N Engl J Med 321:425, 1989.

Perez A, Vela P, Masnilk GS, and Potter R: First ovulation after childbirth, Am J Obstet Gynecol 114:1041, 1972.

Sharman A: Postpartum regeneration of the human endometrium, J Anat 87:1, 1953.

Sharman A: Menstruation after childbirth, J Obstet Gynaecol Br Commonw 58:440, 1951.

Simpson-Herbert M and Huffman SL: The contraceptive effect of breast-feeding, Stud Fam Plann 12:125, 1981.

Williams JW: Regeneration of the uterine mucosa after delivery with especial reference to the placental site, Am J Obstet Gynecol 22:664, 1931.

42

Michael P. Hopkins

Diseases of the vulva

Objectives

RATIONALE: Ignoring or improperly evaluating vulvar symptoms often delays treatment of vulvar neoplasia. Early recognition and diagnosis will improve outcome and may obviate the need for extensive surgery.

The student should be able to:

A. Demonstrate a knowledge of the approach to the patient with vulvar symptoms.

B. List methods of diagnosis of vulvar diseases.

C. Describe characteristics of the typical patient at risk for vulvar neoplasia.

D. Recognize vulvar malignancies.

E. Define principles of management of benign and malignant vulvar diseases.

A great variety of developmental, trophic, inflammatory, and neoplastic disorders occur in the vulvar skin and its appendages. The following list includes some of the more common vulvar disorders:

1. Epidermis and dermis—the common dermatologic diseases, allergies, infections, nevi, dystrophies, and malignant neoplasms
2. Skin appendages—folliculitis, sebaceous cysts, hidradenomas, and Paget's disease
3. Adjacent structures—lipomas, hemangiomas, fibromas, and sarcomas
4. Development—vulvovaginal cysts and ectopic breast tissue

5. Hormones—atrophic changes occurring as a result of loss of estrogen stimulation after menopause

There often is a long delay in arriving at an accurate diagnosis of vulvar disease even though vulvar disorders occur frequently, the lesions can be inspected and palpated without difficulty, material can be obtained for culture directly from the lesions, and biopsy is simple. Too many physicians treat vulvar symptoms rather than vulvar disease, often without even a superficial examination.

The *symptoms* most often produced by vulvar lesions are *pruritus* and *irritation*. Abscesses, other acute infections, and acute ulcerative lesions can cause *severe localized pain,* but most other lesions do not. *Bleeding,* except from ulcerated lesions of invasive cancer and that caused by trauma from injury or scratching, is unusual. An accurate diagnosis can usually be made by inspection, palpation, bacterial culture, and biopsy.

BENIGN CONDITIONS

The most common benign vulvar lesions are as follows:

I. Inflammatory lesions
   A. Common skin infections
   B. Vulvitis associated with vaginal infections
      1. Trichomoniasis
      2. *Candida albicans*
      3. Atrophic vaginitis
   C. Sexually transmitted diseases
      1. Herpesvirus vulvitis
      2. Condylomata acuminata
      3. Molluscum contagiosum
      4. Chancroid
      5. Granuloma inguinale
      6. Lymphogranuloma venereum
      7. Syphilis
   D. Contact vulvitis
   E. Gland infections
      1. Bartholin's gland infection
      2. Minor vestibular gland infection
II. Ulcers
   A. Simple acute ulcer
   B. Tuberculosis
III. Atrophy
IV. White lesions
   A. Pigment defects
      1. Leukoderma
      2. Vitiligo
   B. Hyperkeratotic lesions
      1. Dystrophies
         a. Lichen sclerosus
         b. Hyperplasia
            (1) Without atypia
            (2) With atypia
V. Benign tumors

A. Cystic tumors
   1. Sebaceous cysts
   2. Bartholin's cysts
B. Solid tumors
   1. Fibroma
   2. Lipoma
   3. Hemangioma
   4. Melanoma
   5. Hidradenoma (may be cystic)
   6. Papilloma

Some of these lesions occur frequently, whereas others are less often encountered. All can be diagnosed without difficulty by using uncomplicated clinical techniques. This classification is incomplete because the rare and unusual lesions have been omitted.

Inflammatory lesions

Common skin infections. The most common skin infections are *intertrigo* and *folliculitis.* They develop in the labial folds and inner surfaces of the thighs of obese women and often in women who wear pantyhose and tight slacks regularly. The basis for the infection is compression of the vulvar structures with decreased evaporation of normal vaginal and vulvar secretions followed by bacterial infection of the macerated skin and the hair follicles.

The basic treatment is to remove the cause by weight reduction in obese women and by substituting loose cotton undergarments and skirts for pantyhose and tight slacks, at least until the infection is eradicated. The vulva should be washed several times daily with bland soap. After it has dried completely, an unmedicated protective powder is applied. Antimicrobial ointments may be helpful in the initial stages of treatment. Itching, which may be intense until the condition improves, can usually be controlled by applying 0.5% to 1.0% hydrocortisone ointment three or four times daily.

Vulvitis associated with vaginal infections. Trichomoniasis, *Candida* vaginitis, and atrophic vaginitis involve the vulva and the vagina secondarily (Fig. 42-1). The initial symptom is pruritus,

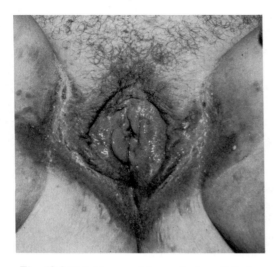

Fig. 42-1 Vulvitis caused by vaginal candidiasis.

which soon becomes intense and constant. Vulvar irritation is a result of changes in the vulvar skin, which is constantly bathed in the profuse discharge from the vagina.

Diagnosis and treatment are discussed in Chapter 43.

Pediculosis pubis, scabies, and other bites. *Pediculosis pubis* is a common infection resulting from invasion of the hair-skin junction by the crab louse, *Pthirus pubis*. The outstanding symptom is pruritus; the skin may be excoriated from constant scratching. The eggs can be seen at the base of the hairs with a magnifying glass. *Scabies* may involve the pubic hair and other hairy areas of the body. Both these conditions can be treated with topical medications that are designed to destroy the parasites. These include lindane shampoo (unless the patient is pregnant) and pyrethrins and piperonyl butoxide. Insect, flea, bedbug, and other bites are treated as they are in other parts of the body.

Sexually transmitted diseases

HERPESVIRUS INFECTIONS. Vulvar lesions resulting from infections with herpes simplex viruses are seen with great frequency. Herpes simplex virus vulvovaginitis is transmitted almost entirely by sexual contact. About 90% of the genital lesions are caused by herpesvirus type 2. These lesions may involve the vulva, the vagina, and the cervix. The remaining 10% result from herpesvirus type 1, the usual cause of herpetic lesions on the upper part of the body, particularly the lips (fever blisters). Genital infections with this organism usually occur only on the vulva.

Herpesvirus type 2 genital tract infections are transmitted by sexual intercourse and involve the vulva, the vagina, and the cervix. Those resulting from herpesvirus type 1 are probably caused by orogenital contact, which may explain their localization primarily on the external structures.

The initial symptoms, intense vulvar pruritus, burning, and paresthesia, usually begin 6 to 10 days after the introduction of the virus. These symptoms are soon replaced by pain, which becomes progressively more intense as the infection advances. This pain and the presence of the lesions usually bring the patient to the physician.

At the onset many small papular and vesicular lesions are scattered over the vulva, the vestibule, the perianal area, and even the inner surfaces of the thighs. The clear fluid in the vesicles soon becomes opaque, and the vesicles rupture, leaving painful ulcers. They may coalesce into large lesions. The vagina and the cervix may also be involved. In the most severe cases, there may be so many lesions and so much reaction in the surrounding tissue that the patient cannot void. At this stage most patients feel ill and have low-grade temperature elevations. As the lesions regress, the pain disappears. There is no residual scarring after the ulcers heal, but, with the first infection, resolution may take 2 to 4 weeks.

The lesions recur after the initial attack in at least 50% of patients. The lesions occur in the same places as did the first ones, but subsequent infections are usually less severe and of shorter duration than the first. The infections may continue to recur periodically for years.

The reason for the recurrences is that there is no effective treatment for herpes simplex virus infections, so the virus cannot be eradicated. The infection involves sensory nerves, and, as the tissues recover from the acute phase, the virus retreats to the sacral sensory nerve ganglia, where it remains dormant until a new attack is precipitated.

Antibodies against herpesvirus types 1 and 2 are produced as a result of an initial infection. These antibodies may offer some protection against subsequent infections. Patients who have developed antibodies against herpesvirus type 1 in childhood may have less severe herpesvirus type 2 infections than do those who have no antibodies against either type.

The clinical diagnosis is usually obvious, but it should be confirmed by culturing the virus from the lesions after rupturing the vesicles or removing the crusts. The social and medical (especially obstetric) implications of this diagnosis are of such magnitude that, whenever possible, the diagnosis should be made with complete accuracy. Thus, a culture should be done whenever possible to confirm the diagnosis definitely. A less accurate method than culture is to demonstrate the presence of intranuclear inclusion bodies and multinucleated giant cells in exudate from the lesions.

Treatment is generally unsatisfactory because no specific systemic medication will eradicate the herpesvirus. Acyclovir (Zovirax 5%) ointment applied directly to the lesions every 3 hours may decrease pain and healing time and, when used during the initial attack, duration of viral shedding. It does not alter the course of recurrent attacks. Local anesthetic ointments may be prescribed during the painful stages of the infection. Oral acyclovir, in doses of 200 mg two to five times daily, reduces the recurrence rate significantly as compared to placebo-treated controls. Long-term treatment for up to 1 year has been reported without undue side effects.

Herpes simplex virus infections during pregnancy are discussed in Chapter 24.

Condylomata acuminata. Condylomata acuminata occur frequently as verrucous growths scat-

tered over the vaginal introitus, the vulva, the perineum, and around the anus. There may be a few discrete lesions or confluent masses with a cauliflower appearance. Condylomata may also develop on the vaginal walls and the cervix. The incidence of clinical condyloma has increased approximately 500% over the last decade.

The etiologic agent is the human *papillomavirus* (usually types 6, 11), one of several related viruses called the *papovavirus group,* all of which produce papillomas in a variety of animals. This virus may also cause the common warts so often found in other parts of the body. The virus is transmitted by direct, usually sexual, contact, and it proliferates in the moist, warm genital tissues. The environment is even more supportive of viral growth if the genitals are constantly bathed by excessive vaginal secretions, particularly those accompanying a vaginitis. The virus also grows much more luxuriantly and spreads more rapidly in women who are pregnant, those with diabetes, and those with altered immunologic states. The lesions rarely spread to other parts of the body, although they have been reported in a number of sites.

The verrucous pattern of the lesions and their characteristic distribution make the diagnosis relatively easy. They must be differentiated from the raised, round or oval, plaquelike lesions of secondary syphilis and from verrucous cancer. If there is any question as to the diagnosis, biopsy is imperative.

Treatment is often unsuccessful because eliminating the underlying cause may be impossible. Conversely, the lesions often disappear spontaneously, as do warts in other parts of the body. This suggests an altered immunologic state as a background.

Small, isolated condylomata can be destroyed by touching each one with *25% podophyllin in tincture of benzoin, or 40% trichloracetic acid;* the surrounding skin must be protected from the medication. The vulva should be washed thoroughly after 6 hours. Podophyllin should not be used to treat large or numerous lesions in the vagina because the local and systemic reactions can be intense. Vaginal ulceration, polyneuritis, and paralysis have occurred after the medication has been applied to vaginal lesions. It should never be used during pregnancy.

Individual condylomata also can be destroyed with *liquid nitrogen, electrocautery, electrodesiccation,* or *cryocautery. Laser therapy* can also be used to destroy individual lesions. After a lesion is destroyed with laser, *papillomavirus* can be detected in the skin in 45% of patients, and the lesion can recur in 67% of the patients with residual virus. The lesion recurs less frequently if the virus cannot be detected in the skin edges; therefore, a wide area of skin surrounding the lesion itself should be vaporized with the laser beam. Additionally, the entire vulva should be treated with enough power to blanch the skin when using the laser to allow for destruction of latent virus present in the vulvar epithelium. Large masses of condylomata can be treated with laser or by excision. The virus particles are present in the vapor particles when the laser is used, and care must be taken not to inhale this plume of smoke. *Alpha interferon* produces excellent results in approximately 60% of patients. It requires three weekly sublesional injections of 1 million units per lesion. A maximum of 4 million units is recommended to minimize the possibility of side effects.

Molluscum contagiosum. This viral disease is thought to be transmitted by contact. The small, raised, umbilicated lesions may occur anywhere on the vulva and the upper thighs. There is little inflammatory reaction, and most patients have few symptoms. The diagnosis can be confirmed by demonstrating the typical cytoplasmic inclusion bodies in excised lesions. Individual lesions are treated by expressing their contents and cauterizing the base of each with trichloroacetic acid.

Other sexually transmitted diseases. Other vulvar diseases that are transmitted by sexual intercourse include chancroid, granuloma inguinale, lymphogranuloma venereum, and syphilis.

CHANCROID. Also known as *ulcus molle* or *soft chancre,* chancroid is an infectious disease that is presumed to be transmitted by sexual contact. The incubation period is 3 to 5 days. The infecting organism, *Haemophilus ducreyi,* can be identified by culture.

The lesion may occur at any point in the vestibule and, when first seen, usually is an irregular ulcer with a purulent base and little surrounding induration. Multiple lesions may occur because of several primary areas or by autoinoculation from the original lesions.

Inguinal adenitis appears about 1 week after the primary lesion is noted. The glands are tender and matted together and may suppurate.

The treatment is either erythromycin, 500 mg four times a day for 10 days, or trimethoprim and sulfamethoxazole, 160/800 mg twice a day for 10 days.

GRANULOMA INGUINALE. This disease may not appear for several months after the contact. The initial lesion is a papule on the vulva or in the vagina. The lesions soon ulcerate; the ulcer has a red, granular base and a sharply defined margin.

The process spreads slowly by continuity and contiguity, forming superficial ulcers. The inguinal lymph nodes are involved by direct spread of the lesion, and a pseudobubo, which is actually a subcutaneous granuloma rather than an abscessed node, may develop in the inguinal area.

The primary lesions are painless at the onset, but the ulcers may be painful because they are secondarily infected. Numerous small ulcers may coalesce into larger ulcerating areas, the bases of which are covered by granulation tissue that bleeds readily with manipulation. These ulcers usually do not heal spontaneously.

The organism that causes granuloma inguinale is the bacillus *Calymmatobacterium granulomatis,* and the diagnosis is made by identifying *Calymmatobacterium* bodies or inclusions in the involved tissue.

The treatment is tetracycline, 500 mg four times daily for at least 14 days. The ulcers heal with appropriate treatment, but there is considerable residual scarring.

LYMPHOGRANULOMA VENEREUM. Lymphogranuloma venereum is a venereal disease that is prevalent in the southeastern United States. Lymphogranuloma venereum is caused by organisms of the *Chlamydia trachomatis* group. After an incubation period of only a few days, a papule or pustule appears on the vulva, but it soon heals and almost always is overlooked. The infection spreads through the lymphatics and involves the inguinal lymph nodes. It may also extend along the lymph channels draining toward the rectum.

The involved inguinal nodes may coalesce and ulcerate. The ulcer is surrounded by an area of edema and fibrous induration.

Lymphatic drainage through the affected lymph channels is obstructed, and the vulvar tissues may be involved in a hyperplastic and hypertrophic lesion, accompanied by lymphostasis and lymphedema. The vulva and perineal area may be ulcerated. Eventually, scar tissue may contract and form vaginal and rectal strictures. Fistula formation is common.

Treatment of acute lymphogranuloma is with tetracycline, 500 mg four times daily for 2 weeks; doxycycline, 100 mg twice a day for 16 days; or erythromycin, 500 mg four times a day for 14 days. Excising the enlarged vulvar structures may be necessary, particularly if ulcers do not heal. Colostomy may be necessary for tight rectal strictures.

Carcinoma of the vulva eventually may develop in the chronically infected scarred tissues and presents an additional reason for removing persistent ulcerated areas.

SYPHILIS. The initial lesion of syphilis, a chancre, may occur on the vulva, but it usually is not recognized because it is transient and produces almost no symptoms. A dark-field examination, the only way syphilis can be diagnosed in its earliest stages, should be performed as part of the investigation of any vulvar ulcer in an attempt to identify spirochetes. The raised, round or oval, plaquelike lesions of secondary syphilis, condylomata lata, should not be confused with condylomata acuminata. The lesions may extend laterally and involve the upper thighs. Pronounced lymphadenopathy is usually present. The serologic test for syphilis generally is positive by the time the secondary lesions appear. Pregnancy complicated by syphilis is discussed in Chapter 24.

Contact vulvitis. Contact vulvitis often represents a local reaction to undergarments made from synthetic materials, to detergents, and to medications. One type of preparation that produces a vulvar reaction is deodorant spray.

The acute symptoms can usually be relieved by using oral antihistaminics or local cortisone ointments, wearing cotton panties rather than those made of synthetic fabrics or wearing none at all, washing underwear in bland soap and rinsing it well, and discontinuing the use of any medication in the vagina or on the vulva.

Bartholin's gland infections. The ducts of the Bartholin's or vulvovaginal glands open on the medial surface of each labium minus at about the 4 and 8 o'clock positions just outside the hymen. An acute bartholinitis can develop in one or both glands. The responsible organisms are most often gonococci, streptococci, and *E. coli.*

The gland becomes swollen and red, and the tissues around it are edematous. If the duct is obstructed, a Bartholin abscess may form. An abscess usually ruptures spontaneously within about 3 days if it is not drained surgically. An abscess is usually extremely painful, and patients present for the relief of the pain.

The early stages of Bartholin's gland infections are usually not seen because patients are unlikely to seek help until the infection has been present for several days. Early acute Bartholin's gland infections can be treated with hot soaks and an antimicrobial agent.

If the infection cannot be controlled and an abscess forms, or if the patient is first examined at this stage, the only logical treatment is surgical drainage. An incision is made over the medial bulging surface of the abscess, and the pus is evacuated. The infection usually subsides promptly.

If a wide opening persists, recurrent infections are not likely to occur, but they are common if the stoma closes.

Vulvar vestibulitis syndrome. Infections in the minor vestibular glands, which are located on the vestibular surface outside the hymen, have recently been recognized as a source of vulvar symptoms. The gland openings, which can be seen best with a magnifying glass, are scattered over the vestibule, with the major concentration being posterolaterally and posteriorly within the fourchette.

The initial symptom is usually pruritus, which is followed by burning, pain, and dyspareunia.

The areas surrounding the gland ostia are reddened, and the erythematous areas may coalesce as more and more glands become involved. In advanced cases the entire vestibule is affected. Pressure on the red areas or brushing them with a cotton swab usually reproduces the symptoms.

The application of 3% acetic acid exposes numerous areas of white epithelium that are similar to flat condylomata on the cervix. Human papillomavirus has been isolated from the lesions. The etiology of this disorder is unclear. The *papillomavirus* has been implicated as a causative agent, but definitive proof is lacking.

The symptoms can be relieved by surgical excision of the posterior hymenal ring, the adjacent vestibule, and the skin over the perineal body. Alternatively, 20% podophyllin in tincture of benzoin can be applied to individual lesions or to the entire vestibule. Carbon dioxide laser vaporization of individual lesions or of the vestibule to a depth of 2 mm can also be used, but discomfort is greater, and healing may not be complete for several weeks. This technique may also have a higher failure rate.

Ulcers

The principal ulcerated vulvar lesions, other than those described previously in the discussion of sexually transmitted disease, are the simple acute ulcers. These may occur in the lower vagina or on the vulva. They often are situated on the medial surface of the labia majora. The ulcerated lesions may be moderately painful.

Atrophy

Atrophy occurs as a normal consequence of decreased estrogen secretion after the menopause. The labia become flatter, and the skin may hang loosely as a result of loss of subcutaneous fat. The epithelium is pale, smooth, and thin. The introitus may become constricted. Atrophic changes cannot be reversed by estrogen, but in most instances they can be prevented when appropriate hormone therapy is started early.

White lesions

The white lesions of the vulva include a variety of conditions, some of which have little relationship to each other except for their color.

Pigment defects. The skin over the vulva may contain no pigment and appear perfectly white. The congenital absence of pigment is called *leukoderma,* and the secondary loss, *vitiligo.* Neither defect produces symptoms or has any clinical significance.

Hyperplastic (hyperkeratotic) lesions. The hyperkeratotic lesions are characterized by a keratin layer thicker than that on normal vulvar epithelium. The hyperkeratotic lesions vary from benign lesions associated with chronic irritation (for example, intertrigo) to epithelial cancer (Fig. 42-2).

Intertrigo is a hyperplastic lesion that occurs in the vulvar skin of obese women and women who wear pantyhose, tight synthetic-fabric underwear, or tight slacks. All compress the vulvar structures

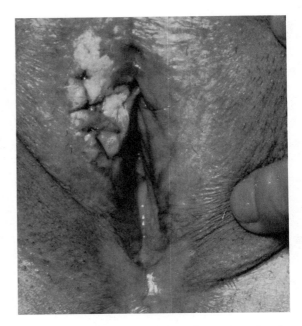

Fig. 42-2 Area of epithelial hyperkeratosis and early cancer.

and prevent evaporation of normal secretions. This and localized infection produce continued irritation. The hyperkeratotic change in the skin reverses if the irritation can be eliminated.

The outstanding symptom of *chronic vulvar dermatitis* is pruritus, which may be intractable. The itching is usually worse at night after the patient has gone to bed than during the day.

The vulva may appear normal except for mild irritation, or it may be pale and edematous. The skin may be thickened and white, and there may be linear excoriations on the surface or in the skin folds. If the itching has been severe, the skin may be excoriated and secondarily infected from constant scratching.

Any of the common skin infections can cause pruritus, scratching, and chronic vulvitis. Other causes include irritation from the discharge produced by long-standing vaginal and cervical infections such as trichomoniasis, candidiasis, atrophic vaginitis, or chronic cervicitis or from secondary infection of areas of contact vulvitis.

A diagnosis of chronic vulvar dermatitis can be made on the basis of the history and clinical findings. Dysplasia and malignancy must be eliminated by biopsy of any suspicious areas before treatment is prescribed.

Chronic vulvar dermatitis cannot be treated successfully without eradicating the basic etiologic factor. The itching can usually be relieved by local application of 0.5% to 1.0% hydrocortisone ointment applied after the vulva is washed with a bland soap and patted dry. Cool sitz baths or cold, wet compresses also afford temporary relief. Vaginitis and cervicitis must be treated appropriately. Topical antibiotic therapy may be helpful if the vulva is secondarily infected.

Surgery rarely is necessary; in fact, the dermatitis will recur after operations unless the causative condition is eliminated.

DYSTROPHIES. The vulvar dystrophies are disorders of epithelial growth characterized by a keratin layer that is abnormally thick, changes in the thickness of the epithelial layer, chronic subepi-thelial inflammatory infiltration, and changes in the subepithelial connective tissue. Almost all are benign, but abnormal hyperplasia does occur in some. The vulvar dystrophies include lichen sclerosus and hyperplastic and mixed dystrophies.

Lichen sclerosus. Lichen sclerosus can occur at any age and in other areas of the body, but it is most often diagnosed in the vulvae of postmenopausal women.

In their earliest stages, the lesions are small, raised, bluish papules that eventually coalesce until they may involve the entire vulvar area and extend laterally to the thighs. In their late stages they are white. The affected skin looks thin, and frequently fissures and excoriations result from continued scratching. As atrophy advances, the tissues shrink, and the introitus may become smaller and smaller.

Lichen sclerosus is basically an atrophic lesion that is characterized by thin, atrophic epithelium covered by a keratin layer that varies in thickness. There is increased collagen formation in the subepithelial layer, and beneath this an infiltration of inflammatory cells.

The principal symptoms are pruritus, and, as atrophy and shrinkage of the tissue progress, dyspareunia.

Lichen sclerosus is not a premalignant lesion unless abnormal hyperkeratosis also is present. Cancer develops in no more that 3% of women with the disorder; as a consequence, vulvectomy is not usually necessary. Before deciding on any treatment, however, multiple biopsies should be obtained to make certain that the condition actually is benign.

Lichen sclerosus probably cannot be prevented by estrogen therapy; although the condition is usually diagnosed in postmenopausal women, it also occurs in women with normal ovarian function and even in children.

Local treatment with *hydrocortisone ointment* usually controls the itching. Cortisone should be used only to provide temporary relief of symptoms. An *ointment of 2% testosterone proprionate in petrolatum* rubbed into the skin two or three times daily usually eliminates the symptoms and reverses many of the tissue changes. An obvious effect may not be apparent until several weeks have passed, but it can be continued indefinitely.

Topical estrogen cream may be used in the vagina to eradicate atrophic vaginitis if it is present. The continuing irritation of the vulva by abnormal vaginal secretions may interfere with treatment of the vulvar disease.

Hyperplastic dystrophies. Epithelial hyperplasia, or the hyperplastic dystrophies, have no specific gross appearance: the lesions vary in color from dusky red when little hyperkeratosis is present to white when it is advanced; they may involve the labial and perineal structures diffusely, or they may be localized to a small area; and the borders may be poorly defined, or they may be distinct plaques that are raised above the surface of the surrounding skin (Fig. 42-2). The lesions often occur as a consequence of chronic irritation, but they may represent primary hyperplastic dysplasia; hence multiple biopsy is essential before treatment is started. *Topical hydrocortisone* is the treatment of choice for the hyperplastic dystrophies. Once the process has been stabilized, maintenance daily applications should be reduced to the minimum amount.

The microscopic changes in the hyperplastic lesions may show varying degrees of chronic dermatitis accompanying the epithelial hyperplasia, but there usually is no evidence of atypicality.

Atypia is classified as mild, moderate, and severe, each grade showing a progressive decrease in cellular maturation as dysplasia becomes more pronounced.

Mixed dystrophies. The mixed dystrophies are those that combine the gross and microscopic characteristics of both lichen sclerosus and a hyperplastic dystrophy. It is these in which cancer may develop.

The evaluation and treatment of the hyperplastic and mixed dystrophies are similar to those described for lichen sclerosus. Even though the symptoms are relieved and the lesions improve,

one must be certain, by repeat biopsies, that the dysplastic change also has reversed.

Diagnosis of vulvar diseases. An accurate diagnosis is essential to successful treatment of vulvar lesions; this requires biopsy. Most vulvar lesions are benign, but, in some cases, premalignant and early malignant changes, which are not obvious by gross inspection alone, can be diagnosed by histologic examination.

The areas selected for biopsy are thickened white plaques, pigmented lesions, fissures, any ulcerated area, and any other area that looks suspicious. Multiple biopsies are essential because carcinoma in situ of the vulva can be multifocal and the true diagnosis can be made only by sampling several areas. Adequate tissue can usually be obtained in the office, using local anesthesia and a 4-mm Keyes dermatologic punch with which a full thickness of skin can be removed. Excisional biopsy of entire small lesions may be appropriate.

The use of toluidine blue to stain the vulvar tissues may be helpful in selecting biopsy sites. The entire vulva is painted with toluidine blue, which is a nuclear stain; after 3 minutes it is removed by dissolution with 1% acetic acid. The intact skin is decolorized by the acetic acid, but a blue stain is retained at breaks in the epidermis. Toluidine blue is not a specific stain for cancer cells; rather, it stains any cells that are exposed by injury or ulceration caused by infection or malignant lesions.

Benign tumors

Cystic tumors. The two most common benign cystic tumors of the vulva are sebaceous cysts and Bartholin's cysts.

Sebaceous cysts of the vulvar skin occur frequently and are exactly like those that arise in other parts of the body. They can be excised if they produce symptoms or repeatedly become infected.

Bartholin's cysts are more properly called Bartholin's duct cysts because the duct rather than the gland itself makes up the cyst wall. The main duct or an accessory duct is occluded. The gland continues its secretory activity, but the secretions cannot be discharged through the closed duct opening. The result is a retention cyst, which continues to enlarge as secretions accumulate.

Bartholin's cysts may follow obvious infections of the gland but more often have no specific antecedent cause.

Most Bartholin's cysts produce no symptoms, and the patient is unaware of their presence. Generally, they are from 3 to 5 cm in diameter, but occasionally they may become much larger. Sometimes they become infected with a resultant abscess.

Asymptomatic Bartholin's cysts need no treatment. Those that interfere with intercourse or are uncomfortable because of their size and those that repeatedly become infected should be treated surgically.

In most instances, *marsupialization* is preferable to excision of the cyst. In marsupialization a linear incision is made over the medial border of the cyst in the region of the occluded duct opening. The cyst lining is sutured to the vulvar skin and allowed to heal. If an incision of adequate length is made, the resultant opening is widely patent, and the cyst does not often recur.

Solid tumors. The solid benign tumors of the vulva include a variety of nevi, hemangiomas, fibromas, lipomas, papillomas, and hidradenomas. Only the first three are common.

The importance of nevi is that the vulva is a site for the development of melanomas. Suspicious nevi should be removed. Hemangiomas occur frequently in infants and may be large enough to produce pronounced distortion of the vulvar structures. The hidradenoma is a tumor arising in apocrine glands. It is a red, raised, often ulcerated, sessile tumor. The treatment is wide local excision.

MALIGNANT LESIONS

About 3% to 4% of primary malignancies of the reproductive organs occur in the vulva. The crude incidence for invasive cancer of the vulva is 1.9 of 100,000 women and for carcinoma in situ

it is 0.7 of 100,000 women. In contrast to carcinoma of the cervix and of the endometrium, there is little difference in incidence between black and white women, the age-adjusted rate being 1.7 in white women and 1.8 in black women.

Invasive carcinoma of the vulva (Fig. 42-2) can occur at any age, but it is basically a disease of older women and occurs most often after the age of 60 years. The period of delay between the onset of symptoms and the first visit to a physician and from first visit to diagnosis is longer than for any other cancer of the genital organs. *The first symptom, usually pruritus, is likely to be ignored by the patient and treated symptomatically by the physician, too often without adequate examination.*

Carcinoma of the vulva is usually of squamous cell origin, but 10% to 15% may be other cell types. These include *melanomas, adenocarcinomas,* and *sarcomas.* Those beginning in Bartholin's gland may be squamous cell (from the duct orifice), transitional cell (from the duct itself), or adenocarcinoma (from the gland). Bartholin's gland cancer is rare. *Basal cell cancer* also develops in vulvar skin.

Carcinoma of the vulva often is associated with carcinoma of the cervix or the vagina. Women who have been treated for carcinoma of the cervix may develop multiple foci of squamous cell cancer in the vagina and vulva. Conversely, women who have been treated for carcinoma of the vulva may develop cervical or vaginal neoplasms.

Carcinoma in situ of the vulva usually occurs in women who are much younger than those with invasive lesions, and it appears to be increasing in frequency. This may be related to the increasing incidence of *papillomavirus* infections because a high percentage of these lesions contain *papillomavirus.* Additionally the verrucous type of carcinoma contains human papillomavirus 6 and 11.

The principal symptom of carcinoma in situ, like that of many other vulvar diseases, is pruritus. The lesions may be single or multiple papules, which may be discrete or coalesced (Fig. 42-3). They often are darkly pigmented, but they

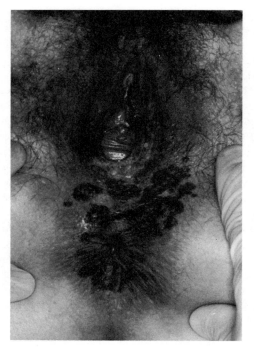

Fig. 42-3 Multiple areas of pigmented carcinoma in situ.

may be white or red. The skin may be hyperkeratotic or scaly and eczematoid. Lesions of the bowenoid type appear as white keratotic islands on a red background.

The diagnosis is made by biopsy. Tissue should be obtained from obviously ulcerated and abnormal areas and from areas that retain toluidine blue stain. Because carcinoma in situ often is a multifocal lesion, multiple biopsies from all areas of the vulva are necessary for accurate evaluation.

If carcinoma in situ is localized to a single area or to several isolated areas, and there are no premalignant changes elsewhere on the vulva, the lesion alone can be removed by wide local excision. This operation preserves the normal vulvar contours. Wide, superficial ("skinning") vulvectomy with skin graft may be appropriate for diffuse multifocal disease. Before closing the wound, the edges can be checked by frozen section to make sure the tumor has been removed completely. In recent years carbon dioxide laser has been used for ablation of vulvar carcinoma in situ. It provides a satisfactory outcome with recurrence rates that are similar to surgical excision. Importantly, the laser allows for preservation of vulvar tissue with less tissue destruction and scarring. Thus it is an ideal surgical approach, especially in the young patient.

Paget's disease

Paget's disease of the vulva arises from apocrine glands. It is a malignant lesion that usually is intraepithelial, but it may be invasive. Grossly, the typical lesions are multifocal and red with white patches and crusting. They have a velvetlike appearance. They may be located any place on the vulva and in the perianal region. The treatment of Paget's disease is wide excision. If invasive adenocarcinoma is found in the excised tissue, a radical vulvectomy with inguinal and femoral lymph nodes is the preferred treatment. Gastrointestinal adenocarcinoma and breast cancer are increased in patients with Paget's disease, and an evaluation for them should be done.

All patients who have been treated for intraepithelial carcinoma of the vulva and Paget's disease must be examined at regular intervals. The lesions may recur in the vulvar skin at any time after the operation. Of even more importance is that women with in situ vulvar cancer have an increased incidence of malignancies in the vagina and cervix.

Invasive cancer

The first symptom of invasive carcinoma of the vulva is persistent itching, which most patients treat with home remedies for several months. As the tumor grows, a lump may become obvious, and eventually the lesion becomes ulcerated. Exophytic lesions also are common. In contrast to in situ lesions, most invasive vulvar cancers are unifocal rather than multicentric. They also occur more often in elderly women than do the intraepithelial tumors.

Many women do not seek treatment until an ulcer or a fungating lesion several centimeters in diameter is present. By this time the tumor often has metastasized to the regional lymph nodes.

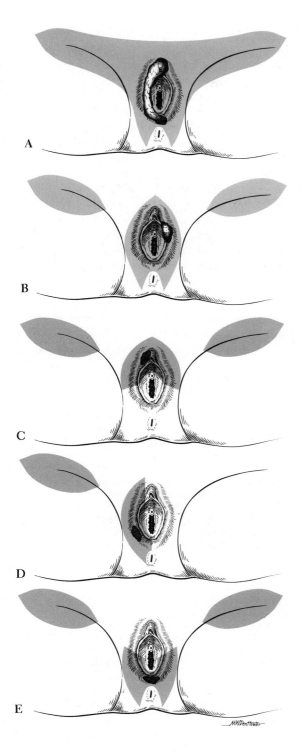

The diagnosis is made by biopsy. The potential for cure of cancer of the vulva is determined by the stage of the lesion when it is diagnosed and the quality of the treatment administered. Small, localized tumors can be eradicated completely; consequently, the cure rate can be improved only by early diagnosis. Early diagnosis is possible only if patients report symptoms at their onset and if physicians make accurate diagnoses rather than merely treat the symptoms produced by the vulvar disease.

Vulvar cancer is staged surgically and the T-N-M system is used (see box on p. 562). The treatment of invasive cancer of the vulva is radical vulvectomy and inguinal, femoral lymph node dissection. Small lesions can be treated with a more limited radical vulvectomy. Utilizing the three separate incision technique, the bridge of skin between the groin and the vulva can be preserved. Unilateral lesions can be treated with unilateral groin node resection. For large lesions, the so-called butterfly radical vulvectomy must be done (Fig. 42-4).

Pelvic radiation therapy is used when the most cephalad inguinal node (Cloquet's node) is involved with metastatic disease. A pelvic node dissection can obviate the need for radiation therapy if the pelvic nodes are negative.

Malignant melanoma

Malignant vulvar melanomas make up 3% to 5% of all melanomas in women, and they occur at all ages. The lesions are pigmented and may be either nodular or superficially spreading tumors.

Fig. 42-4 Surgical approaches to radical vulvectomy. **A,** En bloc butterfly. **B,** Three separate incisions with preservation of skin bridges. **C,** Upper hemivulvectomy for midline anterior malignancy. **D,** Unilateral hemivulvectomy and unilateral grain node dissection for unilateral malignancy. **E,** Posterior hemivulvectomy for midline posterior malignancy.

FIGO STAGING SYSTEM FOR VULVAR CANCER

Tumor
T 1 ≤2 cm
  2 >2 cm
  3 Spread to lower urethra, vagina, anus
  4 Involving upper urethra, bladder, rectum, fixed to bone

Node status

N 0	Negative nodes
1	Unilateral regional node metastasis
2	Bilateral regional node metastasis

Metastases

M 0	No metastases
1	Distant metastases (including pelvic nodes)
Stage I	T1 N0 M0
Stage II	T2 N0 M0
Stage III	T1 2 N1 M0
	T3 N0 1 M0
Stage IVA	T1 2 3 N2 M0
	T4 Any N M0
Stage IVB	Any T Any N M1

liative therapy was appropriate. In the second time period, the incidence of patients seen with far advanced lesions has decreased to only 5%. This represents greater attention paid to the diagnosis of this lesion. The survival rate is significantly influenced by the stage of the disease: stage I and II, 90%; stage III, 40%; and stage IV, 25%. The lymph node status is a significant predictor of survival, and the incidence of positive lymph nodes increases in proportion to the stage of the disease. Patients with negative lymph nodes had a 93% survival, whereas those with positive lymph nodes had a 40% survival. Thus the overall survival for this disease is excellent when diagnosed early. Now, with further refinements of radical surgery, less radical procedures are necessary when it is diagnosed early.

The edges usually are irregular, and they may ulcerate and bleed. A pigmented lesion that enlarges rapidly may be a melanoma. The treatment is wide local excision or vulvectomy, with lymph node sampling or dissection, depending on the extent of the lesion. The prognosis is determined by the size of the tumor and the depth of invasion.

Prognosis. In a collective experience covering more than 50 years at the University of Michigan Medical Center, involving approximately 450 patients with invasive squamous cell cancer of the vulva, the overall survival was 72%. Two separate time periods were studied during this review: 1935 to 1975 and 1975 to 1988. During the first time period, 21% of the patients were seen with vulvar malignancies so far advanced that only pal-

SUGGESTED READING

Baker DA, Blythe JG, Kaufman R, Hale R, and Portnoy J: One-year suppression of frequent recurrences of genital herpes with oral acyclovir, Obstet Gynecol 73:84, 1989.

Buscema J, Woodruff JD, Parmley TH, and Genadry R: Carcinoma in situ of the vulva, Obstet Gynecol 55:225, 1980.

Choo YC and Morley GE: Multiple primary neoplasms of the anogenital region, Obstet Gynecol 56:365, 1980.

Collins CG, Hansen LH, and Theriot E: A clinical stain for use if selecting biopsy sites in patients with vulvar disease, Obstet Gynecol 28:158, 1966.

Douglas JM and others: A double-blind study of acyclovir for suppression of recurrences of genital herpes simplex virus infection, N Engl J Med 310:1551, 1984.

Fenn ME, Morley GW, and Abell MR: Paget's disease of vulva, Obstet Gynecol 38:660, 1971.

Ferenczy A and others: Latent papilloma virus and recurring genital warts, N Engl J Med 313:784, 1985.

Friedrich EG Jr: Lichen sclerosus, J Reprod Med 17:147, 1976.

Friedrich EG Jr: The vulvar vestibule, J Reprod Med 28:773, 1983.

Friedrich EG Jr, Wilkinson EJ, and Fu YS: Carcinoma in situ of the vulva: a continuing challenge, Am J Obstet Gynecol 136:830, 1980.

Growdon WA and others: Pruritic vulvar squamous papillomatosis: evidence for human papilloma virus etiology, Obstet Gynecol 66:564, 1985.

Jaramillo BA and others: Malignant melanoma of the vulva, Obstet Gynecol 66:398, 1985.

Kaufman RH and Woodruff JD: Historical background in developmental stages of the new nomenclature, J Reprod Med 17:133, 1976.

Morley GW: Infiltrative carcinoma of the vulva: results of surgical treatment, Am J Obstet Gynecol 124:874, 1976.

Straus SE and others: Suppression of frequently recurring genital herpes: a placebo-controlled double-blind trial of oral acyclovir, N Engl J Med 310:1545, 1984.

Wilkin JK: Molluscum contagiosum venereum in a women's outpatient clinic: a venereally transmitted disease, Am J Obstet Gynecol 128:531, 1977.

Woodruff JD and Parmley TH: Infection of the minor vestibular gland, Obstet Gynecol 62:609, 1983.

43

J. Robert Willson

Diseases of the vagina

Objectives

RATIONALE: Vaginal discharge, vaginal irritation, and vaginitis are among the most common symptoms for which women seek treatment. One must understand the source of normal vaginal secretions as well as the causes of vaginitis to diagnose and treat vaginal infections appropriately.

The student should be able to:

   A. Describe the sources, character, and

chemistry of normal vaginal secretions and the changes that may occur during normal menstrual cycles.

B. Describe the etiology, symptoms, methods of clinical diagnosis, and treatment of vaginitis caused by *Candida, Trichomonas vaginalis,* and bacterial vaginosis infections and allergic and atrophic vaginitis.

Leukorrhea, a term applied to any nonbloody discharge from the vagina, may consist of physiologic secretions, or it may be produced in response to irritation or infection of the genital organs. A certain amount of vaginal discharge, made up of secretion of the cervical glands, endometrial debris, effusions from the vaginal mucosa, and exfoliated vaginal epithelium, is always present; but it is not obvious to most women. Normal secretions are nonirritating and usually are not profuse.

The adult vagina is lined by stratified squamous epithelium, the activity, thickness, and glycogen content of which are controlled primarily by variations in the level of estrogenic hormone. *The pH of the vaginal secretions* in the adult is between 3.5 and 4.5, the acidity being produced by the conversion of cellular glycogen to lactic acid by Döderlein's bacilli, which are normal vaginal inhabitants. Before the menarche and after the menopause, when estrogen production is low, the epithelium is inactive and only a few cell layers thick; the cells contain no glycogen, the Döderlein bacilli are absent, and the pH is between 6 and 7 (Table 43-1). The inactive unstimulated mucosa is especially susceptible to infection by an

TABLE 43-1 Changes in vaginal epithelium, flora, and secretions at various ages

	Newborn	Childhood	Premenarche	Adult midcycle	After menopause
Estrogen	High	Minimal	Increasing	High	Minimal
pH	3.5-5	6-8	4-5	3.5-4.5	6-7
Flora	Lactobacilli	Mixed	Mixed, lactobacilli	Lactobacilli	Mixed
Vaginal epithelium	Thick	Thin	Thickness increasing	Thick	Thin
Predominant cytology	Cornified squamous	Parabasal cells	Intermediate squamous	Cornified squamous	Parabasal cells
Glycogen	High	Absent	Increasing	High	Absent

organism like *Neisseria gonorrhoeae,* whereas the estrogen-stimulated vagina during the years of menstruation is rarely invaded by pathogenic bacteria.

The *volume of secretions* in the normal vagina varies throughout the menstrual cycle. In the immediate postmenstrual phase, when the estrogen level is low, the mucosa is thin and relatively inactive, and there is little secretion from the cervical cells. As estrogen production increases, the vaginal cells proliferate and exfoliate more rapidly, and the cervical cells secrete more and more mucus. At ovulation, when estrogen production is maximal, cervical mucus is profuse and watery, and vaginal desquamation reaches a peak. Some women are aware of discharge only at this time. The secretions then diminish until just before the onset of menstruation.

Secretions of the genital organs are also influenced by psychologic stimuli. Many women are aware of increased vaginal discharge during periods of emotional stress. The most powerful psychologic stimulant to genital tract secretion is sexual excitement. Before Masters's studies of coital physiology, vaginal lubrication before and during coitus was believed to come from an outpouring of secretions from cervical and Bartholin glands. Masters observed the formation of a smooth, shiny, lubricating covering for the vagina during sexual stimulation that started as a transudation of droplets of fluid from the vaginal wall during the excitement phase and rapidly coalesced into a uniform coating.

Abnormal discharge is most often caused by infection of the vagina or the cervix, but it can be the result of chronic irritation, hyperemia, or endocrine disorders that are accompanied by excessive estrogen production. Diagnosis of a specific cause for a vaginal discharge cannot be made by gross inspection alone. The evaluation of these women requires a pH evaluation of the vaginal secretions, a microscopic examination of secretions in a saline and 10% potassium hydroxide solution, and, occasionally, bacterial culture.

TRICHOMONIASIS

Vaginitis caused by *Trichomonas vaginalis* is a common cause of leukorrhea in adults, but it is seldom encountered during the prepubertal period. The presence of trichomonads does not always indicate active infection because they can be demonstrated in the vaginal secretions of some women who have no symptoms.

The methods by which the infection is acquired are not always obvious, but since trichomoniasis can be produced by introducing organisms into normal women, it must be assumed that the organism is usually implanted in the vagina during sexual intercourse. Trichomonads have been found in the male urethra and prostate, and the highest incidence of positive cultures occurs in women who have had frequent exposure to numerous sexual partners.

The primary complaint of most women with trichomoniasis is of moderate to profuse discharge accompanied by intense itching and irritation of the vagina and vulva. They can have a vaginal burning sensation, and intercourse can be uncomfortable. The initial symptoms often begin during or immediately after a menstrual period; after the infection is established, both the discomfort and the discharge usually increase during the premenstrual phase of each cycle.

The vulva, vagina, and cervix are intensely inflamed, and punctate red "strawberry spots" can sometimes be seen scattered over the vaginal and cervical mucosa. The vagina contains a large amount of discharge that characteristically is foul smelling and thin, greenish yellow, and bubbly in appearance. The vaginal pH is higher than 5.

The diagnosis is confirmed by identifying trichomonads in the secretion. A drop of the vaginal secretions is mixed with a small amount of warm saline solution in a test tube, and 2 or 3 drops of the suspension are placed on a clean glass slide and examined under the microscope at once without staining. Numerous motile trichomonads and pus cells can be seen. There are few epithelial cells.

Metronidazole (Flagyl), a trichomonacidal drug, is effective when taken orally and will kill the organisms in both men and women. The trichomonads can be eradicated with more certainty if partners also are treated because the infection often will recur unless foci in the male urethra and prostate are eliminated. A single dose of 2 g of the drug or 250 mg three times a day for 7 days will eradicate at least 90% of infections in women. If it does not, it can be repeated.

If the infection persists after the second dose, a more detailed evaluation is in order. One must consider the possibility of reinfection rather than treatment failure and examine and treat infected sexual partners. If this is not the case, the possibility of more resistant trichomonads needs to be considered. A dosage of 3 g of metronidazole a day should be prescribed orally for 7 days. If the patient cannot tolerate this, he or she will have to be admitted for intravenous therapy.

Although there have been no reports of anomalies in infants whose mothers were treated with metronidazole during pregnancy, local therapy is preferable in the first trimester, but oral therapy can be prescribed after that.

Patients should not drink alcohol during treatment. Metronidazole enhances the systemic effects of alcohol and has an Antabuse-like effect.

Transient relief from itching can be obtained with acid douches of vinegar (2 tablespoonfuls in 1 quart of warm water) once or twice daily. Although local agents are less effective than is metronidazole, clotrimazole vaginal cream used twice daily eradicates the infection in about 50% of women. It may be used in women who cannot tolerate metronidazole or during the first trimester of pregnancy.

Local treatment must be continued during menstruation because exacerbations usually occur at this time. Treatment should be continued for at least three menstrual cycles, even though the symptoms disappear and no organisms can be identified in the secretions. Patients should be advised to resume local therapy during each of the first three or four menstrual periods after daily treatment is stopped.

CANDIDIASIS

Candidiasis, which is also called *moniliasis* or *yeast infection,* occurs most frequently during pregnancy, in women using oral contraceptives or antibiotics, and in those who have diabetes. *Candida albicans* is responsible for almost all vaginitis of this type. Thrush in infants may be contracted during delivery if vaginal contents containing the organisms enter the mouth.

The typical symptoms are watery discharge and intense itching of the vagina and vulva. The external genitals usually are edematous, intensely inflamed, and irritated, and the vagina is fiery red and contains a considerable amount of thin, watery discharge as well as a thick, white, cheesy exudate that may be adherent to the vaginal walls.

The diagnosis is confirmed by culture or by

demonstrating mycelia and spores in a wet preparation. The addition of a drop or two of 10% potassium hydroxide to the wet preparation is of help in identifying yeastlike organisms. This chemical destroys most of the white blood and epithelial cells, leaving the mycelia clearly visible.

A simple and accurate culture method consists of the inoculation of a commercially prepared slant of Nickerson's medium with a specimen of discharge picked up on a dry, sterile cotton applicator (Fig. 43-1). The cap is replaced, and the inoculated tube is kept at room temperature. If yeastlike organisms are present, they will appear as isolated brown or black colonies within 48 hours.

The most effective treatment for *Candida* vulvovaginitis is to instill *miconazole* (Monistat) or *clotrimazole* (Gyne-Lotrimin) *cream* into the vagina nightly for 3 to 7 days. *Clotrimazole,* 200-mg vaginal tablets, inserted daily for 3 days is effective in nonpregnant patients. Two percent *buconazole vaginal cream* instilled nightly for 3 nights eradicates the organism in at least 90% of patients. The cream can also be applied to the vulva several times a day during the first 2 or 3 days of treatment.

Women who have regularly recurring infections, particularly those who are pregnant or using oral contraceptives, can usually keep them under control by instilling cream two or three times a week or by starting to use it as soon as the itching is felt. Before recommending this, one must be certain that the recurrences really are *Candida* infections. Antifungal treatment need not be prescribed prophylactically just because antibiotic therapy is necessary. However, it can be used if *Candida* vulvovaginitis recurs inevitably whenever antibiotics are used.

Recurrent vaginal candidiasis may come from a reservoir in the intestine. In young women with repeated infections, *Candida* organisms can usually be recovered from feces when they are present in the vagina. The obvious implication is that feces should be cultured in women with recurrent vaginal candidiasis that is resistant to treatment.

Mycotic infections can be *transmitted between sexual partners,* but the male reproductive tract is not necessarily the source. In a study of couples with recurrent vulvovaginitis, Horowitz, Edelstein, and Lippman found reservoirs of infection in the oral cavity in 36%, in the rectum in 33%, and in the male ejaculate in only 15%. Restriction of sexual contact with the reservoirs resulted in cure.

Povidone-iodine gels and douches are often prescribed for women with *Candida* vulvovaginitis, but they are less effective than are other agents. In addition, they may have undesirable side effects. The iodine is absorbed readily, and serum concentrations of free and inorganic iodine are increased as much as fifteenfold from povidone-iodine preparations in the vagina. Thyroid hormonogenesis may be suppressed. *Povidone-iodine products should not be used during pregnancy; the absorbed iodine can induce goiter and hypothyroidism in the fetus.*

BACTERIAL VAGINOSIS OR NONSPECIFIC VAGINITIS

Bacterial vaginosis in the past was called nonspecific vaginitis because trichomonads, yeastlike organisms, and other common causes could not

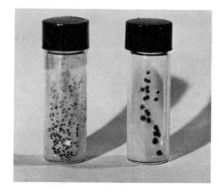

Fig. 43-1 Yeastlike organisms growing in Nickerson's medium.

be identified. *Gardnerella vaginalis* has been established as the cause, but there may also be an overgrowth of anaerobic bacteria.

The usual complaint of women with bacterial vaginosis is a discharge with a disagreeable odor. There usually is no irritation as there is in other common forms of vaginitis. There is little, if any, evidence of vaginitis other than a gray exudate with a pH of 5 or more.

The diagnosis can be suspected by the symptoms and by the appearance of the vagina. It is confirmed by recognizing a *fishy amine odor* when a drop of 10% potassium hydroxide is added to fresh vaginal exudate on a glass slide and by identifying characteristic *"clue cells"* in a saline suspension of the vaginal secretion. Clue cells are vaginal epithelial cells with a stippled appearance and rather vague borders. The stippling is caused by many adherent short rods. Other bacteria can also adhere to epithelial cells, but most are gram positive in contrast to gram-negative *Gardnerella vaginalis*. The cause can also be suspected by the paucity of white blood cells, which usually cover the slide in trichomoniasis and candidiasis. When all the clinical evidences of bacterial vaginosis are present, the diagnosis can be made without difficulty. When vaginosis is suspected but cannot be proven, Gram stain or culture may be helpful.

The infection responds to systemic therapy. Metronidazole, 250 mg three times daily for 7 to 10 days, will usually eradicate it. Ampicillin, 500 mg four times daily for 5 days, also is effective, although with a lower cure rate.

Haemophilus vaginitis is a venereal infection; hence it may recur. Treatment of sexual partners whenever possible would seem appropriate, although it does not improve cure rates. As an alternative, the male can be counseled to use a condom.

Bacterial vaginosis during pregnancy may be associated with complications that include chorioamnionitis, premature rupture of membranes, premature labor, and postpartum endomyometritis.

ATROPHIC VAGINITIS

The pale, thin, smooth atrophic epithelium that lines the vagina in postmenopausal women is easily infected; even minor injuries may permit the entry of bacteria.

The patient usually complains of irritating vaginal discharge, pruritus, and, often, swelling and pain. The vagina is red and inflamed and may be covered with "strawberry spots" similar to those observed with trichomoniasis. The discharge is purulent and often profuse; in some women it is blood tinged. *If the patient has a bloody discharge, cancer must be suspected even though the physician can see a vaginal source for the bleeding.*

Estrogenic therapy will convert the atrophic epithelium to a thick, stratified squamous layer that is resistant to infection. Ordinarily, no other medication is necessary. Local treatment with an estrogenic vaginal cream nightly for 3 weeks will usually be effective, or oral estrogen can be used. Infection may recur as the epithelium returns to its pretreatment atrophic state, but it will respond to retreatment. Recurrences can usually be prevented by using the estrogenic material two or three times a week. There may be some systemic effect from vaginal applications of estrogen because estrogen is absorbed readily from the vagina.

If atrophic vaginitis is not treated, the vagina may become almost completely obliterated by atrophy and adhesions between denuded areas.

CHEMICAL AND ALLERGIC VAGINITIS

The vagina may become irritated in response to the introduction of certain chemicals. Some, such as creosote or potassium permanganate, which once were used as douches to induce abortion, can produce extensive tissue destruction. Chemical vaginitis can also be produced by medications being used to treat specific forms of vaginitis. Substances used in commercial douche powders, vulvar lotions, or aerosol sprays may cause allergic reactions in susceptible women. An occasional woman is allergic to the ejaculate of her male sexual partner.

This type of vaginitis should be suspected whenever the introduction of a substance into the vagina is followed by irritation that gradually subsides but recurs in response to reintroduction of the same material. The appearance of the vagina is determined by the tissue response to the irritant. Strong concentrations of creosote or potassium permanganate, for example, may produce deep ulcerations and bleeding. With allergic reactions the vagina is reddened and edematous, and secretions are usually thin and watery. They may become purulent if infection is superimposed.

Treatment of chemical vaginitis consists of recognizing the cause and discontinuing the use of the irritating preparation. Warm, plain water or saline solution douches may aid in relieving irritation. An antihistamine preparation, either taken orally or applied locally as ointment, may be helpful if the reaction is primarily an allergic one. Hydrocortisone ointment will relieve vulvar itching and irritation. If the allergy is to the male ejaculate, the use of a condom is helpful.

OTHER CAUSES OF LEUKORRHEA

Cervicitis, one of the most common causes of leukorrhea in adults, is discussed in Chapter 44, and herpesvirus infections in Chapter 42. Among the less common causes are foreign bodies (for example, tampons and pessaries); carcinoma of the cervix, endometrium, or tube; and certain rare infections of the genital organs.

TUMORS

Benign tumors. *Vaginal inclusion cysts* may develop at the site of injuries that occur with delivery. They frequently develop along the episiotomy scar. Inclusion cysts rarely cause symptoms and need not be treated.

Gartner duct cysts are residual remnants of the paramesonephric ducts that do not atrophy. They usually are found in the lateral vaginal fornices or along the lateral walls of the upper third of the vagina. They rarely cause symptoms and, as a general rule, need no treatment.

Condylomata acuminata may involve the vagina as well as the vulvar structures. During pregnancy they may grow luxuriantly and actually fill the vagina. Extensive involvement may preclude vaginal delivery. The lesions often regress during the puerperium.

The use of podophyllin to destroy vaginal lesions during pregnancy is contraindicated, but isolated small condylomata can be treated with 40% trichloroacetic acid. The lesions often regress when vaginitis is eradicated or after delivery. Large lesions can be destroyed by electrodessication or by laser.

Vaginal adenosis may develop in young women who were exposed to diethylstilbestrol during embryonic and fetal life. A few may progress to clear cell adenocarcinoma. This lesion is discussed in Chapter 3.

Malignant tumors. *Primary squamous cell carcinoma* of the vagina is an unusual lesion. It may develop in the upper third of the vagina of women who have been treated for carcinoma of the cervix or of the vulva.

The diagnosis can be suspected by a report of an abnormal cytologic study, particularly in women who have been treated for cervical cancer or after hysterectomy.

The diagnosis is confirmed by biopsy of any obvious lesion or by multiple biopsies of the vagina if the cytology is abnormal but no lesion can be seen.

Vaginectomy is usually adequate treatment for carcinoma in situ of the vagina. The vagina can be reconstructed by vaginoplasty.

Invasive cancer is treated by radium application and external radiation. In some patients, particularly those in whom radiation has failed to eradicate the tumor, pelvic exenteration can be considered.

SUGGESTED READING

Ansel R and others: Nonspecific vaginitis. Diagnostic criteria and microbial and epidemiologic associations, Am J Med 74:14, 1983.

Buxton CL, Weinman D, and Johnson C: Epidemiology of *Trichomonas vaginalis* vaginitis, Obstet Gynecol 12:699, 1958.

Eschenbach DA and others: Diagnosis and clinical manifestations of bacterial vaginosis, Am J Obstet Gynecol 158:819, 1988.

Horowitz BJ, Edelstein SW, and Lippman L: Sexual transmission of candida, Obstet Gynecol 69:883, 1987.

Masters WH: The sexual response cycle of the human vagina; vaginal lubrication, Ann NY Acad Sci 83:301, 1959.

Muller M and others: Three metronidazole-resistant strains of *Trichomonas vaginalis* from the United States, Am J Obstet Gynecol 138:808, 1980.

Sobel JD, Schmitt C, and Meriweather C: Clotrimazole treatment of recurrent and chronic candida vulvovaginitis, Obstet Gynecol 73:330, 1989.

Symposium Vulvovaginal candidiasis: current views, Am J Obstet Gynecol 158:985, 1988.

Thomason JL and Gelbart SM: Trichomanas vaginalis, Obstet Gynecol 74:536, 1989.

Vorherr H, Vorherr UF, Mehta P, Ulrich JA, and Messer RH: Vaginal absorption of povidone-iodine, JAMA 244:2628, 1980.

44

Michael P. Hopkins

Benign and malignant diseases of the cervix

Objectives

RATIONALE: As with many malignancies, detection of the preinvasive lesion reduces the mortality associated with carcinoma of the cervix. An understanding of the approach to the patient with a cervical lesion is important for all physicians.

The student should be able to:

A. List the symptoms and physical findings of cervicitis and neoplasia.

B. Devise an approach to the patient with an abnormal Pap smear.

C. List the histologic categories and risk factors.

D. Describe the course of cervical neoplastic disease, including common complications.

E. Explain diagnostic methods for women with cervical diseases.

F. Differentiate benign and malignant cervical diseases.

The relative ease with which the cervix can be exposed has permitted a study of the changes that occur normally throughout life. Its position also permits detailed study of pathologic conditions by direct inspection, colposcopy, biopsy, and chemical and microbiologic study of the secretions. It is exposed to a variety of foreign substances throughout a woman's lifetime, and that a variety of abnormalities affect this structure is therefore not surprising.

NORMAL CERVIX

The cervix, the most inferior part of the uterus, is derived from the fused caudal portions of the müllerian ducts. During reproductive life, it protrudes into the vaginal canal at the apex of the vagina, where the vaginal walls blend into the epithelial covering of its external surfaces. After the menopause, the cervix atrophies as estrogen is gradually withdrawn until it is flush with the vaginal vault. The part of the cervix that lies above the level at which the vaginal wall is attached is the *supravaginal cervix,* and that below the attachment is the *portio vaginalis.* The supravaginal cervix is surrounded by pelvic fascia laterally and anteriorly and by the cul-de-sac peritoneum posteriorly. The *cervical canal,* which is fusiform and 2 to 3 cm long, provides a passageway between the vagina and the uterine cavity.

The portio vaginalis of the normal cervix is covered by pink, smooth, stratified squamous epithelium much like that which lines the vagina. The cervical canal is lined by mucus-secreting columnar epithelium that is thrown into folds and grooves that form complex branching clefts and tunnels called *crypts.* The caudal end of the canal is constricted to form an opening into the vagina, the *external cervical os* (Fig. 44-1). The opening is round and centrally placed in nulliparous women. It is more likely to be represented by a transverse slit in those who have had children. The upper end of the canal also is constricted at the opening into the uterine cavity called the *internal os.*

In contrast to the body of the uterus, which is principally a muscular organ, the cervical stroma is predominantly collagenous connective tissue with some elastic fibers and a few smooth muscle cells. The change, which may be abrupt or gradual, occurs just above the internal os in an area known as the *isthmus.* The epithelium overlying the isthmus is more like the lining of the uterine cavity than like that of the cervical canal.

The cervical epithelium responds to changes in ovarian hormone concentrations, but the responses of the stratified squamous epithelium on the portio are different from those of the columnar cells in the canal. The squamous cells proliferate under the stimulus of rising estrogen concentrations during the first half of the cycle and respond to progesterone after ovulation, as do vaginal epithelial cells.

The columnar cells are also affected by changes in hormone concentrations, but the results are more obvious because these cells secrete mucus. After a menstrual period, the cervical mucus is thick and sticky, but it changes from day to day under the stimulus of increasing concentrations of estrogen. At about the time of ovulation, the mucus is profuse, watery, and transparent and can be drawn out in strands 10 to 15 cm long (spinnbarkheit). After ovulation the mucus becomes thick and tenacious in response to progesterone. The pH at ovulation is 7 to 8 as compared with about 4.5 early and late in the cycle.

Arborization, or ferning, of cervical mucus is induced by the effect of estrogen and is inhibited

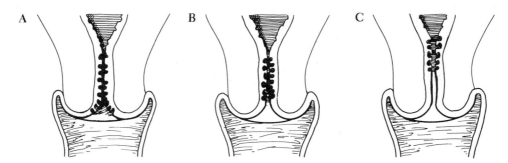

Figure 44-1 Location of squamocolumnar junction according to age. The location where the endocervical glands meet the squamous epithelium becomes progressively higher with age. **A,** Puberty. **B,** Reproductive years. **C,** Postmenopause.

by progesterone. Ferning is absent in estrogen-deficient states, minimal during the postmenstrual phase of the cycle, maximal at the time of ovulation, and absent as progesterone secretion increases after ovulation and during pregnancy (Chapter 2).

Squamocolumnar junction

The point at which the squamous epithelium that covers the portio joins the columnar epithelium of the cervical canal is the *squamocolumnar junction* (Figs. 44-1 and 44-2). The junction can be identified as the line of demarcation between the pale pink squamous epithelium that covers the portio and the bright red columnar epithelium that lines the canal. The division may be at the external os, on the surface of the portio lateral to the opening, or within the cervical canal. The columnar epithelium often extends well beyond the external os in the diseased cervix and *quite normally* in newborn infants and during puberty and adolescence. In postmenopausal women, the squamocolumnar junction may be high in the canal where it cannot be seen. Visualization of the squamocolumnar junction is critical when colposcopy is done. Many of the neoplastic changes that occur in the cervix do so at this junction.

BENIGN DISEASE
Cervicitis

Acute cervicitis does not often occur as an isolated entity; rather, it accompanies an acute infection in some other part of the reproductive system. The acute infections that most often involve the cervix are those caused by *Trichomonas vaginalis*, *Haemophilus vaginalis*, genital herpesvirus, *Chlamydia* infections, and gonorrhea. Acute cervicitis can also develop when foreign bodies such as menstrual tampons are left in the vagina for long periods of time. Acute cervical infections occur regularly as part of puerperal and postabortion uterine infections.

The cervix is congested, edematous, and inflamed, and there usually is a profuse, purulent exudate from the canal. The vagina may also be inflamed. The cervix is tender, and the parame-

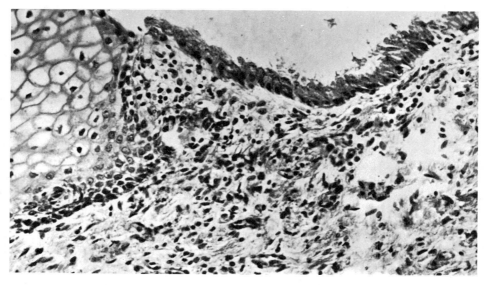

Fig. 44-2 Section through squamocolumnar junction. Squamous epithelium on left adjacent to tall columnar epithelium of endocervix. (×279.)

trial areas may be indurated and tender when palpated. The cause of the infection can be determined by bacterial culture of the exudate.

Chronic cervicitis occurs more often than does any other infection of the female reproductive organs. Almost all women who have delivered babies or had abortions have histologic evidence of chronic cervicitis. The vast majority of these infections cause no symptoms and are of no consequence. There is no known relationship between chronic cervicitis and cervical cancer.

The major involvement, *endocervicitis,* is in the cervical canal. Here the infection involves both the columnar epithelium lining the crypts and the underlying stroma. The secretion from the infected columnar epithelium is white, yellow, or green and thick and purulent in contrast to the normal clear mucus these cells usually secrete. In mild cases the portio may be completely covered by normal-appearing squamous epithelium, the only evidence of infection being the purulent secretion coming from the canal. In some instances the process extends outward from the canal, and one may see an irregular reddened area surrounding the external os. It may not be evident until the exudate is wiped away.

With the most severe infections, the squamous epithelium that usually covers the portio is replaced by friable granulation tissue, and the cervix is edematous and hypertrophied. There may even be an associated parametritis as the process extends laterally through the lymphatic channels. These lesions often bleed after the slightest touch and can be differentiated from cancer only by biopsy.

Women with only histologic evidence of infection usually have no symptoms. Those with more extensive lesions may be annoyed by the discharge, which is present constantly but which usually increases at midcycle and premenstrually. Some have so much secretion that they must wear perineal pads to protect their clothing. Other symptoms such as lower abdominal pain, dyspareunia, and backache may accompany infections that extend beyond the cervix, but they are unusual.

Treatment. The treatment of *acute cervicitis* is determined by identifying the causative organism. Culture and sensitivity studies indicate the appropriate medication.

Small areas of *chronic cervicitis* can be treated by *thermal cautery* or by *freezing (cryosurgery).* The effect of both methods is to destroy the abnormal tissue, which is followed by healing and reepithelization. The entire surface of the visible lesion and at least the lower 1 to 2 cm of the endocervical canal are treated. Nabothian cysts are usually destroyed in the process. The annoying discharge from the sloughing cervical tissue can be controlled with vinegar douches and the daily instillation of an antibiotic cream, which may be discontinued after 7 to 10 days.

Regeneration and healing may not be complete for 6 to 8 weeks; consequently, repeat treatment should be delayed at least that long. *Lesions that do not heal after adequate treatment should be biopsied to eliminate cancer as a cause of the failure.*

Local treatment of chronic cervicitis with douches and antibiotic creams or with chemical cautery (silver nitrate) almost always fails because the lesion is relatively deep-seated in the tissue, and medications applied to the surface have no appreciable effect. Systemic antibiotics also are ineffective in the treatment of chronic cervicitis.

Ectropian

Ectropian is an extension of the columnar epithelium that lines the cervical canal outward across the vaginal face of the cervix. The squamocolumnar junction is at the periphery of the lesion rather than in the region of the external cervical os. It is common at birth and in young girls and is seen frequently during adolescence, but most disappear as the reproductive organs and their functions mature.

The glandular areas become epithelialized as the medial border of squamous epithelium advances toward the os by a process of metaplasia. The metaplastic epithelium is gradually transformed to a more mature squamous type. The stimulus for the replacement is unknown but may

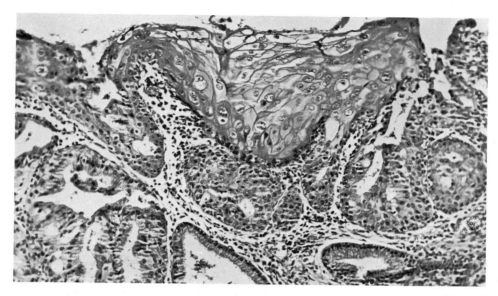

Fig. 44-3 Section showing squamous metaplasia of endocervical mucosa and contiguous crypts. (×164.)

be estrogen, which increases before puberty, or the resultant reduced pH. Areas of columnar cells may be trapped beneath the advancing squamous epithelium as the lesion heals (Fig. 44-3).

They generally produce no symptoms, but some women may be aware of excessive, clear, nonirritating, mucoid secretions, which may be most obvious during the midcycle peak of estrogen stimulation.

Nabothian cysts

As squamous epithelium proliferates and replaces columnar epithelium that has extended onto the portio, areas of columnar epithelium may become isolated beneath the advancing metaplastic squamous layer. The columnar cells continue to secrete mucus. Because there is no opening to the surface, the secretion accumulates, forming nabothian cysts. These structures are usually no larger than 1 to 2 mm in diameter. They are filled with normal-appearing cervical mucus, which does not become infected. Nabothian cysts cause no symptoms.

Diagnosis of cervical lesions

Diagnostic procedures are relatively simple. Most benign lesions can be recognized with reasonable accuracy by gross inspection of the cervix, but all available diagnostic aids should be used if there is any question of the diagnosis, particularly when a cervical lesion resembles cancer.

Polyps

Cervical polyps occur frequently. These small, pedunculated lesions arise in the endocervical canal and consist almost entirely of columnar epithelium with or without squamous metaplasia. They vary in size from a few millimeters up to 2 to 3 cm. They are soft, red, and friable. If cervical polyps are present, bleeding may be induced by the slightest trauma to the cervix. They rarely undergo carcinomatous change.

Cervical polyps are often responsible for episodes of slight vaginal bleeding. If the physician assumes that the polyp alone is responsible for the bleeding and does not perform an endometrial and endocervical curettage, a carcinoma may go undetected, particularly in postmenopausal women, when the bleeding may actually be from an abnormal endometrium.

Polyps can be removed in the office if there has been no abnormal bleeding. Although they rarely are malignant, they should be examined histologically.

Hypertrophy

Both the diameter and the length of the cervix may increase severalfold. Usually the increase in diameter results from edema that accompanies a long-standing chronic infection. Vaginal relaxation and prolapse of the uterus, however, are frequently associated with a hypertrophy and lengthening of the supravaginal portion of the cervix. The weight of the cystocele and rectocele pulling on the cervix gradually stretches this portion of the uterus to several times its normal length. If the uterine supports remain reasonably intact, the cervix may elongate so that it protrudes far beyond the introitus, even though the uterus descends only slightly.

The treatment of hypertrophy alone depends a great deal on the accompanying pathologic findings and the age and physical condition of the patient. Rarely, a high cervical amputation and a vaginal plastic operation may be all that is necessary if the uterus is normal and well supported. If the uterine supports are stretched, a vaginal hysterectomy and vaginal plastic repair are the procedures of choice.

Stenosis

Stenosis of the cervical canal is caused by scar tissue contracting and by the agglutination of raw surfaces within the endocervix. Stenosis may follow cauterization, conization operations, cervical amputations, and intrauterine cesium applications.

The major symptoms are related to menstruation. The flow may be scant, painful, and prolonged because of the stricture of the cervical canal. An acquired dysmenorrhea after cervical operations strongly suggests cervical stenosis. Obstruction may be complete in rare instances, with hematometra resulting. These woman present

with cyclic monthly cramps but without bleeding. An enlarged uterus suggests the diagnosis, and ultrasound is used to confirm the clinical findings. Severe cervical stenosis occasionally prevents cervical dilation during labor and makes cesarean section mandatory.

The uterus and cervix atrophy after the menopause. Contraction and stenosis may so completely close the endocervix that secretions from the atrophic endometrial cavity have no way to escape. The secretions and cellular debris accumulating within the cavity of the uterus may eventually become infected, and *pyometra* results. Pyometra may also occur with endometrial carcinoma or with cancer of the cervix that obliterates the cervical canal.

Treatment consists of dilation of the cervix and culture of the escaping purulent material. Appropriate antibiotics may be needed, although it is usually unnecessary. The cervix must be kept open by the passage of a 3- or 4-mm dilator once a week until the point of stricture remains open without force, about four to six dilations. In rare instances, patency cannot be maintained, and hysterectomy is indicated if the stenosis recurs. *Diagnostic curettage is essential in women with pyometra because it is associated with uterine cancer in approximately 50% of cases.*

Benign new growths

In addition to the common polyp previously discussed, myomas can involve the cervix. They are considered in Chapter 45. Likewise, endometriosis, although infrequent in the cervix, does occur and is discussed in Chapter 11.

MALIGNANT DISEASES

Approximately 10% of all invasive cancers in women occur in the uterus; of these, about 30% arise in the cervix. In 1989, about 13,000 new invasive cancers of the cervix were diagnosed and 7000 women died of the disease. The crude annual incidence of invasive carcinoma of the cervix is 17.3 of 100,000 women of all ages and 27 of 100,000 women over the age of 20 years. In addition to the invasive lesions, at least 45,000 non-invasive carcinomas of the cervix were also detected.

Although cancer of the cervix can occur at any age, invasive lesions are most often diagnosed in women between the ages of 35 and 65 years. Noninvasive lesions are diagnosed in women about 10 to 15 years younger.

Epidemiologic factors

Carcinoma of the cervix and sexually transmitted diseases have many similarities, sexual intercourse being an almost essential factor in the development of both.

Rothkin, studying 400 women with cervical cancer and an equal number of matched control subjects, found the most significant difference in the two groups to be the *age of first coitus*. Those with cancer started intercourse before the age of 20 years, many in their early teens. Related influences that appear to be important in the genesis of early cancer are *the number of sexual partners, the number of contacts of their male partners with other women, frequency of intercourse, and the number of marriages*. Although most carcinomas of the cervix develop in parous women, the number of pregnancies seems to be less important than age at first coitus and the number and sexual habits of partners. Cervical cancer is unusual in nuns and virgins.

Carcinoma of the cervix occurs more often in women of *low socioeconomic status* than in those who are more affluent. Although socioeconomic status has been linked, it is related to the previously mentioned factors and not social status per se. Cancer of the cervix also occurs more often in black than in white women. The age-adjusted rate for invasive cervical cancer in black women is 33.6 of 100,000 as compared with 15 of 100,000 for whites. A similar ratio holds for carcinoma in situ: 62.6:32.5. The difference, which is at least partly caused by socioeconomic factors, may be eliminated as the age at which sexual activity is initiated decreases and as frequency of intercourse and number of partners in all races increase. Re-

cently, cervical cancer has been associated with *smoking*.

The incidence of cervical cancer is not increased in women whose first intercourse occurred after age 20, even though other factors are similar to those for women who had intercourse early. One possible explanation is that a stimulus introduced during coitus induces anaplastic proliferation in the immature metaplastic epithelial cells of the transformation zone. Columnar epithelium, which often extends over the entire portio in young girls, undergoes a normal metaplastic change induced by the altered biochemical environment in the vagina after puberty. If the process continues without being disturbed, the metaplastic cells are converted to a mature squamous epithelium with the squamocolumnar junction near or just within the external cervical os. A mitogen introduced repeatedly before the conversion occurs and to which mature squamous epithelium is not particularly susceptible may induce an anaplastic reaction in the immature cells.

A *sexually transmitted carcinogen* is a unifying factor that can explain all of the epidemiologic factors associated with cervical cancer. A sexually related infection that may play a role in the development of cervical cancer is that caused by *human papillomavirus 16, 18, 31, 33, and 35.* Reid and co-workers were able to demonstrate *papillomavirus* in the cervix in 88% of uteri removed for cervical dysplasia and in 95% of those removed because of invasive cancer. Only 12.5% of control specimens were positive. *Papillomaviruses* have been identified in condylomata acuminata of the vulva and vagina and in warty growths in other parts of the body. Cervical condylomata are flat rather than sessile and are not usually visible on gross inspection. They are obvious, however, using the colposcope after 30% acetic acid has been applied to the cervix.

Although a recent increase in cervical condylomata has been assumed to coincide with earlier onset of coitus and more frequent sexual activity in teenagers, this may not be true. Bernstein and co-workers reexamined 1264 cervical biopsy specimens that had been obtained in 1972 and found changes consistent with human *papillomavirus* in 36.5%; only 0.7% had been reported as positive on the initial examinations. Of 965 biopsies obtained in 1982, 34% showed viral changes. Therefore, the frequency of cervical condylomata seems likely not to have changed much.

Further evidence that the viruses are sexually transmitted is that penile condylomata can often be identified in the sexual partners of women with cervical condylomata and cervical intraepithelial neoplasia.

Although Papillomavirus has not been proved to be a direct cause of cervical cancer, the two conditions are definitely related. Evidence also suggests that Herpesvirus hominis type 2 may be a cofactor that induces abnormal cervical cell growth. Catalano and Johnson identified *Herpesvirus hominis* type 2 antibodies in 35.7% of women who subsequently developed carcinoma in situ of the cervix but in only 7.1% of matched control subjects who did not develop carcinoma in situ during the observation period. Antibodies were identified in 42% of patients with proven carcinoma in situ and in 17.7% of matched controls. Naib and co-workers observed 245 women with active *Herpesvirus* genital infections for 5 or more years. Anaplastic cervical lesions developed in 58 (23%), including four with invasive cancer and 12 with carcinoma in situ. Anaplasia occurred in 1.6% with only one noninvasive and no invasive lesions in a matched control group without *Herpesvirus* infection.

The relationship between coitus and the development of cervical cancer and especially of the possibility of a *male factor* is strengthened by Kessler's study of 1087 second wives of men whose former partners had been treated for carcinoma of the cervix and 659 present wives of men whose former partners had not had the disease. Carcinoma in situ or invasive cancer was detected in 29 (2.7%) of the study group and seven (1.1%) of the control subjects. Cervical cancer or an abnormal cytologic study occurred in 14% of the study group and 8% of the controls.

Although male factors seem likely to be responsible for inducing the cellular changes that

precede invasive cervical cancer, they have not been precisely identified. Once again, the HPV virus is a unifying factor and could be transferred from the male.

The common benign lesions of the cervix have long been suspected to be precursors of cancer, but the relationship has never been proven. Peyton and colleagues reported on the results of 38 years of ablation of abnormal cervical tissue by office cautery. Of the 6533 patients who were not cauterized, 81 (27 of 1000) developed in situ or invasive cancer. In contrast, the only malignancies diagnosed in the 6364 who underwent cauterization of the cervix were three carcinomas in situ (0.5 of 1000).

Premalignant lesions

Dysplasia is the earliest recognizable cellular alteration that may be a forerunner of invasive cancer. The arrangement of the undifferentiated basal cells is disorderly. They vary in size and shape, and many mitotic figures can be identified. The abnormal changes occur in single or multiple focal areas. In some but not all women, the dysplastic change becomes progressively more severe as the cells take on more of the characteristics of malignancy. Because telling in advance whether the lesion will progress or regress is impossible, dysplasia must be considered a step toward the development of cancer, hence the designation *cervical intraepithelial neoplasia (CIN)*.

Because cervical intraepithelial neoplasia is oftentimes associated with human *papillomavirus* infections, the cellular changes caused by the virus can often be identified in biopsy specimens. The most characteristic of these is the presence of *koilocytes*, which are squamous cells with dense, hyperchromatic, pyknotic nuclei surrounded by a clear cytoplasmic halo (Fig. 44-4).

With *mild dysplasia, or CIN I*, the undifferentiated cells are confined to the lower one third of the epithelial layer. The cells become progressively more differentiated toward the surface. In *moderate dysplasia, or CIN II* (Fig. 44-5), the lower 50% to 75% of the epithelial layer is re-

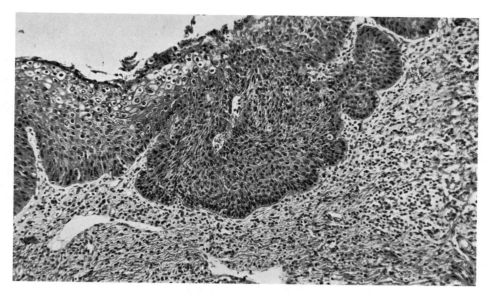

Fig. 44-4 Section showing dysplastic change. Prominent koilocytes in the superficial layers are characteristic of papillomavirus infection. (×255.)

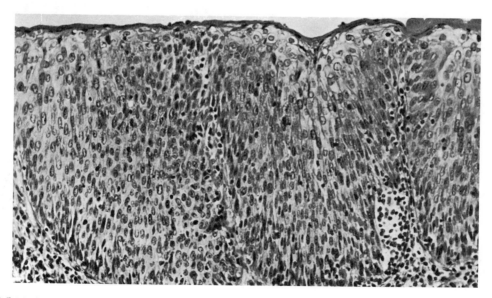

Fig. 44-5 Moderate to severe dysplasia. Cells are closely packed, and arrangement is fairly orderly. Upper half of epithelial surface shows maturation with some keratin production on surface. (×255.)

placed by undifferentiated cells, but the superficial layer are fairly well differentiated. The entire thickness of the epithelium is replaced by anaplastic cells in *carcinoma in situ,* and there is no surface cornification (Fig. 44-6). Perceiving the difference between severe dysplasia and carcinoma in situ may be impossible; hence they are usually considered as a single entity, CIN III.

Dysplasia should be considered as a continuum rather than a series of individual lesions. Any dysplastic lesion may regress to normal epithelium, but regression is more likely to occur with CIN I than with the more advanced lesions; the latter are likely to progress to invasive cancer.

Conversion of dysplasia to unmistakable carcinoma in situ usually takes about 4 years. The time interval between the diagnosis of dysplasia and of carcinoma in situ is determined by the severity of the dysplastic process when it is first recognized. It may take 5 or more years for mild dysplasia to become recognizable carcinoma in situ but only a few months for the more advanced lesions to progress to carcinoma in situ.

Most but not all carcinomas in situ continue to proliferate and eventually grow through the basement membrane to invade the cervical stroma. The exact period between the development of CIN and invasive cancer is not known but is probably between 10 and 15 years. One cannot rely on a specific time period, however, because more aggressively growing lesions may progress from dysplasia through carcinoma in situ to invasion within 1-year. Rarely, they may progress so rapidly that dysplasia and carcinoma in situ are not recognized. These fast-progressing cancers have been associated with human papillomavirus 16 and 18.

Symptoms

Dysplasia or early carcinoma of the cervix has no symptoms. An abnormality usually is first indi-

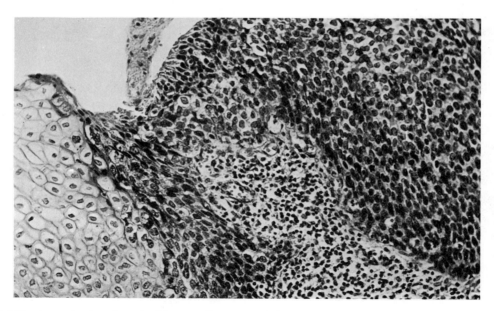

Fig. 44-6 Carcinoma in situ of cervix. Mature cells occur on left with abrupt change to complete loss of maturation of right, with intact basement membrane.

cated by a *watery discharge followed by bleeding,* which characteristically is painless, bright red, intermenstrual or postmenopausal, and prone to follow trauma such as coitus or douching. *Postcoital bleeding is a hallmark symptom of cervical cancer and usually indicates that a friable tumor is present on the cervix.* Thus a tumor is not evident by palpation and gross inspection of the cervix until there is an ulcerative cervical lesion. With further growth, bleeding increases and may be constant and profuse.

Pain occurs only when the tumor has extended far enough to invade the pelvic nerves in the lateral pelvic wall and the nerve roots. Pain therefore usually indicates far advanced disease.

Because the bowel is not often involved until the tumor is in an advanced stage, most women with cervical cancer remain well nourished. Weight loss occurs only during the late stages of the disease.

Diagnosis

Cervical carcinoma can be suspected if abnormal cells are found in a cytologic examination or by visual inspection, but it can be diagnosed with certainty only by biopsy.

Screening cytologic examination is an essential part of the periodic examination of presumably well women. It is usually performed at intervals of 12 to 18 months in women who have had several normal studies and are not likely candidates for cervical cancer. It should be performed more frequently in women who have been treated for dysplasia and in those who are at risk of developing cancer of the cervix.

Carcinoma of the cervix cannot be diagnosed with certainty by cytologic examination, but the presence of abnormal cells in the screening cytology alerts the physician to the need for a more complete investigation.

Cytology is not absolutely accurate in detecting either CIN lesions or invasive cancer. The false-negative rate associated with screening cytology is at least a 10 to 30%. The false-negative rate is actually higher with invasive tumors. This fact

suggests that lesions with the characteristics of cervical cancer should be biopsied, even though malignant cells may not detected on the cytology.

Advanced invasive cancer can be suspected by visual inspection of the cervix, but benign conditions, particularly chronic cervicitis, can look almost exactly like malignant lesions, and a cervix containing an extensive invasive cancer may appear normal.

The *characteristic malignant lesion* is either an ulcer or an exophytic growth. In both instances the tissue is friable and usually bleeds readily when sponged with a cotton ball. A lesion that begins within the cervical canal may not be accompanied by bleeding and may not be visible. Such tumors often are far advanced when they are detected.

Abnormal epithelium can be identified by its failure to stain with iodine *(Schiller's test).* The reaction is based on normal, glycogen-containing epithelial cells staining deep brown when Lugol's iodine solution is applied. Abnormal epithelial cells contain little or no glycogen and do not stain when iodine is applied. The absence of glycogen is not infallible evidence of cancer; it only indicates an area of abnormal epithelium. Normal cervical and vaginal squamous cells in postmenopausal women contain little glycogen and may not stain.

Carcinoma of the cervix can be diagnosed with certainty only by tissue biopsy. This confirmatory examination is essential before treatment is started. Tissue can be obtained by office punch biopsy or conizaton; the choice depends on the location and extent of the lesion.

Multiple punch biopsy is an appropriate step for an obvious cervical lesion. Bits of tissue are taken from several areas around the periphery of the lesion with punch biopsy forceps. Samples from the squamocolumnar junction, if it can be identified, are important. If invasive cancer is found, the physician may proceed directly to treatment. *If only CIN is diagnosed, more adequate biopsy is essential.*

The accuracy of punch biopsy, particularly if

the lesion is small or is not obvious, can be increased by the use of the *colposcope,* an instrument that provides a light source and binocular magnification of 10 to 40. Lesions on the portio and vagina can be studied easily, but those in the cervical canal are more difficult to see, especially when the external os is stenotic and the squamocolumnar junction lies within the canal.

Colposcopic examination is inconclusive unless the entire transformation zone or the squamocolumnar junction can be seen. Although experienced colposcopists can usually assess lesions accurately on the basis of their physical characteristics, the impression should be confirmed by colposcopic-directed biopsy before treatment is initiated. All abnormal areas should be sampled, and an *endocervical curettage* should be performed. The latter is particularly important if the upper edge of the lesion in the canal cannot be seen and biopsied.

Conization (cone biopsy) is an accurate method for studying the portio of the cervix and the entire cervical canal when invasive cancer is suspected because of abnormal cytology, colposcopic-directed biopsy does not confirm the diagnosis, or the upper limits of an endocervical lesion cannot be seen. The accuracy of conization is determined by how many sections of the specimen the pathologist examines.

Conization is mandatory when (1) the upper limit of the lesion in the cervical canal cannot be seen, (2) CIN is diagnosed in tissue removed by endocervical curettage, (3) biopsy does not confirm invasive cancer suggested by colposcopy or cytologic examination, and (4) microinvasion is diagnosed on punch biopsy.

Treatment

Dysplasia. The justification for treating cervical dysplasia vigorously is that it may be a precursor to cancer. Eradication of the areas of abnormal cell growth reduces the likelihood of this occurring.

The first step is to map the abnormal areas by colposcopic examination, biopsy, and endocervical curettage.

Small lesions that have been diagnosed as CIN I or II and that are confined to the portio of the cervix and the lower cervical canal can be destroyed by *laser vaporization or cryocautery.* The tissue destruction must be deep enough (5 mm) to destroy lesions that involve the cervical clefts and tunnels and must include the entire involved area. More extensive lesions can be eliminated by *conization,* which should be wide and deep enough to remove any abnormal tissue on the portio and as much of the cervical canal as possible. The advantage of conization is that multiple sections can be made and the entire lesion studied. Severe dysplasia usually should be treated in the same manner as carcinoma in situ.

If the entire lesion is not removed or destroyed, the remaining abnormal tissue may continue to proliferate. Even though the lesion is completely removed, it may recur because the abnormal stimuli responsible for its growth may continue. Women who have been treated for dysplasia must be observed closely with regular cytologic examinations for life, even though the original lesion has been eradicated.

Carcinoma in situ. The justification for treating carcinoma in situ (CIN III) is that it is the immediate predecessor of invasive cancer. There generally is an interval of months or years between its development and invasion.

Wide conization, laser vaporization, and cryosurgery are acceptable alternatives to hysterectomy. Although they preserve menstrual and even childbearing functions, they provide less certain assurance of complete removal of the lesion than does hysterectomy.

Conization alone carries a risk of recurrence, even though the lesion is completely removed. The risk of recurrence after conization appears to be from 2% to 3%, but rates as high as 20% have been reported when cone margins are not free.

Laser vaporization, with which lesions in the lower cervical canal as well as those on the portio can be eradicated, can destroy CIN III. Large lesions can be effectively treated, as the lesion can be visualized with the colposcope. The failure rate may be as high as 15%

with the first treatment, but it can be reduced to less than 5% by a second attempt.

Cryocautery is effective in treating CIN III, but failure rates as high as 25% have been reported, probably because of failure to destroy the entire lesion on the portio, because the freeze in the canal does not penetrate deeply enough, or because the upper part of the lesion is not frozen. This technique is better for small lesions; if the size of the lesion covers more than 40% of the cervix, laser vaporization or conization is preferred. Furthermore, after cryocautery the squamocolumnar junction may retreat to a position within the cervical canal where it cannot be seen through the colposcope, and adequate follow-up then becomes difficult.

These forms of treatment are appropriate for women who are willing to return at regular intervals for examination. All are more effective for small lesions on the portio or for those that extend only a short distance up the cervical canal than for those that are more extensive.

Dysplasia during pregnancy represents a specific situation when temporization until the pregnancy is completed is desired. The transformation zone is usually easy to identify during pregnancy because the cervical canal is everted and clearly visible. Colposcopic-directed biopsies can be taken, although bleeding is greater than in nonpregnant women. Conization during pregnancy carries a significant risk of hemorrhage and abortion. It is therefore indicated only to exclude an invasive cancer. The extent of the lesion can almost always be determined by colposcopy, alleviating the need for conization in most women.

The patient in whom invasive cancer has been ruled out is observed closely throughout the prenatal period. Cytologic smears are obtained every 4 to 6 weeks, and colposcopy is repeated at 36 weeks. Progressive changes constitute an indication for complete reassessment.

There is no evidence to suggest that vaginal delivery influences the course of carcinoma in situ adversely. Cesarean delivery is necessary only for obstetric indications.

Reevaluation of the lesion and definitive treatment can usually be delayed until involution is complete.

MALIGNANT LESIONS
Cell types

Most cervical carcinomas begin in the labile transformation zone. Subcylindrical (reserve) cells, which are found beneath the columnar epithelium at the squamocolumnar junction, form the metaplastic cells in the transformation zone. They proliferate, undermining and raising the columnar epithelium, as they advance across the portio. Metaplastic cells are normal and are usually transformed into mature epithelium, but in some instances they become atypical, a change that precedes dysplasia and cervical cancer.

About 90% of cancers of the cervix are of squamous cell origin, and about 10% arise in columnar epithelium (adenocarcinoma). Rarely, sarcoma, mixed mesodermal tumors, malignancies of the lymphoid series (for example, reticulum cell sarcoma or malignant lymphoma) or small cell neuroendocrine tumors may be primary in the cervix.

Microinvasion, as the term suggests, is the earliest stage at which extension of the cancer beneath the basal epithelial layer can be recognized. Microinvasion is diagnosed when neoplastic cells invade the cervical stroma to a depth of no more than 3 mm below the base of the epithelium and when no obvious blood vessel or lymphatic invasion has occurred.

A band of carcinoma in situ and possibly another of dysplasia usually surround an area of invasive cancer. Random punch biopsies may be inaccurate in assessing the extent of the tumor because the tissue removed may not be representative of the entire lesion; thus colposcopy, directed biopsies, or cone biopsy is necessary for diagnosis. Microinvasive cancer of the cervix can be diagnosed only by cone biopsy. When punch biopsy shows microinvasion, a cone biopsy must be performed to ensure that deeper invasion is not present.

Clinical stages

The extent to which the cervix and surrounding structures are involved with cancer is referred to as the *clinical stage of the disease.* This factor definitely influences prognosis or the 5-year survival rate. Small, early lesions that are confined to the cervix have the best prognosis, whereas those that extend beyond the cervix have less chance of a cure.

Carcinoma of the cervix spreads by direct extension and through the lymphatics. Hence, the pelvic lymph nodes must, of necessity, be invaded as the tumor grows. Brunschwig and Daniel identified cancer in the pelvic lymph nodes in 13% of women with stage I lesions, 30% in stage II, 46% in stage III, and 53% in stage IV.

The *ureter* is particularly vulnerable in cervical malignancy because it passes through the parametrium just lateral to the cervix. Some degree of ureteral obstruction can be demonstrated in about two thirds of women with advanced invasive cancer of the cervix. The tumor grows laterally from the cervix and around the ureter, but the ureteral wall usually is not invaded. *Distant metastases are uncommon,* but they can occur in any part of the body.

The clinical stage or extent of the lesion must be determined before treatment is started. Appropriate treatment differs, depending on the stage. Also, clinical staging permits a comparison of treatment results.

The clinical stage of an individual tumor is determined by inspection, vaginal and rectal palpation, and biopsy. Obviously, clinical staging is not always accurate because involved lymph nodes and other extensions of the disease cannot always be recognized.

The most widely accepted clinical staging classification of cervical cancer is that of the International Federation of Gynecology and Obstetrics (Fig. 44-7).

Invasive cancer of the cervix is most often treated by radiation therapy, but operation may be preferable for some. Patients with microinvasion, certain patients with stage I lesions, and those whose lesions either did not respond to radiation or recurred can be treated surgically (see box on p. 585).

Cancer of the female reproductive organs is best treated in centers that are equipped to pro-

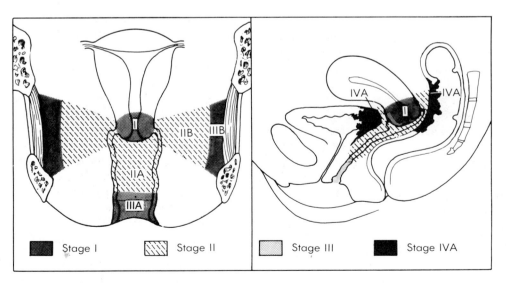

Fig. 44-7 Staging system for carcinoma of cervix uteri according to International Federation of Gynecology and Obstetrics (FIGO).

FIGO STAGE AND TREATMENT

Stage	Description	Treatment
0	In situ	Cryotherapy, laser ablation, cone biopsy
IA$_1$	Microinvasion	Total abdominal hysterectomy
IA$_2$	No greater than 5 mm deep and 7 mm wide	Total abdominal hysterectomy for less than 3 mm and without capillary/lymphatic involvement
		Radical hysterectomy, pelvic lymph node dissection deeper than 3 mm or capillary/lymphatic involvement
IB	Confined to cervix	Radical hysterectomy, pelvic lymph node dissection, bilateral salpingo-oophorectomy, optional depending on age
IIA	Upper ⅔ vagina involved; parametrium free	Radiation therapy preferred; radical hysterectomy for smaller lesions
IIB	Parametrium involved but not to side wall; IV pyelogram normal	Radiation therapy
IIIA	Extension to lower ⅓ vagina, not to side wall	Radiation therapy
IIIB	Extension to one or both pelvic side walls or obstructed ureter on IV pyelogram	Radiation therapy
IVA	Extension to bladder/rectum	Radiation therapy
IVB	Distant metastases	Chemotherapy, palliative care

vide all forms of cancer therapy. A therapeutic team made up of gynecologic oncologists and radiation oncologists should be responsible for evaluating and directing the treatment of all women with invasive cancer. Survival figures for groups of patients treated in this manner are significantly better than for those who are treated by individual practitioners who have had limited experience in cancer therapy.

Pretreatment investigation includes examination of the urinary tract by cystoscopy and intravenous pyelography to establish functional capacity and to detect any encroachment on the structures by the tumor. The bowel is studied by sigmoidoscopy, and a chest x-ray film examination is obtained. Basic laboratory studies include hemoglobin and hematocrit, white blood cell count, blood urea nitrogen and serum creatinine concentrations, and urine examinations. Lymphangiograms or CT scans may be helpful in determining the extent of lymph node involvement.

Radiation therapy

If radiation therapy is selected, the radiation oncologist calculates the dose in gray (1 cGy = 1 rad) to be delivered to the cervical tumor, the parametria, and the lateral pelvic wall, where most of the lymph nodes are situated. Radiation is usually delivered as a combined modality—external and internal. Supervoltage is delivered to the pelvis through its walls *(external therapy)* by linear accelerator, and cesium is placed in the cervical canal and upper vagina *brachytherapy)*.

Cesium is inserted into the cervical canal in tubes that are designed to provide afterloading of the radioactive sources. The effects of radiation from the cervical tandems are concentrated on the local lesion in the cervix because its penetrating power is limited. Additional sources are from ovoids placed lateral to the cervix in each lateral vaginal fornix. These are held in place by an applicator and tight vaginal packing to increase the distance from the bladder. The effects of radiation from the vaginal containers is on the cervix medially, the parametrium adjacent to the cervix superiorly, and the va-

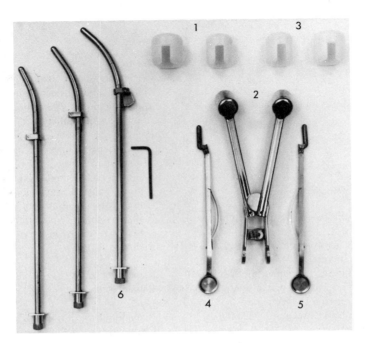

Fig. 44-8 Applicators used in intracavity radium therapy. *1* and *3*, Large and medium sleeves to fit over basic Fletcher applicator *(2)*; *4* and *5*, steel tandems; *6*, uterine tandems.

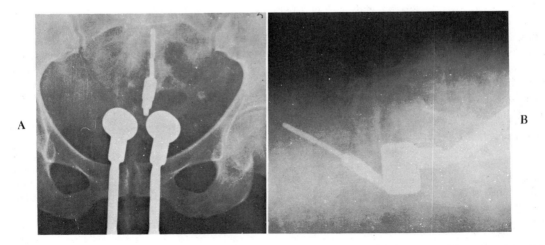

Fig. 44-9 Intracavity radium tandem in uterine canal and vaginal applicator with its two ovoids against lateral fornices. **A,** Anteroposterior view. **B,** Lateral view.

ginal wall and more distal parametrium laterally. One type of cesium applicator with its ovoids for the vaginal sources and tandems for insertion into the cervical canal is shown in Fig. 44-8. An x-ray film of the applicator in place is shown in Fig. 44-9.

The major effect of internal radiation is on the tumor in the cervix and in the nearby parametrium. An effective dose cannot be delivered to the lateral pelvic wall by brachytherapy alone. Radium was used in previous years but has been replaced by cesium (^{137}Cs). The cesium sources can be loaded once the patient has returned to her hospital room, thus decreasing unnecessary exposure to health care workers.

External radiation is delivered to the pelvic structures through an anterior portal over the abdomen and a posterior portal over the lower back. The external radiation increases the dose delivered to the central portion of the lesion by the cesium and also delivers a cancericidal dose to the lateral pelvis, where the tumor may have spread.

The total dosage of radiation delivered by the two sources is planned to destroy the tumor wherever it is in the pelvis. Unfortunately, there is no accurate way to predict the response of individual tumors to radiation; some may respond to relatively small amounts, whereas others are much less easily affected. In most treatment plans a maximum of 10,000 cGy is delivered to the central lesion by combined internal and external therapy and approximately 5000 cGy to the lateral pelvic wall. The latter is almost entirely from the external source.

Because the beneficial effect of radiation is produced by tissue destruction and the radiation cannot be restricted to the tumor cells alone, normal tissue must inevitably be injured during radiation therapy. Fortunately, the *reactions* from well-planned and supervised treatment are usually not serious. Most women experience *diarrhea,* which starts after several days of treatment and is caused by irritation of the rectosigmoid. Generally, it is easily controlled with a low-fiber diet and antidiarrheal medication. Others may have some *bladder irritation* from the same source and, in addition, from urethrocystitis, which develops during cesium implantation. It is treated with appropriate antimicrobial drugs.

Patients should be examined weekly while they are under treatment to evaluate the effects of the radiation.

Surgical therapy

The radical operation, which Wertheim introduced in 1898, now consists of removing the uterus, paracervical, parametrial, and upper paravaginal tissue, the upper vagina, and the pelvic lymph nodes (Fig. 44-10). This procedure was used extensively until radiation therapy was improved enough to provide better results. Meigs revived radical hysterectomy and added regular complete and meticulous lymphadenectomy during the early 1940s. His total 5-year survival rate for women with stage I and II lesions was 78%; involvement of the lymph nodes reduced the survival to 26%, the same as for radiation in his clinic. Brunschwig and Daniel detected lymph node involvement of 13% in clinical stage I patients, 30% in clinical stage II patients, and 46% in clinical stage III patients. Therefore, well-designed radiation therapy seems preferable to primary operation except for early lesions.

Operation is preferable for patients with *microinvasion,* in which focal areas of invasion do not extend more than 3 mm into the stroma, and with which there is no evidence of lymphatic or vascular involvement. These women can be treated adequately with extrafascial total abdominal hysterectomy without lymphadenectomy. Those with *small invasive clinical stage I lesions* can be treated by radical hysterectomy and pelvic lymph node dissection, with results comparable to those with radiation. Because the ovaries can be preserved and the inevitable destructive effects of radiation on normal tissue avoided, operation is particularly appropriate for young women with limited lesions. The other cell types such as adenocarcinoma or sarcoma should be treated with either radical hysterectomy or radiation therapy as there is no clear definition of microinvasion for these cell types.

Radical surgical procedures are also appropriate when radiation therapy fails to halt tumor growth. Women who have undergone radiation therapy must be examined at 3-month intervals. If the cytologic analysis remains positive and tumor growth continues, an operation should be considered. Under these circumstances the operation may be a *radical hysterectomy or a far more extensive procedure, depending on the extent of the lesion.*

In a few patients, particularly those with recurrent disease, *pelvic exenteration* operations may be performed. With this operation, the uterus, vagina, bladder, and rectum are removed. A colostomy and urinary

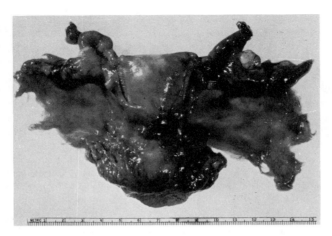

Fig. 44-10 Radical hysterectomy. Wide and deep dissection was necessary to remove parametrium and supporting structures.

diversion are necessary. Morley and colleagues reported exenterations with a surgical mortality of 2%. The 5-year survival rate in this group of patients, all of whom would otherwise have died of their tumors, was 68%; the 3-year survival rate was 71%.

Complications

Problems incident to surgery for carcinoma in situ or microinvasive cervical cancer are no different from those encountered with hysterectomy for other disease. Operative and postoperative complications resulting from radical hysterectomy and lymph node dissection for invasive cervical cancer are higher than for standard hysterectomy. Hemorrhage, infection, and urinary fistula formation are the most common problems encountered.

Radiation therapy also is attended by complications. For the most part, these affect the skin, large and small bowel, urinary tract, and fistula formation. Complications, whether associated with surgery or radiation, occur least often when treatment is carried out in a well-equipped center staffed by qualified, well-trained cancer therapists.

Follow-up care

Women who have been irradiated or operated on for cervical cancer require medical observation for the remainder of their lives.

Patients should be examined at 6 and 12 weeks after completing treatment to assess the initial effect of radiation on the tumor and then every 3 months for 1 year. If the cancer is resistant to radiation, cytologic smears remain positive, and there is palpable and perhaps visible evidence of continuing tumor growth. Induration in the paracervical areas, the uterosacral ligaments, and the base of the broad ligaments increases. Failure of response must be recognized early so that an attempt can be made to remove the tumor surgically before it becomes inoperable.

The majority of women treated for cervical cancer show satisfactory response at the end of the first 6 months. Their cytologic smears are normal and the cervix small, somewhat more mobile, and flush with the vaginal fornices. The supporting structures and paracervical and paravaginal areas are smooth and fibrotic.

The time between follow-up appointments is then gradually lengthened, so that after 2 years from the completion of treatment, examinations are on a semiannual basis. Even though the initial response to therapy is satisfactory, the follow-up examiner must remain vigilant. Recurrence or regrowth may appear at any time.

The semiannual follow-up examination of a treated cancer patient should include an interval historic note and a reasonably complete physical examination. Taking a smear for cytologic evaluation is essential.

Women who are followed after treatment for one malignant growth have a 5% to 8% probability of developing another primary cancer. As many as five primary malignant lesions have been seen in a woman treated for pelvic cancer.

Result of treatment

According to the 1982 FIGO report, the survival rates for 12,497 women treated for squamous cell cancer of the cervix in 82 institutions were:

	Radiotherapy only (%)	Surgery alone or combined with radiotherapy (%)
Stage I	70.4	84.2
Stage II	52.4	68.6
Stage III	28.3	42.3
Stage IV	8.2	20

The survival for patients with adenocarcinoma was less for each stage. Because these figures were derived from a number of different institutions that had variations in the quality of the treatment, they do not represent what can be achieved under the best of circumstances. Many clinics in the United States report higher survival rates, at least for the earlier stages of the disease.

Pregnancy and cervical cancer

Screening cytologic examination should be a part of each first prenatal examination, even though carcinoma of the cervix occurs only about once in every 2000 pregnant women. The procedure for further studies when the cytologist identifies abnormal cells is identical to that described for nonpregnant women: colposcopic-directed biopsies unless a lesion is obvious, when direct biopsy may be appropriate. Conization is not often necessary and should be avoided if possible. Bleeding is profuse and difficult to control, and the membranes may be perforated during the operation or may rupture later, perhaps because of their proximity to the infected granulating cervix. The operation does not interfere with cervical dilation during labor.

The physician may temporize in treating carcinoma in situ or microinvasion during pregnancy until after delivery, but prompt treatment is essential for invasive lesions.

Invasive cancer diagnosed during early pregnancy is treated as though the patient were not pregnant and without regard for preserving the pregnancy. Lesions that are thought to be confined to the cervix can be treated by an appropriate surgical operation. Those that are more extensive are treated with radiation.

When external radiation therapy is begun during the first 20 weeks of gestation, the fetus usually dies during the second or third week of treatment and is expelled from the uterus. External therapy is completed, and cesium is applied after some involution has taken place.

If labor does not begin spontaneously, the uterus should be evacuated to permit proper cesium application and because of the teratogenic effects of intensive radiotherapy.

If the pregnancy is so advanced that the infant has a reasonable chance of surviving, it should be delivered by classical cesarean section before radiation treatment is started. This procedure prevents fetal damage and prevents laceration of the lower uterine segment, which may be involved with tumor.

The results of treating carcinoma of the cervix during pregnancy are determined by the extent of the disease and the quality of the treatment rather than by the pregnancy. In most instances the outcome is the same or only slightly less successful than that in nongravid women.

Care of patients with advanced disease

Little can be done for patients in whom radiation or radical surgical procedures or both have failed to control the cancer. As the disease advances, it invades the nerve roots, particularly the sciatic plexus, and constricts the ureters and possibly the rectosigmoid. Continued growth in the cervix itself produces a necrotic crater that may bleed with the slightest irritation. Death usually occurs from uremia caused by ureteral obstruction, infection, hemorrhage, or combinations of the three. Chemotherapy has a limited role in this disease. Cisplatinum has activity in squamous cell cancer of the cervix and can be used for metastatic disease. It can provide an objective response in approximately 30% of patients treated but is only palliative in nature.

At this stage, the physician should prescribe whatever medications are needed to relieve pain and keep the patient reasonably comfortable. There is no place for heroic measures simply to prolong life.

PREVENTION

Invasive carcinoma of the cervix is a preventable disease. The proof of this statement is that the incidence of invasive cancer of the cervix decreased by 58% between the time of the second National Cancer Survey in 1947 and the third in 1970. There has been an even greater decrease in deaths. Bayes, Worth, and Anderson reported that in British Columbia the incidence of invasive cancer of the cervix in women over age 20 was reduced from 28.4 of 100,000 in 1955 to 7.6 of 100,000 in 1977, and that deaths declined from 11.4 to 3.8 of 1000,000 during the same period.

The reduction has resulted principally from the increasing availability of screening cytologic analysis, which permits diagnosis of the disease in its earliest stages when it is more amenable to therapy.

The responsibility for early diagnosis rests with (1) communities and public health services, which must make screening facilities readily available, particularly to those women who are at greatest risk of developing the lesion; (2) physicians, who must provide the services for their patients; and (3) patients themselves, who must learn to assume responsibility for their own health.

The controllable factors, in addition to periodic screening, include improved socioeconomic status, more concern for personal hygiene and cleanliness, and expanded sex education that should stress the relationship between coitus and cancer as well as between coitus and the other sexually transmitted diseases. Unless each individual assumes responsibility for minimizing the chances of developing cancer of the cervix and of detecting it in its earliest stages if it does develop, there will continue to be too many preventable deaths.

SUGGESTED READING

Bayes DA, Worth AJ, and Anderson GH: Experience in cervical cancer screening in British Columbia, Gynecol Oncol 12:143, 1981.

Bernstein SG, Voet RL, Guzick DS, and others: Prevalence of papillomavirus infections in colposcopically directed biopsy specimens in 1971 and 1982, Am J Obstet Gynecol 151:577, 1985.

Briggs RM: Dysplasia and early neoplasia of the uterine cervix: a review, Obstet Gynecol Surv 45:70, 1979.

Brunschwig A and Daniel WW: The surgical treatment of cancer of the cervix, Am J Obstet Gynecol 82:60, 1961.

Burghardt E and Ostor AG: Site and origin of squamous cell cancer: a histomorphologic study, Obstet Gynecol 62:117, 1983.

Catalano LW and Johnson LD: Herpesvirus antibody and carcinoma in situ of the cervix, JAMA 217:447, 1971.

Dorman SA, Leigh MD, Wilson DJ, and others: Detection of chlamydial cervicitis by Papanicolaou stained smears and cultures, Am J Clin Pathol 79:421, 1983.

FIGO: Annual report of the results of treatment in gynecologic cancer, vol 18, Stockholm, 1982, Radiumhemmet.

Hacker NF, Berek JS, and Lagasse LD: Carcinoma of the cervix associated with pregnancy, Obstet Gynecol 58:735, 1982.

Hopkins MP, Schmidt R, Roberts DA, and Morley GW: Gland cell (adenocarcinoma of the cervix), Obstet Gynecol 72:789, 1988.

Kessler II: Venereal factors in cervical cancer, Cancer 39:1912, 1977.

Linhartova A: Extent of columnar epithelium on the ectocervix between the age of 1 and 13 years, Obstet Gynecol 52:451, 1978.

Meigs JV: Wertheim operation for carcinoma of the cervix, Am J Obstet Gynecol 49:542, 1945.

Morley GW, Hopkins MP, Lindenauer SM, and Roberts JA: Pelvic exenteration: University of Michigan 100 patients at five years, Obstet Gynecol 74:934, 1989.

Naib ZM, Nahmais AJ, Josey WE, and Kramer JH: Genital herpetic infection: association with cervical dysplasia and carcinoma, Cancer 23:940, 1969.

Nelson JH, Jr., Averette HE, and Richart RM: Dysplasia, carcinoma in situ, and early invasive cervical carcinoma, CA 344:306, 1984.

Papanicolaou GN and Traut NF: Diagnosis of uterine cancer by vaginal smears, New York, 1943, The Commonwealth Fund.

Peyton FW, Peyton RR, Anderson VL, and Pavnica P: the importance of cauterization to maintain a healthy cervix, Am J Obstet Gynecol 131:374, 1978.

Reid R, Stanhope CR, Herschman BR, and others: Genital warts and cervical cancer. I. Evidence of an association between subclinical papilloma-viral infections and cervical malignancy, Cancer 50:377, 1982.

Review of cervical cancer, Semin Oncol 9:entire issue, 1982.

Rotkin ID: Epidemiology of cancer of the cervix. III. Sexual characteristics of a cervical cancer population, Am J Public Health 57:815, 1967.

Roy M, Morin C, Casas-Cordero M, and Meisels A: Human papillomavirus and cervical lesions, Clin Obstet Gynecol 26:949, 1983.

Sadeghi SB, Hseih EW, and Gunn SW: Prevalence of cervical intraepithelial neoplasia in sexually active teenagers and young adults, Am J Obstet Gynecol 148:726, 1984.

Shingleton HM, Gore H, and Austin JM Jr: Outpatient evaluation of patients with atypical Papanicolaou smears: contribution of endocervical curettage, Am J Obstet Gynecol 126:122, 1976.

Syrjanen KJ: Current concepts of human papillomavirus infections in the genital tract and their relationship to intraepithelial neoplasia and squamous cell carcinoma, Obstet Gynecol Surv 39:252, 1984.

45

Michael P. Hopkins

Benign and malignant diseases of the uterus

Objectives

Uterine Leiomyomata

RATIONALE: The uterine myoma is the most common gynecologic neoplasm and is often asymptomatic. Physicians are often called upon to distinguish myomas from other pelvic masses which may need more immediate management.

The student should be able to:

A. Demonstrate a knowledge of the symptoms and physical findings of uterine leiomyomata.

B. List methods to confirm the diagnosis.

C. Discuss indications for both medical and surgical treatment.

Adenomyosis

RATIONALE: Adenomyosis is a frequent cause of secondary dysmenorrhea in women over age 35.

The student should be able to:

A. Describe the symptoms and physical findings of adenomyosis.

B. Name problems in the diagnosis.

C. Discuss the medical and surgical management.

Endometrial Carcinoma

RATIONALE: Endometrial carcinoma is a major concern for women using estrogen replacement therapy. As with other neoplasms, early diagnosis will improve long-term survival.

The student should be able to:

A. Demonstrate a knowledge of the: approach to the patient with postmenopausal bleeding.

B. List risk factors for endometrial carcinoma.

C. Discuss the symptoms, and physical findings.

D. Describe methods to diagnose and stage endometrial carcinoma.

E. Explain the course of the disease.

Diseases of the uterus are numerous. Hysterectomy, one of the most common operations performed in the United States, is usually performed for benign disorders such as menorrhalgia, dysmenorrhea, or leiomyomata. It is also employed for uterine cancer, which is the most common gynecologic malignancy.

BENIGN DISEASES

The benign lesions that most often enlarge the uterus are leiomyomas and adenomyosis. Of these, leiomyomas are by far the most common.

Leiomyomas

Benign uterine leiomyomas, also called *myomas, fibromyomas,* or, more commonly, *fibroids,* can be found in the uteri of 30% to 50% of all women past 30 years of age. They occur more often, appear at an earlier age, and grow more luxuriantly in black than in white women. Although they are often encountered in nulliparas and can be a cause of infertility, many women with fibroids conceive without difficulty.

Pathologic findings. The tumors probably develop from immature smooth-muscle cells of the uterine wall. The smallest ones are made up almost entirely of muscle, but strands of fibrous tissue appear between the bundles of unstriated muscle as the tumor enlarges. In some tumors the fibrous tissue predominates. Leiomyomas, although well circumscribed, have no true capsule; a layer of compressed uterine muscle surrounding each neoplasm forms a pseudocapsule.

The tumors may occur singly, but more often they are multiple. They vary in size from those visible only under the microscope to huge masses that almost fill the abdominal cavity. They may occupy any portion of the uterine wall. When sectioned, they are firm and white, and the whorled, trabeculated muscular bundles are characteristic.

The tumor types are designated according to their position in the uterine wall (Fig. 45-1). *Sub-*

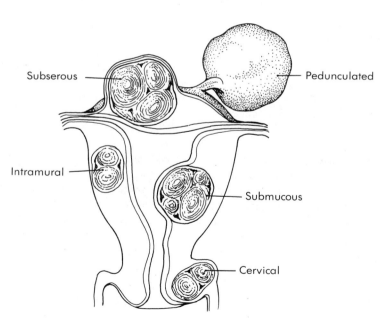

Fig. 45-1 Types of fibroid tumors.

mucous tumors lie beneath the endometrium and protrude into the uterine cavity. *Intramural or interstitial* tumors occupy the central portion of the uterine wall, whereas those of the *subserous* variety lie beneath the peritoneal covering and protrude into the abdominal cavity. If the tumors are predominantly intramural or subserous, they may grow to a remarkable size without altering the size and shape of the uterine cavity. However, intramural tumors that grow toward the center of the uterus rather than toward the peritoneal surface may enlarge and distort the endometrial cavity as much as do the subserous types. *Cervical* fibroids develop from the musculature of the cervical portion of the uterus. Tumors that grow laterally between the leaves of the broad ligament are called *intraligamentous*.

Submuous, subserous, and cervical myomas, particularly those located near the surface, can become *pedunculated* as they gradually grow away from the myometrium. Occasionally, a subserous growth loses its connection to the uterus completely and becomes a *parasitic* fibroid, deriving its blood supply from the omentum or some other extrapelvic source.

DEGENERATIVE CHANGES. The blood supply, which comes through the pseudocapsule from the vessels in the uterine wall rather than by way of a single blood vessel, frequently becomes inadequate as the tumor enlarges; as a result degenerative changes are common. In *hyaline degeneration,* the type most often observed, the fibrous and muscle tissues are partially or completely replaced by hyaline tissue, which grossly is smooth, relatively soft, and lacks the usual whorl-like appearance. Under the microscope the hyalinized areas are homogeneously pink stained and may be completely acellular. *Cystic degeneration* or *liquefaction* occurs when the hyaline material breaks down from a further reduction in blood supply. With *calcification,* which occurs most often after the menopause, the tumor may be stonelike because of a deposition of calcium; this type of tumor can often be detected by x-ray film examination (Fig. 45-2). *Fatty degeneration* is rare.

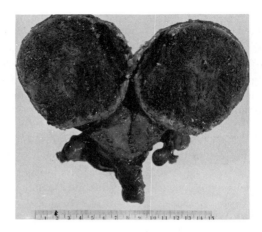

Fig. 45-2 Large, hard, calcified fibroid.

Necrosis of a tumor may occur if its blood supply is compromised. This situation is most often encountered when pedunculated tumors twist on their pedicles, which completely occludes the vessels, but it may also happen in rapidly growing leiomyomas of other types. Necrotic submuous tumors often become secondarily *infected.*

Red or *carneous degeneration* can occur during pregnancy and affects at least half of all fibroids in gravid women. When sectioned, the tumor bulges out of its bed, and the characteristic dark red color produced by hemorrhage into the tissue is obvious.

Sarcomatous degeneration occurs in about 1 of 1000 (0.1%) of leiomyomas. The cut surface is pink and soft and has been compared to the appearance of raw pork. Later the tissue may become friable, with ragged cavitation in the center.

Etiologic factors. The cause of leiomyomas is unknown, but the growth of the tumor is in some way related to stimulation by estrogen. This theory is supported by the fact that the tumors do not often occur before the ovaries have functioned for several years and that growth usually ceases after the menopause. In addition, rapid enlargement of leiomyomas occurred in some women who were taking the early oral contraceptive pills, which contained relatively large amounts of estrogen. It rarely happens with the present low-dosage forms.

Signs and symptoms. Symptoms vary with the size and location of the tumors. Some huge growths cause no discomfort or disturbance of the menstrual pattern, whereas much smaller ones may produce severe pain or exsanguinating hemorrhage.

BLEEDING. An alteration in menstrual bleeding is the most frequent single symptom produced by uterine fibroids. *The characteristic bleeding pattern associated with leiomyomas is excessive or prolonged flow or both, with little if any change in the cycle.* As the tumors enlarge, the amount of bleeding increases, but the change may occur so gradually that the patient is not aware of the increasing flow.

Abnormal bleeding is almost always caused by submucous or intramural tumors that enlarge and distort the uterine cavity. Subserous tumors, even the largest ones, which do not alter the size and shape of the endometrial cavity, are ordinarily not accompanied by abnormal bleeding.

The source of the bleeding is the endometrium, and the mechanism is the same as that responsible for menstruation in the normal uterus. The endometrial glands and stroma respond to the changes in ovarian hormone levels in the same manner as in normal women. The excessive bleeding is at least in part caused by the increased endometrial surface in the uterus containing a number of large submucous tumors. The endometrial surface area may increase from about 15 cm^2 in normal uteri to as much as 200 cm^2 in those with myomas. An additional factor is an increase in the number and size of endometrial veins in association with submucous tumors. They may be a result of abnormal hormone stimulation or of pressure from the tumors.

Acyclic bleeding can occur in women with myomas as a result of infected or ulcerated submucous tumors, hormonal disturbances (dysfunctional bleeding), or cervical or endometrial cancer; however, *uncomplicated leiomyomas do not cause intermenstrual or postmenopausal bleeding.*

PRESSURE AND PAIN. Many women experience increasing pressure on the bladder and frequency of urination as the tumors grow. Occasionally a large tumor in the anterior uterine wall will push the fundus posteriorly into the cul-de-sac and rotate the cervix anteriorly beneath the pubis, where it compresses the vesicle neck. As the tumor grows, it becomes progressively more difficult to initiate urination, and finally complete obstruction may occur. Large posterior wall tumors may fill the cul-de-sac and make evacuating the rectum difficult.

Pain may indicate that the tumor itself is degenerated, twisted, or infected or that it is pressing on another organ or on the pelvic nerve roots. Small tumors may cause more symptoms than large ones if they are located where they can exert pressure on sensitive areas.

DYSMENORRHEA. Severe, cramping, laborlike pains may occur as the uterus attempts to expel a pedunculated submucous tumor. However, dysmenorrhea is not usually a characteristic symptom of fibroid.

INFERTILITY. Many women with leiomyomas are infertile, but the presence of the tumors cannot always be related to the failure to conceive because other women with tumors of equal size or larger are normally fertile. Occasionally, growths in the cornual areas distort the fallopian tubes or disturb their function, but more often the lumina are patent. Some women experience long periods of infertility before small fibroids are first detected, making the presence of the tumors an unlikely etiologic factor.

Spontaneous abortion occurs more frequently in those who do conceive, perhaps because the implantation site is near or on a submucous myoma where the endometrium cannot respond appropriately. *Premature delivery* also occurs more often.

Diagnosis. The diagnosis is made by abdominal and bimanual palpation of the uterus, which is enlarged and nodular as a result of the presence of numerous leiomyomas. The tumors vary in size from some that are too small to be detected by physical examination to those that are 15 to 20 cm or more in diameter. Individual myomas are smooth, firm, and nontender unless they have degenerated. The uterine mass may be fixed or freely movable, depending on the size and location of the neoplasm.

DIFFERENTIAL DIAGNOSIS. Several pelvic lesions are at least superficially similar to uterine fibroids.

Cancer. Endometrial and cervical carcinomas cause irregular intermenstrual bleeding and develop in fibroid uteri as often as in those that are normal. Benign uterine tumors do not predispose to the development of cancer. Necrotic, bleeding, pedunculated, submucous tumors protruding through a normal but dilated external os may look much like cervical carcinoma. Malignancy should be excluded by cytologic examination, dilation and curettage, and cervical biopsy in women with irregular or postmenopausal bleeding before they are treated for fibroids.

Pregnancy. Large, soft leiomyomas, particularly large single tumors growing on the fundus of the uterus, may simulate pregnancy, and women with uterine fibroids may conceive. Most errors in diagnosis are made because the history of amenorrhea and the softening of the cervix and the lower part of the uterus are ignored. Even a remote possibility of pregnancy should be eliminated by pregnancy test or sonography before surgery (Chapter 24).

Ovarian neoplasms. These tumors usually are separate from the uterus, but differentiating a pedunculated fibroid from a solid ovarian neoplasm may be difficult. The symptoms produced by either an ovarian neoplasm or a pedunculated leiomyoma twisting on its pedicle are similar, and degenerated or cystic fibroids situated in the lateral uterine wall or those that are pedunculated may simulate cystic ovarian tumors. Neoplasms of the ovary usually do not alter the menstrual cycle, whereas increased bleeding occurs frequently with uterine fibroids.

Treatment. Of the several methods for treating women with uterine fibroids, the one selected will be determined by the age, parity, and physical condition of the patient; the size of the tumors; and the symptoms they produce. Cancer must always be suspected if the bleeding is irregular, intermenstrual, or postmenopausal; it can be excluded by dilation and curettage and cervical biopsy. Anemia can be corrected by iron therapy or, if it is profound enough, by blood transfusion.

OBSERVATION. As a general rule, leiomyomas of almost any size need not be treated unless they are producing symptoms because they do not predispose to malignancy, seldom undergo malignant degeneration, and do not interfere with the functions of other pelvic organs. Active treatment can be instituted at any time if symptoms develop or if the tumors begin to enlarge rapidly. In the majority of cases, active treatment never becomes necessary. If the enlarged uterus fills the pelvic cavity, it may exert pressure on the ureters. X-ray film pyelography should be ordered if large tumors are to be observed.

Observation is especially appropriate for women near the menopause because, after ovarian function ceases, bleeding will stop and the uterine mass will no longer grow and may become smaller. Fibroid tumors in postmenopausal women rarely need to be removed unless they continue to grow.

The schedule of periodic examinations for women known to have uterine fibroids need not be changed after the menopause. No special examinations are necessary unless the tumors continue to grow or symptoms appear. Conversely, if a pelvic tumor is found in a postmenopausal woman whom the physician has never examined before, a more precise diagnosis must be made. Physical examination alone cannot differentiate a benign uterine fibroid from an ovarian neoplasm. Sonography may be helpful; if not, a diagnostic laparoscopy usually provides the necessary information.

SURGICAL REMOVAL. Large fibroids, those that

increase in size over a short observation period, and those that produce symptoms should usually be removed.

Myomectomy, or the removal of individual tumors from the uterine wall, should be considered for young women in whom maintaining both menstruation and reproductive function is desirable. This operation is of particular value in the management of pedunculated, subserous, and submucous tumors. Myomectomy occasionally corrects infertility, but it should be reserved for those in whom all other possible factors have been eliminated. Myomectomy should be considered for young women who have had no children and who do not plan to become pregnant for several years. If the tumors are not removed, they may grow enough to be a factor in infertility or to increase the risk of pregnancy complications.

The removal of the tumors alone, except the pedunculated submucous variety in an otherwise normal uterus, may not alter excessive bleeding. If bleeding occurs irregularly, and if endometrial biopsy a few days before an anticipated period of bleeding is productive of proliferative endometrium or of benign hyperplastic endometrium (dysfunctional bleeding), hysterectomy is a preferred procedure because the bleeding is probably caused by an endocrine disorder rather than by the tumors.

Although most myomectomies are performed through abdominal incisions, small submucous tumors can sometimes be removed by *hysteroscopic resection.* Obviously, such operations should be attempted only by those with considerable experience in hysteroscopic surgical procedures.

Leiomyomas recur—or those that are overlooked grow—in about 15% of women after myomectomy. About 10% of these require treatment, either repeat myomectomy or hysterectomy. Treatment usually is not necessary when myomectomy has been performed after ages 35 to 40. The remaining tumors grow slowly, and they probably will not cause symptoms before the menopause occurs.

Hysterectomy, or removal of the uterus, is the operative procedure most often selected for the treatment of fibroid tumors. It is indicated for large and multiple tumors producing considerable distortion of the uterine cavity, for those that have grown rapidly, for those accompanied by profuse and irregular bleeding, and for those producing pressure symptoms. In young women, one or both ovaries should be left in place if they appear normal.

Medical management. The medical management of fibroids is a very attractive alternative to surgery. Progesterones have been tried with limited results. A GnRH agonist (Lupron) can decrease the size of leiomyoma by as much as 50%. The continuous use of this substance leads to decreased ovarian stimulation and decreased estrogen. Thus a postmenopausal-like state is achieved with the resultant decrease in size of the leiomyoma. This medical management, however, is usually temporary, as a prolonged estrogen-deficiency state has significant side effects leading to the discontinuation of this therapy. Additionally, it is not as effective on large leiomyoma.

Special problems in treatment

PEDUNCULATED SUBMUCOUS FIBROIDS. Pedunculated submucous fibroids occasionally grow to a diameter of 10 to 12 cm, and they often undergo necrosis and become infected. The patient may experience laborlike pains and profuse bleeding during the menses as the uterus attempts to expel the tumor. If the infected tumor protrudes through the dilated cervix, it should usually be removed vaginally after preliminary treatment with an antibiotic preparation and, when necessary, blood transfusion. If no other fibroids are in the uterus, further treatment may not be necessary; if hysterectomy is required, it usually should not be performed until the residual uterine infection has been eliminated.

DEGENERATION AND INFECTION. Degenerative changes and subsequent infection usually develop because of interference with the blood supply to the tumor. If the blood flow is obstructed, antibiotic preparations cannot reach the tumor. Consequently, removal is necessary before the surrounding intraabdominal structures become involved in the inflammatory process.

SARCOMATOUS DEGENERATION. Malignant degeneration in a fibroid tumor seldom occurs, but it should be suspected whenever a rapid increase in size is detected. Prompt removal of rapidly growing tumors is indicated.

Contraception. Although estrogen appears to be the responsible factor in the growth of leiomyomas, their presence does not contraindicate the use of *oral contraceptives* with low estrogen content.

Adenomyosis

Adenomyosis, a benign uterine condition in which endometrial glands and stroma are found deep in the myometrium, is often considered to be a form of endometriosis, but they probably are not related disorders. The frequency with which adenomyosis is diagnosed depends largely on how many sections of uterine wall are studied. The reported incidence varies from about 10% of all hysterectomies to about 90%. It is diagnosed most often in women between the ages of 40 and 50.

The histogenesis is not entirely clear, but adenomyosis is related in some way to estrogen stimulation, particularly when the action of estrogen is unopposed by progesterone. The cells in the basal portions of the endometrial glands grow downward between the myometrial muscle bundles and may lose their connection to the uterine cavity. The lesions are usually diffuse, with patches of endometrial tissue scattered throughout the entire thickness of the uterine wall. The process may be extensive enough to enlarge the uterus but not often beyond a size comparable to a pregnancy of 8 to 10 weeks. Occasionally, the process may be more circumscribed with the formation of a distinct nodule, an *adenomyoma,* but this is much less common than is diffuse involvement. Adenomyosis is often associated with uterine fibroids.

The ectopic endometrial tissue responds to variations in ovarian estrogen concentration, but, like the epithelium in the bases of the glands from which it originates, it is less active than are the more superficial portions of the endometrial glands and stroma. It does not often undergo a progestational change.

The most frequently reported symptoms are *colicky secondary dysmenorrhea* and *abnormal bleeding,* but many women with adenomyosis have no symptoms. The pain is caused by first swelling and then hemorrhage in the uterine wall as the confined patches of endometrium grow under the stimulus of a rising estrogen concentration

and then disintegrate and bleed as the stimulus is withdrawn. Excessive bleeding may reflect the expanding endometrial surface as the uterus enlarges. Increased and irregular bleeding may also occur because of ovulatory failure (dysfunctional bleeding).

The diagnosis is suspected in a woman over 40 who complains of increasingly severe dysmenorrhea and excessive bleeding if the uterus is enlarged and tender. Oral contraceptives relieve the pain of ordinary dysmenorrhea and that associated with endometriosis, but these preparations have little effect on the pain associated with adenomyosis.

The only uniformly successful treatment for adenomyosis is hysterectomy. However, operation is not necessary if the menopause can be expected to occur soon and if the dysmenorrhea can be controlled. The symptoms disappear after ovarian hormone secretion ceases. Replacement estrogen therapy is not contraindicated.

MALIGNANT DISEASES

Carcinoma of the body of the uterus (endometrial carcinoma) is the most common gynecologic cancer diagnosed in the United States. Approximately 37,000 new invasive cancers of the body of the uterus are diagnosed annually, compared to approximately 14,000 new cases of cervical cancer and 18,000 new cases of ovarian cancer.

Although carcinoma of the endometrium can occur at any age, it is most common in women past age 50, with the median age approximately 61; 75% of women with corpus cancer are postmenopausal. By contrast, cervical cancer occurs in younger women.

Because endometrial cancer occurs in an older age group, it often is complicated by medical conditions such as hypertensive cardiovascular disease, obesity, and diabetes. These and other medical complications add to the problem of establishing an adequate treatment program.

Etiologic factors. The etiologic factors responsible for the development of endometrial carcinoma are largely related to unopposed estrogen stimulation. *Estrogen* is implicated in the pathogenesis of carcinoma of the endometrium, but its exact role has not been clarified. Endometrial cancer develops more often in women with *estrogen-secreting ovarian neoplasms* and in young women with *polycystic ovarian disease* than in women with normally functioning ovaries. In each of these conditions, the effects of estrogen are unopposed by progesterone.

The coincidence of the increase in estrogen use by perimenopausal and postmenopausal women and a steady rise in the incidence of endometrial cancer prompted numerous investigators to seek a connection. Most reports indicated that estrogen does increase the risk of developing endometrial cancer at least three to four times and as much as tenfold. These studies also indicated that the cancer rate increased only after estrogen had been used for from 3 to 5 years. Before this the incidence was similar to that for nonusers of the same age. Both patients and doctors became concerned, and estrogen use decreased. This was followed by a nationwide fall in the incidence of endometrial cancer in the late 1970s.

Other observations support the role of estrogen in the genesis of uterine cancer. Endometrial cancer is reported to develop in women with gonadal dysgenesis who have taken estrogenic substances for many years. Peterson, studying 32 women under age 40 with endometrial cancer, found that 26 were obese, 16 had never been pregnant, and 26 had grossly irregular or anovulatory bleeding. Many of these women must have had long exposures to excessive and unopposed estrogen stimulation.

The fact that estrogen stimulates benign and adenomatous hyperplastic changes in normal-appearing endometrium is well known. These changes usually regress when the stimulus is withdrawn. Because similar hyperplastic changes precede frank endometrial cancer, estrogen seems likely to be able to induce a malignant change if the endometrium is biologically prepared to respond to the stimulus. Estrogen is probably not the "cause" of endometrial cancer, but its long-term stimulation may well induce the lesion in certain susceptible women.

The prototypical woman who is most likely to develop endometrial cancer is said to be obese, hypertensive, and diabetic. *All studies implicate obesity as the principal metabolic disturbance in women with endometrial cancer.* Because fat is a major site in which androgenic steroids are converted to estrogen, obese women are subjected to higher levels of estrogen than are those at or below normal weight. Obesity also predisposes to diabetes and hypertension, which is why these medical disorders are likely associated with endometrial cancer.

The woman most likely to develop carcinoma of the endometrium might then be suspected to be postmenopausal and obese. She may have had a long history of ovarian dysfunction, as indicated by infertility and abnormal bleeding associated with anovulation. She may also have hypertension or diabetes, but these probably are coincidental, as the greatest risk is from obesity. The results of most studies suggest that the *major risk factor is long-term unopposed exposure to estrogen. Cancer is less likely to develop in those whose endometria are stimulated periodically by progesterone.*

The relationship between long periods of unopposed estrogen stimulation and endometrial abnormalities seems to be fairly well established. Regular intervals of progesterone stimulation followed by endometrial shedding are likely to reduce its incidence. The cyclic administration of progesterone to women with polycystic ovarian disease and anovulatory bleeding (Chapter 8) and during postmenopausal estrogen therapy (Chapter 47) reduces the incidence of uterine cancer. If abnormal changes already have developed, they may not be reversible. Although the administration of progesterone can sometimes convert abnormal endometrium to a normal pattern, continuing hormone therapy for many years may not be logical, for example, in women with endometrial dysplasia diagnosed near or after menopause. Under these circumstances, hysterectomy is indicated. Conversely, progesterone therapy might be appropriate in young women with a reason to preserve the uterus temporarily. Women who have recurrent bleeding after dilation and curettage during the climacteric or postmenopausal periods, particularly those who have an endometrial abnormality, are best treated by hysterectomy.

Pathologic findings. Cancer of the endometrium, like malignant lesions in other anatomic areas, is preceded by abnormal cell changes.

Endometrium obtained during bleeding episodes preceding the development of endometrial carcinoma indicates a progression from normal-appearing proliferative endometrium through *cystic hyperplasia* to *adenomatous hyperplasia* (Fig. 45-3). With the latter lesion the gland cells are overactive, and the glands, which lie back to back, may be dilated or irregularly shaped, with papillary projections into the lumina. The individual cells are fairly well oriented to each other, but the nuclei may be hyperchromatic, and mitoses may be present.

As the process advances, more cellular evidence of malignancy can be detected. At the stage of *atypical hyperplasia,* or *carcinoma in situ* (Fig. 45-4), the cells are larger and more disoriented, and the nuclei often are eccentrically placed and irregular in size and staining characteristics. The stromal cells are not affected. This change is followed by invasive cancer.

With few exceptions, malignancy of the uterine body is an *adenocarcinoma*. This lesion may be so anaplastic that glandular pattern is completely lost. Conversely, some are so well differentiated that differentiating them from atypical hyperplasia may be difficult.

Although most endometrial cancers are pure adenocarcinomas, increasing numbers with a squamous component are being recognized. The squamous epithelium apparently develops as a

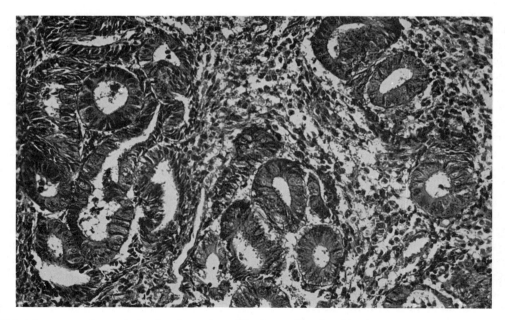

Fig. 45-3 Adenomatous hyperplasia of endometrium. Glands are dilated and in their characteristic back-to-back position.

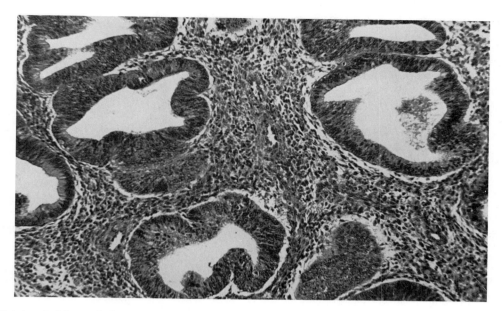

Fig. 45-4 Atypical hyperplasia, or carcinoma in situ, of endometrium. Glands are well formed, show no secretory activity, and have large cells, some cellular disorientation, and disparity in size.

metaplastic change in glandular basal cells. Adenosquamous tumors in which benign-appearing squamous epithelium is mixed with adenocarcinoma are called *adenoacanthomas.* Those in which both components are malignant are called *mixed* or *adenosquamous carcinomas.* Most reports suggest that mixed carcinomas are more aggressive and respond less well to treatment than do pure adenocarcinomas. The *papillary serous* type is a more aggressive type that spreads in a diffuse pattern throughout the abdomen.

Secondary carcinoma of the corpus uteri may develop from metastases from carcinoma of the ovary, breast, or gastrointestinal tract. Women with carcinoma of the stomach can present with no other symptoms than uterine bleeding from a metastatic lesion.

SARCOMA. Sarcoma of the uterus is rare and may arise either in fibroids or in otherwise normal muscle. No more than 0.1% of myomas undergo this type of malignant change.

Müllerian stroma is capable of giving rise to highly malignant tumors with a variety of histologic patterns. For this reason, they can be grouped together and referred to as tumors of *mixed mesodermal origin.* The homologous type consists of tissue normally found in the uterus, whereas the heterologous type contains foreign tissue such as cartilage and skeletal muscle.

Stromatosis is a term to designate a rare, slow-growing tumor with a monotonous cellular pattern not unlike endometrial stroma. These growths should be regarded as sarcomatous, but they are much less aggressive than the usual *stromal sarcomas.*

Clinical stages

The surgical stages of endometrial cancer are presented in the box on p. 602. Tumor cells can *invade the myometrium* directly and, in fact, may grow completely through to the serosal layer. *Lymphatic spread* is less predictable in that the tumor may invade the periaortic lymph nodes without involving those on the pelvic wall. The metastatic patterns of tumors that develop near the cervix may be more like those of primary cervical le-

FIGO STAGE AND TREATMENT FOR UTERINE CANCER

FIGO stage	Description	Treatment
IA G1, 2, 3	Confined to endometrium	TAH/BSO + RT for G3
IB G, 2, 3	Less than 50% myometrial invasion	TAH/BSO + RT for G3
IC G1, 2, 3	Greater than 50% myometrial invasion	TAH/BSO + RT
IIA	Endocervical gland involvement	TAH/BSO + RT
IIB	Cervical stromal invasion	TAH/BSO + RT
IIIA	Uterine serosal or adnexal involvement	TAH/BSO + RT
IIIB	Vaginal metastases	Preoperative RT + TAH/BSO
IIIC	Positive pelvic or paraaortic lymph nodes	TAH/BSO + RT
IVA	Extension to rectum or bladder	Preoperative RT + TAH/BSO
IVB	Distant metastatic or inguinal node involvement	TAH/BSO + systemic therapy

TAH/BSO = total abdominal hysterectomy bilateral salpingo-oophorectomy; RT = radiation therapy; G1 = well differentiated; G2 = moderately differentiated; G3 = poorly differentiated.

sions. *Hematogenous spread* can produce distant metastases, particularly to lung, pleura, and liver.

Symptoms

Endometrial cancer often produces early symptoms, the first of which usually is a *serous, malodorous discharge*. Frequently it is not regarded seriously by the patient. The watery leukorrhea is soon replaced by a *bloody discharge, intermittent spotting of blood,* or *steady bleeding.* If these symptoms are disregarded, the bleeding ultimately becomes frank hemorrhage. The increasing blood loss indicates progressive growth of the cancer and enlargement of its area of ulceration.

Differential diagnosis

The possibility of carcinoma of the corpus is immediately suggested when irregular uterine bleeding occurs near the menopause or when postmenopausal bleeding occurs. The symptom of bleeding usually brings the patient to medical attention. Occasionally the patient does not know from which orifice she is bleeding. An evaluation for bladder or rectal cancer should also include the uterus as a possible source.

Although only 20% of postmenopausal bleeding is caused by pelvic carcinoma, the physician cannot afford to disregard this important early sign of the lesion. Assuming that a cervical polyp, a fibroid, atrophic vaginitis, or any other benign lesion is the cause of abnormal bleeding is unwise. *The physician cannot make a definite diagnosis until a fractional curettage has been performed and a biopsy of the cervix has been done.*

Exfoliative cytologic studies are less helpful in diagnosing endometrial cancer than cervical lesions. The cytologic examination reveals positive findings in no more than 50% of women with invasive endometrial cancer.

The diagnosis can be made by *outpatient endometrial biopsy* if malignant tissue is removed with the curet or by suction. *Dilation and curettage* is essential, however, if the tissue is normal or if only hyperplasia, dysplasia, or carcinoma in situ is identified in the biopsy specimen. An area of invasive tumor may have been missed.

Treatment

SURGERY. Abdominal hysterectomy and bilateral salpingo-oophorectomy with pelvic and paraaortic node sampling is the operation most frequently indicated and is the most important part of the treatment of endometrial carcinoma. Vaginal hysterectomy may be preferable to an abdominal operation in extremely obese women, but it may be difficult to evaluate the lymph nodes and to remove the tubes and ovaries if the structures are atrophic.

Primary hysterectomy alone is most appropriate for women with early, well-differentiated, superficially invasive endometrial cancer (Fig. 45-5). Radiation therapy is added postoperatively for high-risk features such as poorly differentiated tumors, deep myometrial invasion, or involved lymph nodes. Radiation may consist of combined external pelvic radiotherapy and vaginal cuff irradiation. In many centers all patients receive at least vaginal cuff irradiation with cesium to decrease the incidence of vaginal cuff recurrence. When cuff irradiation is given preoperatively or postoperatively, the incidence of vaginal cuff recurrence decreases from a reported 10% to 1%.

POSTOPERATIVE RADIATION. Far-advanced carcinoma of the endometrium may extend directly through the uterus at any point. Generally, it occurs near the lower uterine segment and involves the parametrial or broad ligament areas or both. It may preclude wide dissec-

tion; in fact, the gynecologist may be forced to cut across the tumor at some point. If extension beyond the uterus is diagnosed preoperatively, whole pelvis irradiation should be given in an attempt to sterilize the parametrium before hysterectomy.

RADIATION. Some women with endometrial carcinoma are poor candidates for any operation, and their entire treatment must be by radiation. A preliminary course of telecobalt therapy followed by intrauterine cesium gives the best result. The 5-year survival rate in patients treated with radiation alone is lower than that with surgery alone or when hysterectomy is combined with radiation.

COMBINED THERAPY. The combination of preoperative intrauterine cesium therapy followed by hysterectomy has a theoretical advantage over either form of treatment alone. Preoperative radiation devitalizes tumor cells, reduces the total mass of bulky tumors, and thus makes the subsequent operation easier. Hysterectomy is performed a few days after cesium implantation.

TREATMENT OF VAGINAL METASTASES. Vaginal metastases often occur because the tumor already has ex-

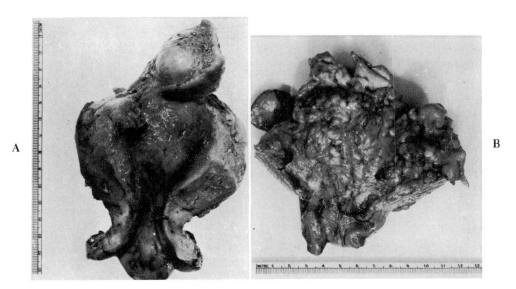

Fig. 45-5 Invasive carcinoma of corpus. **A,** Circumscribed adenocarcinoma; superficial raised area 2.5 cm in diameter is at right cornu. **B,** Diffuse, superficial carcinoma.

tended beyond the uterus by the time the operation is performed or because live tumor cells are disseminated during the operation. One of the benefits of adjuvant radiation is that the incidence of postoperative vaginal metastases is less than that after a primary surgical procedure alone.

TREATMENT WITH PROGESTOGENS. High doses of progesterone have been used in the treatment of metastatic endometrial carcinoma. The effect of progesterone in producing remission is most pronounced in pulmonary metastases, but control of local pelvic recurrence also has been observed. Well-differentiated tumors are more likely to respond favorably than are more anaplastic lesions. Response to progestins appears to be determined by the presence of cytoplasmic progesterone receptors. Well-differentiated tumors contain more progesterone receptors that do those that are anaplastic, which may explain the lack of response in the latter. Progesterone therapy must be considered as palliative rather than curative. Unfortunately the adjuvant use of progesterone for high-risk features has not proven to be of benefit.

RESULTS OF TREATMENT. The prognosis is determined by the clinical stage of the disease when it is diagnosed, the depth of penetration, the histologic pattern, and the degree of differentiation of the tumor. The 5-year survival of women with stage IA grade 1 disease is approximately 95 to 98% and decreases to 60% for stage IC grade 3. Treatment failures increase with more advanced lesions. Many failures reflect the condition of the patients, as well as the disease and its treatment. Many women with endometrial cancer are poor risks for any form of treatment, and others have disease that is too extensive to eradicate.

SUGGESTED READING

Bird CC, McElin TW, and Manalo-Estrella P: The elusive adenomyosis of the uterus—revisited, Am J Obstet Gynecol 112:583, 1972.

Ehrlich, CE, Cleary RE, and Young PCM: Which endometrial cancers respond to progestin therapy? Contemp Obstet Gynecol 15:139, 1980.

Farrer-Brown G, Beilby JOW, and Tarbit MH: Venous changes in the endometrium of myomatous uteri, Obstet Gynecol 38:743, 1971.

Gallup DG and Stock RJ: Adenocarcinoma of the endometrium in women 40 years of age or younger, Obstet Gynecol 64:417, 1984.

Gambrell RD Jr, Bagnell CA, and Greenblatt RB: Role of estrogens and progesterone in the etiology and prevention of endometrial cancer: review, Am J Obstet Gynecol 146:696, 1983.

Gusberg SB: The individual at high risk for endometrial carcinoma, Am J Obstet Gynecol 126:535, 1976.

Hammond CB, Jelovsek FR, Lee KL, Creasman WT, and Parker RT: Effects of long-term estrogen replacement therapy. II. Neoplasia, Am J Obstet Gynecol 133:537, 1979.

Hausknecht RU and Gusberg SB: Estrogen metabolism in patients at high risk for endometrial carcinoma. II. The role of androstenedione as an estrogen precursor in postmenopausal women with endometrial carcinoma, Am J Obstet Gynecol 116:98, 1973.

Henriksen E: The lymphatic dissemination in endometrial carcinoma, Am J Obstet Gynecol 123:570, 1975.

Jick H, Watkins RN, Hunter JR, Dinan BJ, Madsen S, Rothman KJ, and Walker AM: Replacement estrogens and endometrial cancer, N Engl J Med 300:218, 1979.

Kelley RM and Baker WH: Progestational agents on the treatment of carcinoma of the endometrium, N Engl J Med 264:216, 1961.

Lucas WE and Yen SSC: A study of endocrine and metabolic variables in postmenopausal women with endometrial carcinoma, Am J Obstet Gynecol 134:180, 1979.

MacDonald PC and Siiteri PK: Relationship between extraglandular production of estrone and the occurrence of endometrial neoplasia, Gynecol Oncol 2:259, 1974.

Neuwirth RS: Hysteroscopic management of symptomatic submucous myomas, Obstet Gynecol 62:509, 1983.

Patanaphan V, Salazar OM, and Chougule P: What can be expected when radiation therapy becomes the only curative alternative for endometrial cancer? Cancer 55:1462, 1985.

Peters WA III, Andersen WA, Thornton WN Jr, and Morley GW: The selective use of vaginal hysterectomy in the management of adenocarcinoma of the endometrium, Am J Obstet Gynecol 146:285, 1983.

Peterson EP: Endometrial carcinoma in young women, Obstet Gynecol 31:702, 1968.

Sehgal N and Haskins AL: The mechanism of uterine bleeding in the presence of fibromyomas, Am J Surg 26:21, 1960.

Soules MR and McCarty KS Jr: Leiomyomas: steroid receptor content. Variation within normal menstrual cycles, Am J Obstet Gynecol 143:6, 1982.

Spellacy WN: Plasma growth hormone and estradiol levels in women with uterine myomas, Obstet Gynecol 40:829, 1972.

Walker AM and Jick H: Declining rates of endometrial cancer, Obstet Gynecol 56:733, 1980.

Wilson EA, Yang F, and Rees ED: Estradiol and progesterone binding in uterine leiomyomata and in normal uterine tissues, Obstet Gynecol 55:20, 1980.

46

Michael P. Hopkins

Ovarian neoplasms

Objectives

RATIONALE: The adnexal mass is a common finding in both symptomatic and asymptomatic patients. The appropriate approach to the patient with adnexal findings results in earlier detection of ovarian malignancy.

The student should be able to:

A. Demonstrate a knowledge of the approach to the patient with an adnexal mass, with special attention to the size

and consistency of the mass and the age of the patient.

B. Describe the characteristics of functional cysts and benign neoplasms.

C. List the symptoms and physical findings, methods of diagnosis and staging, and the histologic classification of carcinoma of the ovary.

The ovary has a tremendous potential for neoplastic growth, probably greater than any other structure in the body. Various neoplastic tumors arise from both glandular and connective tissues and from embryonic remnants that often are present within normal ovaries. An understanding of the changes that occur in the ovary during a normal menstrual cycle is essential to understanding the normal functional nature of particular ovarian cysts. Delineating functional ovarian enlargements that usually need no treatment from neoplastic malignant changes for which the proper treatment is surgery is important.

ADNEXAL MASS

The *adnexa* refers specifically to the tube or ovary. An *adnexal mass* usually means an undiagnosed enlargement on the left or right side of the pelvis. The symptoms and differential diagnosis of the adnexal mass are important aspects of a full gynecologic evaluation.

Symptoms

Most ovarian neoplasms produce no symptoms and are found during examination of women who are asymptomatic. As the tumor is growing, the patients may experience *pressure in the pelvis* but even this may be absent if the tumor can move freely within the peritoneal cavity. Large tumors cause *enlargement of the abdomen,* but even then these generally grow slowly and thus the patient may not appreciate or complain specifically of this enlargement. Fixed or incarcerated tumors may produce *painful micturition, painful defecation, tenesmus, or pain during coitus. Menstrual disturbances* occur in approximately 15% of women with benign ovarian neoplasms.

Acute episodes of pain may occur if the ovarian neoplasm twists on its pedicle (ovarian torsion). Torsion occurs most often with tumors of moderate size, 8 to 12 cm in diameter. Larger tumors are usually not mobile enough to rotate, and the smaller ones are not heavy enough. The twisting usually occurs suddenly and is accompanied by sharp pain in the pelvis. The pain occasionally subsides spontaneously if the twisting is reversed and the circulation to the ovary is restored. The pain becomes progressively more severe if the obstruction is not relieved. Many patients have transitory recurrent attacks of mild pain before the final episode. Should the vascular obstruction persist, the tumor becomes necrotic and hemorrhagic. At this point, it is exceedingly tender to palpation. Eventually, peritoneal irritation appears, and the treatment at this point is prompt surgical removal.

Diagnosis. Ovarian neoplasms can usually be diagnosed by pelvic examination except in early stages when they are too small to palpate. An ultrasound examination done because of vague abdominal symptoms can confirm a clinical suspicion that an ovarian neoplasm is present. Neoplasms develop in retained ovaries after hysterectomy at the same rates that they do with the uterus in place; hence, regular examinations are important after hysterectomy. Ovarian tumors should also be suspected as the cause of vague pelvic discomfort and of mild GI distress. When the examiner suspects an enlarged ovary, the patient should be examined after a cleansing enema and at the end of a menstrual period, when physiologic cysts are not likely to be present. If the di-

---

DIFFERENTIAL DIAGNOSIS OF THE ADNEXAL MASS

Gastrointestinal
Colon cancer (sigmoid, cecal, rectal)
Diverticulitis/diverticular mass
Appendiceal abscess
Impacted feces
Genitourinary
Distended bladder
Pelvic kidney
Bladder cancer
Urachal cyst
Retroperitoneal
Lymphoma
Fibrosis
Metastatic
Breast
Stomach

---

agnosis is still uncertain, diagnostic ultrasound may be helpful. A diagnostic laparoscopy is justified if sonography is inconclusive.

Differential diagnosis. Differential diagnosis of an adnexal mass includes the GI and GU systems, as well as infectious causes and metastatic lesions. A differential diagnosis is presented in the box above.

Evaluation of the adnexal mass should be based on the patient's age and symptoms, as well as the pelvic examination. A small mobile mass in a young woman rarely needs an extensive metastatic workup, as bowel cancer is extremely unusual in young women. At the other end of the spectrum, in a postmenopausal woman with a fixed, solid pelvic mass and postmenopasual bleeding, the mass could represent anything from an endometrial cancer to a metastatic breast cancer. Thus, in this patient, a complete metastatic workup including mammogram, upper GI, barium enema and/or colonoscopy, IVP, and endometrial biopsy and/or D&C would be obtained prior to exploratory laparotomy. An IVP and a barium enema are probably the two most common diagnostic tests ordered preoperatively. The IVP is done to ensure that both kidneys are functioning, determine the presence or absence of a double collecting system, and ensure that a pelvic kidney simulating an adnexal mass is not the etiology. A barium enema is performed to ensure that a sigmoid colon cancer on the left side or a cecal cancer on the right side is not the etiology for the adnexal mass. When the metastatic workup is negative, surgical exploration should be performed and the exact nature of the adnexal mass determined by both frozen section as well as permanent section.

NONNEOPLASTIC CYSTS

Normal ovaries of newborn infants contain 1 to 2 million primordial follicles. Many of these degenerate before menarche. During active reproductive life, several follicles begin to grow under the stimulus of FSH during the preovulatory phase of each menstrual cycle. One or occasionally two or more follicles mature and produce ova that are capable of being fertilized. The rest become atretic. Ovulation occurs about 14 days before menstruation begins, and a corpus luteum develops and persists until just before the next menstrual period. The cycle is repeated except during pregnancy until a climacteric phase of life.

Functional cysts

The so-called functional cysts are related to the normal cycling ovary. A follicular cyst occurs with each normal menstrual cycle. A follicle reaches its maximum size just before ovulation, when the ovary may be 4 to 5 cm in diameter. The cyst then disappears with ovulation due to rupture of the cyst. Occasionally the follicle fails to rupture and may continue to grow, sometimes reaching 8 to 10 cm in diameter. These persistent follicular cysts are thin-walled and contain clear, serous fluid. Granulosa theca cells can be identified in the walls of a smaller cyst, but as the cyst enlarges the cells flatten. Histologically, they are frequently described as *simple cysts*. The large, persistent follicular cyst usually produces no hormones, although the fluid in the normal follicle contains a high concentration of estrogen. The *normal corpus luteum is a cystic structure* and may enlarge the ovaries slightly. Rarely the corpus luteum may fail to involute. It continues to

secrete progesterone, thus delaying the onset of menses. These cysts may continue to enlarge, and the *corpus luteum cyst* may produce pain as it expands or if it ruptures intraperitoneally. The combination of a delayed period, pain, and bleeding may thus simulate an ectopic pregnancy. Persistent corpus luteum cysts do not occur often in the absence of pregnancy. In fact, undiagnosed pregnancy may be the cause of a persistent corpus luteum. Women are usually unaware of the presence of normal follicles and corpora lutea or even large follicular cysts because they produce no symptoms unless a complication develops.

These so-called functional cysts of the ovary occur frequently and usually need no treatment. They can be recognized by the relationship to the menstrual cycle, with a follicular cyst occurring before ovulation and a corpus luteum cyst just before menstruation. Thus whenever a small ovarian cyst is discovered, the patient should be reexamined before definitive treatment such as laparotomy is considered. The most appropriate time for reexamination is at the end of the menstrual period when ovarian activity is at a minimum. If the enlargement has disappeared, the physician can assume that a functional cyst was present. The patient should be examined again in 2 to 4 months. Should the enlargement be present after menstruation but less than 5 cm in diameter, the patient should be reexamined just after her next menses. Two to three cycles of oral contraceptives can be utilized if the ovary is still slightly enlarged after menstruation. Small, persistent follicular cysts may regress when pituitary gonadotropin secretion is inhibited.

Ultrasound may sometimes be helpful in the management of these cysts. The clinical diagnosis is corroborated when ultrasound is utilized and a unilocular fluid-filled cystic structure is present. Definitive diagnosis, however, can be made only by sequential exams with resolution of the cyst or a tissue diagnosis.

A functional cyst that requires surgery because of enlargement or failure to regress under observation is usually single, thin-walled, and unilocular, with smooth lining and filled with clear, serous fluid. Oophorectomy is usually not necessary; a cystectomy is adequate therapy.

Occasionally when ovulation occurs, a blood vessel on the surface of the ovary is torn. The amount of bleeding from the *ruptured ovarian follicle* is determined by the size of the blood vessel. The scant bleeding that occurs normally may produce no symptoms, but occasionally extensive intraperitoneal bleeding causes the patient to develop the typical signs of hemorrhagic shock. While the clinical picture of intraperitoneal hemorrhage is identical to ruptured ectopic pregnancy, the clinical situation, however, is different from ectopic pregnancy. The ruptured follicular cyst usually occurs at midcycle after a normal menstrual period and usually with no vaginal bleeding. No treatment is necessary for the ruptured follicular cyst unless bleeding from the ovary is excessive or does not stop spontaneously. Laparoscopy with cauterization of the involved blood vessel can be accomplished, although laparotomy may be necessary in an acute situation. Oophorectomy is rarely necessary.

Theca-lutein cysts. Excessive production of chorionic gonadotropin (hCG) overstimulates the theca-lutein cells and produces theca-lutein cysts. They are composed of many follicles of varying sizes surrounded by luteinized theca cells. These cysts characteristically develop in women with hydatidiform moles, but they may occur with multiple pregnancy and Rh sensitization. They also follow ovarian overstimulation by gonadotropins given to induce ovulation. Theca-lutein cysts are bilateral and may be as large as 20 to 25 cm in diameter. They are usually asymptomatic unless they undergo torsion. These cysts regress when the hCG stimulation is withdrawn at delivery.

Luteoma. A luteoma probably develops from hyperplastic overgrowth of luteinized theca cells. They occur during normal pregnancy and are less likely to be bilateral than are theca-lutein cysts although luteomas may be 15 to 20 cm in diameter. They usually produce no symptoms and are generally diagnosed as an incidental finding at ultrasound or at cesarean delivery. Approximately 25% of women with luteomas are virilized because of the large amounts of androgen steroid produced by the luteinized cells. The female fetus may be born with clitoromegaly and fused labia. Both the theca-lutein cysts and luteomas regress after the pregnancy is terminated and thus the only indication for their removal is torsion.

Polycystic ovarian disease, in which multiple small cysts develop, is discussed in Chapter 9. *Endometriomas* are discussed in Chapter 11 and should not be confused with endometrioid ovarian neoplasm.

NEOPLASTIC: BENIGN OR MALIGNANT

A neoplastic process may be benign or malignant; therefore, the term *ovarian neoplasm* indicates a growth in the ovary. Whether it is malignant or not depends on the final pathology review.

Ovarian neoplasms occur less often than do the functional cysts, but they are far more important. They may grow to a large size, can secrete hormones that alter normal physiologic functions, and may be malignant. Small malignant tumors may not be palpated, and by the time they are large enough to be palpated, the disease may have spread throughout the peritoneal cavity. Any ovary larger than 5 cm in diameter at any age may well contain a neoplasm and thus cannot be ignored. The neoplasms of germ cell origin usually occur before the age of 30; those of epithelial origin generally occur beyond the age of 30. There are many classifications of ovarian neoplasms. A common one is that described by Abell (see box on p. 609).

The incidence of carcinoma of the ovaries has been increasing steadily and now accounts for approximately 5% of all cancers in women. About 18,000 new cancers of the ovary were diagnosed in 1989, and approximately 12,000 women died of the disease. It is the fourth leading cause of cancer death in women. Cancer of the ovary is unusual before the age of 20 but increases

OVARIAN CLASSIFICATION SYSTEM

I. Neoplasms of germ cell origin
  A. Dysgerminoma
  B. Embryonal teratoma (embryonal carcinoma)
  C. Partially differentiated teratoma (malignant teratoma, solid teratoma)
  D. Mature teratoma (benign cystic teratoma)
  E. Mixed germ cell neoplasms (teratocarcinoma)
  F. Carcinoma or sarcoma arising in a mature teratoma
II. Neoplasms of celomic (germinal) epithelium and its derivatives
  A. Serous (tubal cell) type
  B. Mucinous (endocervical) type
  C. Endometroid (endometrial cell) type
  D. Brenner tumors
  E. Mixed and unclassified cell types
III. Neoplasms of specialized gonadal stroma (sex cords and mesenchymal)
  A. Granulosa-theca cell group
    1. Granulosa cell tumor
    2. Theca cell tumor
    3. Granulosa-theca cell tumor
  B. Sertoli-Leydig cell group
    1. Sertoli cell tumor
    2. Leydig cell tumor (hilus cell)
    3. Arrhenoblastoma
  C. Luteomas

From Abell MR: Can Med Assoc J 94:1102, 1966.

steadily thereafter with approximately 1 in 100 women developing ovarian cancer sometime during their lives. The average age at which it is diagnosed is about 50 years. It occurs somewhat more often in white than in black women.

The *symptoms* are usually related to the GI tract and include mild gastrointestinal disturbances, dyspepsia, and a slight increase in girth. The only current method for detecting ovarian cancer is periodic abdominal and pelvic examinations, and thus the malignancies are usually diagnosed in an advanced state.

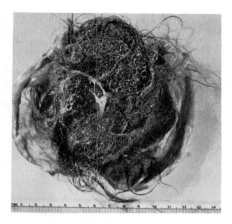

Fig. 46-1 Opened benign cystic teratoma, contents of which are mainly hair and sebaceous material.

Germ cell tumors

A variety of ovarian neoplasms can arise from germ cells.

Cystic teratomas (dermoids). Benign cystic teratomas, or dermoid cysts, which arise from primordial germ cells, comprise approximately 20% of all ovarian neoplasms. They occur at any age and account for about 60% of benign ovarian neoplasms in females under age 15. They are the second most common ovarian neoplasms in women of all age groups and are outnumbered only by serous cystadenomas. Benign cystic teratomas usually are between 5 and 10 cm in diameter when they are diagnosed, but occasionally a dermoid may be 15 cm or larger in diameter. Approximately 10% are bilateral.

These tumors are gray, glistening, smooth, and tense. They are cystic, usually a single cavity filled with oily, sebaceous fluid and a mass of matted hair (Fig. 46-1). There usually is a solid prominence in the tumor wall adjacent to the ovary. The prominent tissue is of ectodermal origin, but endodermal and mesodermal structures can be identified. Tissues most often recognized are skin and its appendages, cartilage, and respiratory and neural elements. Importantly, all the tissues are mature, and occasionally teeth can be

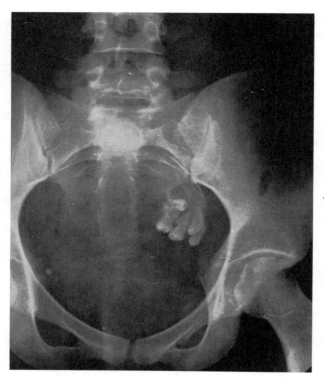

Fig. 46-2 Well developed teeth within benign cystic teratoma demonstrated by x-ray film examination.

seen on flat plate x-ray film examination (Fig. 46-2). Teratomas can give rise to an area of malignancy that develops in an otherwise benign teratoma. It is almost always squamous cell carcinoma.

Immature teratoma. An immature teratoma is a germ cell tumor that contains elements similar to a benign cystic teratoma, but the tissues have undergone a malignant differentiation. The usual tissue is of neural origin. Formerly these tumors were highly malignant and usually fatal, but with the advent of multiagent chemotherapy they now have a favorable prognosis.

Dysgerminoma. Dysgerminomas are malignant germ cell tumors, 80% of which are diagnosed during the early reproductive years, usually in teenagers. The tumor is smooth, gray-tan, and usually of a firm, rubbery consistency. The size varies from a small nodule to a mass that fills the entire abdomen. There usually are no symptoms except for abdominal enlargement. Although dysgerminomas have no endocrine activity, they may occur in association with ambiguous sexual development. Dysgerminomas are usually unilateral.

The treatment is usually unilateral salpingo-oophorectomy unless widespread metastases are present, in which case further removal of reproductive organs may be necessary. These tumors have been reported to secrete LDH; when they do so, the LDH is oftentimes elevated dramatically to the 10,000 to 15,000 range. These tumors are very radiosensitive and can be effectively treated with external radiation. In the young woman desiring to save reproductive function, encouraging results have been reported using multiagent chemotherapy, consisting of cisplatin, bleomycin, and VP-16.

Epithelial tumors

The most common epithelial neoplasms are the *serous or mucinous cystadenomas,* which account for approximately 50% of all benign ovarian neoplasms. The epithelial neoplasms have a spectrum of differentiation. The cystadenoma is a benign process and is highly treatable by cystectomy or oophorectomy. On the opposite end of the spectrum is a poorly differentiated serous or mucinous cyst, adenocarcinoma. A borderline lesion has been described that has also been given the name *ovarian tumor of low malignant potential.* This entity, although not completely benign, has a more favorable prognosis and tends to recur late with an excellent survival in almost all stages of disease.

Serous cystadenoma. These tumors occur more frequently than do the mucinous types. They are diagnosed more often between the ages of 20 and 50 years, with a peak incidence during the fourth decade of life. The surface is pearly gray, glistening, and lobulated because of its multilocular interior (Fig. 46-3). The lining may be smooth or covered with papillary projections. Similar excrescences are often seen on the surface of the tumor. The fluid is thin and pale unless there has been hemorrhage into the cavity of the tumor. The incidence of bilateral serous cystadenomas is approximately 25%.

The cells lining the cyst cavity may represent germinal epithelium but more characteristically are secretory and ciliated like those of the lumen of the normal fallopian tube. Small calcified granules, called *psammoma bodies (calcospherites),* are sometimes present in the cyst wall. They represent degeneration and subsequent calcification of small papillae. Psammoma bodies serve to differentiate serous from mucinous cystadenomas, as the psammoma bodies do not occur in the latter. Psammoma bodies are also seen in serous cystadenocarcinomas.

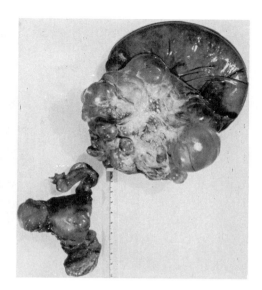

Fig. 46-3 Multilocular serous cystadenoma.

Mucinous cystadenoma. Differentiating mucinous cystadenomas from serous cystadenomas by gross inspection may be impossible. Mucinous cystadenomas are likely to be larger (Fig. 46-4). Mucinous cysts are usually multilocular and contain thick, straw-colored, viscous fluid. Papillary growths occur less often than with the serous cystadenomas. Only about 5% of mucinous cystadenomas are bilateral. Cells lining the cyst cavity are tall and columnar with clear cytoplasm and dark nuclei located close to the basement membrane. The cells resemble those normally seen in the endocervix.

Brenner tumor. Brenner tumors are unusual solid tumors in which massive epithelial cells grow in connective tissue stroma. They rarely become malignant and secrete no hormones. Approximately one third of them are discovered in association with another tumor, often a mucinous cystadenoma, in the opposite ovary. The diagnosis is usually made by histologic examination.

Malignant epithelial neoplasms. Both *serous and mucinous cystadenomas* can be malignant from their onset or undergo malignant change af-

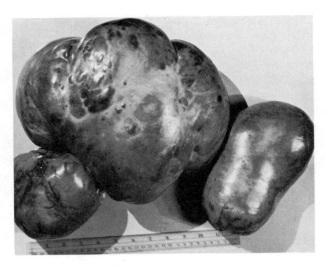

Fig. 46-4 Bilateral, multilocular mucinous cystadenoma.

ter many years. They account for two thirds of all malignant ovarian tumors; almost all are carcinomas. The *endometrioid type* is the other common epithelial tumor, and these cells are similar to the endometrial cells lining the uterine cavity. From 30% to 40% of serous tumors are malignant (serous cystadenocarcinoma) in contrast to only 5% to 10% of the mucinous variety (mucinous cystadenocarcinoma). About half of all ovarian adenocarcinomas are of the serous type, and 15% are mucinous. The remainder are largely composed of the endometrioid type. Rarely, a Brenner tumor is malignant.

Stromal tumors

These neoplasms of specialized gonadal stroma often secrete either estrogen or an androgen, and the hormone can produce its characteristic effect on the patient.

Granulosa theca cell tumors. These tumors may be made of predominantly granulosa cells, theca cells, or a combination of both. Many of these neoplasms secrete estrogen, and thus are called *feminizing tumors.* The name is not completely accurate, however, as virilization may occur in some women. Granulosa cell tumors are diagnosed most frequently during the climacteric and postmenopausal period, although they may develop in premenarchal girls. Approximately 10% are bilateral. The principal symptoms of feminizing tumors are those resulting from estrogen. In young females, the estrogen stimulates breast and general maturation and uterine bleeding (isosexual precocious puberty). Postmenopausal women with estrogen-secreting tumors may experience postmenopausal bleeding. When this tumor is present, a coexistent endometrial cancer may also be present.

Thecomas. Thecomas that arise from stromal cells are solid, benign, and almost always unilateral. They occur less often than do granulosa cell tumors, but they can secrete estrogen.

Sertoli-Leydig cell tumor. These rare gonadal stromal tumors usually have a virilizing effect. The so-called *arrhenoblastomas* occur in women between the ages of 20 and 40 years and are rare in children. The principal effect is defeminization, followed by virilization. The first evidence is usually amenorrhea and decreased breast size. This stage is followed by increased hair growth of male distribution, deepening of the voice, coarsening of the skin with acneform eruption, and hypertrophy of the clitoris. Some arrhenoblastomas are hormonally inert. The diagnosis is usually suspected when virilization is occurring and when an ovarian tumor is also visualized. Usually removal of the ovary is all that is necessary.

Fibroma. This neoplasm occurs most frequently during the fifth and sixth decades of life. Fibromas usually are unilateral, and they are not often malignant. Meigs described an interesting association of ascites and hydrothorax with ovarian fibromas *(Meig's syndrome)*. Ascites and hydrothorax can also occur in the presence of other ovarian neoplasms. *The physician should consider the possibility of an ovarian neoplasm in anyone with ascites and a pleural effusion.* Feeling the tumor may not be possible until the fluid has been removed. Ultrasound provides an easy method of diagnosis in the woman with ascites, as the ovaries are better visualized in the presence of the fluid medium.

TREATMENT

The diagnosis and management of ovarian neoplasms usually involve surgery; when malignancy is present, surgery is mandatory for staging. The benign germ cell and stromal cell tumors should be treated with conservative surgery in the young woman and with at least oophorectomy in the elderly woman. Attention must be paid to future fertility in the young woman and thus a cystectomy is the usual therapy. In the perimenopausal or postmenopausal patient, a bilateral salpingo-oophorectomy and hysterectomy is usually appropriate, in addition to removal of the benign process. The critical determination is that of malignancy.

Ovarian cancer is staged surgically as presented in Table 46-1. A unilateral salpingo-oophorectomy can be performed for the young woman with unilateral disease; however, all of the other staging procedures must also be performed. In patients whose fertility is not an issue, a total abdominal hysterectomy, bilateral salpingo-oophorectomy, omentectomy, pelvic and paraaortic node biopsies, pelvic washings throughout the abdomen, and biopsies of all adhesions are the critical initial step in therapy. When the results from the surgical staging are complete, the therapy is then guided according to the pathologic features as well as the clinical stage (box on p. 614).

The prognosis is directly related to the stage of the disease. Patients with advanced-stage disease have a poor 5-year survival. Patients with stage III disease have an approximate 15% 5-year survival, whereas those with stage IV disease have a 0% 5-year survival. The differentiation of the tumor also influences survival. Patients with a poorly differentiated tumor have decreased survival, stage for stage, compared to those with a well-differentiated tumor.

In patients with epithelial tumors and stage I disease or early stage II disease, a single-agent alkylating agent or intraperitoneal chromic phosphate (P32) is adequate therapy. For advanced-stage disease, multiagent chemotherapy is usually necessary. Patients without any residual disease can be treated with chemotherapy or whole abdomen radiation. Once a serous epithelial ovarian neoplasm has been diagnosed, a CA-125 serum level can be obtained to follow the course of the disease. When this tumor marker is elevated, it provides an adequate marker to follow the course of the disease as well as its response to chemotherapy.

The benign germ cell tumors as well as the stromal tumors can be adequately treated with unilateral salpingo-oophorectomy; in the perimenopausal or postmenopausal patient, the remaining pelvic organs can be removed at the time of surgery. In the younger patient, cystectomy alone is adequate therapy. The malignant germ cell tumors should be treated with unilateral salpingo-oophorectomy as well as staging. They usually occur in younger women, and thus fertility is an issue. They can be effectively treated with adjuvant chemotherapy, providing a chance for salvage of childbearing potential.

POSTMENOPAUSAL PALPABLE OVARIES

After the menopause, the ovaries become progressively smaller and should not be palpated. Approximately 5 years after menopause, the ovaries should be approximately 0.5 by 0.5 cm in size. If the ovary can be palpated, particularly if it has not been palpated previously, a neoplasm should be suspected. Usually an ultrasound can

STAGING FOR OVARIAN CANCER AND TREATMENT

FIGO stage	Description	Treatment
IA	Confined to one ovary Capsule intact No tumor on surface	G1, 2: TAH/BSO No further treatment G3: P32 or chemotherapy
IB	Confined to both ovaries	G1, 2: TAH/BSO No further treatment G3: P32 or chemotherapy
IC	Sames as 1A or 1B with positive ascitic fluid or washings, intraoperative rupture/spillage of tumor, extension of tumor through capsule.	TAH/BSO P32 or chemotherapy
IIA	Extension to uterus/tubes	TAH/BSO P32 or chemotherapy
IIB	Extension to other pelvic structure	TAH/BSO P32 if no residual or chemotherapy
IIC	Sames as IIA or IIB with positive ascitic fluid or washings, intraoperative rupture/spillage of tumor, extension of tumor through capsule.	TAH/BSO P32 if no residual or chemotherapy
IIIA	Intraabdominal spread microscopically	TAH/BSO Multiagent chemotherapy, or whole abdomen radiation
IIIB	Intraabdominal spread Macroscopically <2 cm	TAH/BSO Multiagent chemotherapy or whole abdomen radiation
IIIC	Intraabdominal spread Macroscopically >2 cm Positive retroperitoneal or inguinal nodes	Multiagent chemotherapy
IV	Disease above the diaphragm or intraparenchymal liver metastasis	Multiagent chemotherapy

The surgical staging includes TAH/BSO, omentectomy, lymph node sampling, washings, and evaluation of all peritoneal surfaces. TAH/BSO = total abdominal hysterectomy, bilateral salpingo-oophorectomy.

confirm the suspicion of the examiner, and an evaluation by laparoscopy or laparotomy is indicated.

Establishing the exact diagnosis is particularly important when the ovary is suspected to be enlarged in a postmenopausal woman. An enlarged ovary has approximately a 20% to 30% chance of containing some type of neoplasm.

SUGGESTED READING

Abell MR: The nature and classification of ovarian neoplasms, Can Med Assoc J 94:1102, 1966.

Barber HRK: Ovarian cancer: diagnosis and management, Am J Obstet Gynecol 150:910, 1984.

Demopoulos RI and others: Characterization and survival of patients with serous cystadenoma of the ovaries, Obstet Gynecol 64:557, 1984.

Evans AT III, Gaffey TA, Malkasian GD, and Annegers JF: Clinopathologic review of 118 granulosa and 82 theca cell tumors, Obstet Gynecol 55:231, 1980.

Fenoglio CM and Richart RM: Mucinous tumors of the ovary, Contemp Obstet Gynecol 9:64, 1977.

Garcia-Bunuel R, Berek JS, and Woodruff JD: Luteomas of pregnancy, Obstet Gynecol 45:407, 1975.

Gordon A, Lipton, and Woodruff JD: Dysgerminoma: a review of 158 cases from the Emil Novak Ovarian Tumor Registry, Obstet Gynecol 58:497, 1981.

Hallatt J, Steele CH Jr, and Snyder M: Ruptured corpus luteum with hemoperitoneum: a study of 173 surgical cases, Am J Obstet Gynecol 149:5, 1984.

Heintz AP, Hacker NF, and Lagasse LD: Epidemiology and etiology of ovarian cancer: a review, Obstet Gynecol 66:127, 1985.

Hibbard LT: Adnexal torsion, Am J Obstet Gynecol 152:456, 1985.

Hopkins MP, Kumar NB, and Morley GW: An assessment of pathologic features and treatment modalities in ovarian tumors of low malignant potential, Obstet Gynecol 70:923, 1987.

Meigs JV: Cancer of the ovary, Surg Gynecol Obstet 71:44, 1940.

Peter A, Heintz M, Hacker NF, and Lagasse L: Epidemiology and etiology of ovarian cancer: a review, Obstet Gynecol 66:127, 1985.

Smith LH and Oi RH: Detection of malignant ovarian neoplasms: a review of the literature. I. Detection of the patient at risk; clinical radiological and cytological detection, Obstet Gynecol Surv 39:313, 1984.

Smith LH and Oi RH: Detection of malignant ovarian neoplasms: a review of the literature. II. Laboratory detection, Obstet Gynecol Surv 39:320, 1984.

Smith LH and Oi RH: Detection of malignant ovarian neoplasms: a review of the literature. III. Immunological detection and ovarian cancer associated antigens, Obstet Gynecol Surv 39:346, 1984.

Tazelaar HD and others: Conservative treatment of borderline ovarian tumors, Obstet Gynecol 66:417, 1985.

J. Robert Willson

Aging

Objectives

RATIONALE: Life expectancy in women is increasing from year to year and many live for 30 or more years after the menopause. Physicians who care for aging women must understand the physical and psychosocial changes that occur with aging and familiarize themselves with methods of helping women cope with these changes.

The student should be able to:

A. Demonstrate knowledge of the physiologic changes in reproductive hormone secretion during the climacteric and postmenopausal phases of life.

B. Discuss the symptoms and physical findings that result from these changes.

C. List the changes in general physiologic functions.

D. Describe the pathologic results of reproductive hormone depletion.

E. Explain emotional responses to the menopause.

F. Name the indications and contraindications for hormone replacement therapy.

G. Outline the risks and benefits of hormone replacement therapy.

The biologic changes that accompany chronologic aging begin early in life, but most of those that occur before the ages of 40 to 45 are of little significance. The most obvious evidence of aging is cessation of menstruation, the menopause, which clearly marks the transition from the reproductive phase of life to senescence. Many other less evident changes are important determinants of physical and emotional health and well-being.

The menopause and the atrophic changes that occur during the postmenopausal period are unique to humans and undoubtedly are attributable to increased longevity. Former generations of women were likely to have died at an early age from complications of repeated pregnancies or from infectious diseases, both of which can now effectively be prevented.

In 1982 about 34 million women in the United States were at least 50 years of age. As life expectancy continues to increase, this segment of the population will expand. Within a few years more than 50 million women will be over age 50, and 57% of them will live for another 30 years. By 2010 about 4.5 million people will be older than 85, and by 2025 almost 59 million people, 20% of the population, will be over age 65. The majority of these elderly people will be women.

It has been customary to think of aging in women only in terms of the menopause, but this is too limited a concept. Aging is a continuing process that begins during embryonic life and ends with death. During the *climacteric* or *perimenopausal phase of life,* reproductive capacity is lost. The climacteric begins several years before the menopause and terminates when ovarian function ceases, usually a year or more after menopause. The *menopause,* an episode in the climacteric period, indicates complete cessation of menstruation. The *postmenopausal phase of life* includes the late climacteric period and the subsequent years during which atrophic changes progress.

CLIMACTERIC

Sometime after the age of 40, the ovaries begin to lose their ability to respond to pituitary gonadotropin stimulation by the orderly sequence of follicle growth, maturation of the ovum, and ovulation, and by the secretion of normal amounts of estrogen and progesterone. This change is directly related to a significant decrease in the number of responsive ovarian follicles. Only about 300,000 of the maximum of 6 to 7 million follicles that are present in the fetal ovary at the twentieth gestational week remain at menarche. They are gradually depleted during the 300 to 350 ovulatory menstrual cycles during the reproductive phase of life. Ovaries removed at the time of hysterectomy in women who were menstruating regularly at the time of the operation contain ten times more follicles than those from women who are perimenopausal. Ovaries removed from postmenopausal women contain almost no follicles.

After the age of 40, ovulation begins to occur

less regularly than it had in the past. The relatively few remaining follicles are less likely to respond appropriately to gonadotropin stimulation. This may be because the estrogen peak necessary to release LH may not be reached or because the most responsive follicles have already been used. As a consequence, anovulatory cycles occur more and more frequently. As the months go by, the diminishing number of remaining follicles produce less and less estrogen, and, finally, when there no longer are any that can respond, both estrogen secretion and bleeding cease.

As ovarian function declines, the concentrations of FSH and LH rise because there is no longer enough estrogen to inhibit their secretion. The reproductive hormone pattern during the early climacteric, therefore, is gradually declining estrogen, almost no progesterone after ovulation no longer occurs, and corresponding rises in FSH and LH. Later, when ovarian function ceases, FSH rises 10-fold to 20-fold and LH about threefold, reaching a maximum in 1 to 3 years (Fig. 47-1).

Menopause

The menopause, the complete cessation of menstruation and the most obvious evidence of termination of reproductive function, is the outstanding event of the climacteric phase of life. Menopause is the antithesis of menarche, an event during adolescence that marks the onset of reproductive capacity. Menopause can be diagnosed after a period of amenorrhea of 1 year.

The average age at which the menopause occurs is about 51. Some women stop menstruating as early as age 35, whereas others may continue until age 55 or even longer. Although both these limits may be normal, they are unusual.

In some women the periods continue to recur at regular intervals until they stop abruptly and permanently. More often the change is gradual. Over a period of 1 to 3 years, the amount of bleeding decreases, the interval between bleeding episodes lengthens, and periods of amenorrhea, which increase in duration, occur. The final periods may

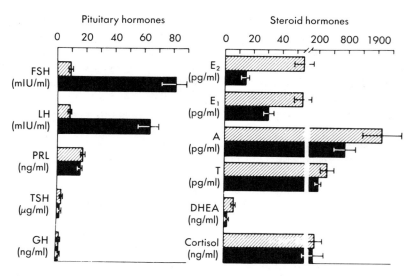

Fig. 47-1 Circulating concentrations of pituitary and steroid hormones in premenopausal women on days 2 to 4 of cycle *(hatched bars)* and postmenopausal women *(solid bars)*. *FSH*, Follicle-stimulating hormone; *LH*, luteinizing hormone, *PRL*, prolactin; *TSH*, thyroid-stimulating hormone; *GH*, growth hormone, E_2, estradiol; E_1, estrone; *A*, androstenedione; *T*, testosterone; *DHEA*, dehydroepiandrosterone. (From Yen SSC: J Reprod Med 18:287, 1977.)

be represented by only slight spotting. The change in bleeding pattern occurs because of a progressive decline in ovarian estrogen secretion. Bleeding ceases permanently when too little estrogen is being produced to cause endometrial growth.

Some women have increased bleeding before the menopause. Periods of bleeding that may recur as often as every 2 to 3 weeks and that may be prolonged and profuse occur because of erratic increases and decreases in estrogen secretion. This is similar to dysfunctional bleeding in younger women. *Increased and irregular bleeding cannot be accepted as a consequence of declining ovarian function until uterine malignancy has been eliminated as a cause.*

Hormone secretion

The concentration of circulating estrogens decreases significantly after the menopause, and there is a reversal of estrogen fractions. Most of

what is available in postmenopausal women is estrone rather than estradiol. Neither the ovary nor the adrenal gland secretes significant amounts of estrogen during the postmenopausal period of life. The major source is peripheral conversion of androstenedione to estrone. Most of the androstenedione is derived from the adrenal cortex, but some comes from ovarian stroma. The ovary also produces testosterone, some of which may be converted to estradiol. The principal site of conversion is fat, although other tissues, especially the liver, do contribute. In some women enough estrone is produced by peripheral conversion to cause endometrial growth, even to the stage of hyperplasia, and bleeding. Because the prototypic candidate for endometrial cancer is obese, one can hypothesize that the exaggerated estrone production in adipose tissue may play a role in the genesis of the tumor.

The menopause can be precipitated by removing the ovaries: *surgical menopause*. In contrast to the natural climacteric, during which ovarian function is reduced slowly, it is terminated abruptly and completely by oophorectomy. The FSH and LH concentrations begin to rise almost immediately and remain elevated indefinitely. If the ovaries are removed, the only source of androgen for conversion is adrenal androstenedione; hence, an estrogen-deficient state develops rapidly.

PHYSIOLOGIC CHANGES ACCOMPANYING AGING

The changes that occur with aging affect all structures and functions of the body.

Changes in reproductive organs

The outstanding physical changes in the reproductive organs after the menopause are directly related to the withdrawal of the tissue-stimulating effects of estrogen. Labial fat is gradually reabsorbed, so the labia majora are flattened and, in elderly women, the skin may hang in folds. The labia minora may actually disappear.

The vagina gradually narrows, the fornices become shallower, and the epithelial lining becomes progressively thinner. The vaginal smear reflects the change; as estrogen secretion diminishes, superficial cornified cells disappear, and eventually the cell type is predominantly parabasal and basal cells with a few of the intermediate type—a typical estrogen-deficient pattern.

Vaginal pH increases from the normal 3.5 to 4.5 in menstruating women to 5.0 or more after the menopause. The change is a result of decreased glycogen production in vaginal epithelial cells and the consequent decreased conversion of carbohydrate to lactic acid by Döderlein lactobacilli. There also is *less vaginal fluid,* which parallels the *decrease in vaginal blood flow.*

The supporting structures of the uterus, bladder, and rectum lose much of their tone and premenopausal strength because of atrophic changes in the tissues themselves, accompanied by a significant decrease in vascularity that further reduces their integrity. These changes and the atrophy of the vaginal wall contribute to the development of cystocele, rectocele, and uterine prolapse. Stress urinary incontinence often increases or may begin after the menopause.

The cervix gradually becomes shorter, but this may not be evident for some years; however, the secretory activity of the cervical glands decreases early in the climacteric. The mucus becomes scant and viscid, and the arborization phenomenon, which is a function of estrogen, is either absent or greatly reduced. Part of the atrophic change is a retreat of the squamocolumnar junction from its normal position on the portio or at the external os to a position well within the cervical canal (Fig. 47-2). Because the changes leading to squamous cell cervical cancer begin at the squamocolumnar junction, material for cervical cytology studies in elderly women should be obtained from the cervical canal as well as by scraping the portio.

The uterus gradually becomes smaller until it

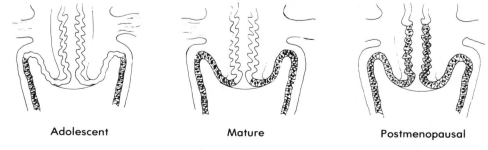

Adolescent　　　　　Mature　　　　　Postmenopausal

Fig. 47-2 Position of squamocolumnar junction at various life stages.

resembles the uterus of the prepubertal girl. The endometrium as a rule becomes thin and atrophic, but various forms of retrogressive hyperplasia may occur in response to extragonadal estrogen stimulation.

General body changes

A variety of changes in many physiologic functions occurs with aging. These physiologic changes include decreased thyroid function, decreased renal function, decreased insulin release in response to glucose challenge, hyperparathyroidism, impairments in thermoregulation, decreased tissue response to catecholamines, increased conversion of androstenedione to estrone, changes in fat distribution, and excessive hair growth. Neurologic changes include loss of memory, confusion, and impairments in balance control, which often result in falls.

Cardiovascular changes. The risk of death from ischemic heart disease in women between the ages of 50 and 75 is about 10,500 of 100,000. The fact that the incidences of coronary artery disease, hypertension, and stroke are lower in premenopausal women than in men of similar ages and that the risk increases after the menopause led to the assumption that estrogen might have a protective effect. Support for this concept is provided by studies that indicate a two- to threefold reduction in risk of death from cardiovascular disease in postmenopausal women who are taking estrogen. Furthermore, there is a sevenfold increase in myocardial infarctions after bilateral oophorectomy in women under age 35 who are not given estrogen replacement therapy. A similar decrease does not occur following hysterectomy with ovarian conservation.

The protective action of estrogen may be a result of its effect on lipoproteins. Low-density lipoprotein cholesterol (LDL-C), which is atherogenic, increases after menopause while the protective high-density lipoprotein fraction (HDL-C) decreases. Estrogen replacement therapy reverses the ratio, increasing HDL-C and decreasing LDL-C.

Hypertension is common in older women and a risk factor for cardiovascular disease. The relationship between estrogen and hypertension is uncertain because estrogen replacement therapy is accompanied by either no change in blood pressure or only a slight increase.

Bone changes. Bone loss begins at about age 30 and is progressive throughout adult life in both sexes. An abrupt acceleration occurs after the menopause, either natural or artificial, and the increasing length of life has compounded the associated problems. Postmenopausal women lose bone at an average rate of 1% to 2% a year. Those in their eighties may have lost half or more of their skeletons. *Osteoporosis* is accompanied by an increased risk of disability and death. The risk of death following osteoporotic fractures in women between the ages of 50 and 75 is about 938 of 100,000.

Osteoporosis occurs more often in white and Asian than in black women, in thin than in fat women, and in smokers than in nonsmokers. It is more prevalent in those who have a family history of osteoporosis, in those receiving glucocorticoid therapy, and in those who, by choice or of necessity, are physically inactive (see box on p. 621).

Bone loss occurs because of bone resorption that is not balanced by reconstruction. Although available calcium may be reduced by inadequate dietary intake, decreased intestinal absorption, and increased renal excretion, all of which may occur in elderly women, the most important factor appears to be estrogen deprivation. Bone mineral densities are significantly reduced in hypogonadal women, in those whose ovaries have been removed early in life, and in those well past the menopause if they are not taking estrogen. Bone loss in estrogen-deficient women occurs at a rate of 1% to 2% a year. The loss can be prevented by estrogen replacement therapy.

Bone loss begins first in trabecular bone and somewhat later in cortical bone. Demineralization of trabecular bone in the dorsal and lumbar vertebrae is followed by compression fractures that may first appear soon after the menopause. About

RISK FACTORS FOR OSTEOPOROSIS

Hereditary
Female gender
Ovarian agenesis
Positive family history
Small bone mass
White or Oriental
Endocrine
Amenorrhea
Diabetes mellitus
Menopause
Thyrotoxicosis
Nulliparity
Adrenal steroid therapy
Nutritional
High alcohol intake
High caffeine intake
High animal protein intake
High sodium intake
High vitamin D intake
Low calcium intake
Life-style
Cigarette smoking
Inactivity
   Bedridden
   Inadequate exercise
   Weightlessness

60% of women over 60 who are not taking estrogen will develop vertebral compression fractures. The only evidence may be gradual loss of height and the development of kyphosis. Pain occurs when nerves are compressed. Fractures through cortical bone occur somewhat later. Women have more long-bone fractures than do men of comparable ages. More than 40% of women will have had a fracture by age 75. At least 80% of women who develop hip fractures after age 40 are at least 75 years old. Most hip fractures are intertrochanteric and in osteoporotic bone.

Symptoms

The most distressing symptoms in aging women begin to appear before the menopause and continue after the periods cease. Not all of the symptoms are directly related to changes in hormone secretion. Many of the same symptoms occur in men. In both sexes they result from the general physical and emotional changes that accompany aging.

Vasomotor symptoms (hot flush). The most characteristic symptom of the menopause is the *hot flush*. The typical hot flush appears suddenly, with the first symptom being a sensation of heat in the chest, neck, and head that increases rapidly and lasts from a few seconds to 3 or 4 minutes. The flush is followed by chilling and diaphoresis, which may be profuse enough to saturate the clothing. Hot flushes occur both at night and during the day, and they are often accompanied by vertigo, palpitation, and a feeling of faintness.

The frequency and duration of the flushes vary. Some women have no vasomotor symptoms, but at least 85% experience flushes. In the majority the flushes are mild and may occur several times a day, but interfere little with usual activities. In the minority they recur many times during the day and at night and are so severe that they are disabling.

The flush follows rapid and localized vasodilation, which often is evident because the face and neck become bright red. Core body temperature decreases slightly, but temperature in the fingers and toes rises because of vasodilation and increased blood flow. Blood pressure is unchanged. Each flush coincides with a pulsatile release of LH, but FSH does not change. No significant changes take place in plasma dopamine, epinephrine, or norepinephrine.

The frequency with which flushes occur and their intensity usually begin to decrease in a few months. Most women are comfortable by 24 to 30 months, except during periods of emotional stress, when flushes usually are more troublesome.

The flushes are related to the decreasing secretion of estrogen as ovarian function declines. They do not occur in preadolescent girls or in women with primary hypogonadism before they are treated with estrogen. However, young women with gonadal dysgenesis who have been treated with exogenous estrogen will develop typical flushes if the medication is stopped. It seems likely that a period of estrogen stimulation followed by withdrawal is an essential factor in the development of hot flushes.

Nervous and psychologic symptoms. Headache, insomnia, vertigo, depression, and feelings of hopelessness, worthlessness, and self-condemnation are often experienced during the climacteric. These symptoms are of emotional origin and are not a direct result of estrogen deficiency. There is no evidence to suggest that psychoses are precipitated by menopause.

Few women understand the physiologic changes that occur during the climacteric and that are responsible for the menopause. Many have bizarre ideas of what to expect. Their fears include obesity, excessive hair growth, and other changes in their bodies that will make them less attractive; loss of sexual appetite; the development of psychoses; and, of course, the undeniable fact that they are getting old.

Many women who have been busy caring for their families find that their children no longer need them and their husbands are preoccupied with their jobs. These women now have less and less to do, and too few know how to make use of the many free hours available to them. Those who are working may realize that there is no hope of advancing to more interesting or responsible positions.

Women often become more sexually active when the fear of pregnancy is removed. Others lose libido completely when menstruation ceases. Sexuality and sexual activity have little relationship to estrogen secretion.

Genital symptoms. Most of the genital tract symptoms in postmenopausal women are caused by the atrophic changes that develop as a result of estrogen deprivation. The principal one is *atrophic vaginitis* (Chapter 43). *Dyspareunia* may occur because of decreased precoital lubrication, vaginitis, or constriction of the vagina or introi-

tus. *Pruritus vulvae* also occurs frequently after the menopause.

The severity of symptoms associated with cystocele, rectocele, and uterine prolapse is determined by the extent of the changes in the supporting structures. Stress urinary incontinence is common in postmenopausal women.

Skeletal symptoms. Pain and stiffness in the joints is a common complaint in climacteric women and is often called *menopausal arthralgia*. Physical and x-ray examinations do not disclose any arthritic changes. The discomfort may be caused by an obscure change in the soft tissues surrounding the joints, or it may arise in muscles and tendons that are not exercised enough.

Osteoporosis involves most of the bone mass. It is particularly noticeable in the spine, with the formation of "dowager's hump" (dorsal kyphosis). Pain occurs only with fractures.

Differential diagnosis

Women who have periods of amenorrhea during the climacteric often fear that they may be pregnant. This can be ruled out by pelvic examination, demonstration of arborization in cervical mucus, and a pregnancy test when other examinations are inconclusive.

Not infrequently, the physician sees women in their forties who are still menstruating regularly but who complain of headache, dizziness, insomnia, fatigue, and some degree of depression. The temptation to blame these symptoms on the menopause is strong. Most often the patient is suffering from a condition that is totally unrelated to estrogen deprivation. The physician should hesitate to make a diagnosis of "climacteric syndrome" in patients who are still menstruating regularly, especially if vasomotor phenomena are not prominent features of the illness.

Treatment of the climacteric patient

It is essential that obstetrician-gynecologists, internists, and family physicians who are responsible for the total care of elderly women be aware of the general physiologic changes of aging as well as the gynecologic problems that may develop.

Because many of the changes attributed to aging are much like those that occur with prolonged periods of reduced physical activity, disuse may play an important role in the aging process. Bone loss is increased significantly by inactivity. Blood pressure, which may be elevated in elderly people, is often decreased by exercise. It seems essential that aging women be encouraged to remain active and that they be instructed in exercise programs that are within their limits of tolerance. The best exercises, particularly to decrease the risk of osteoporosis, are those that stress bone; walking and aerobic exercises are excellent.

Dietary instruction is important. Many elderly women are undernourished because they cannot afford nutritious food, because they have no interest in preparing meals if they live alone, because they are edentulous or have poor dentures and cannot chew solid food, or because they are unaware of their nutritional needs. A particularly important dietary ingredient is calcium. An intake of 1500 mg of calcium is recommended to help decrease postmenopausal bone loss. This can be reduced to 1000 mg in women who are taking estrogen.

Because *excessive alcohol intake* and *cigarette smoking* increase the risk of both cardiovascular disease and osteoporosis, elderly women should be encouraged to drink moderately and to stop smoking completely.

Periodic examinations are even more important for women during the climacteric and after the menopause than in younger women. The incidence of many malignancies increases, as do degenerative changes in other organ systems. Emotional problems that may have caused little discomfort while a woman was busy caring for her family may become far more serious and even disabling as physical discomfort increases and responsibilities decrease. The symptoms may be magnified by her children leaving home and by the death of her husband.

The examination should be designed to detect the disorders that first appear or that are more prevalent in older than in younger women. For example, pregnancy, genital herpes, and gonorrhea rarely occur during the climacteric period, but cancer, both genital and extragenital, hypertension, obesity, degenerative diseases, diabetes, nutritional deficiencies, and anemia are common. Young women have little concern for death and aging, but these are of great importance after the menopause.

An *appropriate periodic examination* for the presumably well elderly woman includes a history update, complete physical examination including tonometry, breast, pelvic, and rectal examinations, and a check for occult fecal blood. Basic laboratory studies should include a Pap test, hemoglobin and hematocrit, white blood cell count, and urine examination. Other laboratory studies are ordered as indicated. A yearly mammogram will help to detect early breast abnormalities. There are no tests comparable to cervical cytology to detect early uterine or ovarian cancer, but if one is able to palpate an ovary in a postmenopausal woman an abnormality should be suspected and investigated. The normal ovary is so small that it cannot often be felt (Chapter 46).

Depression is almost universal in elderly people, and physicians often do not recognize the less obvious forms. Loss of memory and episodes of mental confusion also may occur. As physical and mental functions deteriorate, day-to-day living becomes more difficult. Physicians must be prepared to recognize these changes and to help patients cope with them.

Psychotherapy. An unhurried discussion of the meaning and manifestation of the menopause is the first and perhaps most important step in therapy for the climacteric patient. This provides authoritative guidance and reassurance to the middle-aged woman who at this time finds herself in need of both. No woman can blithely disregard the change in her appearance and the prospect of progressive aging.

A well-adjusted, emotionally secure woman can be encouraged to draw psychologic strength from her past successes and to turn her resources and energies to new pursuits. Reeducation, reassurance, and mild manipulation of the patient's environment constitute the methods of superficial psychotherapy that are available to all interested physicians. Such measures will be sufficient for the vast majority of climacteric women. The patient with profound changes in personality or who becomes extremely depressed should be referred to a psychiatrist for more specialized treatment.

Hormone therapy. Because the symptoms and physiologic alterations that accompany the menopause occur in women whose ovarian function is failing, it seems logical to assume that ovarian hormone replacement therapy should be beneficial. This assumption is true. Although psychotherapy and other measures are appropriate and may be helpful, they do not often eliminate the symptoms caused by estrogen deficiency.

ESTROGENS. The principal reasons for prescribing estrogen therapy are *to eliminate hot flushes, to prevent or delay atrophy of the genital structures, to reduce the risk of cardiovascular disease,* and *to prevent osteoporosis.*

There are many effective estrogen preparations that differ in their derivation, potency, duration of action, and cost. The dosage is regulated by the degree to which hot flushes are relieved, insomnia corrected, and a feeling of well-being produced. The amount required to accomplish this usually also prevents genital atrophy and unusual bone loss.

The preparations most often used are sodium estrone sulfate, in daily dosages of 0.625 to 1.25 mg, and ethinyl estradiol, 0.05 to 0.2 mg orally. Estrogen may also be administered percutaneously from skin patches, which provide good control of symptoms.

Unopposed estrogen stimulation appears to be an important factor in the induction of endometrial cancer, but the risk can be reduced substantially if a progestogen is added during the last 10 to 14 days of the treatment cycle. Estrogen does produce about a twofold increase in the risk of cholelithiasis, but there is no evidence that it alters carbohydrate metabolism or disturbs the blood-clotting mechanism. The overall mortality in postmenopausal women who are taking estrogen is lower than in those who are not.

The initial dose of estrogen should be the lowest that might be expected to control symptoms while still preventing atrophic changes in the reproductive organs and bone loss. In most women *0.625 mg of sodium estrone sulfate (Premarin) daily during the first 25 days of each month* will accomplish these aims. The frequency and severity of flushes are either decreased significantly or eliminated. If the symptoms persist, 1.25 mg can be prescribed. It is unusual that a dose larger than this is needed.

The prescription of *10 mg of medroxyprogesterone acetate* (Provera) daily starting on the thirteenth day of the treatment cycle will reduce the risk of abnormal endometrial hyperplasia. Unfortunately, the combination of estrogen and progesterone often stimulates withdrawal bleeding. This, together with the possibility that the combination will produce symptoms like those during the premenstrual phase of the normal cycle, fluid retention, breast tenderness, and depression makes many women reluctant to continue the regimen. Withdrawal bleeding may continue until age 60 or longer.

An alternative method, which reduces the likelihood of significant bleeding while still offering the protective effect of a progestogen, is to prescribe combined treatment to be taken continuously. Conjugated estrogens, 0.625 mg, and Provera, 2.5 mg, are given daily. There usually is some irregular spotting for 3 or 4 months, but it stops. The endometrium becomes atrophic, which should protect against malignancy.

In the past, limiting the duration of estrogen use was thought necessary, but, because of the beneficial effects on bone metabolism, it probably should be continued indefinitely. An even more important reason for long-term estrogen replacement therapy is the protection it provides against cardiovascular disease. Although progestogens, particularly the 19-nortestosterone preparations, tend to counteract the beneficial effects of estrogen on lipoproteins, there is little evidence of a deleterious effect from medroxyprogesterone in the doses now being used.

One of the important indications for estrogen therapy is *atrophic vaginitis*. It is better managed by estrogenic cream applied to the vagina than by oral estrogen. The vaginal cells are stimulated to proliferate and cornify, which permits them to overcome the infection without the use of other agents. *Estrogen is absorbed from the vagina and may produce systemic effects*. Atrophic vaginitis is discussed in detail in Chapter 43.

Estrogen may also be helpful in controlling *stress urinary incontinence* that begins after the menopause. The atrophy of the tissues and the loss of vascularity in the structures surrounding the vesicle neck may permit them to relax enough to interfere with urinary control. The symptoms may be relieved by vaginal applications of estrogen cream. Estrogen will have no effect in premenopausal women, nor can it be expected to correct incontinence that is associated with extensive vaginal relaxation nor that caused by unstable bladders. Pubococcygeus exercises should also be recommended (Chapter 39).

There is little evidence to support the concern that estrogen plays a role in the genesis of cancers of the cervix or ovary or of malignancies in other parts of the body, particularly when it is administered with a progestogen. The major concern is for breast lesions. Although there is no solid evidence that unopposed estrogen increases the risk of breast cancer, a definitive answer must await further study.

Uterine bleeding. Most women who take estrogen-progestogen preparations cyclically have withdrawal bleeding, which may continue in decreasing amounts until about age 60. After that it decreases, but in some bleeding will continue as long as progestogen is administered. Those who are taking estrogen-progestogen continuously usually have no bleeding after the first few months.

No investigation is necessary if the bleeding occurs only after progestogen withdrawal. Conversely, if bleeding occurs at any other phase of the cycle, endometrial biopsy or curettage is essential to determine the cause.

CONTRAINDICATIONS. Estrogens are contraindicated in women with *acute liver disease* or *whose liver function is significantly reduced,* those who have had severe *thrombophlebitis* or *thromboembolism,* those with *estrogen-dependent malignant neoplasms,* or those with *abnormal vaginal bleeding for which the cause has not yet been determined.*

Progesterone. Medroxyprogesterone acetate may be used to control hot flushes when estrogen is contraindicated. It may be given orally as Provera, 10 to 20 mg daily, or by injection as Depo-Provera, 150 to 200 mg every 4 to 6 weeks. Although progesterone may eliminate flushes, it is not a complete substitute for estrogen. Progesterone may have a depressive effect on some women.

Nonhormonal treatment. There are alternative methods of treating climacteric symptoms in women who do not want to take estrogen or those in whom it is contraindicated. Mild symptoms can often be ameliorated by superficial psychotherapy and the prescription of small doses of phenobarbital or tranquilizers. These drugs have a limited effect on women who are disabled by the flushes. The antihypertensive agent clonidine may reduce the severity of the flushes.

SUGGESTED READING

Bartuska DG: Physiology of aging: metabolic changes during the climacteric and menopausal periods, Clin Obstet Gynecol 20:105, 1977.

Bider D, Mashiach S, Serr DM, and Ben-Rafael Z: Endocrinological basis of hot flushes, Obstet Gynecol Survey 44:495, 1989.

Bortz WM II: Disuse and aging, JAMA 248:1203, 1982.

Bush TL and Barrett-Connor E: Noncontraceptive use and cardiovascular disease, Epidemiol Rev 7:80, 1985.

Bush TL, Barrett-Connor E, Cowan LD, and others: Cardiovascular mortality and noncontraceptive use of estrogen in women: results from the Lipid Research Programs Follow-up Study, Circulation 75:1102, 1987.

Gambrell RD: The menopause: benefits and risks of estrogen-progestogen replacement therapy, Fertil Steril 37:457, 1982.

Gambrell RD: Sex steroid hormones and cancer, Curr Probl Obstet Gynecol 7:1, 1984.

Hammond CB and Maxson WS: Current status of estrogen therapy for the menopause, Fertil Steril 37:5, 1982.

Hassager C and Christensen C: Blood pressure during oestrogen/progestogen substitution therapy in healthy postmenopausal women, Maturitas 9:315, 1988.

Hassager C, Riis BJ, Strøm V, Guyene TT, and Christiansen C: The long-term effect of oral and percutaneous estradiol on plasma renin substrate and blood pressure, Circulation 76:753, 1987.

Judd HL, Cleary RE, Creasman WT, Figge DC, Kase N, Rosenwaks Z, and Tagatz GE: Estrogen replacement therapy, Obstet Gynecol 58:267, 1981.

Lapidus L, Bengtsson C, and Lindquist O: Menopausal age and risk of cardiovascular disease and death, Acta Obstet Gynecol Scand (Suppl) 130:37, 1985.

Lindsay R, Hart DM, and Clark DM: The minimum effective dose of estrogen for prevention of postmenopausal bone loss, Obstet Gynecol 63:759, 1984.

Lindsay R, Hart DM, MacLean A, Clark AC, Kraszewski A, and Garwood J: Bone response to termination of oestrogen treatment, Lancet 1:1325, 1978.

Lobo RA and others: Depo-medroxyprogesterone acetate compared with conjugated estrogens for the treatment of postmenopausal women, Obstet Gynecol 63:1, 1984.

Matthews KA, Meilahn E, Kuller LK and others: Menopause and risk factors for coronary heart disease, New Engl J Med 321:641, 1989.

Natl Inst Health Consensus Conference Statement: Osteoporosis, Bethesda, 1984, National Institute of Arthritis, Diabetes, and Digestive and Kidney Diseases.

Persson I: The risk of endometrial and breast cancer after estrogen treatment: a review of epidemiologic studies, Acta Obstet Gynecol Scand (Suppl) 130:59, 1985.

Richardson SJ, Senikas V, and Nelson JF: Follicular depletion during the menopausal transition: evidence for accelerated loss and ultimate exhaustion, J Clin Endocrinol Metab 65:1231, 1987.

Rigg LA, Hermann H, and Yen SSC: Absorption of estrogens from vaginal creams, N Engl J Med 298:195, 1978.

Rosenberg L, Hennekens CH, Rosner B, Belanger C, Rothman KJ, and Speizer FE: Early menopause and the risk of myocardial infarction, Am J Obstet Gynecol 139:47, 1981.

Schiff I, Tulchinsky D, Cramer D, and Ryan KJ: Oral medroxyprogesterone in the treatment of postmenopausal symptoms, JAMA 244:1443, 1980.

Semmens JP: Estrogen deprivation and vaginal function in postmenopausal women, JAMA 248:445, 1982.

Sherwin BH and Gelfand MM: A prospective one-year study of estrogen and progestin in postmenopausal women: effects on clinical symptoms and lipoprotein lipids, Obstet Gynecol 73:759, 1989.

Tulandi T and Lal S: Menopausal hot flush, Obstet Gynecol Surv 40:553, 1985.

Index

NOTE: *f* indicates illustration; *t* indicates table.